ONCOGENE-DIRECTED THERAPIES

CANCER DRUG DISCOVERY AND DEVELOPMENT
Beverly A. Teicher, Series Editor

ONCOGENE-DIRECTED THERAPIES

Edited by

JANUSZ RAK, MD, PhD

Henderson Research Centre, McMaster University
Hamilton, Ontario, Canada

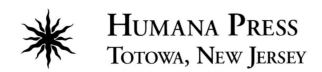

HUMANA PRESS
TOTOWA, NEW JERSEY

© 2003 Humana Press Inc.
999 Riverview Drive, Suite 208
Totowa, New Jersey 07512

www.humanapress.com

This publication is printed on acid-free paper. ∞
ANSI Z39.48-1984 (American Standards Institute)
Permanence of Paper for Printed Library Materials.

Cover illustration: Image representing fibroblasts transformed with the HER-2/neu oncogene stained for expression of intracellular protein vimentin. Original image provided by Dr. Alicia Viloria-Petit. Final collage designed by Danuta Rak.

Production Editor: Tracy Catanese
Cover design: Patricia F. Cleary

For additional copies, pricing for bulk purchases, and/or information about other Humana titles, contact Humana at the above address or at any of the following numbers: Tel.: 973-256-1699; Fax: 973-256-8341; E-mail: humana@humanapr.com; or visit our Website: **www.humanapress.com**

Printed in the United States of America. 10 9 8 7 6 5 4 3 2 1

Library of Congress Cataloging in Publication Data

Oncogene-directed therapies / edited by Janusz Rak
        p. ; cm. -- (Cancer drug discovery and development)
    Includes bibliographical references and index.
    ISBN 0-89603-982-X (alk. paper); 1-59259-313-5 (e-book)
    1. Oncogenes. 1. Cancer--Molecular aspects. 3. Cancer--Gene therapy. 4. Biological response modifiers. I. Rak, Janusz. II. Series.
    [DNLM: 1. Oncogenes. 2. Neoplasms--therapy. QZ 202 O5414 2003]
RC268.42.O5196 2003
616.99'4042--dc21

                                                                                2002068918

PREFACE

Through experience we know only appearances ..., but not the modum noumenon ..., not things as they are in themselves.

—*Immanuel Kant*

Could cancer be treated, perhaps cured, by targeting and effectively removing its "cause"? A possible answer to this question is often as difficult to conceptualize as is the very essence of this life-threatening disease. In this regard, a reductionist viewpoint emphasizes properties of a "cancer cell" *(1,2)* or evolving and transformed clones of such cells *(3)*, each of these entities typically equated with a "unit of malignancy." On the other hand, cancer can also be viewed as a heterogeneous "society" of freely interacting but phenotypically altered cells and cell subpopulations. Each of such co-existing cell subsets, in and of itself, does not define the malignant process as a whole, but rather such definition is encoded in the (aberrant) functional interplay between its constituents *(4)*. An even more "holistic" approach invokes a contribution of deregulated host responses, which either fail to control the "spontaneous" emergence of cancer cells (e.g., immunity) *(5)*, or become subverted by the latter to support unrestricted tumor growth, invasion, and metastasis (e.g., angiogenesis) *(6)*. In the latter instance, the vascularized, multicellular conglomerate involving both transformed and nontransformed (stromal) cells could be viewed as a different type, more complex tumorigenic "unit" *(1,7)*. Could these vastly diverse concepts accommodate a common denominator, a unifying "causal" influence that drives multifaceted pathological processes and is responsible for the multitude of clinical manifestations of malignancy? Could such influence(s) be controlled therapeutically?

Breathtaking developments in cancer genetics over the last two to three decades seem to suggest that the answer to this crucial question may be affirmative. Indeed, intrinsic genetic lesions in cancer cells are now thought to be the *primum movens* behind expression of all major "hallmarks of cancer" *(1)*, including formation of the vascular tumor stroma. In this sense, "cancer-causing" mutant genes are ultimately responsible for the development and progression of the malignant disease as we know it *(2)*. It is, of course, possible that such overt genetic changes are preceded by more subtle epigenetic events affecting tissue or cellular homeostasis. It is also possible that the "cancer-causing" effects of mutant genes may be either direct or indirect in nature. Nevertheless, once they occur, the biological impact of "broken genes" transcends cellular boundaries, and emanates into the local and systemic realms of cancer-associated pathology.

Up to seven independent genetic "hits" are thought to be associated with development and progression of an overt malignant tumor *(8)*. However, recent studies suggest that abnormal expression of only three genes might be sufficient, at least in some cases, for a complete conversion of normal human cells into their cancerous counterparts *(9)*. Incidentally, all three of the "cancer-causing" genes implicated in such a process (i.e., *H-ras, hTERT, SV40-LT*) are known to induce "gain-of-function" type changes and thereby could be traditionally classified as dominant acting, transforming *oncogenes* *(1,2)*. Moreover, inactivation of even a single oncogene (e.g., mutant *ras*) in the context of a full-blown malignant tumor in vivo, can result in profound growth inhibition and/or tumor regression *(10,11)*. Thus, despite a multitude of genetic and epigenetic influences and complexities associated with tumor formation, at least in some cases, sustained expression of certain oncoproteins is clearly functionally important, nonredundant, and virtually indispensable for continued tumor growth and "maintenance" (*10,11*). Indeed, it is difficult to formulate a better definition of an (almost) ideal therapeutic target.

In recent years, oncogenes have attracted a great deal of interest as prospective molecular targets for anticancer therapy. The tremendous amount of work and thought that went into exploration of this concept culminated in the recent FDA approval of at least two oncogene-targeted anticancer agents—Herceptin/trastuzumab and STI571/Gleevec—with several other compounds and approaches still in the "pipeline." All of these efforts hold great promise, but there are also challenges ahead. These challenges have to be fully understood to be properly met in the future. For these various reasons, it is difficult to imagine a more appropriate time for the publication of a comprehensive overview on *Oncogene-Directed Therapies*. In the past, cancer *research* and cancer *treatment*, although motivated by similar long-term goals and objectives, have been developing along somewhat different trajectories influenced by their respective focus on either current or future challenges in dealing with human malignancies. In 2002, we can claim with some degree of credibility that with regards to the rational, causality-based, scientifically sound cancer treatment, "the future is now." The advent of new Protein Kinase Inhibitors (PKI), Farnesyltransferase Inhibitors (FTIs), and other types of "anti-oncogenic" signal transduction antagonists heralds a significant change in the practice of oncology by bringing together the results of basic, translational, and clinical research. It continues to be a fascinating pursuit and many more potential targets for oncogene-directed therapies still remain unexplored (Table 1).

Although the nominal focus of this book is on targeting *oncoproteins*, it is important to realize that traditionally, antithetical concepts of "oncogenes" and "tumor suppressor genes" are gradually being replaced by more sophisticated models in which cellular transformation and tumor progression can be explained more accurately by analysis of interactive molecular circuitry involving protein products of both types of genes. We attempted to highlight this conceptual shift in this book.

Oncogene-Directed Therapies is a result of the concerted effort of a number of devoted individuals who have made significant contributions to this promising field of cancer research. The content of the book is composed in such a way as to give readers a balanced blend of fundamental science, basic research, experimental therapeutics, and early clinical experiences. The first section (Chapters 1–7) is devoted to the "concept" of an *oncogene* and *oncogenesis*. The reader will be presented with a series of up-to-date overviews on "how" and "why" certain proteins can acquire the ability to transform eukaryotic cells, and under what conditions. The many mechanisms, pathways, and complexities of the cell transformation process will be the main themes of this section. Chapters 8–13 are meant to introduce the crucial biological consequences of the oncogenic transformation, particularly for cellular mitogenesis, survival, differentiation, migration, proteolysis, or angiogenic competence. This is meant to open the discussion on how oncogene-directed therapies may work to obliterate essential elements of cancer pathogenesis. Chapters 14–22 are devoted to premises, principles, techniques, and approaches to oncogene targeting in vari-

Table 1

Functional Classification of Oncoproteins [adapted from R. Hesketh *(12)*].

Oncoproteins	Biological functions	Examples
Class 1	Growth factors	HSTF1, INT2, PDGFB/SIS, WNT1-3
Class 2	Tyrosine kinases	HER-2/NEU, EGFR, ABL-1, TRK, SRC,
Class 3	Non-kinase receptors	MAS, MPL
Class 4a	Membrane G-proteins	H-RAS, K-RAS, N-RAS, TC21, $G_{\alpha 12}$, $G_{\alpha 13}$
Class 4b	Guanine nucleotide exchange proteins	SDC25, OST
Class 4c	RHO/RAC binding proteins	BCR, DBL, TIAM1, VAV, TIM, ECT2
Class 5	Cytoplasmatic protein serine kinases	BCR, MOS, RAF, PKC , CLK, TPL-2
Class 6	Protein series, threonine (and tyrosine) kinases	AKT1, AKT2, STY
Class 7	Cytoplasmatic regulators	BCL1, CRK, NCK, PEM, ODC1
Class 8	Cell cycle regulators	INK4A, INK4B, INK4C, CyclinD1, CDC25
Class 9	Transcription factors	ETS, JUN, FOS, MYC, REL, TAL-1, E2F1
Class 10	Transcription elongation factors	ELL
Class 11	Intracellular membrane factors	BCL2
Class 12	Nucleoporins	NUP98, NUP214
Class 13	Adapter proteins	SHC
Class 14	RNA binding proteins (Translation factors)	EWS (eIF-4E)
Class 15	Unknown function	MEL, MAF, DAN, DLK, LBC

ous types of human cancer by using signal transduction inhibitors, immunological targeting methods, and/or antisense gene therapy. These chapters also review the results of preclinical and clinical testing of some of the most advanced therapeutic agents already developed (e.g., Gleevec, Herceptin, IMC225). It is also noteworthy that inhibition of oncoprotein activity could sensitize cancer cells to more traditional forms of anticancer therapy (e.g., radio- or chemotherapy) and, possibly, to inhibitors of angiogenesis. Therefore, oncogene targeting agents are likely to be used not instead of, but rather in addition to, already established treatment modalities. The discussion on each of these subjects is supported by an extensive survey of the relevant literature, providing a resource to those seeking more detailed information.

Many individuals have made their mark on this book and deserve thanks and gratitude. In particular, I am deeply indebted to all the contributors to this volume for their outstanding work and cooperation, to the publisher for a great deal of patience, to my colleagues, particularly Drs. Petr Klement and Jeffrey Weitz, for their encouragement and support, to my daughter Anna and wife Dana for their forgiveness and help, as well as to my mother Stanislawa for pretty much everything.

I would like to include another personal note. While this volume was in preparation, someone posed to me the following question: Why would an expert in a particular field of research contribute a book chapter these days? Why would such an individual risk the somewhat longer publication cycle and forgo the instant relief and gratification of much faster publication in a scientific journal? My experience, with this book and otherwise, has taught me that scientists who agree, or else can be persuaded, to write a book chapter are a different breed. Perhaps these are the people who believe that in today's reality often illuminated by limelights of scientific "fashion," flashes of information snapshots, and the glow of ever changing research headlines, something qualitatively different is also needed. Working on a book inherently entails a more collegial process and results in something more lasting, more complete and comprehensive, and perhaps more mature than the "last minute" research report. Books are more about ideas and directions than about "hot" results. We hope that *Oncogene-Directed Therapies* will possess at least some of these lasting qualities and that it will help to accurately reflect the emerging new "climate" in oncology. We believe such understanding will benefit academics, students, physicians, and ultimately, the patients.

Janusz Rak

REFERENCES

1. Hanahan D and Weinberg RA. The hallmarks of cancer. *Cell* 2000; 100:57–70.
2. Bishop JM. Cancer: the rise of the genetic paradigm. *Genes Dev* 1995; 9:1309–1315.
3. Nowell PC. The clonal evolution of tumor cell populations. *Science* 1976; 194:23–28.
4. Heppner GH. Tumor cell societies. *J Natl Canc Inst* 1989; 81:648–649.
5. Burnet FM. The concept of immunological surveillance. *Prog Exp Tumor Res* 1970; 13:1–27.: 1–27.
6. Folkman J. Angiogenesis in cancer, vascular, rheumatoid and other disease. *Nature Med* 1995; 1:27–31.
7. Rak J. Possible role of tumour stem - end cell interaction in metastasis. *Med Hypoth* 1989; 29:17–19.
8. Fearon ER and Vogelstein B. A genetic model for colorectal tumorigenesis. *Cell* 1990; 61:759–767.
9. Hahn WC, Counter CM, Lundberg AS, Beijersbergen RL, Brooks MW, and Weinberg RA. Creation of human tumour cells with defined genetic elements. *Nature* 1999; 400:464–468.
10. Shirasawa S, Furuse M, Yokoyama N, and Sasazuki T. Altered growth of human colon cancer cell lines disrupted at activated Ki-ras. *Science* 1993; 260:85–88.
11. Chin L, Tam A, Pomerantz J, Wong M, Holash J, Bardeesy N, Shen Q, O'Hagan R, Pantginis J, Zhou H, Horner JW, Cordon-Cardo C, Yancopoulos G.D, and DePinho RA. Essential role for oncogenic Ras in tumour maintenance. *Nature* 1999; 400:468–472.
12. Hesketh R. *The Oncogene and Tumor Suppressor Gene Facts Book*, second ed., Academic Press, New York, 1997.

CONTENTS

CONTRIBUTORS

JAMES L. ABBRUZZESE, MD • *Department of Gastrointestinal Medical Oncology, M.D. Anderson Cancer Center, The University of Texas, Houston, TX*

JANE ARBOLEDA, PhD • *Division of Hematology-Oncology, Department of Medicine, UCLA School of Medicine and Jonsson Comprehensive Cancer Center, Los Angeles, CA*

ERIC J. BERNHARD, PhD • *Department of Radiation Oncology, University of Pennsylvania, Philadelphia, PA*

DANIEL P. CAHILL, MD, PhD • *Johns Hopkins Oncology Center, Baltimore, MD*

ANN F. CHAMBERS, PhD • *Departments of Oncology and Medical Biophysics, University of Western Ontario, and London Regional Cancer Centre, London, Ontario, Canada*

GERHARD CHRISTOFORI, PhD • *Institute of Biochemistry, University of Basel, Switzerland*

ELIZABETH COHEN-JONATHAN, MD, PhD • *Institut Claudius Regaud, Toulouse, France*

CLAUDIO J. CONTI, DVM, PhD, MD • *Anderson Cancer Center, Science Park, Smithville, Texas*

FINBARR E. COTTER, PhD, FRCP, FRCPATH • *Department of Experimental Haematology, St. Bartholomew's and the Royal London, Queen Mary School of Medicine and Dentistry, London, UK*

ADRIENNE D. COX, PhD • *Departments of Radiation Oncology and Pharmacology, University of North Carolina at Chapel Hill, Chapel Hill, NC*

CHANNING J. DER, PhD • *Department of Pharmacology, Lineberger Comprehensive Cancer Center, University of North Carolina at Chapel Hill, Chapel Hill, NC*

SUSAN J. DONE, MA, MB, BCHIR, PhD, FRCPC • *University Health Network, Ontario Cancer Institute, and the Departments of Laboratory Medicine and Pathobiology, and Medical Biophysics, University of Toronto, Ontario, Canada*

BRIAN J. DRUKER, MD • *Oregon Health & Science University Cancer Institute, Portland, OR*

DEAN A. FENNELL, MD • *Department of Experimental Haematology, St. Bartholomew's and the Royal London, Queen Mary School of Medicine and Dentistry, London, UK*

JORGE FILMUS, PhD • *Department of Medical Biophysics, University of Toronto, Sunnybrook and Women's College Health Sciences Centre, Toronto, Ontario, Canada*

AMATO J. GIACCIA, PhD • *Division of Radiation and Cancer Biology, Department of Radiation Oncology, Stanford University School of Medicine, Stanford, CA*

ABHIJIT GUHA, MD, FRCSC, FACS • *Division of Neurosurgery, Arthur & Sonia Labatts Brain Tumor Centre, Hospital for Sick Children, University of Toronto, Ontario, Canada*

ANJALI K. GUPTA, MD • *Department of Radiation Oncology, University of Pennsylvania, Philadelphia, PA*

STEPHEN M. HAHN, MD • *Department of Radiation Oncology, University of Pennsylvania, School of Medicine, Philadelphia, PA*

MICHAELA HERZIG, PhD • *Research Institute of Molecular Pathology, Vienna, Austria*

ERIC C. HOLLAND, MD, PhD • *Departments of Cell Biology, Neurosurgery, and Neurology, Memorial Sloan-Kettering Cancer Center, New York, NY*

ROBERT S. KERBEL, PhD, • *Department of Medical Biophysics, University of Toronto, Sunnybrook and Women's College Health Sciences Centre, Toronto, Ontario, Canada*

SAMIR N. KHLEIF, MD • *Cancer Vaccine Clinic, NCI-Naval Hospital Bethesda, National Cancer Institute, Bethesda, MD*

MARK H. KIRSCHBAUM, MD • *Department of Biological Regulation, the Weizmann Institute of Science, Rehovot, Israel*

GIANNOULA KLEMENT, MD • *Sunnybrook and Women's College Health Sciences Centre, Toronto, Ontario, Canada*

GOTTFRIED E. KONECNY, MD • *Division of Hematology-Oncology, Department of Medicine, UCLA School of Medicine and Jonsson Comprehensive Cancer Center, Los Angeles, CA*

EDWARD H. LIN, MD • *Department of Gastrointestinal Medical Oncology, The University of Texas M.D. Anderson Cancer Center, Houston, TX*

JOSEPH A. LUCCI, III, MD • *University of Texas Medical Branch, Galveston, TX*

MINA D. MARMOR, PhD • *Department of Biological Regulation, the Weizmann Institute of Science, Rehovot, Israel*

FRANK MCCORMICK, PhD • *UCSF Cancer Center/Cancer Research Institute, San Francisco, CA*

W. GILLIES MCKENNA, MD, PhD • *Department of Radiation Oncology, University of Pennsylvania, School of Medicine, Philadelphia, PA*

GRETCHEN A. MURPHY, PhD • *Department of Pharmacology, Lineberger Comprehensive Cancer Center, University of North Carolina at Chapel Hill, Chapel Hill, NC*

RUTH J. MUSCHEL, MD, PhD • *Department of Pathology and Laboratory Medicine, University of Pennsylvania, Philadelphia, PA*

MICHAEL E. O'DWYER, MD • *Oregon Health & Sciences University Cancer Institute, Portland, OR*

MARK PEGRAM, MD • *Division of Hematology-Oncology, Department of Medicine, UCLA School of Medicine and Jonsson Comprehensive Cancer Center, Los Angeles, CA*

JANUSZ RAK, MD, PhD • *Henderson Research Centre, Department of Medicine, McMaster University, Hamilton, Ontario, Canada*

MARCELO L. RODRIGUEZ-PUEBLA, PhD • *College of Veterinary Medicine, North Carolina State University, Raleigh, NC*

KIRILL ROSEN, PhD • *Sunnybrook and Women's College Health Sciences Centre, Toronto, Ontario, Canada*

TAKEHIKO SASAZUKI, MD, PhD • *Research Institute, International Medical Center of Japan, Tokyo, Japan*

ADRIAN M. SENDEROWICZ, MD • *National Institute of Dental and Craniofacial Research, NIH, Bethesda, MD*

SENJI SHIRASAWA, MD, PhD • *Department of Pathology, Research Institute, International Medical Center of Japan, Tokyo, Japan*

DENNIS J. SLAMON, MD, PhD • *Division of Hematology-Oncology, Department of Medicine, UCLA School of Medicine and Jonsson Comprehensive Cancer Center, Los Angeles, CA*

JEREMY A. SQUIRE, PhD • *University Health Network, Ontario Cancer Institute, and the Departments of Laboratory Medicine and Pathobiology, and Medical Biophysics, University of Toronto, Ontario, Canada*

HEMANTH J. VARGHESE, BSC • *Department of Medical Biophysics, University of Western Ontario, and London Regional Cancer Centre, London, Ontario, Canada*

YOSEF YARDEN, PhD • *Department of Biological Regulation, The Weizmann Institute of Science, Rehovot, Israel.*

GELAREH ZADEH, MD • *Arthur & Sonia Labatts Brian Tumor Centre, Hospital for Sick Children, University of Toronto, Ontario, Canada*

I BASIC CONCEPTS IN ONCOGENE RESEARCH

1

Genetic Basis of Cancer Progression

Susan J. Done, MA, MB, BCHIR, PhD, FRCPC and Jeremy A. Squire, PhD

CONTENTS

1. INTRODUCTION

The current paradigm for the development of cancer is that it is a genetic disease, with the malignant phenotype resulting from an accumulation of genetic alterations. This model was first postulated by Cavenee et al. *(1)* and further developed by Fearon and Vogelstein *(2)*. In the simplest situation of a hematologic neoplasm, such as chronic myeloid leukemia (CML), neoplasia arises as a direct result of the formation of the Philadelphia chromosome *(1)*. This primary aberration is observed recurrently in CML, and the onset of the more aggressive acute phase of the disease is usually heralded by the acquisition of secondary chromosomal changes *(3)*. Many hematologic neoplasms and sarcomas are characterized by the presence of consistent primary chromosomal rearrangements. However, for most carcinomas, a more complex pattern of acquisition of genomic aberration takes place. An advanced carcinoma may have undergone multiple genetic alterations involving both simple mutations in tumor suppressor genes and oncogenes, as well as extensive karyotypic aberrations. Genetic changes are accompanied by a spectrum of phenotypic changes, and, as the number of genetic aberrations increases, there appears to be a more marked histologic phenotype. Through studies of colon cancer, we understand that colorectal neoplasia arises as a result of the mutational activation of oncogenes coupled with the mutational inactivation of tumor suppressor genes (for a review *see* ref. *2*). It is believed that the total number of genetic changes, rather than the sequence in which they occur, is a primary

From: *Oncogene-Directed Therapies*
Edited by: J. W. Rak © Humana Press Inc., Totowa, NJ

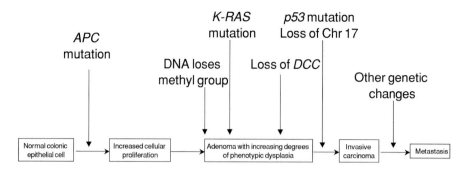

Fig. 1. Genetic changes associated with progression in colon cancer (modified from ref. 2).

factor in the development of malignancy. Vogelstein and coworkers found that at least five distinct genetic events were required for colon cancer to develop (2). In this malignancy, the specific genetic changes that lead to the production of invasive carcinoma have been clearly identified: the combination of adenomatous polyposis coli (APC) gene mutations; methylation status alterations; K-ras mutations; DCC (deleted in colon cancer) gene mutations; and p53 mutations. Invasive carcinoma has more genetic alterations than a benign lesion like an adenoma, and, in turn, an adenoma has more genetic alterations than histologically normal epithelium (Fig. 1). This particular model has guided much of our current thinking about how cancer arises.

Alterations in specific normal cellular functions appear to be prerequisites for malignancy to develop: lack of a requirement for outside growth signals, loss of sensitivity to growth inhibitory signals, avoidance of apoptosis, failure to repair DNA damage appropriately, and limitless replicative potential. In addition, tumor cells require the ability to establish a blood supply and the ability to invade and metastasize (4). Genes altered in cancer cells can broadly be divided into two groups, oncogenes and tumor suppressor genes (see Chapter 6). Although many oncogenes are involved in the control of normal growth and development, a persistent high level of oncogene activation in cancer cells results in uncontrolled growth. Tumor suppressor genes act in the opposite direction to prevent uncontrolled growth, and it is their inactivation that allows cancer to develop. The activation and inactivation of these genes can occur in a variety of ways, including mutation, loss of chromosomal material, and transcriptional up-regulation or silencing. Normal somatic cells are dependent on external stimuli to control cell cycle checkpoints. Cells become committed only toward the end of the G1 phase of the growth cycle. Multiple proteins exert positive and negative regulatory influences on a family of cyclin dependent kinases (cdks)(5). Any disturbance of this interplay can result in unchecked proliferation.

New techniques used in the study of in vitro and in vivo models of cancer have shown the tremendous complexity of these genetic alterations, although distinct systematic patterns are beginning to emerge. Evidence in support of the Vogelstein model comes from a variety of sources, including analysis of chromosomal alterations, methylation analysis of tumor DNA, and the study of mutations of known oncogenes, tumor suppressors, and mismatch repair genes. The extraordinary success in the understanding of the genetic basis of progression of complex tumors, such as colon cancer, has been a direct result of an increasing number of sensitive assays capable of screening and analyzing tumors for consistent genomic alteration. In this chapter, we will review some of the key technologies that have improved our understanding of genetic perturbations in tumors, and will then review some of the evidence supporting current models of cancer causation and progression and recent developments in this area.

2. DETECTION OF GENETIC PERTURBATIONS IN THE DEVELOPMENT OF CANCER

Advances in techniques for the analysis of genetic material have fueled improvements in our understanding of the genetic basis of cancer. Studies have shown an increasing number of genetic aberrations accompany the development of cancer. The first techniques to be developed were for the study of whole chromosomes. Techniques evolved to allow the study of segments of DNA and, more recently, to study DNA of the whole genome.

2.1. Cytogenetics

Karyotyping was one of the first techniques employed to study chromosomal alterations in human cancers. With the ability to see inside cells and visualize their chromosomes, came the recognition that certain consistent patterns of chromosomal alterations could be found in particular tumors. One of the first consistent chromosomal alterations to be detected was the translocation between chromosomes 9 and 22, t(9;22), called the Philadelphia chromosome (Fig. 2), which is seen in CML. This translocation brings the oncogenes *BCR* and *ABL* together. The BCR/ABL protein product has elevated tyrosine kinase activity and phosphorylates many cellular substrates *(6)*. Karyotyping has proven very helpful for diagnosis in several other leukemias and lymphomas, where recurrent well-defined translocations have been found. However, traditional karyotyping methods, such as Geimsa (G)-banding, have been less successful in many types of solid tumors, since it is difficult to prepare good quality metaphase chromosomes, and the results are often complex and ambiguous.

2.2. Fluorescence In Situ Hybridization

Cancer cytogenetics has become more accessible as fluorescence *in situ* hybridization (FISH) has been applied systematically *(7)*. Specific FISH probes can assay for subtle chromosomal changes that would have been impossible to detect by conventional G-banded analysis. Target preparations for FISH analysis include metaphase and interphase cells derived from standard cytogenetic preparations as well as archived formalin-fixed paraffin-embedded (FFPE) histological material and fixed cytological preparations. To detect gene amplifications, translocations, or microdeletions, there are a number of commercial unique sequence gene probes that can readily identify recurrent chromosomal aberrations. FISH is one of the techniques used clinically to detect increased copy number of *Her2/neu* in breast cancer and *c-myc* in neuroblastoma. Amplification of *Her-2/neu,* also known as *c-erbB-2*, has been found in several solid tumors, most notably breast. Amplification of this oncogene appears to correlate with poor prognosis in some patients and predicts response to chemotherapy *(8)*. With the recent introduction into the clinic of the humanized monoclonal antibody directed against HER-2/neu protein (Herceptin trastuzumab), there has been an increased need for assessment of HER-2/neu status as only those with amplification (usually measured by FISH) or overexpression (usually measured immunohistochemically) are believed

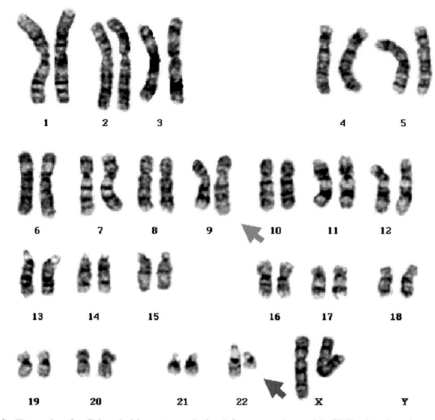

Fig. 2. Example of a G-banded karyotype derived from a patient with CML showing the transloca-tion between chromosomes 9 and 22 (arrowed) leading to the production of the small Philadelphia chromosome.

to respond *(9).* In neuroblastoma, a solid tumor of childhood, the *myc* oncogene may be amplified. Amplification of *myc* can be seen by FISH as extrachromosomal material (Fig. 3) with the number of copies present having prognostic value *(10).*

Useful probes for detecting terminal rearrangements are the telomere-specific probes. Whole chromosome-specific paint probes can be very helpful for confirming the identity of rearrangements in which G-banding has proved inconclusive. Recently, some sensitive and highly specific screening FISH techniques utilizing differentially labeled chromosome-specific paints *(11)* have been developed. These allow the full chromosome complement to be analyzed to identify unknown karyotype aberrations. Increasingly, the use of multicolor FISH painting techniques (called spectral karyotyp-ing [SKY] or multicolor FISH [M-FISH]) is proving invaluable as a general cytoge-netic screening method to detect the more complex classes of chromosomal rearrangements that characterize the karyotypes of advanced malignancies.

2.3. Comparative Genomic Hybridization

Comparative genomic hybridization (CGH) is a technique that allows gene copy number comparison between two genomes (Fig. 4a). One of the chief advantages of

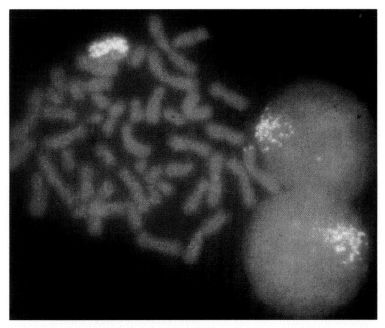

Fig. 3. Example of FISH analysis of a neuroblastoma cell line with 50 copies of the *N-myc* onco-gene. In the panel, one metaphase cell has a large homogeneously staining region (HSR) exhibiting multiple yellow signals as a result of *N-myc* FISH. In the two interphase nuclei, the HSR generates a large speckled yellow domain in each nucleus as a result of *N-myc* amplification.

CGH is that it is only necessary to obtain DNA from a tumor to derive cytogenetic information concerning genomic imbalances. This means that DNA collected over many years can be used for retrospective CGH analysis. In typical experiments, labeled DNA fragments from the tissue of interest are used to probe normal metaphase chromosomes competitively against normal DNA fragments labeled with a different colored fluorochrome. CGH offers the advantage of allowing a whole genome scan in one experiment. However, the benefit of gaining a whole genome overview comes at the cost of resolution. The smallest region of gain or loss that can be detected is 5–10 Mb of DNA. Although, when high copy number amplification (>10-fold) is present, it is possible to detect changes in the order of a few hundred kilobases of DNA. The development of strategies that allow the CGH analysis of FFPE tissues has increased the types of lesions amenable to analysis. Unfortunately, several hundred nanograms of DNA are needed. For high quality CGH, the labeled probes need to be 0.5–3 kb; thus, the starting material should contain a large propor-tion of high molecular weight DNA fragments (4–20 kb). Whole genome amplifica-tion methods, such as degenerate oligonucleotide-primed polymerase chain reaction (DOP-PCR), primer-extension preamplification PCR (PEP-PCR), and improved PEP-PCR (I-PEP-PCR) are making CGH possible using much smaller microdis-sected samples *(12)*. CGH analysis is being increasingly applied to microarray tar-gets to overcome the resolution limitations of metaphase chromosome targets.

A

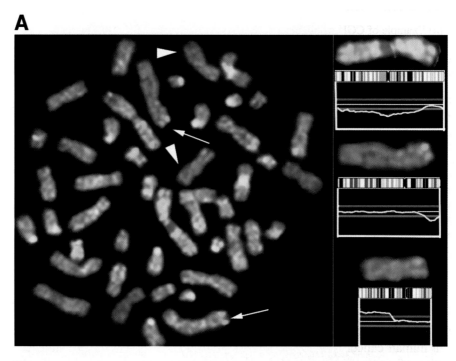

B

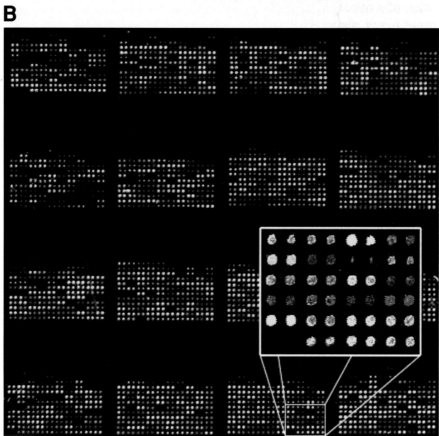

Fig. 4. (a) Example of CGH using DNA derived from a neuroblastoma. Note the intense small area of green signal on the short arm of chromosome 2 (arrows) resulting from *N-myc* gene amplification, in contrast to the red signal generated on most of the long arm of chromosome 6 (arrow heads) caused by deletion of part of this chromosome. To the left of this panel are profiles from chromosomes 1 (upper), 2 (middle), and 6 (lower). When the yellow trace of red:green ratio is present close to the green line, it indicates gain. If it is in between the red and green lines, there is no net DNA imbalance in the tumor, and if the trace moves to the red line, then DNA loss or deletion is indicated. In these examples, most of chromosome 1 is gained. There is high copy number amplification in the region containing *N-myc*, and most of the long arm of chromosome 6 is deleted. **(b)** Microarray analysis of prostate cancer gene expression using tumor RNA with reference to RNA derived from normal prostate tissue. In this analysis, cDNAs were differentially labeled with Cy5 and Cy3 fluorophores, respectively, and hybridized to a human cDNA microarray. For a list of the cDNA collection used for this array and protocols used for array construction, please refer to the University Health Network Microarray Centre Web site (http://www.uhnres.utoronto.ca/services/microarray). Differential gene expression can be recognized as duplicate spots showing strong green (inset upper left) or red intensity signals (inset lower right).

2.4. Loss of Heterozygosity

Loss of heterozygosity (LOH) analysis is used to study and localize genetic alterations in human cancer. As loss of a portion of a chromosome is one mechanism of inactivation of a tumor suppressor gene, LOH studies have been used to pinpoint the positions of tumor suppressor genes *(1)*. A large number of chromosomal loci can be studied by assembling a panel of microsatellite markers (di-, tri-, or tetra nucleotide repeats in noncoding regions) and reactions can be multiplexed. This technique has been popular because selection of primer pairs amplifying short fragments of the order of 150–300 bp has allowed the study of FFPE tissues. If an individual has inherited detectably different genomic fragments from each of their parents, and one fragment is absent in tumor tissue or lesional tissue from this individual, the tumor or lesion is said to exhibit LOH. Although there are several methods of measuring LOH, the term usually refers to the study of PCR-amplified highly polymorphic genetic markers *(13)*. Sites for study are chosen that have a high frequency of heterozygosity, i.e., there are many alleles at a selected locus, such that there is a high likelihood that an individual will inherit alleles of different lengths from each parent. Having determined that an individual is informative at a selected locus, i.e., they possess two alleles of different lengths when normal tissue is studied, one can then study lesional tissue. LOH is said to exist if only one of the two alleles can be detected in the lesional tissue, or there is loss of intensity of one of the alleles below a predetermined threshold. A difference in intensity could reflect differential amplification of one allele over the other rather than complete loss. For this reason, some investigators prefer the term "allelic imbalance", as it is more strictly correct. In practice, LOH is the term that is more widely used and encompasses either loss or amplification of one allele over the other.

2.5. Mutation Screening

Single-strand conformation polymorphism (SSCP) is a commonly used technique for screening for mutations in cancer genes *(14)*. This technique detects regions with various types of DNA changes, including single base substitutions. It relies on the property of single-stranded DNA, having a tendency to adopt complex conformational structures stabilized by weak intramolecular hydrogen bonds. When a mutation is present in the DNA, it will affect the conformation of that sequence and will result in a different electrophoretic mobility relative to the wild-type sequences, typically referred to as "shifts".

Another useful screening technique for detecting mutations in DNA is heteroduplex analysis. This method identifies mismatched bases formed when complementary strands of a mutant and its normal sequence are allowed to hybridize to form a double-stranded heteroduplex molecule *(14)*. This PCR-based technique can detect single base substitutions in a large tract of DNA; however, owing to its efficiency and simplicity, it has been more widely used in the detection of nucleotide insertions and/or deletions in heterozygous individuals. Heteroduplex formation is carried out by subjecting PCR products to heat denaturation, during which PCR molecules are separated into their single-stranded forms, followed by a cooling down step where single-stranded molecules reanneal to form double-stranded molecules. Compared to homoduplex molecules, where base pairing between the strands is complete, the mismatched heteroduplex molecules migrate much more slowly in polyacrylamide gels owing to their shape, thus, enabling the detection of mutations. Since both heteroduplex analysis and SSCP do not provide information about the nature of the change found, DNA sequencing must be performed on the abnormal regions of the gene to determine the nature of the mutation.

2.6. Methylation, Imprinting, and Epigenetics

Alterations in DNA methylation are widespread in cancers. Evidence is now accumulating that methylation changes may occur progressively during carcinogenesis *(15)*. In addition, differential methylation can be associated with the natural process of transcriptional silencing of alleles of specific genes, in a process termed genomic imprinting. Often, the genes that appear to be imprinted are growth factors or are involved in growth control, and there are several examples of loss of imprinting associated with specific types of tumors. To detect genomic DNA that is differentially methylated or imprinted, it is common to use methylation-dependent restriction endonuclease digestion and Southern analysis. Methylation and imprinting can also be associated with alterations to the overall chromatin structure in large domains of genomic DNA encompassing several hundred kilobases of DNA. It is probable that more sensitive assays capable of scanning these intriguing regions of the genome will soon be available. DNA methylation of promoter-associated CpG islands is an alternate mechanism to mutation in silencing gene function and has been shown to affect tumor-suppressor genes, such as *p16* and *RBl*, growth and differentiation controlling genes, such as *IGF2,* and many others *(16)*.

2.7. Microarrays

Prospects for whole genome scanning in the future lie with microarrays. The development of microarrays comprising hundreds or thousands of different cDNAs, bacterial artificial chromosomes (BACs), or oligonucleotides dotted onto glass slides is allowing analysis of gene expression patterns *(17),* sequence analysis *(18),* and comparative genomic hybridization *(19)* (Fig. 4b) on a vastly greater scale than has been possible before. It will be possible to simultaneously analyze samples for hundreds of separate parameters, allowing for a much richer understanding of gene interactions. The challenge is now to develop statistical approaches that will permit us to make sense of the vast amounts of data that this technology will generate. In addition, tissue arrays have also been developed that allow as many as 1000 cylindrical tissue biopsies (of diameter of 1 mm or less) from individual FFPE blocks, to be placed into a single paraffin block. This enables the parallel analysis of *in situ* DNA, RNA, and proteins in histologically defined tissue *(20)*.

2.8. Tissue Microdissection

Improvements in PCR technologies have allowed the analysis of smaller and smaller amounts of starting template. This has permitted the study of genomic material in single cells or groups of cells. Initially, tissue microdissection was performed by excavating material from paraffin-embedded tissue blocks. However, owing to the destructive nature of this technique, methods have been developed to allow study of samples dissected from standard tissue sections of the order of 5 μm thick. Depending on the size of the lesion of interest, the tissue can be removed by either manual microdissection using a stereomicroscope or, for smaller lesions, a laser-capture microdissection (LCM) system can be used. In one of the most widely used LCM systems, a cap coated with adhesive material is placed directly over the lesion of interest. Firing of a laser beam through the tissue melts the tissue to the cap allowing precise removal of the lesion *(21)* for genetic analysis of DNA, RNA, and/or protein.

3. EVIDENCE IN SUPPORT OF GENETIC MODELS OF CANCER PROGRESSION

Evidence in support of the genetic basis of cancer comes from a variety of sources (reviewed in ref. *4*). Many years ago, it was recognized that most carcinogens are mutagens. Later studies showed that the susceptibility to certain carcinogens is dependent on the ability of particular cellular enzymes to convert them to the DNA damaging mutagenic form. Additional support is found in the study of situations of increased DNA damage, including aging and exposure to radiation. Defects in DNA repair increase the probability of an individual developing cancer, and acquired mutations in DNA repair proteins are found in some classes of tumors. Ionizing radiation is capable of causing both single- and double-strand breaks in DNA. Studies of atomic bomb survivors in Hiroshima and Nagasaki *(22)* have shown an increased incidence of cancer, suggesting that increasing the frequency of genetic alterations shifts the incidence curve. Following radiation, an increase in mutation rate can be seen in the next generation in both germline and somatic cells *(23)*. Consistent genetic alterations observable at a karyotypic level in specific tumors, provides strong evidence in support of the genetic basis of cancer *(3)*. The most direct evidence is the strong association between the presence of somatic mutations in cellular oncogenes and tumor suppressor genes.

Additional evidence in support of the model of cancer resulting from an accumulation of genetic events comes from age incidence data of cancer *(24)*. Most common cancers, e.g., lung, breast, and colon, become increasingly common to age 80. This age-dependence is to be expected if the genetic perturbations that lead to cancer are considered as stochastic events. With an increasing amount of time, an increasing number of events will occur.

Table 1
Genes Involved in Inherited Cancer Syndromes *(42,43)*

Syndrome	Gene
Retinoblastoma	*RB1*
Li Fraumeni	*p53*
Wilm's tumor	*WT1*
Neurofibromatosis type 1	*NF1*
Neurofibromatosis type 2	*NF2*
Von Hippel Lindau	*VHL*
Multiple endocrine neoplasia type 1	*MEN 1*
Multiple endocrine neoplasia type 2	*MEN 2(ret)*
Cowden syndrome	*PTEN*
Breast cancer	*BRCA1, BRCA2*
Familial adenomatous polyposis	*APC*
Dysplastic nevus syndrome	*p16 (CDKN2A)*
Gorlin-Goltz syndrome	*PTC*
Tuberose sclerosis	*TSC1, TSC2*
Juvenile polyposis	*SMAD4*
Familial gastric cancer	*E-cadherin*
Peutz-Jeghers syndrome	*LKB1*
Xeroderma pigmentosa	*XP-A to G*
Ataxia telangiectasia	*ATM*
Bloom syndrome	Helicase gene
Hereditary non-polyposis colon cancer (Lynch) syndrome	*hMSH2, hMLH1, hPMS1, hPMS2, hMSH6*
Werner syndrome	RNA helicase gene
Fanconi's anemia	*FAA, FAC, FAD*

3.1. Familial Cancer

Some of the most convincing evidence in support of a genetic model of cancer development comes from studies of familial cancer syndromes. The genetic basis of many inherited cancer syndromes has been elucidated and is listed in Table 1. Familial cancer tends to occur at an earlier age, consistent with some of the key alterations being present at birth and, thus, less somatic genetic alterations being required for its development. Familial tumors are more likely to be multiple, consistent with the stochastic model of disease progression. As one of the key transformative genetic events has already occurred, there is an increased risk for tumor development. Various approaches are being taken to discover genes that play a role in the development of cancer. One approach is to study the inheritance patterns in families that have a higher frequency of cancer than would be expected from the general population risk. Confounding this approach is the fact that tumors in inherited cancer syndromes can also be found in sporadic cases. In the past, linkage analysis was used to identify affected individuals within familial cancer kindreds. More recently, many of the genes responsible for these syndromes have been identified, allowing the delineation of the specific mutation present within a family.

One of the first familial cancers to be studied was retinoblastoma. Retinoblastoma is an eye tumor of young children, caused by inactivation of the retinoblastoma *(RB)* gene on

13q14. In 40% of individuals, mutations are inherited in an autosomal dominant fashion with a penetrance of 90–95%, and the remaining approx 60% of children have sporadic tumors. From the work of Alfred Knudson on hereditary retinoblastoma, we understand that in order to develop, a cancer must have lost both copies of the relevant tumor suppressor gene either by mutagenesis, deletion of a small region, or loss of a chromosomal arm (25). Based on Knudsen's "two hit hypothesis" of tumorigenesis, it is plausible that after inactivation of one allele of a tumor suppressor gene by mutation, the other may be lost through genomic deletion. Indeed, it was recognized, when cytogenetic analysis was first applied to both heritable or sporadic retinoblastoma tumors, that 70% of tumors have undergone karyotypic deletions or LOH affecting band 13q14 (1). This observation led to the molecular mapping and cloning of the *RB* gene, permitting a better understanding of how tumor suppressor genes function. Significantly, *RB* mutations were found not only in retinoblastoma tumors, but also as acquired mutations in diverse tumor types. The retinoblastoma protein is intimately involved in cell cycle control, and it appears to be frequently subject to mutation as part of cancer progression.

Studies of large breast cancer kindreds by linkage analysis and positional cloning, led to the discovery of two familial breast cancer genes, *BRCA1* and *BRCA2*. Together, germline mutations in these two genes account for a significant proportion of familial breast cancer. Female mutation carriers have a lifetime breast cancer risk of 60–80% and tend to develop breast cancer at a younger age. Germline mutations in *BRCA1* have been found in 60–80% of women with a family history of both breast and ovarian cancer (26). *BRCA1* and *BRCA2* are large genes, and many different inherited mutations have been described throughout the genes (27). Recurrent mutations have been described in particular populations. Inherited mutations in *BRCA2* typically give rise to breast cancer (male as well as female), although prostate, pancreas, and ovarian cancer have also been reported (28). A germline defect in *BRCA1* or *BRCA2* is usually followed by LOH of the wild-type allele (seen in about 85% of informative tumors), supporting their role as tumor suppressor genes (29). In contrast to *RB*, the role of *BRCA1* and *BRCA2* in sporadic breast cancer remains unclear. This is perhaps reflective of the number of genetic events that need to occur for a breast carcinoma to develop, as compared to a tumor with its origin in an embryonal tissue such as retinoblastoma (30).

4. DEVELOPMENT OF THE GENETIC MODEL OF CANCER PROGRESSION

4.1. Preinvasive/Field Effect

Early stages in cancer development may not be observable in terms of tissue changes. There is growing evidence that genetic alterations often precede phenotypic changes. For example, mutations in the *p53* tumor suppressor gene have been described in benign breast tissues (31). Molecular alterations have been noted in histologically normal epithelium surrounding invasive breast cancer, suggesting that the tumor arose from a field or zone of epithelium containing genetic alterations (32). For these alterations to be detectable, they must be present in a substantial number of cells. As the same alteration is present in a group of cells, it most likely arose from a single cell and, thus, represents a clone that has propagated. Therefore, even lesions that have previously been considered benign can be clonal and, hence, neoplastic. These studies are forcing a reevaluation of the definitions of neoplasia and malignancy.

4.2. Aging, Telomere Erosion, and Genomic Instability

As discussed previously, the incidence of cancer is strongly associated with age. It was, thus, of great significance when it was recognized that age-dependent telomere erosion may lead to genomic instability and tumorigenesis. Telomeres are specialized stabilizing structures at chromosome ends, whose shortening with each replication is thought to serve as a mitotic clock in humans, defining the number of divisions a cell can go through before it reaches senescence. Bypass of senescence, leads to critical telomere shortening ("crisis"), resulting in genomic instability including formation of dicentrics, ring chromosomes, bridge-breakage-fusions, and aneuploidy. Abrogation of crisis and immortalization has been linked in many cell systems to the process of tumorigenesis. Cells from primary tumors have, in general, shorter telomeres than normal counterpart somatic cells, reflecting a greater number of cell divisions these cells undergo prior to reactivation of telomerase. Telomerase, an enzyme that elongates telomeric ends, is inactive in differentiated tissues, but its presence can be detected in germ and stem cells as well as in over 80% of cancers. In cancer cells, it maintains a minimal telomere length required for indefinite cell proliferation. There are some examples of the importance of telomerase activity and cancer progression. In neuroblastomas with high telomerase activity, other genetic changes (e.g., *N-myc* amplification) and an unfavorable prognosis have been observed, whereas tumors with low telomerase activity have acquired less genetic alterations and have a more favorable prognosis *(33)*.

4.3. Gatekeepers and Caretakers

It appears that most tumor suppressor genes can be broadly divided into two groups that have been termed "gatekeepers" and "caretakers" *(34)*. Gatekeepers are, in general, genes that directly regulate the growth of tumors by promoting apoptosis. Loss of function of both alleles of a gatekeeper, such as *RB,* is required to produce tumors. In contrast, inactivation of caretakers does not directly promote growth of tumors. Rather, loss of caretaker function leads to genomic instability, which indirectly promotes tumor growth by increasing the somatic mutation rate in the developing tumor. We probably have more knowledge of gatekeeper function in tumorigenesis at present, but there is increasing interest in understanding cellular processes that control genomic integrity during tumor progression.

It has recently been proposed that cancer can develop by two distinct pathways: chromosomal instability (CIN) or microsatellite instability (MIN). MIN appears to play a role in the development of a proportion of familial colon cancers. Defects in mismatch repair genes result in errors in DNA replication being propagated. CIN may be more important in the development of most human cancers. The basis for CIN is not yet clear, but could be owing to mutations in cell cycle control genes, genes involved in spindle formation, chromosome stability genes, or defects in the centrosome, which lead to abnormal cell division and chromosome missegregation *(35,36)*.

In colon cancer, individuals with the familial type of disease, tend to develop tumors at an earlier age and show increased rates of multiple tumors. Inherited tumors have been found to be owing to defects in mismatch repair genes. Mutations accumulate because of uncorrected misalignments between template and daughter DNA strands during replication. Errors occur particularly during replication of repetitive sequences. This phenomenon is termed microsatallite instability (MIN). Defects in these genes are diagnosed clinically by the analysis of a panel of microsatellite markers. Amplified fragments differ in length in affected individuals.

One of the most frequently altered genes in human cancer is the tumor suppressor gene, *p53*. p53 is a negative regulator of cell growth, and loss of p53 function results in failure to undergo apoptosis and increased cell proliferation *(37)*. Many functions have been proposed for p53, including transcriptional activation and repression, non-transcriptional activation of apoptosis, signal transduction, and a role as a replication factor. Cellular stressors, such as cytokines, hypoxia, genotoxic damage, and metabolic damage, activate p53 to produce coordinated responses, resulting in growth arrest, apoptosis, or adaptation *(38)*. *p53* has been called the "guardian of the genome", because normal cell cycle arrest associated with DNA damage is altered in cells with mutant *p53*, and DNA amplification of a reporter gene can occur up to several hundredfold in cells containing mutant *p53 (39)*.

Alteration of certain key genes within the cell leads to the loss of normal homeostatic controls of genetic material. Subsequent to this, more general genetic alterations may occur, producing a wide range of diversity within the population of cells that make up a tumor. Many of these secondary changes will make the cells unstable and, thus, will be selected against. Only certain cells will acquire the genetic changes necessary for invasion and metastasis, and it is these cells that will gradually comprise the bulk of the tumor *(40)*.

5. SUMMARY

The results from the application of new genetic and molecular biological tools continue to expand our understanding of the genetic basis of cancer progression. If the current paradigm holds true, namely that cancer is a genetic disease with the malignant phenotype resulting from an accumulation of genetic alterations, then in theory, it should be possible to identify critical events in this pathway to invasion. With enhanced understanding will come the opportunity to diagnose tumors at earlier and potentially curable stages and also help in the development of new therapeutic modalities, such as gene therapy. Array technology seems likely to change the way we diagnose and treat cancer. Molecular profiling of tumors *(41)* will produce very detailed portraits of individual tumors. The genetic pathways thus identified will provide new information for more targeted drug development and increased antineoplastic activity. This will allow more accurate prognostic information to be given and also permit therapies to be customized.

REFERENCES

1. Cavenee WK, Dryja TP, Phillips RA, Benedict WF, Godbout R, Gallie BL, et al. Expression of recessive alleles by chromosomal mechanisms in retinoblastoma. *Nature* 1983; 305:779–784.
2. Fearon ER, Vogelstein B. A genetic model for colorectal tumorigenesis. *Cell* 1990; 61:759–767.
3. Heim S, Mitelman F. Cancer Cytogenetics. 2nd ed. Wiley-Liss, New York, 1995.
4. Hanahan D, Weinberg RA. The hallmarks of cancer. *Cell* 2000; 100:57–70.
5. Sandhu C, Slingerland J. Deregulation of the cell cycle in cancer. *Cancer Detect Prev* 2000; 24:107–118.
6. Sattler M, Griffin JD. Mechanisms of transformation by the BCR/ABL oncogene. *Int J Hematol* 2001; 73:278–291.
7. Blancato JK. Fluorescence in situ hybridization. In: Gersen SL, Keagle MB, eds. *The Principles of Clinical Cytogenetics.* Humana Press, *Totowa,* 1999, pp. 443–472.
8. Yamauchi H, Stearns V, Hayes DF. When is a tumor marker ready for prime time? A case study of c-erbB-2 as a predictive factor in breast cancer. *J Clin Oncol* 2001; 19:2334–2356.

9. Schnitt SJ. Breast cancer in the 21st century: neu opportunities and neu challenges. *Mod Pathol* 2001; 14:213–218.

10. Minard V, Hartmann O, Peyroulet MC, Michon J, Coze C, Defachelle AS, et al. Adverse outcome of infants with metastatic neuroblastoma, MYCN amplification and/or bone lesions: results of the French society of pediatric oncology. *Br J Cancer* 2000; 83:973–979.

11. Bayani J, Squire J. Advances in the detection of chromosomal aberrations using spectral karyotyping. Clin Genet 2001; 59:65–73.

12. Dietmaier W, Hartmann A, Wallinger S, Heinmoller E, Kerner T, Endl E, et al. Multiple mutation analyses in single tumor cells with improved whole genome amplification. *Am J Pathol* 1999; 154:83–95.

13. Dracopoli NC. *Current Protocols in Human Genetics.* John Wiley & Sons, New York, 2001.

14. Ausubel FM, Brent R, Kingston RE, Moore DD, Seidman JG, Smith JA, et al. *Current Protocols in Molecular Biology.* John Wiley & Sons, New York, 2001.

15. Baylin SB, Esteller M, Rountree MR, Bachman KE, Schuebel K, Herman JG. Aberrant patterns of DNA methylation, chromatin formation and gene expression in cancer. *Hum Mol Genet* 2001; 10:687–692.

16. Feinberg AP. DNA methylation, genomic imprinting and cancer. *Curr Top Microbiol Immunol* 2000; 249:87–99.

17. DeRisi J, Penland L, Brown PO, Bittner ML, Meltzer PS, Ray M, et al. Use of a cDNA microarray to analyse gene expression patterns in human cancer. *Nat Genet* 1996; 14:457–460.

18. Kozal MJ, Shah N, Shen N, Yang R, Fucini R, Merigan TC, et al. Extensive polymorphisms observed in HIV-1 clade B protease gene using high-density oligonucleotide arrays. *Nat Med* 1996; 2:753–759.

19. Pollack JR, Perou CM, Alizadeh AA, Eisen MB, Pergamenschikov A, Williams CF, et al. Genome-wide analysis of DNA copy-number changes using cDNA microarrays. *Nat Genet* 1999; 23:41–46.

20. Kononen J, Bubendorf L, Kallioniemi A, Barlund M, Schraml P, Leighton S, et al. Tissue microarrays for high-throughput molecular profiling of tumor specimens. *Nat Med* 1998; 4:844–847.

21. Simone NL, Bonner RF, Gillespie JW, Emmert-Buck MR, Liotta LA. Laser-capture microdissection: opening the microscopic frontier to molecular analysis. *Trends Genet* 1998; 14:272–276.

22. Ron E, Preston DL, Mabuchi K, Thompson DE, Soda M. Cancer incidence in atomic bomb survivors. Part IV: Comparison of cancer incidence and mortality. *Radiat Res* 1994; 137(2 Suppl):S98–S112.

23. Dubrova YE, Plumb M, Gutierrez B, Boulton E, Jeffreys AJ. Transgenerational mutation by radiation. *Nature* 2000; 405:37.

24. National Cancer Institute of Canada. *Canadian Cancer Statistics* 2001.

25. Knudson AG. Hereditary cancer, oncogenes, and antioncogenes. *Cancer Res* 1985; 45:1437–1443.

26. Nathanson KL, Wooster R, Weber BL, Nathanson KN. Breast cancer genetics: what we know and what we need. *Nat Med* 2001; 7:552–556.

27. Gayther SA, Mangion J, Russell P, Seal S, Barfoot R, Ponder BA, et al. Variation of risks of breast and ovarian cancer associated with different germline mutations of the BRCA2 gene. *Nat Genet* 1997; 15:103–105.

28. Goggins M, Schutte M, Lu J, Moskaluk CA, Weinstein CL, Petersen GM, et al. Germline BRCA2 gene mutations in patients with apparently sporadic pancreatic carcinomas. *Cancer Res* 1996; 56:5360–5364.

29. Arason A, Jonasdottir A, Barkardottir RB, Bergthorsson JT, Teare MD, Easton DF, et al. A population study of mutations and LOH at breast cancer gene loci in tumours from sister pairs: two recurrent mutations seem to account for all BRCA1/BRCA2 linked breast cancer in Iceland. *J Med Genet* 1998; 35:446–449.

30. Knudson AG. Hereditary cancer: two hits revisited. *J Cancer Res Clin Oncol* 1996; 122:135–140.

31. Millikan R, Hulka B, Thor A, Zhang Y, Edgerton S, Zhang X, et al. p53 mutations in benign breast tissue. *J Clin Oncol* 1995; 13:2293–2300.

32. Deng G, Lu Y, Zlotnikov G, Thor AD, Smith HS. Loss of heterozygosity in normal tissue adjacent to breast carcinomas. *Science* 1996; 274:2057–2059.

33. Hiyama E, Hiyama K, Yokoyama T, Matsuura Y, Piatyszek MA, Shay JW. Correlating telomerase activity levels with human neuroblastoma outcomes. *Nat Med* 1995; 1:249–255.

34. Vogelstein B, Kinzler KW. The *Genetic Basis of Human Cancer.* McGraw-Hill, New York, 1998.

35. Cahill DP, Kinzler KW, Vogelstein B, Lengauer C. Genetic instability and darwinian selection in tumours. *Trends Cell Biol* 1999; 9:M57–M60.

36. Cahill DP, Lengauer C, Yu J, Riggins GJ, Willson JK, Markowitz SD, et al. Mutations of mitotic checkpoint genes in human cancers. *Nature* 1998; 392:300–303.

37. Elledge RM, Allred DC. The p53 tumor suppressor gene in breast cancer. *Breast Cancer Res Treat* 1994; 32:39–47.

38. Hall PA, Meek D, Lane DP. p53—integrating the complexity. *J Pathol* 1996; 180:1–5.

39. Davidoff AM, Humphrey PA, Iglehart JD, Marks JR. Genetic basis for p53 overexpression in human breast cancer. *Proc Natl Acad Sci USA* 1991; 88:5006–5010.

40. Shackney SE, Shankey TV. Genetic and phenotypic heterogeneity of human malignancies: finding order in chaos. *Cytometry* 1995; 21:2–5.

41. Liotta L, Petricoin E. Molecular profiling of human cancer. *Nat Rev Genet* 2000; 1:48–56.

42. Prime SS, Thakker NS, Pring M, Guest PG, Paterson IC. A review of inherited cancer syndromes and their relevance to oral squamous cell carcinoma. *Oral Oncol* 2001; 37:1–16.

43. Lindblom A, Nordenskjold M. The biology of inherited cancer. *Semin Cancer Biol* 2000; 10:251–254.

2

The Molecular Basis of Chromosomal Instability in Human Cancer Cells

Daniel P. Cahill, MD, PhD

1. INTRODUCTION

Aneuploidy, the presence of numerical aberrations in chromosome complement, is characteristic of the vast majority of epithelial solid tumors. This phenotype of human cancer has been well described throughout the long history of careful microscopic and karyotypic scrutiny of human tumors *(1,2)*. More recently, this tradition has been complemented by molecular and cellular analyses of tumor cell aneuploidy. These analyses have shown that tumor cell aneuploidy is the result of a persistent chromosomal instability (CIN). In human cancer cells, CIN appears to be the manifestation of an intrinsic defect in the chromosome segregation machinery. As a result of this defect, CIN drives the continual generation of aneuploidy in human tumors. But what is the molecular genetic basis, if any, for the CIN phenotype? Recent work has demonstrated that some aneuploid cancers have alterations in mitotic checkpoint genes that affect their ability to direct the appropriate segregation of chromosomes in cell division. Future work is aimed at the identification of the genes involved in these processes that are altered in human cancers.

2. WHY ARE HUMAN CANCERS ANEUPLOID?

Recent studies have shown that aneuploidy, or numerical aberrations in chromosome complement, is seen at the earliest stages of tumor development *(3–5)*. However, the underlying reason why aneuploidy is observed early in tumor evolution is not yet clear.

From: *Oncogene-Directed Therapies*
Edited by: J. W. Rak © Humana Press Inc., Totowa, NJ

One theory *(6,7)* suggests that aneuploidy is the spontaneous and self-maintaining result of catastrophic divisions early in tumorigenesis. According to this hypothesis, aneuploidy begets further aneuploidy, thus, CIN is both a cause and a result of tumor cell aneuploidy. The self-generating phenomenon is initiated by chance environmental interactions that turn a normal diploid cell down the path that inexorably leads to aneuploid instability.

There are several predictions that arise from this proposal. The most striking is that specific molecular genetic alterations are not necessary to drive CIN and the resultant aneuploidy. Rather, the discovery of genetic alterations of instability genes will be the exception, not the rule. In most cases, this theory predicts that no molecular genetic cause for CIN will be found. The cause of CIN can be thought of as an unfortunate "episodic" occurrence early in the process of tumor evolution.

Alternatively, there is a mutational theory for tumor cell aneuploidy *(8)*. Perhaps, the vast majority of tumor cell aneuploidy is the direct phenotypic result of genetic alterations in genes controlling chromosome segregation. One key to further molecular analysis of tumor cell aneuploidy lies in the cellular studies done to detail the exact nature of the CIN phenotype. The descriptive characterization of tumor cell CIN provides critical guidance to the molecular analyses of this phenotype. A series of experiments performed with aneuploid cancer cells helps to delineate the phenotypic characteristics of tumor cell aneuploidy *(9)*.

3. CHARACTERISTICS OF HUMAN TUMOR CELL ANEUPLOIDY

First, by scoring the number of chromosome gains and losses that accumulate in tumor cells passaged through a defined number of generations, Lengauer et. al calculate the absolute rate of mis-segregation events that occur per division. As it turns out, the rate of errors in chromosomal segregation in aneuploid tumor cells versus diploid cells is approx 100-fold higher than the rate of these errors in normal diploid cells, leading to a nondisjunction event on the order of once every five cell divisions in tumor cells *(9)*.

Next, analysis of a series of fusion cell clone experiments performed by Lengauer et al. *(9)* identifies the key phenotypic traits of chromosomal instability. First, consider a stable diploid cell line fused to a second stable diploid cell line, artificially inducing tetraploidy at the chromosomal level. Based on studies in yeast *(10,11)*, some have hypothesized that there is an episode of tetraploidization during tumor development that serves as a "first step" towards the degeneration into chromosome instability and aneuploidy. It is easy to appreciate how this model would not require a specific genetic alteration to initiate instability, but rather a single flawed mitosis could lead to the precursor of eventual CIN. According to this proposal, CIN represents an inherent difficulty of the normal chromosomal segregation machinery when confronted with too many chromosomes; therefore, this tetraploid fusion should degenerate into chromosomal instability. Strikingly, though, this fusion has exactly the same level of chromosome stability as the diploid parent fusions *(9)*. Thus, one relatively common conjecture for an episodic (or nongenetic) cause of CIN can be excluded with experimental data.

However, one can argue that this fusion experiment may have been too simplistic. Perhaps CIN can ensue only when there is a loss of chromosomal symmetry *(11)*, that is to say, diploidy (2 copies of each chromosome) or tetraploidy (4 copies) will be stable, but triploidy (3 copies) will be unstable. To address this possibility, a stable diploid line to which a single extra chromosome had been added was examined. This line has the normal diploid chromosome complement with a single additional chromosome added by microsomal fusion techniques, therefore 47 chromosomes in all and a loss of symmetry due to three copies of the added chromosome. Notably, this line is neither CIN across the full complement of chromosomes nor CIN for the additional chromosome *(9)*. All three copies of the added chromosome stably segregate to the daughter cells during division at a rate directly comparable to that of diploid cells. This result suggests that the isolated gain of a single chromosome does not destabilize the segregation machinery.

The most informative experiment, however, is the fusion between a stable diploid cell and a CIN cell. The phenotype of this fusion line should provide insight into the nature of the defect responsible for CIN. For example, if the CIN phenotype were owing to recessive inactivating mutations, then the phenotype of the resulting fusion should be wild-type, since these inactivating mutations would be complemented by the wild-type copies contributed by the stable diploid parent of the fusion. Strikingly, however, the CIN phenotype persists in this fusion line *(9)*. Thus, the CIN defect was not complemented by the wild-type chromosome segregation phenotype of the stable diploid line. The simplest interpretation of this observation is that, at least in this line, the CIN phenotype is dominant, and accordingly, the genetic basis of the CIN phenotype has molecular features of a dominant mutation. From the point of view of Mendelian genetics, this leads to the hypothesis that the CIN gene mutation is equivalent to a classically defined oncogenic or single-hit mutation.

4. TUMOR CELL ANEUPLOIDY IS A PRODUCT OF GENOMIC INSTABILITY

An oncogene has been described as any single-allele gain-of-function alteration in a gene that provides a selection advantage during tumor evolution *(12)*. Practically speaking, most think of oncogenes as those genes which, when genetically altered in human tumors, directly affect the growth and differentiation characteristics of the cancer cell, such as ras or myc. However, the cell fusion studies support the proposal that the CIN seen in human tumors may be the result of a single-hit mutation in genes that control the proper segregation of chromosomes *(8,13)*. Thus, at the molecular level, the hypothetical class of mutations that drive CIN in human cancers act in an oncogenic manner, as single allele alterations that promote the development of the tumor.

An important theory *(14–16),* informing the work on CIN, was the proposal that there is a class of genes that are distinct from classical growth-controlling tumor suppressor and oncogenes, which are responsible mainly for preventing the accumulation of genetic alterations in the genome. Initially, this theory focused on simple elevation of the nucleotide mutation rate through inactivation of repair genes and the role of the elevated mutation rate in the process of tumor evolution. Loeb termed these genes mutators, and a great deal of molecular evidence has arisen in the decades since to support the role of an increased mutation rate driving the tumorigenic process *(14,16)*.

At first, the evidence was best developed in the heritable cancer syndromes. In hereditary nonpolyposis colon cancer (HNPCC), inactivating mutations in the genes responsible for nucleotide mismatch repair (MMR), inherited in the germline, give rise

Two Pathways for Instability

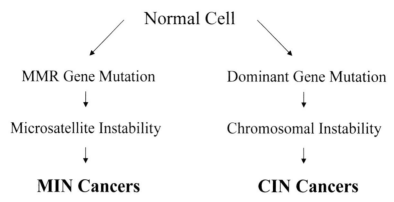

Normal Cell

MMR Gene Mutation   Dominant Gene Mutation

↓   ↓

Microsatellite Instability   Chromosomal Instability

↓   ↓

MIN Cancers   **CIN Cancers**

Fig. 1. Two pathways to tumor cell instability. Colorectal cancers appear to develop one of (at least) two distinct pathways of genetic instability. MIN cancers, which are seen in patients with the HNPCC syndrome and in a small percentage of sporadic nonfamilial cases, have nucleotide instability. This instability is cause by genetic alteration of one of the MMR genes. Alternatively, CIN cancers, which represent the vast majority of sporadic tumors, have CIN. This CIN has been shown, in some cases, to be due to dominant mutations in mitotic checkpoint genes that affect the fidelity of chromosome segregation.

to colon cancers solely as a result of the increased mutation rate in the precancerous adenomas. The MMR genes, when inactivated, also cause a characteristic nucleotide instability in microsatellite repeats, referred to as microsatellite instability (MIN). This focused role of preventing nucleotide instability leads this class of genes to be referred to as caretakers *(17,18)*. Myriad other inherited cancer syndromes (e.g., hereditary breast cancer *(19)*, Bloom's syndrome *(20)*, Werner's syndrome *(21)*, ataxia telangeictasia *(22)*, Nijmegen breakage syndrome *(23,24)*) have now been described where the key role of the inherited mutant gene in driving cancer formation seems to be an elevation of the effective mutation rate.

A significant minority of nonhereditary sporadic colon cancers contain somatic inactivation of MMR genes *(25)*. Thus, the caretaker's role does not appear to be limited to heritable syndromes, but can also impact sporadic disease. However, the nucleotide MMR type of instability is typical of only a minor fraction of epithelial tumors. In aggregate, most sporadic tumors seem to have CIN. CIN may thus represent an alternative instability that arises more frequently in sporadic tumors (Fig. 1). Are there genetic alterations that could account for the CIN phenotype?

5. MOLECULAR BASIS OF TUMOR CELL ANEUPLOIDY

There are two approaches possible to pursue the identity of a putative CIN gene mutation. The first, and most direct, is positional. Using the above described diploid (stable) to aneuploid (unstable) fusion experimental design as a model, one could establish a system whereby defined portions of the CIN cell's genome are added to the background of a stable line, and the resulting clones screened for CIN. Since the hypothesis detailed above suggests that the genetic mutation should act dominantly, similar to a classical

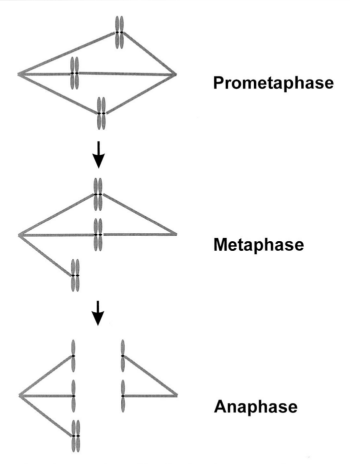

Prometaphase

Metaphase

Anaphase

Fig. 2. Nondisjunction after metaphase with a lagging chromosome. One sequence of events that leads to the generation of aneuploidy is an isolated nondisjunction event during the normal process of mitosis. The two copies of each of the 46 human chromosomes align at the metaphase plate during chromosome congression in late prometaphase. Occasionally, due to chance, a chromosome will lag during this process, not aligning appropriately before the initiation of anaphase, thus leading to the gain of a chromosome in one of the daughter cells of the division and the concomitant loss of a chromosome in the other daughter.

oncogene, theoretically, this approach would have similarities to the classical genome transfer approaches used to identify ras *(26)* or RAG1 and RAG2 *(27,28)*.

A second, and parallel, approach would mirror the effort used to attack the problem of cloning the MIN genes. In that case, a clear cellular phenotypic correlate was established with recognition of the presence of microsatellite repeat instability *(29)*. A series of experiments was able to show that this cellular phenotype of MIN was present in model organisms that had inactivated a gene in the pathway controlling DNA mismatch repair. Following this clue, investigators were able to identify the human counterparts (or homologs) of lower organism MMR genes and then test these homologs for mutation in MIN tumors *(30–32)*. This strategy of phenotypic characterization in model organisms implicating a pathway of genes and then candidate testing of the human homologs in human disease proved successful. Thus, much as with the example set forth from the work with MIN, we look to model systems to identify the genetic components of these processes to guide our molecular analysis of human tumors.

The phenotypic correlate in the case of CIN is the gain and loss of chromosomes during cell division (Fig. 2). The detailed description of this phenotype becomes particularly important when considering corresponding pathways of genes from model organisms as potential targets of genetic alteration. For example, genes that when mutated lead to increased rates of tetraploidization are not candidates that best typify the CIN phenotype in human cancer. This particular example is important, because a number of checkpoint genes involved in either the replication of DNA or the appropriate timing of entry and exit from mitosis have this phenotype when inactivated in lower organisms *(33)*. While many of these genes are classically thought of as the "guardians of the genome", they do not seem to fit as candidates for CIN genes.

The observations of the dynamics of human cancer karyotypes suggest that there is a defect in the basic mechanics of cell division that contributes to the aneuploidy seen in tumor karyotypes. What is known about the basic biology of cell division that can inform our investigations into CIN in cancer? As it turns out, the answer is "A great deal"—the study of the genetics of mitotic cell division is one of the most active areas of basic biological investigation. Work has detailed many of the structural components necessary for cell division in the yeast *Saccharomyces cerevisiae (34,35),* the importance of mitotic protein kinase networks *(36–39),* and control of mitotic motor proteins in the alignment of chromosomes *(40–42).*

6. MITOTIC CHECKPOINTS

The phenotype of yeast cells that have alterations in genes involved in mitotic spindle assembly *(34,35)* is probably most directly analogous to the CIN of human cancer cells. Genetic screens in yeast have led to the discovery of several genes that can disrupt the mitotic checkpoint and lead to CIN phenotypes *(43,44).* Perhaps the best studied pathway leading to chromosome instability, yeast cells with alterations of these genes, have an increased rate of single chromosome gain and loss, thus developing aneuploidy in a process similar to human tumors. In addition, there is a subset of these genes that is more specifically involved in a spindle assembly checkpoint that monitors for the alignment of chromosomes on the metaphase plate (Fig. 3), including BUB1, 2, 3, MAD1, 2, 3, and MPS1, some of which bind to the kinetochore, and all of which are required for a normal mitotic delay in response to spindle disruption *(45–50)* (Fig. 4). Subsequent work has detailed other important protein components of this pathway and has provided insight into how the interactions between these components propagate the inhibitory signal.

These checkpoints are typically assessed after treatment of cells with microtubule-disrupting agents, which prevent spindle assembly during mitosis (mitotic checkpoints) *(43).* Cells with intact checkpoints sense that kinetochores are not attached properly to the spindle and delay chromosome decondensation, nuclear membrane reformation, and other events that would normally initiate interphase at the completion of mitosis (Fig. 5). Cells with defective checkpoints do not recognize the presence of a lagging chromosome and, subsequently, undergo much less of a delay and exit mitosis prematurely *(51),* leading to gains or losses of chromosomes *(52–54).* Elegant cytological experiments by Li and Nicklas have shown that a single lagging chromosome can gen-

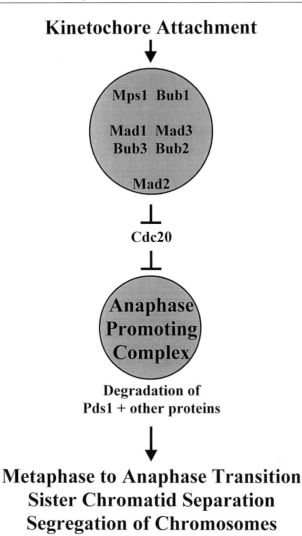

Kinetochore Attachment

Mps1 Bub1

Mad1 Mad3
Bub3 Bub2

Mad2

Cdc20

Anaphase Promoting Complex

Degradation of Pds1 + other proteins

Metaphase to Anaphase Transition
Sister Chromatid Separation
Segregation of Chromosomes

Fig. 3. Mitotic checkpoint pathway genes. The genes in the mitotic checkpoint that monitors for the alignment of chromosomes on the metaphase plate include BUB1, 2, 3, MAD1, 2, 3, and MPS1. These genes are involved in the generation of an inhibitory signal that delays the onset of metaphase to allow the lagging chromosome time to align correctly. This signal appears to be mediated through the Cdc20 protein and its interactions with the anaphase-promoting complex (APC), which prevents the breakdown of Pds1 and other proteins involved in sister chromatid adhesion.

erate an inhibitory checkpoint signal that arrests mitosis at metaphase *(51,55)*. Thus, the proposed mechanism for aneuploidy is that loss of the mitotic checkpoint leads to a premature initiation of metaphase and a nondisjunction event for the lagging chromosome (Fig. 2).

6.1. Mitotic Checkpoint Gene Mad2

The first piece of evidence supporting the involvement of the spindle checkpoint in human cancers was a key observation from Li and Benezra *(56)*, in their initial descrip-

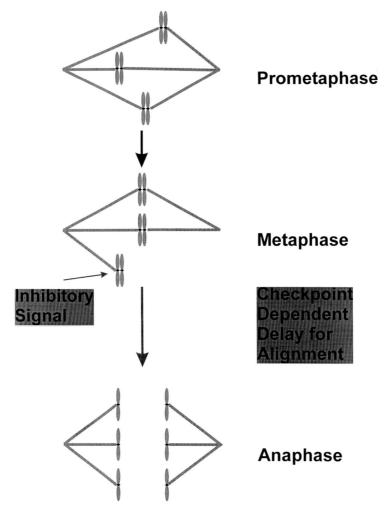

Fig. 4. Normal mitotic checkpoint. Some of the mitotic checkpoint genes bind to the kinetochore of a lagging chromosome during metaphase and activate the propagation of an inhibitory signal that delays the onset of metaphase to allow the lagging chromosome time to align correctly and ensure mitosis proceeds with both daughter cells receiving equivalent contributions from the parent cell.

tion of the human homolog of the mitotic spindle checkpoint gene Mad2. The protein product of this gene appears to be required in stoichiometric amounts to prevent the onset of anaphase when chromosomes are not properly aligned at the metaphase plate *(57–62)*. As a result, when Li and colleagues microinjected antibodies to this protein into cells exposed to microtubule depolymerizing agents, the normal mitotic arrest phenotype is abrogated. In a survey of expression levels of this gene in a small set of cancer cell lines, these investigators showed a decreased level of Mad2 expression in a breast cancer cell line by Western blot analysis. With the above hypothesis in mind, this decreased level of expression could be the basis for chromosome instability in this tumor. This raised the possibility that underlying alterations in expression of the Mad2 protein could contribute to CIN.

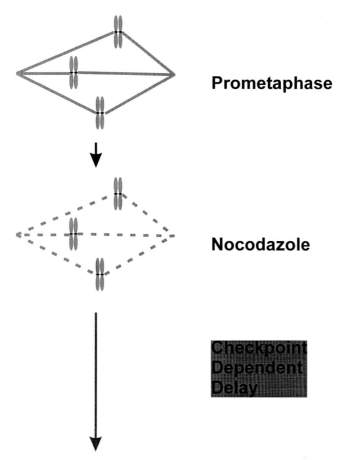

Prometaphase

Nocodazole

Checkpoint
Dependent
Delay

Fig. 5. Mitotic checkpoint assay. Spindle microtubules form the basic structural elements of the mitotic spindle. When these microtubules are depolymerized with antimicrotubule agents such as nocodazole or colcemid, all mitotic chromosomes fall off alignment on the metaphase plate. Since each of these chromosomes represents a "lagging" chromosome, this treatment generates a strong inhibitory signal in cells with intact mitotic checkpoints. This signal enforces chromosome condensation and prevents further progression through the cell cycle, attempting to delay mitotic progression until the microtubules can properly assemble the chromosomes to divide equally among the two daughter cells.

Subsequently, Dobles et al. demonstrated that a murine homozygous knock-out of the Mad2 gene is lethal at the organismal level *(63)*. The knock-out cells display markedly aberrant chromosome segregation with high levels of nondisjunction. Importantly, these results demonstrate that unlike in the yeast, where checkpoint pathways are not essential for survival in normal growth conditions, inactivation of the mitotic checkpoint is lethal in mammalian multicellular systems. Inactivating knock-outs of the homologous Mad2 gene in the yeast divide under normal conditions, but die when challenged with microtubule depolymerizing agents. However, the mammalian version of this gene seemed to be required for normal mitosis to proceed.

Interestingly, heterozygous knock-out of Mad2 in human and mouse cells induces a low but significant level of chromosomal instability *(64)*. It will be interesting to see if the heterozygous Mad2 instability phenotype can contribute to tumorigenesis in these mice.

These data in model systems cast a new light on the role of Mad2 in human cancers. Indeed, recent studies have documented decreased expression levels of Mad2 *(65),* or in one case heterozygous mutation of the gene *(66),* in human cancers. Whether this class of mutants is the cause of instability in these tumors is an important question for future investigation.

6.2. Mitotic Checkpoint Genes Bub1 and BubR1

To begin to elucidate the genetic mechanisms underlying the checkpoint defect in CIN cells, we chose to evaluate the human homologue of *S. cerevisiae* BUB1. BUB1 is the prototype member of the mitotic spindle checkpoint gene family *(45–50).* This gene is at or near the top of the mitotic spindle checkpoint signal cascade in yeast by epistasis analysis *(67).* It has an interesting domain structure, the N terminus of the protein appears to be responsible for localization to a lagging chromosome's kinetochore, while the C terminus contains a kinase domain that is thought to be involved in the generation of the inhibitory checkpoint signal. Interestingly, it had been shown that in vitro-generated variants of murine BUB1 can exert a dominant negative effect, allowing cells to exit mitosis prematurely *(68).* These investigators generated a truncated version of the protein that separated the N-terminal localization domain from the C-terminal kinase domain. This truncated protein acts in a dominant negative manner, localizing to the lagging kinetochore region and inactivating the mitotic spindle checkpoint when overexpressed in mammalian cells.

This dominance was intriguing in light of the demonstration that the CIN phenotype is dominant in cell fusions between stable and CIN cells *(9).* The BUB1 gene is not only a key component of the mammalian mitotic spindle checkpoint, but it is possible for truncating mutations to act dominantly, a potential feature consistent with the previous cell fusion data about the dominant maintenance of CIN at the cellular level. There are two human homologs of the yeast BUB1 gene, Bub and BubR1 (which has been referred to as Mad3L by some investigators *(69).*

Mutational evidence implicating the spindle checkpoint pathway came with the identification of mutations in the checkpoint genes Bub1 and BubR1 *(70).* These mutations were heterozygous, which was consistent with the notion that some genetic alterations responsible for CIN might function as dominant negative mutations and be heterozygous in the cancer cells. Functional characterization of the mutant proteins was necessary to prove they acted in a dominant manner. Both transient transfection experiments *(70)* and stable inducible versions of these mutations inactivate the mitotic checkpoint to a level seen in typical CIN cancers. In addition, these mutations cause true CIN when reintroduced into stable diploid cell lines in an inducible system. Subsequent studies have shown that mutations in Bub1 and BubR1 occur at a low level in tumors *(71–78).*

6.3. Mitotic Checkpoint Gene Mad1

Additional evidence for the role of the mitotic spindle checkpoint pathway came from studies of the mammalian homolog of the mitotic spindle checkpoint gene Mad1 *(79).* The endogenous Mad1 protein is bound and inactivated by the human T-cell leukemia virus protein tax. These data suggests that this inactivation is a contributing factor in the development of chromosomal instability that precedes the development of T-cell leukemias. The recent description of mutations in BUB1 and BubR1 in T-cell leukemias strongly supports the role of checkpoint inactivation in the causal development of these cancers *(74)*.

7. CONCLUSIONS

The mutations described in the mitotic spindle checkpoint pathway thus far are all heterozygous single allele alterations. Functional data for some of the heterozygous mutants suggests that these alterations represent oncogenic mutations. Is this heterozygous spectrum of mutation indicative of the underlying biology of CIN? One explanation for this observed spectrum could be that single hit mutations causing CIN are simply a reflection of the mutational space that is favored statistically *(8)*. According to this reasoning, we observe many more tumors with CIN rather than with nucleotide instability; because there are more opportunities for a random mutational load to affect chromosomal segregation processes with a single allele mutation than nucleotide repair pathways, which are usually disrupted with biallelic inactivating mutations. Evidence in favor of this argument comes from the recent completion of the human genome project. There appear to be hundreds of genes that are potentially involved in chromosome segregation vs a smaller number directly involved in the mechanics of nucleotide MMR.

A second reason for the mutational spectrum is that perhaps it represents a reflection of the selective pressures on tumors *(80)*. Given the balance of selective pressures in tumor evolution, perhaps single hit mutations are seen because there is a selective pressure against complete abrogation of the mitotic checkpoint pathway. Accordingly, we can explain the spectrum of mutation with a balanced principle, whereby some genomic instability is necessary for tumor evolution, but too severe a mutation leads to catastrophic cell death. Only a mutation that is just right will lead to the right amount of increased instability, and, thus, increased rate of evolution of the tumor cell lineage without too much cell death.

At the level of the germline, the murine Mad2 knock-out experiments *(63)* suggests drive further studies to find the molecular basis for human inherited CIN syndromes. For example, defective mitotic checkpoints have been observed in the rare congenital disease mosaic variegated aneuploidy *(81)*. Is it possible that inherited syndromes can be found that are segregating aneuploidizing mutations? Based on a single-hit model of CIN, it might seem unlikely that such a mutation could exist and give rise to viable offspring. However, the murine heterozygous knock-out studies *(64)* demonstrate the possibility of heritable CIN disease. It will be interesting to see what future investigation in this area will reveal.

As we look to the future, it is important to keep in mind the significant differences in the mechanics of mitosis between mammalian cells and *S. cerevisiae*. It is likely that the mitotic checkpoint pathways are more complex in mammalian cells, with more genes playing important roles in monitoring the correct segregation of chromosomes. Work with nonhuman organisms can identify potential instability gene candidates, but can also provide powerful ways to explore their biochemical and physiological mechanisms of action.

Indeed, experiments in *Drosophila melanogaster* have identified novel genes for which there are no counterparts in yeast that appear to work in a parallel mitotic checkpoint pathway to the canonical spindle checkpoint. These experiments highlight the differences between the mechanisms of mitosis in yeast and human and stress the importance of not drawing overly broad connections between these two systems. For example, the genes zw10 and rod, which were first identified in *D. melanogaster (82,83)*, have been shown to be involved in the accurate segregation of chromosomes in mitosis *(84)*. There are no yeast homologs of these genes, and our understanding of these parallel pathways of instability depends almost solely on the elegant genetic analyses that have been carried out in *Drosophila*. These genes seem to function in a mitotic checkpoint pathway *(85,86)*, but this pathway is genetically distinct from the Bub/Mad mitotic checkpoint genes *(87)*. Since these genes cause a characteristic CIN when inactivated, and there are known human homologs *(88)*, it will be interesting to examine their involvement in human tumors.

The most direct interpretation of recent work is that the aneuploidy characteristic of the vast majority of epithelial solid tumors is the result of alterations in genes involved in mitotic checkpoint pathways like the spindle checkpoint. There are a number of genes that have been identified in model organisms, which appear to control various aspects of this process in mammalian cells. The evolutionary trip from yeast to human has spawned a series of parallel control pathways that effect the same result during the mammalian cell division. It is likely that genes more critical to driving aneuploidy in tumors will be found in the not-so-distant future. Indeed, perhaps the most significant contribution of the work in model organisms is to serve as a framework for the analyses of the genetic basis of CIN and aneuploidy in human cancers. These discoveries will lead us to a more fundamental understanding of this phenotype so unique and characteristic of the tumor formation process.

REFERENCES

1. Boveri T. *Zur Frage der Enstehung Maligner Tumoren, Vol. 1.* Gustav Fischer Verlag, Jena, 1914.
2. Mitelman F, Johansson B, Mertens F. *Catalog of Chromosome Aberrations in Cancer. 5th ed.* 2 v. Wiley-Liss, New York, 1994, pp. xxix,4252.
3. Bomme L, Bardi G, Pandis N, Fenger C, Kronborg O, and Heim S. Clonal karyotypic abnormalities in colorectal adenomas: clues to the early genetic events in the adenoma-carcinoma sequences. *Genes Chromosom Cancer* 1994; 10:190–196.
4. Bomme L, Bardi G, Pandis N, Fenger C, Kronborg O, and Heim S. Cytogenetic analysis of colorectal adenomas: karyotypic comparisons of synchronous tumors. *Cancer Genet Cytogenet* 1998; 106:66–71.
5. Shih IM, Zhou W, Goodman SN, Lengauer C, Kinzler KW, and Vogelstein B. Evidence that genetic instability occurs at an early stage of colorectal tumorigenesis. *Cancer Res* 2001; 61:818–822.
6. Duesberg P, Rausch C, Rasnick D, and Hehlmann R. Genetic instability of cancer cells is proportional to their degree of aneuploidy. *Proc Natl Acad Sci USA* 1998; 95:13692–13697.
7. Duesberg P, Rasnick D, Li R, Winters L, Rausch C, and Hehlmann, R. How aneuploidy may cause cancer and genetic instability. *Anticancer Res* 1999; 19:4887–4906.
8. Lengauer C, Kinzler KW, Vogelstein B. Genetic instabilities in human cancers. *Nature* 1998; 396:643–649.
9. Lengauer C, Kinzler KW, Vogelstein B. Genetic instability in colorectal cancers. *Nature* 1997; 386:623–627.
10. Mayer VW, Aguilera A. High levels of chromosome instability in polyploids of Saccharomyces cerevisiae. *Mutat Res* 1990; 231:177–186.
11. Giaretti W. A model of DNA aneuploidization and evolution in colorectal cancer. *Lab Invest* 1994; 71:904–910.

12. Bishop JM. Molecular themes in oncogenesis. *Cell* 1991; 64:235–248.
13. Cahill DP, Kinzler KW, Vogelstein B, and Lengauer C. Genetic instability and Darwinian selection in tumours. *Trends Cell Biol* 1999; 9:M57–M60.
14. Loeb LA, Springgate CF, Battula N. Errors in DNA replication as a basis of malignant changes. *Cancer Res* 1974; 34:2311–2321.
15. Nowell PC. The clonal evolution of tumor cell populations. *Science* 1976; 194:23–28.
16. Loeb LA. Mutator phenotype may be required for multistage carcinogenesis. *Cancer Res* 1991; 51:3075–3079.
17. Kinzler KW, Vogelstein B. Lessons from hereditary colon cancer. *Cell* 1996; 87:159–170.
18. Kinzler KW, Vogelstein B. Cancer-susceptibility genes. Gatekeepers and caretakers. *Nature* 1997; 386:761–763.
19. Haber D. Roads leading to breast cancer. *N Engl J Med* 2000; 343:1566–1568.
20. Ellis NA, German J. Molecular genetics of Bloom's syndrome. *Hum Mol Genet* 1996; 5:1457–1463.
21. Yu CE, Oshima Y, Fu H, Wijsman EM, Hisama F, Alisch R., et al. Positional cloning of the Werner's syndrome gene. *Science* 1996; 272:258–262.
22. Rotman G, Shiloh Y. ATM: from gene to function. *Hum Mol Genet* 1998; 7:1555–1563.
23. Carney JP, Maser RS, Olivares H, Davis EM, Le Beau M, Yates JR, et al. The hMre11/hRad50 protein complex and Nijmegen breakage syndrome: linkage of double-strand break repair to the cellular DNA damage response. *Cell* 1998; 93:477–486.
24. Varon R, Vissinga C, Platzer, M, Cerosaletti KM, Chrzanowska KH, Saar K, et al. Nibrin, a novel DNA double-strand break repair protein, is mutated in Nijmegen breakage syndrome. *Cell* 1998; 93:467–476.
25. Liu B, Nicolaides NC, Markowitz S, Willson JK, Parsons RE, Jen J, et al. Mismatch repair gene defects in sporadic colorectal cancers with microsatellite instability. *Nat Genet* 1995; 9:48–55.
26. Shih C, Weinberg RA. Isolation of a transforming sequence from a human bladder carcinoma cell line. *Cell* 1982; 29:161–169.
27. Schatz DG, Baltimore D. Stable expression of immunoglobulin gene V(D)J recombinase activity by gene transfer into 3T3 fibroblasts. *Cell* 1988; 53:107–115.
28. Schatz DG, Oettinger MA, Baltimore D. The V(D)J recombination activating gene, RAG-1. *Cell* 1989; 59:1035–1048.
29. Strand M, Prolla TA, Liskay RM, and Petes TD. Destabilization of tracts of simple repetitive DNA in yeast by mutations affecting DNA mismatch repair. *Nature* 1993; 365:274–276.
30. Leach FS, Nicolaides, NC, Papadopoulos N, Liu B, Jen J, and Parsons, R, et al. Mutations of a mutS homolog in hereditary nonpolyposis colorectal cancer. *Cell* 1993; 75:1215–1225.
31. Nicolaides NC, Papadopoulos N, Liu B, Wei YF, Carter KC, Ruben SM, et al. Mutations of two PMS homologues in hereditary nonpolyposis colon cancer. *Nature* 1994; 371:75–80.
32. Papadopoulos N, Nicolaides NC, Wei YF, Ruben SM, Carter KC, Rosen CA, et al. Mutation of a mutL homolog in hereditary colon cancer. *Science* 1994; 263:1625–1629.
33. Itzhaki JE, Gilbert CS, Porter AC. Construction by gene targeting in human cells of a "conditional" CDC2 mutant that rereplicates its DNA. *Nat Genet* 1997; 15:258–265.
34. Hoyt MA, Stearns T, Botstein D. Chromosome instability mutants of *Saccharomyces cerevisiae* that are defective in microtubule-mediated processes. *Mol Cell Biol* 1990; 10:223–234.
35. Spencer F, Gerring SL, Connelly C, and Hieter P. Mitotic chromosome transmission fidelity mutants in *Saccharomyces cerevisiae*. *Genetics* 1990; 124:237–249.
36. Adams RR, Carmena M, Earnshaw WC. Chromosomal passengers and the (aurora) ABCs of mitosis. *Trends Cell Biol* 2001; 11:49–54.
37. Ohi R, Gould KL. Regulating the onset of mitosis. *Curr Opin Cell Biol* 1999; 11:267–273.
38. Nigg EA, Polo-like kinases: positive regulators of cell division from start to finish. *Curr Opin Cell Biol* 1998; 10:776–783.
39. Glover DM, Hagan IM, Tavares AA. Polo-like kinases: a team that plays throughout mitosis. *Genes Dev* 1998; 12:3777–3787.
40. Hunter AW, Wordeman L. How motor proteins influence microtubule polymerization dynamics. *J Cell Sci* 2000; 113:4379–4389.
41. Endow SA. Microtubule motors in spindle and chromosome motility. *Eur J Biochem* 1999; 262:12–18.
42. Abrieu A, Kahana JA, Wood KW, and Cleveland DW. CENP-E as an essential component of the mitotic checkpoint in vitro. *Cell* 2000; 102:817–826.
43. Rudner AD, Murray AW. The spindle assembly checkpoint. *Curr Opin Cell Biol* 1996; 8:773–780.
44. Paulovich AG, Toczyski DP, Hartwell LH. When checkpoints fail. *Cell* 1997; 88:315–321.

45. Hoyt MA, Totis L, Roberts BT. *S. cerevisiae* genes required for cell cycle arrest in response to loss of microtubule function. *Cell* 1991; 66:507–517.

46. Li R, Murray AW. Feedback control of mitosis in budding yeast. *Cell* 1991; 66:519–531.

47. Roberts BT, Farr KA, Hoyt MA. The *Saccharomyces cerevisiae* checkpoint gene BUB1 encodes a novel protein kinase. *Mol Cell Biol* 1994; 14:8282–8291.

48. Hardwick KG, Murray AW. Mad1p, a phosphoprotein component of the spindle assembly checkpoint in budding yeast. *J Cell Biol* 1995; 131:709–720.

49. Weiss E, Winey M. The *Saccharomyces cerevisiae* spindle pole body duplication gene MPS1 is part of a mitotic checkpoint. *J Cell Biol* 1996; 132:111–123.

50. Hardwick KG, Johnston RC, Smith DL, and Murray AW. MAD3 encodes a novel component of the spindle checkpoint which interacts with Bub3p, Cdc20p, and Mad2p. *J Cell Biol* 2000; 148:871–882.

51. Nicklas RB. How cells get the right chromosomes. *Science* 1997; 275:632–637.

52. Spencer F, Hieter P. Centromere DNA mutations induce a mitotic delay in *Saccharomyces cerevisiae*. *Proc Natl Acad Sci USA* 1992; 89:8908–8912.

53. Pangilinan F, Spencer F. Abnormal kinetochore structure activates the spindle assembly checkpoint in budding yeast. *Mol Biol Cell* 1996; 7:1195–1208.

54. Wells WA, Murray AW. Aberrantly segregating centromeres activate the spindle assembly checkpoint in budding yeast. *J Cell Biol* 1996; 133:75–84.

55. Li X, Nicklas RB. Mitotic forces control a cell-cycle checkpoint. *Nature* 1995; 373:630–632.

56. Li Y, Benezra R. Identification of a human mitotic checkpoint gene: hsMAD2. *Science* 1996; 274:246–248.

57. He X, Patterson TE, Sazer S. The *Schizosaccharomyces pombe* spindle checkpoint protein mad2p blocks anaphase and genetically interacts with the anaphase-promoting complex. *Proc Natl Acad Sci USA* 1997; 94:7965–7970.

58. Li Y, Gorbea C, Mahaffey D, Rechsteiner M, and Benezra R. MAD2 associates with the cyclosome/anaphase-promoting complex and inhibits its activity. *Proc Natl Acad Sci USA* 1997; 94:12431–12436.

59. Hwang LH, Lau LF, Smith DL, Mistrot CA, Hardwick KG, Hwang ES, et al. Budding yeast Cdc20: a target of the spindle checkpoint. *Science* 1998; 279:1041–1044.

60. Kim SH, Lin DP, Matsumoto S, Kitazono A, and Matsumoto T. Fission yeast Slp1: an effector of the Mad2-dependent spindle checkpoint. *Science* 1998; 279:1045–1047.

61. Fang G, Yu H, Kirschner MW. The checkpoint protein MAD2 and the mitotic regulator CDC20 form a ternary complex with the anaphase-promoting complex to control anaphase initiation. *Genes Dev* 1998; 12:1871–1883.

62. Kallio M, Weinstein J, Daum JR, Burke DJ, and Gorbsky, GJ. Mammalian p55CDC mediates association of the spindle checkpoint protein mad2 with the Cyclosome/Anaphase-promoting complex, and is involved in regulating anaphase onset and late mitotic events. *J Cell Biol* 1998; 141:1393–1406.

63. Dobles M, Liberal V, Scott ML, Benezra R, and Sorger, PK. Chromosome missegregation and apoptosis in mice lacking the mitotic checkpoint protein Mad2. *Cell* 2000; 101:635–645.

64. Michel LS, Liberal V, Chatterjee A. MAD2 haplo-insufficiency causes premature anaphase and chromosome instability in mammalian cells. *Nature* 2001; 409:355–359.

65. Wang X, Jin DY, Wong YC, Cheung AL, Chun AC, Lo AK, et al. Correlation of defective mitotic checkpoint with aberrantly reduced expression of MAD2 protein in nasopharyngeal carcinoma cells. *Carcinogenesis* 2000; 21:2293–2297.

66. Percy MJ, Myrie KA, Neeley CK, Azim JN, Ethier SP, and Petty EM. Expression and mutational analyses of the human MAD2L1 gene in breast cancer cells. *Genes Chromosom Cancer* 2000; 29:356–362.

67. Hardwick KG, Weiss E, Luca FC, Winey M, and Murray AW. Activation of the budding yeast spindle assembly checkpoint without mitotic spindle disruption. *Science* 1996; 273:953–956.

68. Taylor SS, McKeon F. Kinetochore localization of murine Bub1 is required for normal mitotic timing and checkpoint response to spindle damage. *Cell* 1997; 89:727–735.

69. Murray AW, Marks D. Can sequencing shed light on cell cycling? *Nature* 2001; 409:844–846.

70. Cahill DP, Lengauer C, Yu, J, Riggins GJ, Willson JK, Markowitz SD, et al. Mutations of mitotic checkpoint genes in human cancers. *Nature* 1998; 392:300–303.

71. Mimori K, Inoue H, Alder H, Ueo H, Tanaka Y, and Mori M. Mutation analysis of hBUB1, human mitotic checkpoint gene in multiple carcinomas. *Oncol Rep* 2001; 8:39–42.

72. Gemma A, Seike M, Seike Y, Uematsu K, Hibino S, Kurimoto F, et al. Somatic mutation of the hBUB1 mitotic checkpoint gene in primary lung cancer. *Genes Chromosom Cancer* 2000; 29:213–218.

73. Jaffrey RG, Pritchard, SC, Clark C, Murray GI, Cassidy J, Kerr KM, et al. Genomic instability at the BUB1 locus in colorectal cancer, but not in non-small cell lung cancer. *Cancer Res* 2000; 60:4349–4352.

74. Ohshima K, Haraoka S, Yoshioka S, Hamasaki M, Fujiki T, Suzumiya J, et al. Mutation analysis of mitotic checkpoint genes (hBUB1 and hBUBR1) and microsatellite instability in adult T-cell leukemia/lymphoma. *Cancer Lett* 2000; 158:141–150.

75. Sato M, Sekido Y, Horio Y, Takahashi M, Saito H, Minna JD, et al. Infrequent mutation of the hBUB1 and hBUBR1 genes in human lung cancer. *Jpn J Cancer Res* 2000; 91:504–509.

76. Myrie KA, Percy MJ, Azim JN, Neeley CK, and Petty EM. Mutation and expression analysis of human BUB1 and BUB1B in aneuploid breast cancer cell lines. *Cancer Lett* 2000; 152:193–199.

77. Imai Y, Shiratori Y, Kato N, Inoue T, and Omata M. Mutational inactivation of mitotic checkpoint genes, hsMAD2 and hBUB1, is rare in sporadic digestive tract cancers. *Jpn J Cancer Res* 1999; 90:837–840.

78. Yamaguchi K, Okami K, Hibi K, Wehage SL, Jen J, and Sidransky D. Mutation analysis of hBUB1 in aneuploid HNSCC and lung cancer cell lines. *Cancer Lett* 1999; 139:183–187.

79. Jin DY, Spencer F, Jeang KT. Human T cell leukemia virus type 1 oncoprotein Tax targets the human mitotic checkpoint protein MAD1. *Cell* 1998; 93:81–91.

80. Breivik J, Gaudernack G. Genomic instability, DNA methylation, and natural selection in colorectal carcinogenesis. *Semin Cancer Biol* 1999; 9:245–254.

81. Matsuura S, Ito E, Tauchi H, Komatsu K, Ikeuchi T, and Kajii T. Chromosomal instability syndrome of total premature chromatid separation with mosaic variegated aneuploidy is defective in mitotic-spindle checkpoint. *Am J Hum Genet* 2000; 67:483–486.

82. Williams BC, Karr TL, Montgomery JM, and Goldberg ML. The *Drosophila* I(1)zw10 gene product, required for accurate mitotic chromosome segregation, is redistributed at anaphase onset. *J Cell Biol* 1992; 118:759–773.

83. Scaerou F, Aguilera I, Saunders, R, Kane N, Blottiere L, and Karess, R. The rough deal protein is a new kinetochore component required for accurate chromosome segregation in Drosophila. *J Cell Sci* 1999; 112:3757–3768.

84. Williams BC, Gatti M, Goldberg ML. Bipolar spindle attachments affect redistributions of ZW10, a *Drosophila* centromere/kinetochore component required for accurate chromosome segregation. *J Cell Biol* 1996; 134:1127–1140.

85. Basto R, Gomes R, Karess RE. Rough deal and Zw10 are required for the metaphase checkpoint in *Drosophila. Nat Cell Biol* 2000; 2:939–943.

86. Chan GK, Jablonski SA, Starr DA, Goldberg ML, and Yen TJ. Human Zw10 and ROD are mitotic checkpoint proteins that bind to kinetochores. *Nat Cell Biol* 2000; 2:944–947.

87. Basu J, Logarinho, E, Herrmann S, Bousbaa H, Li Z, Chan GK. Localization of the *Drosophila* check-point control protein Bub3 to the kinetochore requires Bub 1 but not Zw10 or Rod. *Chromosoma* 1998; 107:376–385.

88. Starr DA, Williams BC, Li Z, Etemad-Moghadam B, Dawe RK, and Goldberg L. Conservation of the centromere/kinetochore protein ZW10. *J Cell Biol* 1997; 138:1289–1301.

3 Signal Transduction Networks

Ras as a Paradigm

Frank McCormick, PhD

CONTENTS

1. INTRODUCTION

Research in signal transduction has changed radically in recent years. Attention has shifted from functions of individual proteins to relationships between proteins and pathways. As pathways have been elucidated, it has become evident that these pathways form complex interactive networks, in which boundaries between pathways become blurred. This chapter discusses some of the implications of this emerging view in terms of understanding the biology and also the prospects for therapy based on signaling networks.

Many of the paradigms on which our current understanding is based derive from study of oncogenes. In the early days of oncogene research, it appeared that individual oncogenes acted alone, causing dramatic effects on normal cells in culture. Later, it was found that oncogenes act in complementation groups and that the normal cells, which they transformed, harbored mutations that supplied complementing functions. The Ras oncogene illustrates these points quite clearly and has special significance as the first oncogene identified from human tumor DNA. This chapter focuses on Ras and its relationship to the Rb, p53, and APC pathways, particularly in human cancer. These are the pathways that are mutated most frequently in human cancer and offer multiple opportunities for rational cancer therapy.

A current view of Ras signaling is shown in Fig. 1. Ras can interact with several effector proteins to generate downstream signals. These proteins appear to have little in

From: *Oncogene-Directed Therapies*
Edited by: J. W. Rak © Humana Press Inc., Totowa, NJ

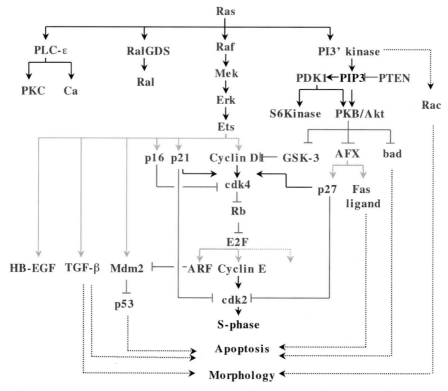

Fig. 1. Pathways downstream of Ras p21. The GTP-bound form of Ras interacts directly with multiple effectors. The consequences of Raf activation and PI 3 kinase activation are best understood: this figure shows some of them and their biological consequences.

common; they have very different biochemical functions and do not have significant sequent homology to one another in the Ras-binding regions. However, structural analysis of Ras proteins bound to Raf, PI 3′ kinase or RalGDS reveals more subtle similarities *(1)*. In addition to multiple direct effectors, Ras proteins cause multiple biological effects. However, it is abundantly clear that these effects are not mediated by distinct effectors, but require cross-talk between effector pathways, as we will discuss in *subheadings.*

The idea that Ras interacts with multiple effectors is now well accepted, but only 10 yr ago, it was thought more likely that Ras interacts with a single downstream target. In contrast, it has been clear for many years *that the receptor tyrosine kinase interacts with* multiple targets simultaneously, since these can be identified in complexes in activated cells. Ras, of course, cannot interact with more than one target at a time, and we assume that the relative abundance of different targets under different conditions determines which is the major signal output, though this issue has been difficult to address.

The biological effects of Ras signaling are complicated and involve changes in cell cycle, cell survival, cell motility, cell senescence, and other phenotypes *(2)*. It is, therefore, not surprising that the endpoints of Ras signaling pathways impinge on pathways regulating each of these biological responses, and the feedback loops sensing these phenotypes regulate Ras signaling output. Ras is well known as a protein that promotes cell proliferation, and its interactions with the cell cycle regulatory proteins and the Rb pathway specifically illustrate how multiple independent biochemical cascades can affect a single protein by distinct mechanisms.

Three major Ras effector pathways have been identified, with several other candidates under investigation (reviewed in ref. 2), including AF6/Canoe and Rin1, which bind to Ras proteins in a GTP-dependent manner, and more recently, protein kinase Cζ (3). Ras activation of Raf kinase is the best known effector function, and the consequent activation of the MAP kinase pathway has been well documented. However, the biochemical mechanisms underlying Ras-dependent activation of Raf kinase activity are still unclear (4) and are beyond the scope of this review.

The Raf/MAP kinase pathway activates transcription of many target genes, through phosphorylation of Ets family members, through Sp1, AP1, and by other means. A gene array analysis of genes induced by artificial activation of Raf kinase has been reported recently (5). This analysis confirmed some well-known targets (cyclin D1, heparin-binding epidermal growth factor [HB-EGF]) and introduced many others. This analysis, along with multiple publications reporting a role for the MAP kinase in transcription of specific target genes, leaves the problem of determining which targets are most critical in normal signaling and in cancer.

2. Ras AND THE Rb PATHWAY

One approach to the problem of identifying critical effectors has utilized the power of mouse genetics, by knocking out major targets of the Ras/MAP kinase pathway and determining effects on normal and neoplastic growth. Analysis of one major target, cyclin D1, has been especially informative. Cyclin D1-deficient mice have been created and are normal in most aspects of their development and physiology, except that they are defective in mammary organ development (6). These data obviously rule out cyclin D1 as an important target of mitogenic signaling during normal growth and development. However, mice lacking cyclin D1 are less prone to carcinogen-induced skin cancers, which is a disease driven by activation of H-ras (7), and are totally resistant to H-Ras-driven mammary carcinomas (8). In contrast, mammary carcinomas driven by wnt and myc still develop in cyclin D1-deficient mice. Cyclin D1 is, therefore, an important target of the Ras and receptor tyrosine kinase oncogenes in this pathological situation, though not in most normal circumstances, and immediately suggests itself as an ideal target for cancer therapy. Unfortunately, it is not at all obvious how this protein could be targeted for therapeutic intervention using current methods of drug discovery. Cdk4 has been a popular target among the pharmaceutical and biotechnology industry, because this kinase is hyperactive in most cancer cells as a result of the loss of Rb, the loss of p16, or the up-regulation of cyclin D1 expression, but drugs targeting cdk4 are less likely to be selective than those targeting cyclin D1.

Cyclin D1 is regulated at the transcriptional level by the Raf/MAP kinase pathway, but the stability of the protein is regulated by PI kinase, itself an effector of activated Ras (9). PI 3′ kinase produces phosphatidyl inositol tris phosphate (PIP3), which activates PDK1 and Akt. Activated Akt has many potential targets, and one of those that is better characterized is glycogen synthase kinase 3 (GSK3), which phosphorylates cyclin D1 and targets it for degradation. Phosphorylation of GSK3 by Akt inhibits its activity, thereby stabilizing cyclinD1 as well as other GSK3 targets. The relative contribution of the Raf/MAP kinase pathway and the PI kinase pathway to expression of cyclin D1 levels is difficult to determine, particularly since Raf activation promotes indirect activation of PI 3′ kinase activity by autocrine production of growth factors, as discussed below.

p21 Cip1 is another target of the MAP kinase pathway, though the mechanism by which this protein is regulated is not clear; evidence for transcriptional and posttranscriptional regulation has been reported. p21 Cip1 is an assembly factor for cyclin D1/cdk4 complexes, but a potent inhibitor of cdk2. Excessive signaling, through expression of high levels of activated Raf kinase or expression of high levels of activated Ras however, causes growth arrest in wild-type cells, though induction of p21. The cdk inhibitor p16 INK4a and the cdk2 inhibitor p27 Kip1 are also induced by high levels of signaling through the Raf/MAP kinase pathway, as reviewed recently *(10)*.

Levels of p27 Kip1 are also regulated by the PI 3′ kinase pathway, which controls p27kip1 degradation *(11)*. As with cyclin D1, the two major arms of the Ras pathway may, therefore, work together: the Raf/MAPK pathway regulating transcription, and the PI 3′ kinase regulating protein stability. This interaction may provide a satisfactory explanation for synergy between Ras effector pathways in transformation assays, originally reported for interactions between Rac and Raf, and later between PI 3′ kinase itself and Raf *(12,13)*.

3. Ras AND Rho

The effects of Ras on cell morphology are equally complex and involve other signaling networks. In the classic studies of *Ridley and Hall,* the effects of Ras on actin stress fibers could be attributed to activation of Rac, which, in turn, activates Rho. However, the extent to which Ras regulates Rho during the process of transformation is less clear. Rho is regulated by G protein-coupled receptors, such as the *lysophosphatidic acid* (LPA) receptor, as well as by multiple other signaling inputs. Recent work from Dr. Chris Marshall and coworkers *(14)* suggests that Rho activity is regulated independent of Ras, but the fates of signals downstream from these GTPases is intertwined. Fig. 2 summarizes some of these relationships. In transformed cells, high levels of Rho. GTP suppress accumulation of p21/Waf1, which is a protein that acts as an assembly factor of Cdk4/cyclin D1 complexes, but inhibits Cdk2 and blocks cell cycle progression at high concentrations. Rho.GTP, therefore, modulates one of the effectors of the Ras/MAP kinase pathway. On the other hand, the Ras/MAP kinase modulates some of the effects of Rho, by suppressing activity of the Rho-regulated kinases ROCK and Rho kinase. These kinases regulate actin stress fiber formation through the LIM kinase. The well-known effects of activated Ras on actin stress fibers (dissolution of stress fibers in transformed cells) appears to be mediated through this interference effects on Rho activity.

The Rho-related protein, Rnd3, may also be involved in the complicated relationship between Ras and Rho *(15)*. Rnd3 appears to function as an inhibitor of Rho function, by acting as a sort of dominant negative mutant: it is locked in the GTP state through changes in the GTPase domain that prevent GTP hydrolysis, and it cannot localize in memberanes, as it lacks a CAAX motif at the C terminus. Rnd3 is induced by activated Raf kinase and appears to be responsible, at least in part, for inhibition of Rho-mediated actin stress fiber formation. Relationships between Ras and Rho are summarized in Fig. 2.

In epithelial cells, alterations in cell morphology and motility following Ras activation may be due additional factors that are not directly related to Rho. Raf induces expression of transforming growth factor (TGF)-β in such cells, and autocrine or

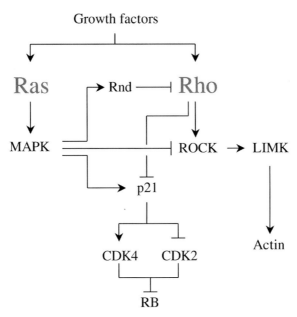

Fig. 2. Crosstalk between Ras and Rho signaling pathways. Both pathways affect cell cycle and cell morphology through effects on Rb and Actin polymerization.

paracrine production of this factor appears to be responsible for increased cell motility *(16)*. TGF-β itself promotes apoptosis in normal epithelial cells. However, cancer cells with activated Ras may be resistant to TGF-β-dependent apoptosis, because Ras also promotes cell survival in the face of numerous pro-apoptotic signals. However, the effects of Ras on survival and apoptosis are just as complicated as effects of Ras on cell morphology and also involve interacting signal transduction pathways.

4. Ras AND PI 3′ KINASE

The best documented role of Ras in survival is mediated through its effects on PI kinase. Epithelial cells are particularly prone to undergo apoptosis when they are removed from their neighbors; this form of cell death even has its name, anoikis. Activated Ras prevents anoikis and allows cells to survive after detachment. This is mediated by PI kinase *(17)*. This may be a major selective advantage to tumor cells, since these cells typically show decreased dependence on normal cell–cell interactions and on increased ability to survive and migrate into inappropriate cellular environments.

The degree to which this effector pathway contributes to Ras' role in human cancer is demonstrated by the observation that loss of the tumor suppressor PTEN and mutational activation of Ras are mutually exclusive, at least in cutaneous melanoma *(18)* and in endometrial cancers *(19)*. PTEN is a phosphatase that degrades PIP3, which is the product of PI 3′ kinase. Loss of PTEN is, therefore, similar biochemically to activation of PI 3′ kinase; both lead to accumulation of PIP3. These data suggest that loss of PTEN is phenotypically equivalent to mutation of Ras and that the major selective advantage of Ras activation is hyperactivation of PI kinase to generate PIP3.

PIP3 activates a large number of substrates, through binding to PH domains and possibly other means. A major target is Akt (also known as protein kinase or PKB). Activation of Akt appears to account for many of the survival effects of PI 3' kinase and PIP3. Activated Akt suppresses anoikis, for example. Akt itself phosphorylates badly and prevents it suppressing apoptosis, and it regulates nuclear import of the transcription factor AFX, which itself may regulate genes involved in apoptosis. These effects may well account for some of Akt's survial properties, but there may be other targets yet to be identified. PIP3 also activates the Rac pathway, and, indeed, activated Rac suppresses apoptosis. We can, therefore, appreciate that the role of the PI 3' kinase/PTEN pathway in survival signaling is complicated, and like the Ras pathway itself, a major challenge is to determine which of the many possible candidates is the more important under physiological or pathological conditions.

The Ras pathway contributes to cell survival and apoptosis through another set of interactions that appear at first sight to be distinct from Ras' role in activating PI 3' kinase to generate PIP3; activated Ras regulates p53. This connection was inferred many years ago when it was discovered that Ras causes growth arrest in certain cells in culture. This was considered astonishing at the time, since Ras was known to be one of the more powerful oncogenes in similar cell culture systems. Growth arrest is now known to be through induction of p21, as described above previously. p21, of course, is a transcriptional target of p53 *(20)*, and it is not surprising that Ras induction of p21, in some cells at least, is p53 dependent. It could also be anticipated that alternative pathways connect Ras to p21 that are p53 independent.

5. Ras AND P53

Ras induction of p53 is mediated by p14ARF, the product of an alternative reading frame within the p16 INK4 locus. p14ARF is expressed at very low levels in normal cells, but can be induced by various oncogenes, including c-myc, Ela, and Ras, *(21–23)*. E2F itself induces p14ARF *(24)*, but it is not yet clear whether this is through direct transcriptional activation. A survey of E2F inducible transcripts recently failed to reveal p14ARF as an E2F target *(25)*. Nevertheless, oncogenes induce p14ARF, and this inhibits *MDM2,* allowing p53 to accumulate (Fig. 3).

MDM2 is a major negative regulator of p53. This has been known for many years, but was made most clear by analysis of mice lacking the mdm2 gene: these mice die in embryo unless p53 is also knock-out *(26)*. In this case, they survive, but get tumors with a similar spectrum to p53 knock-out animals. However, this does not mean that MDM2 is the only major negative regulator of p53. Mice lacking the MDM2-related protein, MDMX, are also rescued by knocking out p53, showing that MDMX is a major regulator, at least in some tissues during development *(27)*.

MDM2 itself is regulated by p53. The P2 promoter within the *MDM2* gene contains a p53-responsive element, and, indeed, *MDM2* mRNA is induced following p53 activation *(28,29)*. This induction provides a feedback loop that results in down-regulation of p53 and inhibition of p53 signaling. However, this feedback loop is by no means the only way that MDM2 levels are regulated. p53-independent regulation of *MDM2* was reported by Oren and coworkers in 1997 *(30)*, and MDM2 transcripts were detected as early inducible targets of fibroblast growth factor (FGF) signaling using microarrays *(31)*. Recently, we pursued this further and found that *MDM2* is a transcriptional target of the Ras/MAPK pathway *(32)*. Ras-responsive elements in the *MDM* promoter were identified and shown to act independently of p53. This explained high levels of MDM2 that we had observed in cancer cells lacking func-

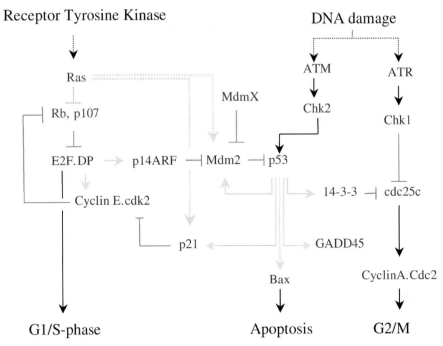

Fig. 3. Crosstalk between mitogenic signaling and DNA damage responses.

tional p53 and also explained an older observation that Ras-transformed cells are resistant to radiation. In these cells, high levels of MDM2 suppress the p53 response to DNA damage.

In normal cells, activated Raf kinase can regulate an inhibitor of MDM2, p14ARF, and transcription of *Mdm2* itself. Activation of the Raf/MAP kinase pathway in normal cells, therefore, has little net effect on p53 *(32)*. However, a large fraction of human cancers, perhaps as many as 40–50% maintain expression of wild-type p53, but fail to express p14ARF. In these cells, p53 is suppressed by MDM2, which is expected to be hyperactive as a result of loss of p14ARF, and highly expressed through activation of the Raf/MAP kinase pathway. In these cancer cells, inhibition of the MEK activity leads to accumulation of p53 as levels of MDM2 fall. This sensitizes cells to killing by DNA-damaging agents or ionizing radiation. Normal cells are not sensitized by MEK inhibitors, because p53 levels are not affected for reasons discussed above. In this example, intersecting signaling pathways can be used to devise selective approaches to cancer therapy.

The question remains as to why the Ras pathway would regulate *mdm2* and p14ARF simultaneously, resulting in no net effect on *MDM2* activity. One explanation may be that these two effects are separated in time. Induction of *mdm2* appears to be an early response to growth factor signaling and may be a mechanism to keep p53 at low levels as cells move from G0 and through the G1 phase of the cell cycle. E2F activity increases as cells approach S-phase, and p14ARF is then able to regulate MDM2 and, thus, regulate levels of p53 as cells enter S-phase. Indeed, an increase in p53 has been noted in quiescent cells approaching S-phase.

Recently, another connection between Ras and MDM2 has been noted: PI 3′ kinase regulates nuclear import of MDM2 through AKT phosphorylation of serine residues on MDM2 itself *(33)*. Activation of both Ras effectors may, therefore, be necessary for maximal effects on MDM2. This duality of function is reminiscent of Ras' effects on cyclin D1 and p27 Kip1 as in *subheading;* the Raf/MAP kinase arm increases transcription and the PI 3′ kinase arm regulates protein stability.

6. Ras AND HB-EGF

One of the first identified targets of the Raf/MAP kinase pathway was HB-EGF *(34)*. A differential display analysis revealed induction of this gene following activation of Raf kinase using an endoplasmic reticulum (ER) fusion protein that renders Raf kinase sensitive to tamoxifen. HB-EGF was also identified as a Raf/MAP kinase target using microarray analysis. Transformation of cells was found to be dependent, at least in part, on HB-EGF expression. These discoveries, like the discovery that Raf activates autocrine production of TGFβ, add another dimension to the complexity of signaling networks. The preceding discussion illustrates the complexity of signaling pathways emitted from a single key regulatory protein. Similar levels of complexity have been described for regulatory proteins such as c-src, Rac and Rho proteins, protein kinase β (PKB), NF-κ B, and many other proteins that have received a similar level of scrutiny. In each case, effects appear astonishingly diverse, typically involving direct interaction.

7. Ras AND APC

The wnt pathway has been implicated for many years in oncogenesis. Increased expression of wnt resulting from proximal integration of mouse mammary tumor virus (MMTV) proviral DNA causes mammary carcinoma in mouse models. Dissection of pathways downstream of wnt was facilitated by analysis of related pathways in *Drosophila* and *Xenopus* and in human cancers *(35)*. Fig. 4 depicts a consensus view of the wnt pathway in mammalian cells. Altered activity of this pathway in human cancers occurs through loss of APC, which is a protein that is necessary for degradation of β-catenin, through mutation of β-catenin itself to make it resistant to degradation. Target genes of the wnt pathway include cyclin D1 *(36)*, and c-myc *(37)*, both of which are proteins involved in growth control and are candidates for targets involved in pathological wnt signaling in cancer. In addition to points of convergence between mitogenic signaling pathways at cyclin D1 and c-myc, and possible connections between the wnt pathway and p53 through E2F and myc regulation of p14ARF *(38)*, another major intersection has been noted. GSK3 is involved in insulin regulation of glycogen storage and in wnt regulation of β-catenin, two seemingly unrelated pathways. Some cells have the capacity to activate both of these pathways simultaneously. In both cases, depression of GSK3 activity promotes downstream signaling, yet inhibition of GSK3 by insulin does not lead to accumulation of β-catenin *(39)*. Nor does wnt affect glycogen. These two pathways appear to be insulated from one another within the cell, presumably through different associated protein complexes.

8. SIGNALING NETWORKS AND DRUG DISCOVERY

This chapter has focused on the Ras pathway as a paradigm for signaling complexity. Perhaps this pathway appears most complex because it is one of the better studied

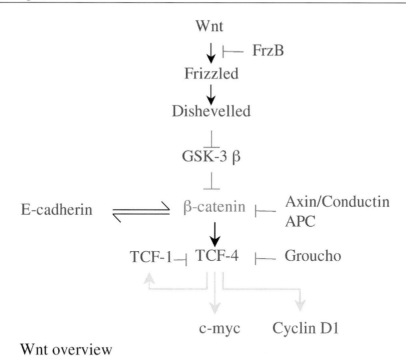

Wnt overview

Fig. 4. The wnt pathway. This pathwy is altered in many human cancers through loss of regulation of β-catenin.

pathways. Examples of cross-talk abound in other areas of signal transduction. For example, there is clear evidence that the JAK/STAT pathway is coregulated with the EGF receptor. *G protein-coupled receptors* use similar signaling pathways to receptor tyrosine kinases, and receptors of these distinct structural classes cross-activate one another. Equally, transcriptional elements receive input from multiple pathways. We have mentioned the cyclin D1 promoter, which is regulated by the MAP kinase pathway and by *T-cell factor (TCF)*. It also receives signals from NFκB *(40),* notched *(41),* Egr-1 *(42),* and probably other sources. This complexity offers unexpected opportunities for therapeutic intervention. For example, in the early days of oncogene research, it appeared likely that differences between signaling in normal and cancer cells were strictly quantitative; mutations in Ras, to pursue this paradigm further, locked the protein in the active state and generated a persistent version of a signal that would normally be transient. Therapies based on these strong persistent signals would be aimed at reducing signal strength by blocking key steps in the cascade. This strategy is likely to be effective at blocking growth of transformed cells, but offers little rational hope of selectivity. However, we now suspect that signaling from activated Ras mutants may be qualitatively different from normal Ras signaling; in normal cells, activation of PI 3′ kinase is only partially dependent on Ras *(43).* Activated receptor tyrosine kinases turn on PI 3′ kinase directly in most cases. However, in Ras transformed cells, PI 3′ kinase is largely dependent on Ras. These discoveries lead to the suggestion that a drug blocking Ras-PI 3′ kinase activation might have selective effects on cancer cells.

Another way in which the complexity of signaling networks might provide opportunities might be based on cross-talk between pathways that are normally isolated from one another. For example, pathways activated by receptor tyrosine kinases following mitogenic stimulation show transient peaks of activation, and downstream products accumulate and disappear with rapid kinetics. In contrast, persistent signaling resulting from mutant signaling proteins leads to sustained production of downstream signals that may now interact.

The discovery that signaling proteins can have multiple effectors raises the problem of determining which effector is most critical to normal and pathologic conditions. On the other hand, if downstream pathways interact synergistically, as shown for Ras, we expect that drugs that block any one pathway will have an indirect effect on the others. Using dominant negative proteins as surrogates for active compounds, we showed that Ras transformation is efficiently blocked by preventing signaling to MAP kinase or to other Ras effectors *(12,44)*. Interacting pathways, therefore, offer opportunities for dramatic therapeutic responses that might not have been expected in earlier days of signal transduction research. Hopefully, these opportunities will soon be translated in the clinic.

REFERENCES

1. Pacold ME, Suire S, Perisic O, Lara-Gonzalez S, Davis CT, Walker EH, et al. Crystal structure and functional analysis of Ras binding to its effector phosphoinositide 3-kinase gamma. *Cell* 2000; 103:931–943.
2. Campbell SL, Khosravi-Far R, Rossman KL, Clark GJ, Der CJ. Increasing complexity of Ras signaling. *Oncogene* 1998; 17:1395–1413.
3. Pal S, Datta K, Khosravi-Far R, Mukhopadhyay D. Role of protein kinase Czeta in Ras-mediated transcriptional activation of vascular permeability factor/vascular endothelial growth factor expression. *J Biol Chem* 2001; 276:2395–2403.
4. Avruch J, Khokhlatchev A, Kyriakis JM, Luo Z, Tzivion G, Vavvas D, et al. Ras activation of the Raf kinase: tyrosine kinase recruitment of the MAP kinase cascade. *Recent Prog Horm Res* 2001; 56:127–155.
5. Schulze A, Lehmann K, Jefferies HB, McMahon M, Downward J. Analysis of the transcriptional program induced by Raf in epithelial cells. *Genes Dev* 2001; 15:981–984.
6. Sicinski P, Weinberg RA. A specific role for cyclin D1 in mammary gland development. *J Mammary Gland Biol Neoplasia* 1997; 2:335–342.
7. Robles AI, Rodriguez-Puebla ML, Glick AB, Trempus C, Hansen L, Sicinski P, et al. Reduced skin tumor development in cyclin D1-deficient mice highlights the oncogenic ras pathway in vivo. *Genes Dev* 1998; 12:2469–2474.
8. Yu Q, Geng Y, Sicinski P. Specific protection against breast cancers by cyclin D1 ablation. *Nature* 2001; 411:1017–1021.
9. Diehl JA, Cheng M, Roussel MF, Sherr CJ. Glycogen synthase kinase-3beta regulates cyclin D1 proteolysis and subcellular localization. *Genes Dev* 1998; 12:3499–3511.
10. McMahon M, Woods D. Regulation of the p53 pathway by Ras, the plot thickens. *Biochim Biophys Acta* 2001; 2:M63–71.
11. Mamillapalli R, Gavrilova N, Mihaylova VT, Tsvetkov LM, Wu H, Zhang H, et al. PTEN regulates the ubiquitin-dependent degradation of the CDK inhibitor p27(KIP1) through the ubiquitin E3 ligase SCF(SKP2). *Curr Biol* 2001; 11:263–267.
12. Qiu RG, Chen J, McCormick F, Symons M. A role for Rho in Ras transformation. *Proc Natl Acad Sci USA* 1995; 92:11781–11785.
13. Gille H, Downward J. Multiple ras effector pathways contribute to G(1) cell cycle progression. *J Biol Chem* 1999; 274:22033–22040.
14. Sahai E, Olson MF, Marshall CJ. Cross-talk between Ras and Rho signalling pathways in transformation favours proliferation and increased motility. *EMBO J* 2001; 20:755–766.
15. Hansen SH, Zegers MM, Woodrow M, Rodriguez-Viciana P, Chardin P, Mostov KE, et al. Induced expression of Rnd3 is associated with transformation of polarized epithelial cells by the Raf-MEK-extracellular signal-regulated kinase pathway. *Mol Cell Biol* 2000; 20:9364–9375.

16. Lehmann K, Janda E, Pierreux CE, Rytomaa M, Schulze A, McMahon M, et al. Raf induces TGFbeta production while blocking its apoptotic but not invasive responses: a mechanism leading to increased malignancy in epithelial cells. *Genes Dev* 2000; 14:2610–2622.

17. Khwaja A, Rodriguez-Viciana P, Wennstrom S, Warne PH, Downward J. Matrix adhesion and Ras transformation both activate a phosphoinositide 3-OH kinase and protein kinase B/Akt cellular survival pathway. *EMBO J* 1997; 16:2783–2793.

18. Tsao H, Zhang X, Fowlkes K, Haluska FG. Relative reciprocity of NRAS and PTEN/MMAC1 alterations in cutaneous melanoma cell lines. *Cancer Res* 2000; 60:1800–1804.

19. Ikeda T, Yoshinaga K, Suzuki A, Sakurada A, Ohmori H, Horii A. Anticorresponding mutations of the KRAS and PTEN genes in human endometrial cancer. *Oncol Rep* 2000; 7:567–570.

20. Levine AJ. p53, the cellular gatekeeper for growth and division. *Cell* 1997; 88:323–331.

21. Zindy F, Eischen CM, Randle DH, Kamijo T, Cleveland JL, Sherr CJ, et al. Myc signaling via the ARF tumor suppressor regulates p53-dependent apoptosis and immortalization. *Genes Dev* 1998; 12:2424–2433.

22. de Stanchina E, McCurrach ME, Zindy F, Shieh SY, Ferbeyre G, Samuelson AV, et al. E1A signaling to p53 involves the p19(ARF) tumor suppressor. *Genes Dev* 1998; 12:2434–2442.

23. Palmero I, Pantoja C, Serrano M. p19ARF links the tumour suppressor p53 to Ras. *Nature* 1998; 395:125–126.

24. Bates S, Phillips AC, Clark PA, Stott F, Peters G, Ludwig RL, et al. p14ARF links the tumour suppressors RB and p53. *Nature* 1998; 395:124–125.

25. Muller H, Bracken AP, Vernell R, Moroni MC, Christians F, Grassilli E, et al. E2Fs regulate the expression of genes involved in differentiation, development, proliferation, and apoptosis. *Genes Dev* 2001; 15:267–285.

26. Montes de Oca Luna R, Wagner DS, Lozano G. Rescue of early embryonic lethality in mdm2-deficient mice by deletion of p53. *Nature* 1995; 378:203–206.

27. Parant J, Chavez-Reyes A, Little NA, Yan W, Reinke V, Jochemsen AG, et al. Rescue of embryonic lethality in Mdm4-null mice by loss of Trp53 suggests a nonoverlapping pathway with MDM2 to regulate p53. *Nat Genet* 2001; 29:92–95.

28. Barak Y, Gottlieb E, Juven-Gershon T, Oren M. Regulation of mdm2 expression by p53: alternative promoters produce transcripts with nonidentical translation potential. *Genes Dev* 1994; 8:1739–1749.

29. Wu X, Bayle JH, Olson D, and Levine AJ. The p53-mdm-2 autoregulatory feedback loop. *Genes Dev* 1993; 7:1126–1132.

30. Shaulian E, Resnitzky D, Shifman O, Blandino G, Amsterdam A, Yayon A, et al. Induction of Mdm2 and enhancement of cell survival by bFGF. *Oncogene* 1997; 15:2717–2725.

31. Fambrough D, McClure K, Kazlauskas A, Lander ES. Diverse signaling pathways activated by growth factor receptors induce broadly overlapping, rather than independent, sets of genes [see comments]. *Cell* 1999; 97:727–741.

32. Ries SJ, Brandts CH, Chung AS, Biederer CH, Hann BC, Lipner EM, et al. Loss of p14ARF in tumor cells facilitates replication of the adenovirus mutant dl1520 (ONYX-015). *Nat Med* 2000; 6:1128–1133.

33. Mayo LD, Donner DB. A phosphatidylinositol 3-kinase/Akt pathway promotes translocation of Mdm2 from the cytoplasm to the nucleus. *Proc Natl Acad Sci USA* 2001; 98:11598–11603.

34. McCarthy SA, Samuels ML, Pritchard CA, Abraham JA, McMahon M. Rapid induction of heparin-binding epidermal growth factor/diphtheria toxin receptor expression by Raf and Ras oncogenes. *Genes Dev* 1995; 9:1953–1964.

35. Bienz M, Clevers H. Linking colorectal cancer to Wnt signaling. *Cell* 2000; 103:311–320.

36. Tetsu O, McCormick F. Beta-catenin regulates expression of cyclin D1 in colon carcinoma cells. *Nature* 1999; 398:422–426.

37. He TC, Sparks AB, Rago C, Hermeking H, Zawel L, da Costa LT, et al. Identification of c-MYC as a target of the APC pathway. *Science* 1998; 281:1509–1512.

38. Damalas A, Ben-Ze'ev A, Simcha I, Shtutman M, Leal JF, Zhurinsky J, et al. Excess beta-catenin promotes accumulation of transcriptionally active p53. *EMBO J* 1999; 18:3054–3063.

39. Ding VW, Chen RH, McCormick F. Differential regulation of glycogen synthase kinase 3beta by insulin and Wnt signaling. *J Biol Chem* 2000; 275:32475–32481.

40. Henry DO, Moskalenko SA, Kaur KJ, Fu M, Pestell RG, Camonis JH, et al. Ral GTPases contribute to regulation of cyclin D1 through activation of NF-kappaB. *Mol Cell Biol* 2000; 20:8084–8092.

41. Ronchini C, Capobianco AJ. Induction of cyclin D1 transcription and CDK2 activity by Notch(ic): implication for cell cycle disruption in transformation by Notch(ic). *Mol Cell Biol* 2001; 21:5925–5934.
42. Guillemot L, Levy A, Raymondjean M, Rothhut B. Angiotensin II-induced transcriptional activation of the cyclin D1 gene is mediated by Egr-1 in CHO-AT1A cells. *J Biol Chem* 2001; 13:39394–39403.
43. Burgering BM, Bos JL. Regulation of Ras-mediated signalling: more than one way to skin a cat. *Trends Biochem Sci* 1995; 20:18–22.
44. Qiu RG, Chen J, Kirn D, McCormick F, and Symons M. An essential role for Rac in Ras transformation. *Nature* 1995; 374:457–459.

4

Oncogenic Receptor Tyrosine Kinases

Mark H. Kirschbaum, MD,
Mina D. Marmor, PhD,
and Yosef Yarden, PhD

CONTENTS

1. INTRODUCTION

Polypeptide growth factors are relatively small and stable molecules that communicate short range signals for cell fate determination. Unlike steroid hormones, which penetrate through the plasma membrane due to their hydrophobic character, these factors must bind a cell surface-localized receptor. In contrast to multispan receptors for neuropeptides and chemical transmitters, growth factor receptors transverse the plasma membrane only once, and their cytoplasmic domains harbor a tyrosine-specific catalytic activity, called protein tyrosine kinase. Ligand binding to a receptor tyrosine kinase (RTK) initiates a cascade of biochemical and phenotypic events known as the pleiotropic response. In addition to ion channels and membrane enzymes, cytoskeletal rearrangements, cytoplasmic enzymes, and adhesive properties of the growth factor-stimulated cell are also modified within seconds to hours. This plethora of surface and cytoplasmic events culminates in the regulation of gene transcription, eventually leading to alterations in cellular behavior ranging from entry into the cell cycle to terminal differentiation (for a specific example of the pleiotropic response to a growth factor see ref. *1*).

Cultured cells experimentally converted from a normal state to a neoplastic phenotype (a process referred to as transformation) share many characteristics with growth factor-stimulated cells; in both cases, cells appear more refractile and rounded, and their actin cables disappear. In addition, transformed cells, as well as cells exposed to a growth factor, lose, in part, their adhesive properties, and some of their metabolic pathways are altered (for a fuller description of the transformed phenotype refer to ref. *2*). The reduced growth factor dependency of cancer cells and the relatedness of the trans-

From: *Oncogene-Directed Therapies*
Edited by: J. W. Rak © Humana Press Inc., Totowa, NJ

formed phenotype to the pleiotropic response were early indications for the significance of growth factors to neoplastic transformation and maintenance of a malignant state. However, these clues solidified only with the findings of parallelism between retroviral oncogenes and cellular genes (proto-oncogenes) encoding molecular components of growth factor signaling. Seminal examples include the discovery in 1983 that *sis,* the oncogene of simian sarcoma virus, encodes an isoform of the platelet-derived growth factor (PDGF)*(3),* and a truncated form of the receptor for another growth factor, the epidermal growth factor (EGF) is encoded by the *erbB* oncogene of the avian erythroblastosis virus *(4).* Altered forms of two additional RTKs, the receptors for the macrophage growth factor (CSF-1 receptor) and the stem cell factor (SCF) are encoded by two feline retroviruses: the Susan McDonough strain (the *v-fms* oncogene) and the Hardy-Zukerman 4 strain (the *v-kit* oncogene), respectively *(5,6).* Retroviruses that carry no oncogene can still transform cells by means of proviral insertional mutagenesis. For example, the avian leukosis virus alters expression of *c-erbB,* a gene driving expression of EGF-receptor (EGFR/ErbB-1) by proviral insertion, whereas the murine leukemia virus similarly affects *c-fms (7).*

However fruitful and strongly influential, isolation of oncogenes through characterization of transforming viruses lacked the resolution power and systematic nature of screening the genome of transformed cells. DNA transfer analyses performed with a transformed donor and a quasinormal recipient cell line (e.g., NIH-3T3 fibroblasts) enabled exhaustive screening for oncogenes in chemically and otherwise transformed cells *(8).* This strategy yielded several more oncogenic forms of RTKs: a point mutant of *neu/erbB-2* was isolated from a carcinogen-induced rat neuroblastoma *(9),* and the *met* oncogene was isolated from a human osteosarcoma cell line transformed in vitro by a chemical carcinogen *(10).* The isolated oncogene turned out to be a fusion between the N terminally truncated kinase of *met,* which is a gene encoding a receptor for the hepatocyte growth factor (HGF), and the *tpr* (translocated promoter region) gene. Similarly, a fusion gene comprised of a truncated *trk,* which encodes a receptor for neurotrophic factors, and the tropomyosin gene was identified in human colon cancer *(11).* Lastly, the *ret* oncogene encoding a receptor for the glial-derived neurotrophic factor (GDNF) was identified by transfection of NIH-3T3 cells with DNA derived from a human T-cell lymphoma *(12).*

Following oncogene identification and biochemical analyses of the encoded proteins, it became clear that the tyrosine kinase portion of the oncoproteins is indispensable for transforming activity. This realization led to attempts to isolate additional RTK genes by using structural and functional similarities to known proto-oncogenes. In this way, for example, genes encoding additional receptors for EGF-like molecules have been detected (i.e., ErbB-3 and ErbB-4), and founder members of the fibroblast growth factor (FGF) receptor and the ephrin receptor families were identified. Moreover, the availability of molecular probes enabled researchers to screen clinical specimens of human malignancies for the presence of mutated forms of RTK-encoding genes. Because many of the newly isolated genes encoded orphan receptors, a parallel effort targeted the unknown ligands. As a result of these combined efforts, the family picture of mammalian RTKs and their respective ligands has been continuously extended and refined *(13,14).* A scheme diagram depicting the major subfamilies of RTKs is presented in Fig. 1. It is likely that the sequencing effort of the Human Genome Project will aid in completing the picture, and gene array techniques will extend the relevance to human cancers and other diseases.

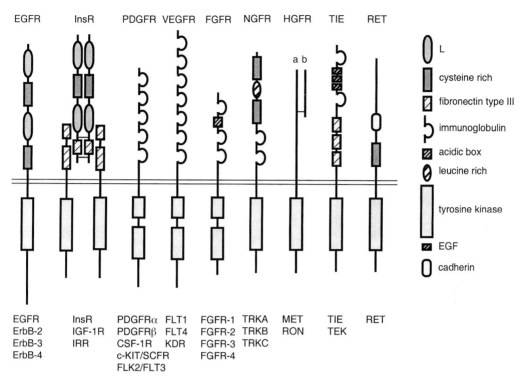

Fig. 1. Schematic illustration of the domain organization of the major RTK subfamilies. The prototype RTK and known members of each subfamily are indicated above and below the diagram, respectively. The horizontal bar represents the plasma membrane. Note the increased structural heterogeneity of the extracellular domains. Abbreviations: EGFR, epidermal growth factor receptor; InsR, insulin receptor; PDGFR, platelet-derived growth factor receptor; VEGFR, vascular endothelial cell-derived growth factor receptor; FGFR, fibroblast growth factor receptor; NGFR, nerve growth factor receptor; HGFR, hepatocyte growth factor receptor; TIE, tyrosine kinase receptor in endothelial cells; IGF-IR, insulin-like growth factor receptor-1; CSF-1R, colony-stimulating factor 1 receptor; SCFR, stem cell factor receptor (c-Kit).

As an introduction to their clinical relevance, this historical perspective is followed by a description of the biochemical function of RTKs. Subsequently, we will concentrate on several subfamilies of RTKs and discuss their significance to specific types of cancers. Other chapters in this volume will introduce the initial therapeutic strategies targeting RTKs and also discuss the features that make these molecules highly attractive for pharmacological intervention.

2. GROWTH FACTORS STIMULATING RTKS

2.1. Common Features of Growth Factors

2.1.1. ISOLATION OF GROWTH FACTORS

Originally, two types of biological sources were used for the isolation of growth factors. Extracts of the salivary glands of mice were used as a starting material for the isolation of EGF *(15)*, whereas brain and pituitary homogenates were shown to contain stimulatory activities for cultured fibroblasts, an observation that led to the isolation of two types of the FGF (reviewed in ref. *16.*) Whereas serum is a poor source for most growth factors, cancer cells or medium conditioned by transformed cells has been a rich source for a myriad of growth factors. In retrospect, the earliest example is the isolation of the neurotrophic growth factor (NGF) from a murine sarcoma *(17)*. Likewise, Sporn and Todaro noted that tumor cells of various origins secrete growth stimulatory activity, which is undetectable in the medium of cultured normal cells *(18)*. Later studies extended this observation and established the notion that one mechanism allowing growth factor autonomy of tumors is self-production of auto-stimulatory ligands. Apparently, the concentration of growth factors in cellular fluids is tightly controlled at the levels of transcription and secretion. After secretion, some growth factors (e.g., the insulin-like growth factor 1 [IGF-1]) bind to specific proteins, either soluble or insoluble, that regulate their availability to target cells. Yet other factors (e.g., transforming growth factor beta [TGFβ]) are secreted in a latent form whose activation requires proteolysis. Hence, growth factor signaling is regulated at a number of critical steps, including transcription, intracellular modification, secretion, and the processes that convey the molecule through intercellular spaces. Dysregulation of any or several of these processes can lead to growth factor overexpression in transformed cells.

2.1.2. Autocrine and Other Stimulatory Loops

Genetic analyses of invertebrates such as worms and insects indicate that growth factors travel only a few cell layers before impinging on the cognate receptor of their target cells. In fact, studies of EGF-like growth factors of *Caenorhabditis elegans* and *Drosophila* provide examples for a direct physical contact between the ligand-synthesizing cell and the responding cell *(19,20)*. The situation in mammals seems similar; unlike classical endocrine hormones, which are secreted by a relatively small number of specialized glands and delivered to their targets through the general circulation, most growth factors are synthesized locally and act as short-range messengers (Fig. 2). The term paracrine loop is reserved for cases in which the growth factor is synthesized by cells within a tissue and acts upon cells in their immediate environment, as is the case for most growth factors signaling through RTKs. A specialized version of paracrine action is the juxtacrine loop, in which a growth factor molecule expressed at the surface of one cell directly binds to a receptor expressed by an adjacent cell *(21)*. Perhaps most relevant to cancer is the autocrine loop, which allows auto-stimulation of a receptor-expressing cell by a self-produced growth factor (Fig. 2). Evidence derived from in vitro studies, animal model systems, and clinical specimens suggest that this type of receptor activation is operative in cancers of several origins (*see Subheading 4.1.1.*).

2.1.3. Families of Growth Factors

In general, growth factor molecules display 3-dimensional structures rich in β pleated sheets and cysteines, and they are grouped into families sharing homologous primary structure. Because each group exhibits some unique features, it is worthwhile reviewing the major groups of ligands for RTKs.

2.1.3.1. EGF and Neuregulins. The EGF motif includes six canonical cysteines that form three bridges and a well conserved protein fold whose β strands are tightly packed (for a review see ref. *22*). The motif is found not only in mitogens acting through EGFR/ErbB-1, but also in a variety of coagulation factors and adhesion molecules. In addition to molecules that bind EGFR, namely EGF, TGFα, amphiregulin, betacellulin, the heparin-binding EGF-like growth factor (HB-EGF), and epiregulin, ligands that bind to ErbB-3 and ErbB-4, and two EGFR-related molecules also contain an EGF

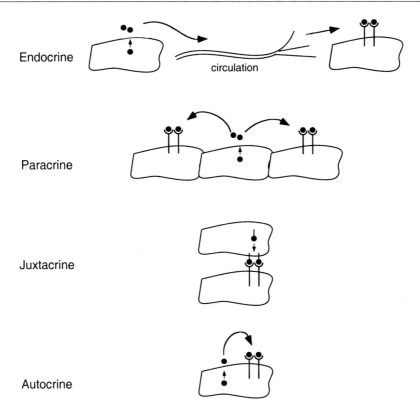

Endocrine

circulation

Paracrine

Juxtacrine

Autocrine

Fig. 2. Different modes of growth factor function. Endocrine action refers to hormone or growth factor dissemination through the circulatory system to act upon cells that are distant from the factor-producing cells. Paracrine action refers to the utilization of growth factors by cells in the immediate vicinity of the factor-producing cells, whereas juxtacrine action refers to the presentation of membrane-bound growth factors to adjacent cells. An autocrine loop indicates the utilization of growth factors by the same cells that produce them.

motif *(23)*. These factors are collectively named neuregulins (NRGs), and they include at least four groups of isoforms generated by alternative splicing (ref. *24* and references therein). A large group of DNA viruses, called pox viruses, encode EGF-like ligands that bind with moderate affinity to ErbB proteins, but their mitogenic activity is unexpectedly high *(25)*. The majority of EGF-like mitogens are synthesized as long transmembrane precursors that undergo cleavage to generate a short ligand molecule comprising an EGF motif, which is often linked to other protein modules *(21)*. Interestingly, an antagonistic ligand, called Argos, was identified in flies *(26)*, but no similar activity has been reported in mammals. The biological reasons for the multiplicity of EGF-like ligands are incompletely understood. Genetic manipulation of mammals indicates that each ligand fulfils a unique set of inductive functions in the development of certain cell lineages. For example, the phenotype of mice lacking expression of TGFα includes abnormal skin, hair, and eye development. Possibly, each ligand binds to different hetero-and homodimers of ErbB proteins, including the ligand-less ErbB-2 *(23,27)*. For example, EGF and TGFα differ in their ability to recruit ErbB-2 into heterodimers, and they also differ in the mode of receptor inactivation *(28)*. These differences may underlie the superiority of TGFα in assays of wound healing, bone resorption, and angiogenesis *(29)*. Finally, protein modules that flank the receptor-binding EGF-like motif may differentially regulate the retention and availability of the various growth factors. An example is provided by HB-EGF, which is a ligand that avidly binds heparan sulfate proteoglycans of the extracellular matrix *(30)*.

2.1.3.2. PDGF and Related Growth Factors. Unlike EGF-like molecules, members of the PDGF family are dimeric molecules with a conserved motif containing eight cysteines. The disulfide-linked dimer includes two chains, PDGF-A and PDGF-B. All three possible homo-and heterodimeric combinations of these chains exist, and they exhibit different receptor binding specificities resulting in marked differences in biological activities and tissue selectivity (reviewed in ref. *31*). In addition, PDGF-A may be expressed in two distinct forms based upon alternative splicing of an exon encoding a C-terminal glycosaminoglycan binding domain *(32)*. Less is known regarding a third chain of PDGF, chain C, whose processing differs from that of the A and B chains. These latter chains are processed by proteolysis at the N termini before binding to target cells. Targets include fibroblasts and smooth muscle cells expressing α and/or β receptors. PDGF is the major mitogen present in human platelets, but its range of biological effects includes also chemotaxis, stimulation of matrix synthesis, and inhibition of cell death.

2.1.3.3. Fibroblast Growth Factors. Two forms of FGFs were initially identified and isolated from various tissue extracts by utilizing the ability of all FGFs to bind with high affinity to the sulfated polysaccharide heparin. Subsequently, two related molecules, Int2 (FGF3) and the androgen-induced growth factor (FGF8), were added to the list of FGFs. These polypeptides are encoded by genes activated by integration of the mammary tumor provirus. Other members of the family were isolated from a Kaposi sarcoma (FGF4) and a glioma (FGF9). Two additional FGFs were isolated by virtue of their strong mitogenic activity toward NIH-3T3 fibroblasts (FGF5) and epithelial cells (FGF7, keratinocyte growth factor). A characteristic of this family of growth factors is the requirement for sulfated polysaccharides of defined length and sequence for activation of their receptors *(33)*. Perlecan and syndecans, along with CD44 and a variety of core proteoglycans, appear to bind FGF molecules and present them to the respective receptors *(34)*.

3. RECEPTORS AND DOWNSTREAM SIGNALING PATHWAYS

The human genome encodes approximately 100 protein tyrosine kinases, of which the number of transmembrane kinases, namely RTKs, is expected to exceed 60 *(13)*. Yet, serine/threonine-specific kinases by far outnumber (by a factor of 5 or more) tyrosine kinases in the genome, and phosphorylated tyrosine represents only a small fraction (less than 0.5%) of the total content of phosphorylated amino acids in cellular proteins. The currently known RTKs fall into 20 subfamilies, sharing structural domains outside of the catalytic region and short homologous sequences within the relatively well conserved catalytic portion. Interestingly, some subfamilies are represented in invertebrates such as *C. elegans,* but only one member of the family exists in worms. For example, a single type I RTK (EGFR/ErbB) exists in worms (denoted Let-23) and in flies (DER), but there are four members in mammals. Hence, it is conceivable that gene duplication, in addition to gene fusion, is responsible for the current complexity of RTKs. The tyrosine kinase domain is the most conserved portion among RTKs, and it is shared with cytoplasmic tyrosine kinases, which lack a transmembrane domain. Nevertheless, in some RTKs (e.g., type III; PDGFR subfamily), the domain is bisected by a variable length hydrophilic sequence, called a kinase insert. Yet in other RTKs (e.g., ErbB-3, Klg/CCK,

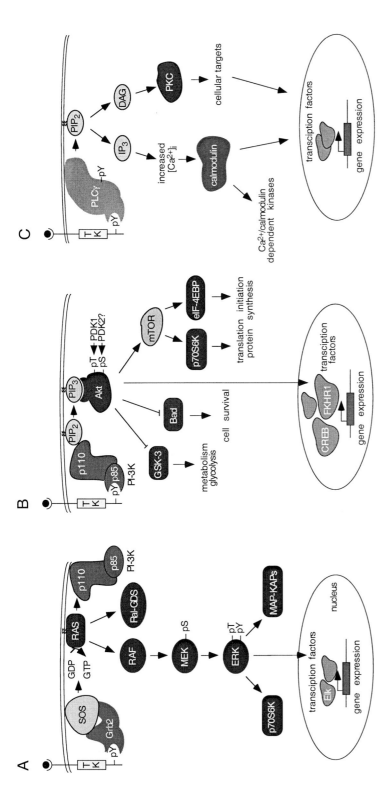

Fig. 3. Major signaling pathways downstream to RTKs. Autophosphorylation of RTKs on tyrosine residues enables the recruitment of multiple adaptor proteins and enzymes containing SH2 or PTB domains. **(A)** Recruitment of Grb2 to activated RTK results in the membrane translocation of associated Sos. Alternatively, the Grb2-Sos complex may be recruited following SH2 domain-mediated binding and subsequent tyrosine phosphorylation of Shc. Sos is a guanine nucleotide exchange factor for Ras, and its membrane translocation serves to activate the Ras GTPase. Downstream effectors of Ras include PI-3K, Ral-GDS, and Raf. Raf then activates a kinase cascade culminating in the activation of Erk1 and Erk2, which phosphorylate p70-S6 kinase, MAP-KAPs, as well as the Elk transcription factor, which regulates transcription from the serum response element. **(B)** The regulatory p85 subunit of PI3K is recruited to the active RTK by SH2 domain-mediated binding to phosphorylated tyrosine residues within the receptor or within adaptor proteins such as IRS or Gab. Recruitment of the p85 subunit activates the catalytic p110 subunit, resulting in the phosphorylation of PIP$_2$ at the 3' position. 3' Phosphorylated phosphoinositides result in the FYVE or PH domain-mediated membrane recruitment of multiple signaling molecules, including Akt. Membrane-localized Akt is subsequently phosphorylated and activated, leading to multiple signaling pathways important for cell survival and proliferation. These pathways include inhibition of the pro-apoptotic function of Bad, inhibition of GSK-3 function, the CREB and FKHR1 transcription factors, and translation initiation and protein synthesis through activation of mTOR, eukaryotic initiation factor 4E, and p70-S6 kinase. **(C)** The SH2 domain-mediated recruitment of PLCγ to RTK and its subsequent tyrosine phosphorylation result in the activation of PLCγ and the hydrolysis of PIP$_2$, thereby generating IP$_3$ and DAG. IP$_3$ results in increases in intracellular calcium concentrations, and the subsequent activation of the calmodulin serine/threonine phosphatase, as well as calcium/calmodulin-dependent protein kinases. DAG and calcium activate PKC, which regulates multiple signaling events.

53

and Ryk/Vik), the catalytic domain contains noncanonical residues that abolish kinase activity. In addition to the kinase domain, all RTKs invariably contain a single hydrophobic stretch of 20–25 amino acids, and the precursors are flanked by a signal peptide, a combination that ensures transmembrane expression. This topology positions RTKs in an orientation suitable for the transmission of extracellular signals to cytoplasmic targets. Hence, it is meaningful to consider RTKs as allosteric enzymes: the extracellular domains bind ligands, which allosterically modulate the cytoplasm-facing enzymatic domain. The key to understanding RTK action is provided by tyrosine autophosphorylation sites localized primarily at the carboxy-terminal tail of the receptor. These sites serve as docking points for a large set of cytoplasmic signaling proteins, the majority of which carry no enzymatic function. These adaptors, however, initiate a series of parallel linear cascades leading to cell activation (Fig. 3).

3.1. Structural Aspects of RTKs

3.1.1. EXTRACELLULAR DOMAINS

The ectodomains may be considered the variable part of RTKs, as they exhibit a variety of structural motifs, including long stretches rich in cysteines, immunoglobulin (Ig)-like domains, kringle motifs, and cadherin-like domains. Monomeric RTKs are catalytically inactive. However, ligand binding to the extracellular domain of a monomeric RTK invariably leads to receptor dimerization and subsequent activation of downstream signaling pathways. Thus, ligand binding and receptor dimerization are closely linked events, whose structural basis is now emerging. Mutagenesis and immunological strategies using monoclonal antibodies that interfere with ligand binding revealed that the binding cleft is comprised of noncontiguous receptor sequences. Thus, the two cysteine-free domains of ErbB-1, which are separated by a long cysteine-rich sequence, contribute to ligand binding (35), and three Ig-like domains of the SCF receptor are needed for high affinity ligand binding (36). Several crystal structures of the ectodomains of RTKs have been reported in the last few years, providing a structural basis for ligand recognition and ligand-induced dimerization of RTKs. The simplest model emerged from studies of Flt-1, which is the receptor for the vascular endothelial growth factor (VEGF) (37), in which the dimeric ligand engages two receptors by binding to Ig-like domain 2 (Ig2). The interface between the ligand and Ig2 is primarily hydrophobic, but limited interaction with Ig3 also exists. Interestingly, Ig4 may be involved in receptor–receptor interactions, in analogy to Ig4 of the SCF receptor, which is dispensible for SCF binding, but essential for receptor dimerization (38). Two ligand-receptor binding sites exist in TrkA, the receptor for NGF; one site is common to all Trk-neurotrophin interactions and the other site determines specificity for a neurotrophin (39). Although two FGF molecules bind to the dimeric receptor, there is no direct contact between the ligands (40), which contrasts with the disulfide-linked monomers of VEGF and NGF. Heparin binding to charged surfaces of the dimeric ligand–receptor complex stabilizes the heterotetrameric structure. Thus, the structural variation exhibited by the RTK family is reflected in a variety of molecular mechanisms enabling ligand recognition and receptor dimerization.

3.1.2. TRANSMEMBRANE DOMAINS

Although the relatively short transmembrane sequences of RTKs show no apparent conservation of structural motifs, the existence of an oncogenic point mutation in the rodent homologue of ErbB-2 (9) raised the possibility that the hydrophobic sequences play a role in receptor dimerization. The mutation, which results in the substitution of a valine for a glutamate, leads to constitutive dimerization and kinase activation. Apparently, the transmembrane domain exists as an α helix, and two adjacent helices interact along a specific surface *(41)*. Several models for ligand-independent dimerization of the two helices have been proposed: a carboxylate group of one helix may hydrogen bond with either the same group *(42)* or with a carbonyl oxygen residing on the other helix *(43)*. Whether or not the transmembrane helices of other RTKs interact with their partners to form ligand-induced dimers is an open question.

3.1.3. CYTOPLASMIC DOMAINS

The intracellular part of RTKs may be divided into three parts: the major and more highly conserved one is the catalytic portion, which is flanked by a juxtamembrane domain and a long hydrophilic tail. Whereas phosphorylation at the juxtamembrane domain is primarily regulatory and may be involved in auto-inhibition *(44)* or in receptor endocytosis *(45)*, phosphorylation of tyrosine residues localized in the carboxyl terminal tail (or in the kinase insert) allows subsequent binding of signaling proteins harboring Src homology-2 (SH2) or phosphotyrosine-binding (PTB) domains. Unlike modification of carboxyl-terminal tyrosines, autophosphorylation at sites located within the catalytic domain activates the enzymatic function. The crystal structure of the catalytic portions of several RTKs have been reported, which resolved a mechanism of *cis*-inhibition coupled to *trans*-activation. The overall architecture of the catalytic domain is similar to that of serine/threonine kinases *(46)*, an amino-terminal lobe rich in β strands is linked to an α helical carboxyl-terminal lobe. ATP binds in the cleft between the two lobes, and the tyrosine-containing peptide substrate binds the carboxy-terminal lobe. Accessibility of substrates to the active site is blocked in the inactive state by the activation loop, which contains between one and three tyrosines. Studies on the insulin receptor kinase domain imply that phosphorylation of these residues takes place upon ligand-induced receptor dimerization, and it occurs *in trans,* namely, in which one receptor within a dimer modifies the activation loop tyrosine of the dimer's mate *(47)*. Stimulation of kinase activity is due to removal of autorepression. In the unstimulated state, the inhibitory tyrosine (Tyr-1162/1163 of the insulin receptor or Tyr-653/654 of FGF-receptor) *(48)* is hydrogen-bonded to conserved residues within the catalytic loop. This obstructs binding of peptide substrates (and ATP, the donor of a phosphate group, in the case of the insulin receptor). Upon phosphorylation, a conformational change repositions the activation loop away from the active site, thereby allowing substrate access. Several oncogenic mutations affecting specific residues within the activation loop (see *Subheading 3.2.1.*) highlight the critical regulatory role of this domain.

3.2. Signaling by RTKs

3.2.1. ACTIVATION BY LIGANDS

In principle, receptor activation is the result of two consecutive phosphorylation events, both initiated upon ligand-induced noncovalent dimerization of monomeric receptors. Dimerization facilitates transphosphorylation of several tyrosine residues localized within (inhibitory tyrosines) and outside (docking site tyrosines) the kinase domain. Ligand-induced dimerization had been first observed with the EGFR *(49,50)* and was then extended to all other RTKs (reviewed in ref. *51*). Dimeric ligands induce dimerization of their surface receptor by virtue of their bivalent structure. However, the situation is less clear when dealing with momomeric ligands such as EGF. Possibly, these ligands contain two nonequivalent binding sites *(52),* which allow them to form complexes with a ligand:receptor ratio of either 2:2 or 1:2 *(53).* In addition to ligand-induced dimerization, conformational alterations may be necessary to properly juxtapose the kinase domains for effective transphosphorylation. The exact nature of the ligand-dependent conformational switches is still unknown.

3.2.2. RECRUITMENT OF ADAPTORS

In addition to phosphorylation of tyrosine residues located within the catalytic domain, receptor activation leads to phosphorylation of multiple tyrosine residues that are positioned in noncatalytic regions such as the juxtamembrane domain, the kinase insert, and the carboxyl-terminal domain. The phosphorylated tyrosine, in the context of several adjacent residues, forms a docking site with high binding specificity for PTB- and SH2-containing proteins *(54).* Only a small fraction of PTB and SH2-containing proteins are enzymes (e.g., kinases, phosphatases, and nucleotide exchange factors). Nevertheless, all are modular proteins carrying motifs recognizing specific lipids (e.g., PH and FYVE domains), proline-rich sequences (WW and SH3 domains), or hydrophobic carboxyl termini of other proteins (PDZ domains). In addition, upon close apposition, many adaptor proteins are phosphorylated by the activated receptor, thereby creating additional phosphotyrosine-based sites for recruitment of signaling proteins. A subset of the group of adaptors, called docking proteins, is characterized by a combination of an N-terminal membrane anchoring motif, either a PH domain (e.g., IRS and GAB), a transmembrane stretch (e.g., LAT), or a myristoylation site (e.g., FRS), and a set of tyrosine phosphorylation sites at the carboxyl-terminal half of the adaptor/docking protein. Hence, receptor activation leads to concerted engagement of multiprotein complexes at specific tyrosine autophoshorylation sites. Because the identity of these sites determines which protein complexes will be recruited to and RTK, it is believed that signaling specificity is encoded by the combination of tyrosine docking sites of each receptor *(55).* Other functions of adaptor proteins seem to be amplification of signaling by providing multiple docking sites for the same target enzyme, and juxtaposition of proteins involved in successive steps of a biochemical pathway (reviewed in ref. *55).*

3.2.3. MAJOR SIGNALING CASCADES

How are signaling cascades initiated? A variety of molecular mechanisms allow the initiation of biochemical processes upon recruitment of an adaptor or an enzyme to a ligand-stimulated receptor. In the case of phospholipase Cγ, tyrosine phosphorylation at specific tyrosine residues is essential for enhanced phospholipid breakdown by the enzyme *(56),* whereas translocation of two other enzymes, PDK-1 and Akt, to the plasma membrane initiates a kinase cascade leading to enhancement of cell survival. Membrane translocation of PDK-1 and Akt is made possible by another enzyme, phosphatidylinositol 3′ kinase (PI3K), which is directly recruited to active RTKs and phosphorylates the 3′ OH group of the inositol ring in phospholipids, which anchor the PH domains of Akt and PDK-1 to the membrane *(57).* Src is maintained in an inactive "closed" state in part by an intramolecular interaction between a C-terminal phopsphotyrosine (tyrosine 527) and an intrinsic SH2 domain. However, upon binding to a phosphorylated receptor's tyrosine, the SH2 domain releases the C-tail, thereby activating the kinase of Src *(58)*. As a result of physical interactions with immediate targets, active RTKs simultaneously initiate a plethora of signaling pathways. These are mediated by small molecule second messengers, such as calcium and lipids, and enzyme cascades (e.g., protein kinases). Here, we review three major pathways activated by RTKs and discuss general signal attenuation processes.

3.2.3.1. Mitogen-Activated Protein Kinase (MAPK) Cascade. Like all GTPases, Ras family members exist in an inactive (GDP-bound) and an active (GTP-bound) conformation. The activation of Ras by RTKs is mediated by a guanine nucleotide exchange factor (GEF) called Sos. Grb2 plays an essential role in coupling ligand-activated RTKs to Sos; by binding to Sos (through its SH3 domains) and to a phosphorylated tyrosine of an RTK (through its SH2 domain), the small adaptor translocates the GEF to the plasma membrane, the site of Ras activity. Indirect recruitment of the Ras/Sos complex to RTKs is possible; the Shc adaptor binds the complex and multiple RTKs in a nonexclusive fashion, and several other adaptors can simultaneously bind an RTK and the GEF via Grb2. RalGDS, PI3K, and Raf1 are all targets of the GTP-bound form of Ras and collectively they start numerous signaling pathways. Raf activation appears to require phosphorylation on one or two tyrosine residues *(59)*, and it takes place at the plasma membrane, probably by Src family members. Once activated, Raf phosphorylates MKK1 and MKK2, two kinases located upstream to the Erk1 and Erk2 MAPKs. The latter are doubly phosphorylated at a Thr-Glu-Tyr sequence within the activation loop in a reaction that is partially ordered with Tyr preceding. Erk favors substrates containing Pro residues at the Pro+1 position. Five protein kinases can be activated by Erks. They are referred to as MAPK-activated protein kinases (MAP-KAPs) and the ribosomal S6 kinase. Another group of substrates is represented by the p62 ternary complex factor (p62^{TCF}/Elk-1), which regulates transcription from the serum response element. Lastly, several cytoskeletal and cytoplasmic proteins are modified by Erks, including Sos-1 and cytosolic phospholipase-A$_2$. Thus, the MAPK cascade regulates several components participating in the response to mitogens: transcription factors, cytosolic enzymes, and cytoskeletal elements.

3.2.3.2. Phosphoinositide Signaling. The preferred substrate of activated PI3Ks is phosphatidylinositol-4,5-bisphosphate (PIP$_2$). This low abundance *polyphosphoinositide* serves as a substrate for another RTK-regulated enzyme, phospholipase Cγ (see below). Upon activation by ligands, RTKs couple to heterodimeric PI3Ks of class IA, whereas activation of G protein-coupled receptors stimulates the related class IB enzymes. RTKs utilize two main mechanisms to recruit and activate the lipid kinase activity of PI3Ks: Ras activation results in the formation of a complex comprising Ras-GTP bound to the p110 catalytic subunit of PI3K. Alternatively, the SH2-containing p85 regulatory subunit of PI3K is physically recruited to specific receptor motifs containing a phosphorylated tyrosine flanked by a methionine. PI3K activation results in rapid production of phosphatidylinositol-3,4,5-trisphosphate (PIP$_3$) and delayed generation of phosphatidylinositol-3,4-bisphosphate. Numerous proteins harboring FYVE or PH domains serve as targets for the lipids modified by PI3Ks. However, from a cell transformation perspective, the most significant target is Akt (also called protein kinase B [PKB]), a cellular homologue of a viral oncogene. The role of Akt in cancer is also illustrated by PTEN, a phosphoinositide-specific phosphatase, which is frequently inactivated in human cancers *(60)*. The PH-containing Akt kinase exists in three isoforms, all of which contain an activation loop Thr-308 and a regulatory Ser-473

residues. The Thr-308 kinase is another PH-containing enzyme, namely the above discussed 3′-phosphoinositide-dependent kinase (PDK-1). Once recruited to the plasma
membrane via binding of its PH domain to PI3K-generated phosphoinositides, Akt
undergoes phosphorylation by PDK-1 and by a still unknown kinase, thereby stimulating translocation of the enzyme to the nucleus *(61)*. The many substrates of Akt are
involved in inhibition of apoptosis and maintenance of steady cell growth. Included in
this list are two transcription factors (CREB and FKHR), the Bcl family member Bad,
and two protein kinases, Raf and glycogen synthase kinase-3 (GSK-3), which are both
inhibited by Akt. Another important substrate of Akt is mTOR, a DNA-dependent protein kinase whose major substrates are two proteins involved in initiation of protein
translation, eukaryotic initiation factor 4E, and the p70 ribosomal S6 kinase. Thus, by
coupling to PI3K and Akt, RTKs enhance cell survival and support cell proliferation
through mechanisms converging on a few critical transcription factors and the protein
translational apparatus.

**3.2.3.3. Signaling Through Phosphoinositide-Specific Phospholipase C and Pro-
tein Kinase C.** The ten mammalian phospholipase C (PLC) molecules specifically
hydrolyze the minor membrane phospholipid PIP_2 to generate two important second
messengers, inositol-1,4,5-trisphosphate (IP_3) and diacylglycerol (DAG) *(62)*. IP_3 activates specific receptors in the endoplasmic reticulum, resulting in calcium release and
activation of Ca^{2+}/calmodulin-dependent protein kinases (e.g., PYK2) and phosphatases (e.g., calcineurin) *(63,64)*. DAG and calcium ions bind to and activate protein
kinase C (PKC). The DAG-PKC complex translocates to the membrane, where PKC
phosphorylates various proteins including RTKs, a process that initiates their inactivation *(45)*. The β type isozymes of PLC molecules are regulated by G proteins. On the
other hand, the γ isozymes serve as targets for many RTKs. This group of enzymes is
characterized by the presence of SH2 and SH3 domains, in addition to PH domains,
and specific tyrosines, whose phosphorylation by active RTKs is essential for maximal
enzymatic activity. Autophosphorylation of RTKs creates docking sites for the SH2
domains of PLCγ and replacement of the tyrosine phopsphrylation sites in EGFR or
PDGF-receptor abolishes growth factor-dependent generation of IP_3. In addition, the
enzyme is indirectly regulated by translocation to the membrane, as well as by PI3K,
which generates PIP_3, an apparent cofactor of PLCγ. Calcium ion mobilization and
PKC activation translate into a large variety of cytoplasmic and nuclear events, including cytoskeletal reorganization and regulation of specific promoters. Nevertheless, the
biological role of PLCγ is not well defined. An "add-back" strategy that reconstituted
the corresponding docking site of the PDGF-receptor on a background of a tyrosine-
less mutant receptor suggested involvement of PLCγ in the Ras pathway, induction of
c-fos and cell proliferation *(65)*. However, direct mutagenesis indicated that coupling to
PLCγ is not essential for mitogenesis by FGF and PDGF *(66,67)*. On the other hand
several studies attributed to PLCγ a positive role in the induction of neurite outgrowth
by cultured neuronal cells *(68,69)*, implying that the multiple signals elicited by this
enzyme are differently interpreted by cells of distinct lineages.

3.2.3.4. Signal Attenuation. An important feature of all signaling pathways is the
kinetics of their inactivation. Studies of the Ras-MAPK pathway revealed that cells
interpret signals arising from this pathway differently according to the kinetics of the
inactivation phase *(70)*. Protein and lipid phosphatases, GTPase activating enzymes, as
well as targeted degradation of activated RTKs by the ubiquitin machinery, seem to be

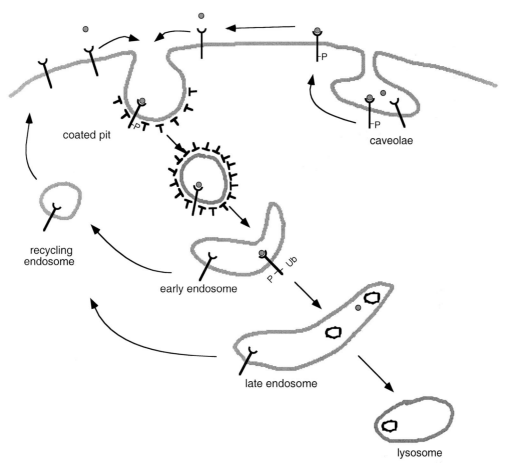

coated pit

caveolae

recycling
endosome

early endosome

late endosome

lysosome

Fig. 4. A model of RTK endocytosis and trafficking. Receptor endocytosis and degradation are important mechanisms for the attenuation and termination of signaling by RTKs. In the absence of ligand, monomeric RTKs may be localized in caveolar or noncaveolar regions of the plasma membrane. Ligand binding induces receptor dimerization, autophosphorylation (marked by P), and migration of caveolar receptors from these membrane domains. Activated receptors internalized via clathrin-coated pits are subsequently sorted through several endosomal compartments and are ultimately degraded in the lysosome. Receptor ubiquitination by Cbl, a ubiquitin-ligase recruited to tyrosine phosphorylated RTK through its SH2 domain, plays a critical role in receptor trafficking and degradation.

important components in refining signal transduction, but how negative signals are integrated in mammals is far from being understood. Genetic analyses of the *Drosophila* EGFR (DER) pathway in flies uncovered a surprisingly complex network of signal inactivation, which is tightly regulated at the transcriptional level. Argos, an inhibitory ligand of DER, Kekkon, a transmembrane protein inhibiting DER oligomerization, Ras-GAP, a GTPase activating protein, d-Cbl, a ubiquitin E3 ligase, and Sprouty, an inhibitor of the Ras-MAPK pathway, have been identified as negative regulators *(26,71)*. The major, and apparently most general, process inactivating RTKs in mammalian cells seems to be endocytosis followed by recycling or degradation of activated receptors *(72)* (see Fig. 4). Most monomeric inactive RTKs may localize to caveolae or to lipid rafts *(73)*. Upon ligand binding, dimeric RTKs are rapidly recruited into clathrin coated pits and endocytose *(74)*. Protein sorting to clathrin-coated invaginations of the plasma membrane is mediated by binding to adaptor protein 2 (AP2), which then recruits clathrin heavy chain. Though hydrophobic motifs on the receptor have been implicated in binding to AP2, ablation of these residues does not block internalization *(75)*, but lessons gained in yeast imply involvement of receptor mono-ubiquitination in targeting receptors to internalization *(76)*. Ubiquitination of target proteins involves three enzymes working in succession: a ubiquitous ubiquitin-activating enzyme (E1), a ubiquitin-conjugating enzyme (E2), and a ubiquitin ligase (E3), which selects a protein for degradation. c-Cbl, a large adaptor protein originally identified as a product of a viral oncogene, has been identified as an E3-specific for active RTKs *(77,78)*. Three Cbl proteins are known in mammals; all three undergo rapid phosphorylation on tyrosine residues and physically associate with many RTKs upon activation (reviewed in ref. *79*). The SH2 domain of c-Cbl mediates receptor binding, and the flanking RING finger recruits a ubiquitin-loaded E2 enzyme, which transfers ubiquitin to the Cbl-bound RTK. Receptor ubiquitination mediated by c-Cbl seems to target RTKs, not only to coated regions of the plasma membrane, but also to subsequent degradation in lysosomes *(80)*. In addition to c-Cbl, Eps-15, RalBP1, c-Src, and Grb2 have been implicated in endocytosis of RTKs, but their exact roles are still obscure.

4. ONCOGENIC MECHANISMS

Unrestrained signals for cell growth may arise when any of the many steps associated with receptor activation is constitutively stimulated. Although in the majority of cases the receptors or components of the downstream pathways are mutated, in a few cases transformation may be attributed only to enhanced availability of specific growth factors. The scope of this review limits the discussion to alterations in receptors and ligands. Two major mechanisms relate to oncogenic transformation by RTK ligands: an autocrine mechanism and a paracrine loop of tumor cell activation. Here, we will deal with several prototypic examples for the respective two mechanisms. Similarly, three main principles underlie transformation by RTKs. First, overexpression of a receptor, which is primarily a result of gene amplification, seems to be the major mechanism, and we will use ErbB-2 as an example. Second, point mutations, which transform a receptor to the active state in the absence of ligand, are exemplified below by c-Kit (SCF-receptor). Last, we use Ret to demonstrate the oncogenic power of point mutations and genomic rearrangements generating constitutively active tyrosine kinases.

4.1. Mechanisms Involving Constitutive Stimulation by Growth Factors

Unlike intrinsic alterations in receptors or effectors, causative relationships between ligand availability and transformation are more difficult to prove in a clinical setting. Nevertheless, experimental model systems provide numerous examples for the oncogenic potential of growth factors in the context of autocrine and paracrine loops. Two examples that we briefly discussed are the induction of PDGF synthesis by the simian sarcoma virus and up-regulation of certain FGF molecules by proviral integration. In addition to direct autocrine pathways, oncogene-transformed cells (e.g., transformation by *ras, mos,* and *raf1*) often exhibit high levels of growth factor in their media. This observation was used to isolate novel EGF-like ligands such as TGFα and NRGs from tumor cells expressing mutant *ras* genes *(81,82)*. Although the necessity of secreted growth factors for transformation by Ras is currently unclear, it is relevant that two ErbB-1 ligands, HB-EGF and amphiregulin, are among the most strongly induced genes in Ras-transformed cells *(83)*. Steroid hormones are other strong inducers of a variety of growth factors in both developing embryos and in cultures. Examples of additional circuits of growth factors have been described, including the regulation of the VEGFs by extracellular agents and hypoxia (reviewed in ref. *84*), and they may reflect physiological networks of cell lineage control. Dysregulation of these secondary mechanisms may also participate in cell transformation.

4.1.1. AUTOCRINE LOOPS

Productive autocrine stimulation requires co-expression of a growth factor and the cognate receptor in the same cancer cell. Although intracellular activation of the receptor, while traveling through the Golgi apparatus, may occur in some tumors, in the majority of cases ligand secretion is essential. Therefore, pharmacological intervention by using extracellular agents (e.g., antibodies, peptidergic ligand antagonists, and soluble receptors) is feasible in most autocrine loops. Because no overexpression of the ligand is necessary for the establishment of an autocrine loop, and usually genes encoding growth factors are weakly transcribed, it is conceivable that many such loops escape immunohistochemical detection in clinical specimens. Nevertheless, an extensive literature exists linking tumoral growth factors with human cancer. Examples include PDGF expression, along with its receptors, in glioblastomas *(85)* and sarcomas *(86)*. Consistent with the transforming potential of autocrine PDGF-BB, most skin tumors of the dermatofibrosarcoma protuberans (DFSB) type express a fusion protein composed of the growth factor and collagen 1A1 *(87)*, which is a combination capable of transforming cultured fibroblasts. Likewise, expression of the HGF in patients with breast or non-small cell lung cancer was shown to be a strong predictor of recurrence and short patient survival *(88)*. Despite these and other examples, causal relationships between ligand-receptor co-expression and transformation are complex and interpretation difficult. To exemplify the issue, we concentrate on ErbB-1 ligands. Early on, co-expression of TGFα and ErbB-1 was noted in many human tumors *(89)*. Overexpression of TGFα in cultured cells rendered them partly transformed due to an autocrine loop involving ErbB-1 *(90)*, and ectopic expression of TGFα in transgenic mice leads to spontaneous squamous papillomas *(91)*, liver and colon hyperplasia, and mammary neoplasia *(92,93)*. Consistent with autocrine stimulation, poorer prognosis of TGFα-expressing tumors, especially those co-expressing ErbB-1, has been reported in lung, ovary, and colon cancer (reviewed in ref. *94*). In prostate cancer, TGFα seems to act in a paracrine fashion at the initial androgen-dependent phase, but it becomes an autocrine factor at the later hormone-independent phase *(95)*. Similarly, expression of TGFα in pancreatic cancer correlates with tumor size and decreased patient survival *(96,97)*. Because over 90% of pancreatic carcinomas exhibit Ki-Ras mutations and transcription from the promoter of TGFα is up-regulated by Ras, overexpression of TGFα in pancreatic cancer may reflect the presence of a mutant Ras gene. Similarly, HB-EGF expression is up-regulated by other ErbB ligands, oxidative stress, and the Raf pathway *(30)*, and the analysis of the TGFα promoter uncovered an EGF-regulated element *(98)*. It is interesting to note that TGFα is nontransforming in transgenic models, but it can dramatically enhance tumorigenicity by other oncogenes *(99)*. However, both Myc and Neu can enhance tumorigenicity of TGFα in transgenic models *(100),* and in TGFα-knock-out mice the incidence of hepatomas was similar to that of wild-type mice *(101).* These observations highlight the complexity of relating an RTK ligand to tumorigenicity; the growth factor may be secondarily induced by a primary oncogene, the stromal component may act as a ligand source, or the ligand may be expressed but unprocessed or sequestered by the extracellular matrix.

4.1.2. PARACRINE LOOPS

Survival, growth, and metastasis of solid tumors depend on a complex network of tumor–stroma interactions. Growth factors synthesized by stromal cells are often necessary for proliferation and migration of tumor cells. On the other hand, tumor-derived molecules seem necessary for the induction of tumor angiogenesis and for the invasive properties of metastasizing cancer cells. The majority of these local and systemic circuits involve RTKs and their ligands. Several such examples are discussed below.

4.1.2.1. Angiogenic Factors. Tumors require continuous blood supply in order to maintain steady mass growth and also metastasize into distant organs by means of the general circulation *(102).* Angiogenic factors secreted by stromal and tumor cells stimulate the migration and proliferation of endothelial cells, thereby initiating sprouting of blood vessels. Vessel density frequently correlates with advanced stage and poor prognosis of glioblastomas *(103).* Similarly, intratumoral vessel count was found to be a prognostic indicator in gastric, breast, and non-small cell lung cancers. The receptors for VEGF, namely Flt-1 and Flk-1/KDR, as well as Tie1 and Tie2/Tek, the receptors for angiopoietins, play a direct role in angiogenesis. Likewise, PDGF, HGF, and FGFs contribute to the angiogenic switch of tumors. Paracrine regulation of angiogenesis by cancer cells has been demonstrated using tumor models in rodents (reviewed in ref. *104),* and ample clinical evidence correlates the level of tumoral VEGF expression with disease stage, metastases, and poor prognosis. Examples of this correlation include pulmonary adenocarcinoma patients whose survival inversely correlates with VEGF expression *(105),* and breast cancer patients, both node-positive and node-negative, displaying poor prognosis and increased microvessel counts in correlation with high VEGF protein and mRNA ref. *106* and references therein). Likewise, expression of Tie2 is markedly up-regulated in highly angiogenic tumors, including glioblastomas and sarcomas (reviewed in ref. *(107)).*

4.1.2.2. Platelet-Derived Growth Factors. PDGF and its receptors are expressed in tumor cells, stroma, and pericytes, and may play a direct or indirect role in tumor angiogenesis. Moreover, many types of tumors, including cancers of the gastrointestinal system, breast, and lung tumors, express PDGF (e.g., see ref. *108),* whereas the juxtaposed stromal fibroblasts almost invariably express the β subtype of the PDGF receptor. This potential paracrine loop is thought to mediate three types of stromal responses. First, tumor-derived PDGF induces proliferation of stromal fibroblasts and pericytes. Second, the growth factor elicits the production of metalloproteinase *(109),* enzymes that degrade the extracellular matrix, and promotes the invasion of metastases through blood vessel walls. Third, the paracrine loop results in an increased interstitial fluid pressure within the stroma, which is an effect thought to block penetration of low molecular weight drugs *(110).* Collectively, the effects of growth factors synthesized by tumor cells may explain why the stroma of tumor cells is often more compact and less penetrable than normal connective tissue.

4.1.2.3. Insulin-Like Growth Factor 1. Although they may be considered endocrine mediators, both insulin and IGF-1 bind to RTKs, and IGF-2 binds a nonkinase surface receptor. Despite their high similarity, the IGF-1 receptor is much more mitogenic than the receptor for insulin, and IGF-1 is involved in several aspects of paracrine tumor regulation. First, paracrine as well as autocrine IGF-1 synthesis is upregulated by mitogens like EGF and PDGF, and tumor suppressors like p53 and WT1, as well as interferons, decrease expression of the IGF-1 receptor (reviewed in ref. *111*). In addition to mitogenic signals, the IGF-1 receptor generates an anti-apoptotic signal, which seems essential for survival of not only normal cells but also transformed cells; receptor-defective cells are refractory to transformation by viral and cellular oncogenes *(112),* and blocking the receptor for IGF-1 by using antisense or immunological strategies can reverse tumorigenesis *(113).* In summary, IGF-1 produced, either locally or in distant organs like the liver, is an essential survival factor for a broad range of tumors. However, because most normal tissues will undergo apoptosis in the absence of IGF-1, potential application of the IGF-1 axis for cancer therapy seems limited.

4.2. ErbB Proteins: Oncogenesis by Overexpression

Immunohistochemical analysis is routinely performed on biopsies or on tumor specimens after surgery. This type of analysis often leads to the observation of unusually high expression of specific antigens. In the case of RTKs, caution must be taken because variation in sample preparation, antibody specificity, and antigen subcellular location may lead to erroneous conclusions. Since, in the majority of tumors, protein overexpression is due to gene amplification, methods that detect amplified genes on specific chromosomes (e.g., fluorescence in situ hybridization [FISH] are preferred over immunohistochemical analyses. Here, we concentrate on ErbB-1 and ErbB-2, two prototypic RTKs, whose overexpression is associated with disease progression in several malignancies.

4.2.1. ErbB-1

Originally, ErbB-1 overexpression was detected in cancer cell lines, including A-431 human epidermoid carcinoma cells. Later analysis of these cells revealed that overexpression was associated with gene amplification and rearrangements *(114).* Further studies detected enhanced expression of ErbB-1 in a variety of carcinomas, including cancers of the lung *(115),* head, and neck *(116).* In addition, high expression is a significant indicator for recurrence in operable breast tumors, and is associated with shorter disease-free and overall survival in advanced breast cancer *(117).* Overexpression of ErbB-1 is also a very frequent genetic alteration in central nervous system malignancies, with amplification of the gene occurring in 40% of gliomas *(118).* Overexpression associates with higher grade, higher proliferation, and reduced survival. In a significant fraction of tumors, gene amplification is accompanied by rearrangements. The most common genetic alteration (type III) of ErbB-1 results in a deletion of amino acids 6–276 of the extracellular domain *(119),* leading to a constitutively active kinase.

4.2.2. ErbB-2

Although an activating mutation of ErbB-2 has been identified in rodent tumor models, no similar alterations have been detected in human tumors. However, as was the case with ErbB-1, gene amplification and protein overexpression were originally observed in cancer cell lines of breast and gastric origin *(120,121).* Subsequently, overexpression of ErbB-2 was identified in several different human malignancies and is frequently associated with negative prognostic features (reviewed in ref. *122*). Tumors most significantly studied in this regard, include those affecting breast, ovary, lung, pancreas, colon, esophagus, prostate, endometrium, and cervix *(120,121)*. The first major link between clinical breast cancer and ErbB-2 was revealed when Slamon and collaborators reported that ErbB-2 gene amplification correlated with poor clinical outcome in node-positive, but not in node-negative patients *(123)*.

One of the factors that makes ErbB-2 a clinically useful prognostic marker is that overexpression is not found in benign breast disease, suggesting that patients with lesion biopsies overexpressing ErbB-2, more than likely require treatment. This matter is relevant for treatment decisions regarding ductal carcinoma in situ (DCIS), a premalignant lesion, increasingly diagnosed as mammography becomes more accessible, but which has a variable risk of developing into invasive cancer. The more aggressive comedo form overexpresses ErbB-2 in up to 90% of cases *(124–28);* overexpression is linked to other cancer related molecular changes *(129–131)*, and consistently correlates with poorly differentiated and more aggressive subtypes in various staging schemes *(132–136)*. The role of ErbB-2 is more complex in invasive ductal carcinoma, where the extent of overexpression drops to around 30% *(123,137)*. In general, several phenomena accompany ErbB-2 overexpression: the primary tumor will be larger *(138)*, of higher grade *(139)*, it will less likely express steroid hormone receptors *(139–141)*, and will have decreased levels of Bcl-2 *(142)*. Histologically, ErbB-2 overexpression is present primarily in invasive ductal histology, and is not found in lobular and other subtypes with better prognosis *(139,143–145)*. As 30% of patients with node-negative disease will suffer a recurrence of their cancer, it is imperative to find markers that might predict which of these tumors need systemic therapy. ErbB-2 may represent such a marker; according to several studies, ErbB-2 overexpression in node-negative disease identifies patients with worse outcome, including shorter relapse-free survival *(146–151)*.

4.2.3. ErbB-2 Overexpression and Chemoresistance

One of the intriguing early clinical findings in studies related to ErbB-2 overexpression was a relationship to chemoresistance *(139,152)* (also reviewed in refs. *153,154*). Patients who have ErbB-2 overexpressing tumors tend to be resistant to chemo-, radio-, and endocrine therapy *(158–161)*. ErbB-2 activates anti-apoptotic machinery, including the up-regulation of Bcl-2 and Bcl-XL *(158)*. Overexpression of ErbB-2 also leads to p21waf1 overexpression *(162)* and hypophosphorylation of Rb *(163)*, which protect cells from genotoxic stress by blocking entry into the cell cycle *(157)*. Conversely, treatment with ErbB-2 blocking antibodies leads to inadequate p21waf1 response in irradiated cells *(164)*. Underlying these defensive pathways may be Akt, which is activated by ErbB-2 and phosphorylates p21waf1 *(165)*. Thus, from a biological perspective, the multiple signaling pathways initiated by the ErbB family RTKs may explain the clinical observation of an invasive metastases-prone and treatment-resistant phenotype that is associated with ErbB-2 overexpression.

4.2.4. How Does an Overexpressed ErbB-2 Transform Cells?

The autocrine and paracrine mechanisms of cell transformation can explain how ErbB-1 overexpression sensitizes cells to one of the EGF-like ligands synthesized locally. Although ErbB-2 overexpression more robustly transforms cultured cells *(166,167)*, a ligand that binds to ErbB-2 with high affinity may not exist *(168)*. Nevertheless, ErbB-2 is preferentially recruited into heterodimers once a ligand binds to one of its family members (169,170). Heterodimerization with ErbB-2 is particularly critical for signaling by ErbB-3, since this receptor is endowed with a catalytically inactive kinase domain (171). Thus, the role of ErbB-2 overexpression in cancer cells may be to bias formation of ligand-induced heterodimers. Consistent with the possibility that the normal developmental role of ErbB-2 is to serve as a heterodimer partner, aspects of the phenotype of ErbB-2 null embryos are shared with animals defective in each of the other ErbB genes (reviewed in ref. 172). In agreement with strong mitogenic signaling, ErbB-2 is coupled to the Ras-MAPK and the PI3K-Akt pathways, and its heterodimers elicits stronger proliferative responses than the respective homodimers of ErbB proteins (173,174). Several functional features underlie the mitogenic superiority of ErbB-2-containing heterodimers. First, ErbB-2 elevates the affinity of heterodimers to the respective ligand by decelerating the rate of ligand dissociation (175). In addition, heterodimers are endowed with broader ligand specificity than the corresponding homodimers (176,177). Last, the kinetics of ErbB-2 desensitization through the endocytic pathway is relatively slow (173,178), and it tends to recycle back to the cell surface after delivering ligands for lysosomal degradation (28,179). In summary, several distinct mechanisms allow prolonged retention of ErbB-2 at the cell surface, thereby extending the duration of signaling by its heterodimeric partners. Hence, by overexpression of ErbB-2, tumor cells may gain increased sensitivity to stromal and autocrine growth factors of the EGF and NRG families.

4.3. Oncogenic Activation of RTKs by Mutations and Gene Rearrangements

Gain of function mutations leading to tonic ligand-independent activation of several RTKs have been detected in human malignancies, as well as in experimental animal systems (reviewed in ref. 13). Examples include mutations in the HGF receptor (Met, in renal cancer), the macrophage growth factor receptor (Fms, in myelomonocytic leukemia), and constitutively dimerized chimeric versions of the receptors for FGF and NGF. Here, we concentrate on two RTKs that are extensively mutated in human cancers, namely: c-Kit, the receptor for SCF, and Ret, which binds the GDNF.

4.3.1. STEM CELL FACTOR RECEPTOR: ONCOGENESIS BY MUTATIONS

Human c-Kit was identified on the basis of a feline viral oncoprotein, v-Kit, which represents a receptor truncated at both extracellular regions and intracellular sequences flanking a bisected tyrosine kinase of the PDGF-receptor family (6). Mapping of the c-kit gene to the murine *White spotting (W)* chromosomal locus led to an understanding of the multiple developmental roles of c-Kit even before SCF had been identified. This ligand–receptor interaction is critically involved in development of several cell lineages, including mast cells, melanocytes, germ cells, and interstitial cells of Cajal (reviewed in ref. 180). Two cytoplasmic domains of c-Kit are major targets for oncogenic mutations in human cancers. These are the activation loop located at the carboxyl-terminal half of the tyrosine kinase (Asp816 in the canonical Asp-Phe-Gly sequence) and an inhibitory α helix located in the juxtamembrane domain (ref. 181 and references therin). Replacement of Asp816 with either a histidine or a valine was identified in germ cell tumors (seminomas and dysgerminomas), adult and atypical pediatric mastocytosis, and in myeloid leukemia. In pediatric and adolescent mastocytosis patients, the disease tends to be more extensive and progressive if patients carry the Asp816 mutation. The mutant receptor displays constitutively high kinase activity and signaling through the PI3K/Akt pathway. The other class of mutations (exon 11) impinge on a short regulatory sequence containing autophosphorylation docking sites specific for c-Src and SHP-1, a tyrosine-specific phosphatase of hematopoietic cells. Apparently, the short α helix is inhibitory for the kinase, and both tyrosines participate in signal attenuation, which is consistent with the tumor suppressive effects of SHP-1 inferred from the phenotype of SHP-1-defective *Motheaten (Me)*-mutant mice. The juxtamembrane domain is mutated in up to 90% of gastroinstestinal stromal tumors (GIST), the most common mesenchymal neoplasm in the human gastroinstestinal tract, and the presence of these mutations predicts worse prognosis *(182)*. In addition, similar germ line mutations and deletions affecting the juxtamembrane α helix exist in families with multiple GISTs. Other types of somatic mutations were detected in various lesions: V559G (valine 559 replaced by a glycine) in mastocytosis, D52N in myeloproliferative disorders, and a variety of intracellular mutations in sinonasal lymphomas *(183)*. How exactly these alterations influence signaling by c-Kit is still unknown, but classification of the mutations and comprehensive understanding of c-Kit activation are crucial for therapy, since several low molecular weight inhibitors of the kinase are now available (e.g., STI571 and SU5416).

4.3.2. GDNF Receptor: Oncogenesis by Gene Rearrangements and Mutations

c-Ret was first inferred by the discovery of an oncogene activated by gene rearrangement *(12)*. The Ret receptor is a rather unique member of the RTK family; one of four glycosyl phosphatidylinositol-linked coreceptors, FGR-α-1 through 4, is essential for ligand binding and subsequent activation of Ret. Two mechanisms of oncogenic activation of Ret were identified in cancer patients: either by somatic gene alterations in radiation-induced or spontaneous papillary thyroid carcinomas, or germ-line mutations in three familial tumor syndromes, multiple endocrine neoplasia type 2A (MEN2A), MEN2B, and familial medullary thyroid carcinoma (FMTC) (reviewed in ref. *184*). Both mechanisms involve constitutive activation of the Ret kinase and downstream signaling. The signaling pathways activated by Ret include Ras-MAPK, PI3K-Akt, Jun N-terminal kinase, and PLCμ, but in vitro studies suggest cell type specificity of signaling by Ret. In contrast with transforming gain of function mutations, loss of function mutations in *ret* lead to Hirschsprung's disease, which is characterized by the absence of enteric autonomous ganglia. Targeted inactivation of the gene in mice confirmed involvement of Ret in development of the enteric system and also revealed its role in kidney development *(185)*.

4.3.2.1. Rearranged Forms of Ret in Papillary Thyroid Cancer. Fusion proteins containing the tyrosine kinase domain of Ret and a variety of N-terminal donor proteins (e.g., H4, ELE1, and ELKS) are frequently detected in human papillary thyroid carcinoma (RET/PTC oncogenes). All chimeric proteins lost the transmembrane domain of Ret, but retained the carboxyl-terminal autophosphorylation region *(186)*. In addition, in each case the N-terminal donor contributes a dimerization function, either a coiled coil domain, or specific cysteine residues forming disulfide bonds. Although the fusion proteins contain no transmembrane domain, a Ret-binding PDZ protein called Enigma seems to recruit the chimera to the inner face of the plasma membrane *(187)*. Hence, activation of Ret is invariably due to constitutive dimerization of the fusion proteins in thyroid carcinomas. Interestingly, thyroid follicular cells can form both follicular and papillary thyroid carcinomas, but RET/PTC fusion proteins were found only in the latter type of cancers, implying specificity of signaling or mutagenic processes. The incidence of RET/PTC activation is relatively low in spontaneous papillary carcinomas of the thyroid, but it increases up to 70% in the radiation-induced lesions. However, the prognostic significance of RET/PTC is currently unclear; whereas some studies associated the rearranged gene with poor prognosis, others correlated it with smaller slow growing and less aggressive tumors. Presumably, the identity of the N-terminal donor gene, technical aspects, environmental factors, and heterogeneity of papillary thyroid carcinomas contribute to the discrepancies.

4.3.2.2. Mutant Forms of Ret in Endocrine Neoplasia Type 2. The *ret* gene has been identified as the susceptibility gene for multiple endocrine neoplasia type 2 disease, which is an inherited cancer syndrome with three subtypes (MEN2A, MEN2B, and FMTC) that are variably characterized by medullary thyroid carcinoma, pheochromocytoma, and parathyroid hyperplasia *(188)*. All germ-line mutations identified in MEN2 families cluster in the cysteine-rich domain (exon 10 and 11) or in the tyrosine kinase domain (exons 13–16). These two classes of mutations differ biochemically, which correlates with different clinical phenotypes; the extracellular mutations (FMTC and MEN2A syndrome) replace a cysteine with a noncysteine residue, thereby converting an intramolecular disulfide bond to an interreceptor bond. On the otherhand, most MEN2B patients carry an M918T mutation that activates the kinase domain without inducing dimers of Ret. In addition to the M918T mutation, FMTC and MEN2B display other recurrent point mutations in highly conserved regions of the kinase domain. Although both extracellular and intracellular mutations in Ret lead to constitutive signaling, only the second type displays responsiveness to ligand, as well as altered substrate specificity and increased signaling via the PI3K pathway *(189)*. In conclusion, future classification of the various *ret* mutations, and detailed understanding of their biochemical effects, will likely lead to improved presymptomatic DNA-based testing and well-reasoned recommendations as to whether or not to perform prophylactic thyroidectomy.

5. CONCLUDING REMARKS

The isolation and molecular cloning of the first RTKs, some 16 yr ago, opened the way for a new era in cell biology and cancer research. Along with the enormous complexity of signaling pathways, the multiplicity of components, and the apparent functional redundancy that have emerged, it is becoming clear that the current experimental tools available to molecular biologists and geneticists are insufficient for deciphering signal transduction in an isolated cell or in a living organism. The richly interconnected networks, their spatial and temporal integration, and the multilayered control circuits call for the application of sophisticated genetic manipulation, as well as parallel computational simulations, which are methodologies that are yet unavailable. Nevertheless, the great strides already achieved in resolving the cell's wiring and in identifying the complete arsenal of the mammalian genome hold promise for the future understanding of RTK signaling. The lessons gained will certainly be applicable to biotechnology and medicine. For example, it is already clear that the multistep nature of cancer development opens the opportunity for reversing a malignant state by inhibiting only one of the accumulated genetic/biochemical alterations. On the other hand, it is becoming clear that RTK signaling plays a significant role in a wider range of cancers than was originally anticipated. Moreover, the relatively deep cleft of the nucleotide binding site of RTKs and the cell surface localization of these receptors offer an attractive target for small molecule inhibitors and antagonistic antibodies. Furthermore, the paucity of tyrosine phosphorylation in intact cells suggests limited adverse effects due to incomplete pharmacological specificity. Compounds with high selectivity for specific RTKs and monoclonal antibodies capable of down-regulating specific receptors are already available for clinical use. Thus, STI571, a compound inhibiting c-Kit, along with PDGF-receptor and Abl tyrosine kinase, effectively inhibits metastiatic gastrointestinal stromal tumors *(190)*, and Herceptin/Trastuzumab, a humanized monoclonal antibody specific for ErbB-2/HER2, is used in combination with chemotherapy in the treatment of metastatic breast cancer patients *(191)*. More target-selective drugs will be designed in the future, as our understanding of RTK signaling and oncogenes deepens.

REFERENCES

1. Carpenter G, Cohen S. Epidermal growth factor. *Ann Rev Biochem* 1979; 48:193–216.
2. Feramisco J, Ozanne B, Stiles C. *Cancer Cells: Growth Factors and Transformation. Vol. 3*. CSH Laboratory Press, Cold Spring Harbor, NY, 1985.
3. Waterfield MD, Scarce T, Whittle N, et al. Platelet-derived growth factor is structurally related to the putative transforming protein of simian sarcoma virus. *Nature* 1983; 304:35–39.
4. Downward J, Yarden Y, Mayes E, et al. Close similarity of epidermal growth factor receptor and v-*erb*-B oncogene protein sequences. *Nature* 1984; 307:521–527.
5. Coussens L, Van Beveren C, Smith D, et al. Structural alteration of viral homologue of receptor proto-oncogene fms at carboxyl terminus. *Nature* 1986; 320:277–280.
6. Yarden Y, Kuang W-J, Yang-Feng T, et al. Human protooncogene c-*kit:* a new cell surface tyrosine kinase for unidentified ligand. *EMBO J* 1987; 6:3341–3351.
7. Varmus HE, Brown PO. Retroviruses. In: Howe M, Berg D, eds. *Mobile DNA*. American Society for Microbiology Publications, Washington, DC, 1989, pp. 53–108.
8. Shih C, Padhy LC, Murray M, Weinberg RA. Transforming genes of carcinomas and neuroblastomas introduced into mouse fibroblasts. *Nature* 1981; 290:261–264.
9. Bargmann CI, Hung MC, Weinberg RA. Multiple independent activations of the *neu* oncogene by a point mutation altering the transmembrane domain of p185. *Cell* 1986; 45:649–657.
10. Cooper CS, Park M, Blair DG, et al. Molecular cloning of a new transforming gene from a chemically transformed human cell line. *Nature* 1984; 311:29–33.
11. Martin-Zanca D, Hughes SH, Barbacid M. A human oncogene formed by the fusion of truncated tropomyosin and protein tyrosine kinase sequences. *Nature* 1986; 319:743–748.
12. Takahasi M, Rich J, Copper MG. Activation of a novel human transforming gene, ret, by DNA rearrangement. *Cell* 1985; 42:581–588.
13. Blume-Jensen P, Hunter T. Oncogenic kinase signaling. *Nature* 2001; 411:355–365.
14. Yarden Y, Ullrich A. Growth factor receptor tyrosine kinases. *Ann Rev Biochem* 1988; 57:443–478.
15. Cohen S. Isolation of a mouse submaxillary gland protein accelerating incisor eruption and eyelid openig in new-born animal. *J Biol Chem* 1962; 237:1555–1562.
16. Burgess WH, Maciag T. The heparin-binding (fibroblast) growth factor family of proteins. *Annu Rev Biochem* 1989; 58:575–606.
17. Levyi-Montalcini R, Hamburger V. Selective growth stimulating effects of mouse sarcoma on the sensory and sympathetic nervous system of the chick embryo. *J Exp Zool* 1951; 116:321–351.
18. Sporn MB, Todaro GJ. Autocrine secretion and malignant transformation of cells. *N Eng J Med* 1980; 308:878–880.
19. Shilo B-Z, Raz E. Developmental control by the *Drosophila* EGF receptor homolog DER. *Trends Genet* 1991; 7:388–392.
20. Sternberg PW, Horvitz R. Signal transduction during *C. elegans* vulval induction. *Trends Genet* 1991; 7:366–371.
21. Massague J, Pandiella A. Membrane-anchored growth factors. *Ann Rev Biochem* 1993; 62:515–541.
22. Groenen LC, Nice EC, Burgess AW. Structure-function relationships for the EGF/TGF-α family of mitogens. *Growth Factors* 1994; 11:235–257.
23. Riese DJ, II, Stern DF. Specificity within the EGF family/ErbB receptor family signaling network. *Bioessays* 1998; 20:41–48.

24. Harari D, Tzahar E, Romano J, et al. Neuregulin-4: a novel growth factor that acts through the ErbB-4 receptor tyrosine kinase. *Oncogene* 1999; 18:2681–2689.

25. Tzahar E, Moyer JD, Waterman H, et al. Pathogenic poxviruses reveal viral strategies to exploit the ErbB signaling network. *EMBO J* 1998; 17:5948–5963.

26. Schweitzer R, Howes R, Smith R, Shilo B-Z, Freeman M. Inhibition of Drosophila EGF receptor activation by the secreted Argos protein. *Nature* 1995; 376:699–702.

27. Tzahar E, Yarden Y. The ErbB-2/HER2 oncogenic receptor of adenocarcinomas: from orphanhood to multiple stromal ligands. *Biochim Biophys Acta* 1998; 1377:M25–M37.

28. Lenferink AE, Pinkas Kramarski R, van de Poll ML, et al. Differential endocytic routing of homo- and hetero-dimeric ErbB tyrosine kinases confers signaling superiority to receptor heterodimers. *EMBO J* 1998; 17:3385–3397.

29. Schreiber AB, Winkler ME, Derynck R. Transforming growth factor α: more potent angiogenic mediator than epidermal growth factor. *Science* 1986; 232:1250–1253.

30. Raab G, Klagsbrun M. Heparin-binding EGF-like growth factor. *Biochem Biophys Acta* 1997; 1333:179–199.

31. Heldin C-H, Wesremark B. Mechanism of action and in vivo role of platelet-derived growth factor. *Physiol Rev* 1999; 79:1283–1316.

32. Andersson M, Ostman A, Westermark B, Heldin CH. Characterization of the retention motif in the C-terminal part of the long splice form of platelet-derived growth factor A-chain. *J Biol Chem* 1994; 269:926–930.

33. Yayon A, Klagsbrun M, Esko JD, Leder P, Ornitz DM. Cell surface, heparin-like molecules are required for binding of basic fibroblast growth factor to its high affinity receptor. *Cell* 1991; 64:841–848.

34. Bennett KL, Modrell B, Greenfield B, et al. Regulation of CD44 binding to hyaluronan by glycosylation of variably spliced exons. *J Cell Biol* 1995; 131:1623–1633.

35. Lax I, Bellot F, Howk R, Ullrich A, Givol D, Schlessinger J. Functional analysis of the ligand binding site of EGF-receptor utilizing chicken/human receptor molecules. *EMBO J* 1989; 8:421–427.

36. Lev S, Blechmann J, Nishikawa S-I, Givol D, Yarden Y. Interspecies molecular chimeras of Kit help define the binding site of the stem cell factor. *Mol Cell Biol* 1993; 13:2224–2234.

37. Wiesmann C, Fuh G, Christinger HW, Eigenbrot C, Wells JA, de Vos AM. Crystal structure at 1.7 A resolution of VEGF in complex with domain 2 of the Flt-1 receptor. *Cell* 1997; 91:695–704.

38. Blechman JM, Lev S, Barg J, et al. The fourth immunoglobulin domain of the stem cell factor receptor couples ligand binding to signal transduction. *Cell* 1995; 80:103–113.

39. Wiesmann C, Ultsch MH, Bass SH, de Vos AM. Crystal structure of nerve growth factor in complex with the ligand-binding domain of the TrkA receptor. *Nature* 1999; 401:184–188.

40. Plotnikov AN, Schlessinger J, Hubbard SR, Mohammadi M. Structural basis for FGF receptor dimerization and activation. *Cell* 1999; 98:641–650.

41. Burke CL, Stern DF. Activation of Neu (ErbB-2) mediated by disulfide bond-induced dimerization reveals a receptor tyrosine kinase dimer interface. *Mol Cell Biol* 1998; 18:5371–5379.

42. Smith SO, Smith CS, Bormann BJ. Strong hydrogen bonding interactions involving a buried glutamic acid in the transmembrane sequence of the neu/erbB-2 receptor. *Nat Struct Biol* 1996; 3:252–258.

43. Sternberg MJ, Gullick WJ. A sequence motif in the transmembrane region of growth factor receptors with tyrosine kinase activity mediates dimerization. *Protein Eng* 1990; 3:245–248.

44. Binns KL, Taylor PP, Sicheri F, Pawson T, Holland SJ. Phosphorylation of tyrosine residues in the kinase domain and juxtamembrane region regulates the biological and catalytic activities of Eph receptors. *Mol Cell Biol* 2000; 20:4791–4805.

45. Bao J, Alroy I, Waterman H, et al. Threonine phosphorylation diverts internalized epidermal growth factor receptors from a degradative pathway to the recycling endosome. *J Biol Chem* 2000; 275:26178–26186.

46. Hubbard SR, Till JH. Protein tyrosine kinase structure and function. *Ann Rev Biochem* 2000; 69:373–398.

47. Hubbard SR, Wei L, Ellis L, Hendrickson WA. Crystal structure of the tyrosine kinase domain of the human insulin receptor. *Nature* 1994; 372:746–754.

48. Mohammadi M, Schlessinger J, Hubbard SR. Structure of the FGF receptor tyrosine kinase domain reveals a novel autoinhibitory mechanism. *Cell* 1996; 86:577–587.

49. Yarden Y, Schlessinger J. Epidermal growth factor induces rapid, reversible aggregation of purified epidermal growth factor receptors. *Biochemistry* 1987; 26:1443–1445.

50. Yarden Y, Schlessinger J. Self-phosphorylation of epidermal growth factor receptor: evidence for a model of intermolecular allosteric activation. *Biochemistry* 1987; 26:1434–1442.

51. Heldin CH. Dimerization of cell surface receptors in signal transduction. *Cell* 1995; 80:213–223.

52. Tzahar E, Pinkas Kramarski R, Moyer JD, et al. Bivalence of EGF-like ligands drives the ErbB signaling network. *EMBO J* 1997; 16:4938–4950.

53. Lemmon MA, Bu Z, Ladbury JE, et al. Two EGF molecules contribute additively to stabilization of the EGFR dimer. *EMBO J* 1997; 16:281–294.

54. Songyang Z, Shoelson SE, Chaudhuri M, et al. SH-2 domains recognize specific phosphopeptide sequences. *Cell* 1993; 72:767–778.

55. Pawson T, Nash P. Protein-protein interactions define specificity in signal transduction. *Genes Dev* 2000; 14:1027–1047.

56. Kim HK, Kim JW, Zilberstein A, et al. PDGF stimulation of inositol phospholipid hydrolysis requires PLC-gamma 1 phosphorylation on tyrosine residues 783 and 1254. *Cell* 1991; 65:435–441.

57. Anderson KE, Coadwell J, Stephens LR, Hawkins PT. Translocation of PDK-1 to the plasma membrane is important in allowing PDK-1 to activate protein kinase B. *Curr Biol* 1998; 8:684–691.

58. Yamaguchi H, Hendrickson WA. Structural basis for activation of human lymphocyte kinase Lck upon tyrosine phosphorylation. *Nature* 1996; 384:484–489.

59. Jelinek T, Dent P, Sturgill TW, Weber MJ. Ras-induced activation of Raf-1 is dependent on tyrosine phosphorylation. *Mol Cell Biol* 1996; 16:1027–1034.

60. Cantley LC, Neel BG. New insights into tumor suppression: PTEN suppresses tumor formation by restraining the phosphoinositide 3-kinase/AKT pathway. *Proc Natl Acad Sci USA* 1999; 96:4240–4245.

61. Toker A, Newton AC. Cellular signaling: pivoting around PDK-1. *Cell* 2000; 103:185–188.

62. Rhee SG, Bae YS. Regulation of phosphoinositide-specific phospholipase C isozymes. *J Biol Chem* 1997; 272:15045–15048.

63. Penta K, Carpenter G. Interaction of phospholipase C-gamma with activated growth factor receptor tyrosine kinases. *Adv Exp Med Biol* 1997; 400B:971–981.

64. Wells A, Ware MF, Allen FD, Lauffenburger DA. Shaping up for shipping out: PLCgamma signaling of morphology changes in EGF-stimulated fibroblast migration. *Cell Motil Cytoskeleton* 1999; 44:227–233.

65. Valius M, Kazlauskas A. Phospholipase Cg and phosphatidylinositol 3 kinase are the downstream mediators of the PDGF receptor's mitogenic signal. *Cell* 1993; 73:321–324.

66. Mohammadi M, Dionne CA, Li W, et al. Point mutation in FGF receptor eliminates phosphatidylinositol hydrolysis without affecting mitogenesis. *Nature* 1992; 358:681–684.

67. Peters KG, Marie J, Wilson E, et al. Point mutation of an FGF receptor abolishes phosphatidylinositol turnover and Ca^{2+} flux but not mitogenesis. *Nature* 1992; 358:678–681.

68. Hall H, Williams EJ, Moore SE, Walsh FS, Prochiantz A, Doherty P. Inhibition of FGF-stimulated phosphatidylinositol hydrolysis and neurite outgrowth by a cell-membrane permeable phosphopeptide. *Curr Biol* 1996; 6:580–587.

69. Stephens RM, Loeb DM, Copeland TD, Pawson T, Greene LA, Kaplan DR. Trk receptors use redundant signal transduction pathways involving SHC and PLC-gamma 1 to mediate NGF responses. *Neuron* 1994; 12:691–705.

70. Marshall CJ. Specificity of receptor tyrosine kinase signaling: transient versus sustained extracellular signal-regulated kinase activation. *Cell* 1995; 80:179–185.

71. Freeman M. Cell determination strategies in the *Drosophila* eye. *Development* 1997; 124:261–270.

72. Ceresa BP, Schmid SL. Regulation of signal transduction by endocytosis. *Curr Opin Cell Biol* 2000; 12:204–210.

73. Mineo C, James GL, Smart EJ, Anderson RG. Localization of epidermal growth factor-stimulated Ras/Raf-1 interaction to caveolae membrane. *J Biol Chem* 1996; 271:11930–11935.

74. Sorkin A. Receptor-mediated endocytosis of growth factors. In: Heldin C-H, Purton M, eds. *Signal Transduction* Chapman & Hall, New York, 1996.

75. Nesterov A, Wiley HS, Gill GN. Ligand-induced endocytosis of epidermal growth factor receptors that are defective in binding adaptor proteins. *Proc Natl Acad Sci USA* 1995; 92:8719–8723.

76. Hicke L. Protein regulation by monoubiquitin. *Nat Rev Mol Cell Biol* 2001; 2:195–201.

77. Joazeiro CA, Wing SS, Huang H, Leverson JD, Hunter T, Liu YC. The tyrosine kinase negative regulator c-Cbl as a RING-type, E2-dependent ubiquitin-protein ligase. *Science* 1999; 286:309–312.

78. Levkowitz G, Waterman H, Ettenberg SA, et al. Ubiquitin ligase activity and tyrosine phosphorylation underlie suppression of growth factor signaling by c-Cbl/Sli-1. *Mol Cell* 1999; 4:1029–1040.

79. Thien BF, Langdon WY. Cbl-Many adaptations to regulate protein tyrosine kinases. *Nat Rev Mol Cell Biol* 2001; 2:294–305.
80. Levkowitz G, Waterman H, Zamir E, et al. c-Cbl/Sli-1 regulates endocytic sorting and ubiquitination of the epidermal growth factor receptor. *Genes Dev* 1998; 12:3663–3674.
81. Holmes WE, Sliwkowski MX, Akita RW, et al. Identification of heregulin, a specific activator of p185*erb*B2. *Science* 1992; 256:1205–1210.
82. Peles E, Bacus SS, Koski RA, et al. Isolation of the neu/HER-2 stimulatory ligand: a 44 kd glycoprotein that induces differentiation of mammary tumor cells. *Cell* 1992; 69:205–216.
83. Schulze A, Lehmann K, Jefferies HB, McMahon M, Downward J. Analysis of the transcriptional program induced by Raf in epithelial cells. *Genes Dev* 2001; 15:981–994.
84. Shibuya M. Structure and function of VEGF/VEGF-receptor system involved in angiogenesis. *Cell Struct Funct* 2001; 26:25–35.
85. Guha A, Glowacka D, Carroll R, Dashner K, Black PM, Stiles CD. Expression of platelet derived growth factor and platelet derived growth factor receptor mRNA in a glioblastoma from a patient with Li-Fraumeni syndrome. *J Neurol Neurosurg Psychiatry* 1995; 58:711–714.
86. Wang J, Coltera MD, Gown AM. Cell proliferation in human soft tissue tumors correlates with platelet-derived growth factor B chain expression: an immunohistochemical and in situ hybridization study. *Cancer Res* 1994; 54:560–564.
87. Simon MP, Pedeutour F, Sirvent N, et al. Deregulation of the platelet-derived growth factor B-chain gene via fusion with collagen gene COL1A1 in dermatofibrosarcoma protuberans and giant-cell fibroblastoma. *Nat Genet* 1997; 15:95–98.
88. Siegfried JM, Weissfeld LA, Singh-Kaw P, Weyant RJ, Testa JR, Landreneau RJ. Association of immunoreactive hepatocyte growth factor with poor survival in resectable non-small cell lung cancer. *Cancer Res* 1997; 57:433–439.
89. Derynck R, Goeddel DV, Ullrich A, et al. Synthesis of messenger RNAs for transforming growth factors alpha and beta and the epidermal-growth-factor-receptor by human tumors. *Cancer Res* 1987; 47:707–712.
90. Rosenthal A, Lindquist PB, Bringman TS, Goeddel DV, Derynck R. Expression in rat fibroblasts of a human transforming growth factor-alpha cDNA results in transformation. *Cell* 1986; 46:301–309.
91. Dominey AM, Wang X-J, King LEJ, et al. Targeted overexpression of transforming growth factor a in the epiderms of transgenic mice elicits hyperplasia, hyperkeratosis, and spontaneous, squamous papillomas. *Cell Growth Differ* 1993; 4:1071–1082.
92. Sandgren EP, Luetteke NC, Palmiter RD, Brinster RL, Lee DC. Overexpression of TGFα in transgenic mice: induction of epithelial hyperplasia, pancreatic metaplasia and carcinoma of the breast. *Cell* 1990; 61:1121–1135.
93. Matsui M, Halter SA, Holt JT, Hogan BLM, Coffey RJ. Development of mammary hyperplasia and neoplasia in MMTV-TGFα transgenic mice. *Cell* 1991; 61:1147–1155.
94. Salomon DS, Brandt R, Ciardiello F, Normanno N. Epidermal growth factor-related peptides and their receptors in human malignancies. *Crit Rev Oncol Hematol* 1995; 19:183–232.
95. Scher HI, Sarkis A, Reuter V, et al. Changing pattern of expression of the epidermal growth factor receptor and transforming growth factor alpha in the progression of prostatic neoplasms. *Clin Cancer Res* 1995; 1:545–550.
96. Friess H, Berberat P, Schilling M, Kunz J, Korc M, Buchler MW. Pancreatic cancer: the potential clinical relevance of alterations in growth factors and their receptors. *J Mol Med* 1996; 74:35–42.
97. Liu N, Furukawa T, Kobari M, Tsao MS. Comparative phenotypic studies of duct epithelial cell lines derived from normal human pancreas and pancreatic carcinoma. *Am J Pathol* 1998; 153:263–269.
98. Awwad R, Humphrey LE, Periyasamy B, et al. The EGF/TGFalpha response element within the TGFalpha promoter consists of a multi-complex regulatory element. *Oncogene* 1999; 18:5923–5935.
99. Sandgren EP, Luetteke NC, Qiu TH, Palmiter RD, Brinster RL, Lee DC. Transforming growth factor alpha dramatically enhances oncogene-induced carcinogenesis in transgenic mouse pancreas and liver. *Mol Cell Biol* 1993; 13:320–330.
100. Muller WJ, Sinn E, Pattengale PK, Wallace R, Leder P. Single-step induction of mammary adenocarcinoma in transgenic mice bearing the activated c-*neu* oncogene. *Cell* 1988; 54:105–115.
101. Russell WE, Kaufmann WK, Sitaric S, Luetteke NC, Lee DC. Liver regeneration and hepatocarcinogenesis in transforming growth factor-alpha-targeted mice. *Mol Carcinog* 1996; 15:183–189.
102. Folkman J. Angiogenesis in cancer, vascular, rheumatoid and other diseases. *Nat Med* 1995; 1:27–31.

103. Wesseling P, van der Laak JA, Link M, Teepen HL, Ruiter DJ. Quantitative analysis of microvascular changes in diffuse astrocytic neoplasms with increasing grade of malignancy. *Hum Pathol* 1998; 29:352–358.

104. Hanahan D. Signaling vascular morphogenesis and maintenance. *Science* 1997; 277:48–50.

105. Takanami I, Tanaka F, Hashizume T, Kodaira S. Vascular endothelial growth factor and its receptor correlate with angiogenesis and survival in pulmonary adenocarcinoma. *Anticancer Res* 1997; 17:2811–2814.

106. Scott PA, Smith K, Poulson R, De Benedetti A, Bicknell R, Harris AL. Differential expression of vascular endothelial growth factor mRNA vs protein isoform expression in human breast cancer and relationship to eIF-4E. Br. J. Cancer 1998; 77:2120–2128.

107. Jones N, Iljin K, Dumont DJ, Alitalo K. Tie receptors: new modulators of angiogenic and lymphogenic responses. *Nat Rev Mol Cell Biol* 2001; 2:257–267.

108. Vignaud JM, Marie B, Klein N, et al. The role of platelet-derived growth factor production by tumor-associated macrophages in tumor stroma formation in lung cancer. *Cancer Res* 1994; 54:5455–5463.

109. Robbins JR, McGuire PG, Wehrle-Haller B, Rogers SL. Diminished matrix metalloproteinase 2 (MMP-2) in ectomesenchyme-derived tissues of the Patch mutant mouse: regulation of MMP-2 by PDGF and effects on mesenchymal cell migration. *Dev Biol* 1999; 212:255–263.

110. Pietras K, Ostman A, Sjoquist M, et al. Inhibition of platelet-derived growth factor receptors reduces interstitial hypertension and increases transcapillary transport intumors. *Cancer Res* 2001; 61:2929–2934.

111. Baserga R, Resnicoff M, Dews M. The IGF-I receptor and cancer. *Endocrine* 1997; 7:99–102.

112. Sell C, Rubini M, Rubin R, Liu JP, Efstratiadis A, Baserga R. Simian virus 40 large tumor antigen is unable to transform mouse embryonic fibroblasts lacking type 1 insulin-like growth factor receptor. *Proc Natl Acad Sci USA* 1993; 90:11217–11221.

113. Kalebic T, Tsokos M, Helman LJ. In vivo treatment with antibody against IGF-1 receptor suppresses growth of human rhabdomyosarcoma and down-regulates p34cdc2. *Cancer Res* 1994; 54:5531–5534.

114. Ullrich A, Coussens L, Hayflick JS, et al. Human epidermal growth factor receptor cDNA sequence and aberrant expression of the amplified gene in A431 epidermoid carcinoma cells. *Nature* 1984; 309:418–425.

115. Gorgoulis V, Aninos D, Mikou P, et al. Expression of EGF, TGF-alpha and EGFR in squamous cell lung carcinomas. *Anticancer Res* 1992; 12:1183–1187.

116. Irish JC, Bernstein A. Oncogenes in head and neck cancer. *Laryngoscope* 1993; 103:42–52.

117. Archer SG, Eliopoulos A, Spandidos D, et al. Expression of ras p21, p53 and c-erbB-2 in advanced breast cancer and response to first line hormonal therapy. *Br J Cancer* 1995; 72:1259–1266.

118. Wikstrand CJ, Reist CJ, Archer GE, Zalutsky MR, Bigner DD. The class III variant of the epidermal growth factor receptor (EGFRvIII): characterization and utilization as an immunotherapeutic target. *J Neurovirol* 1998; 4:148–158.

119. Wong AJ, Ruppert JM, Bigner SH, et al. Structural alterations of the epidermal growth factor receptor gene in human gliomas. *Proc Natl Acad Sci USA* 1992; 89:2965–2969.

120. King CR, Kraus MH, Aaronson SA. Amplification of a novel v-*erb*B-related gene in a human mammary carcinoma. *Science* 1985; 229:974–976.

121. Yamamoto T, Ikawa S, Akiyama T, et al. Similarity of protein encoded by the human c-*erb*B-2 gene to epidermal growth factor receptor. *Nature* 1986; 319:230–234.

122. Klapper LN, Kirschbaum MH, Sela M, Yarden Y. Biochemical and clinical implications of the ErbB/HER signaling network of growth factor receptors. *Adv Cancer Res* 2000; 77:25–79.

123. Slamon DJ, Clark GM, Wong SG, Levin WJ, Ullrich A, McGuire WL. Human breast cancer: correlation of relapse and survival with amplification of the HER-2/*neu* oncogene. *Science* 1987; 235:177–182.

124. Allred DC, Clark GM, Molina R, et al. Overexpression of HER-2/Neu and its relationship with other prognostic factors change during the progression of *in situ* to invasive breast cancer. *Hum Pathol* 1992; 23:974–979.

125. Lodato RF, Maguire HC Jr, Greene MI, Weiner DB, LiVolsi VA. Immunohistochemical evaluation of c-erbB-2 oncogene expression in ductal carcinoma in situ and atypical ductal hyperplasia of the breast. *Mod Pathol* 1990; 3:449–454.

126. Barnes DM, Bartkova J, Camplejohn RS, Gullick WJ, Smith PJ, Millis RR. Overexpression of the c-erbB-2 oncoprotein: why does this occur more frequently in ductal carcinoma in situ than in invasive mammary carcinoma and is this of prognostic significance? *Eur J Cancer* 1992; 28:644–648.

127. van de Vijver M, Peterse JL, Mooi WJ, et al. Neu-protein overexpression in breast cancer. Association with comedo-type ductal carcinoma *in situ* and limited prognostic value in stage II breast cancer. *N Engl J Med* 1988; 319:1239–1245.

128. Ho GH, Calvano JE, Bisogna M, et al. In microdissected ductal carcinoma in situ, HER-2/neu amplification, but not p53 mutation, is associated with high nuclear grade and comedo histology. *Cancer* 2000; 89:2153–2160.

129. Shpitz B, Bomstein Y, Zehavi T, et al. Topoisomerase IIalpha expression in ductal carcinoma in situ of the breast: a preliminary study. *Hum Pathol* 2000; 31:1249–1254.

130. Quinn CM, Ostrowski JL, Harkins L, Rice AJ, Loney DP. Loss of bcl-2 expression in ductal carcinoma in situ of the breast relates to poor histological differentiation and to expression of p53 and c-erbB-2 proteins. *Histopathology* 1998; 33:531–536.

131. Fiche M, Avet-Loiseau H, Maugard CM, et al. Gene amplifications detected by fluorescence in situ hybridization in pure intraductal breast carcinomas: relation to morphology, cell proliferation and expression of breast cancer-related genes. *Int J Cancer* 2000; 89:403–410.

132. Zafrani B, Leroyer A, Fourquet A, et al. Mammographically-detected ductal in situ carcinoma of the breast analyzed with a new classification. A study of 127 cases: correlation with estrogen and progesterone receptors, p53 and c-erbB-2 proteins, and proliferative activity. *Semin Diagn Pathol* 1994; 11:208–214.

133. Moreno A, Lloveras B, Figueras A, et al. Ductal carcinoma in situ of the breast: correlation between histologic classifications and biologic markers. *Mod Pathol* 1997; 10:1088–1092.

134. Mack L, Kerkvliet N, Doig G, O'Malley FP. Relationship of a new histological categorization of ductal carcinoma in situ of the breast with size and the immunohistochemical expression of p53, c-erb B2, bcl-2, and ki-67. *Hum Pathol* 1997; 28:974–979.

135. Kanthan R, Xiang J, Magliocco AM. p53, ErbB2, and TAG-72 expression in the spectrum of ductal carcinoma in situ of the breast classified by the Van Nuys system. *Arch Pathol Lab Med* 2000; 124:234–239.

136. Iwase H, Ando Y, Ichihara S, et al. Immunohistochemical analysis on biological markers in ductal carcinoma in situ of the breast. *Breast Cancer* 2001; 8:98–104.

137. Lipponen HJ, Aaltomaa S, Syrjanen S, Syrjanen K. c-erbB-2 oncogene related to p53 expression, cell proliferation and prognosis in breast cancer. *Anticancer Res* 1993; 13:1147–1152.

138. Schimmelpenning H, Eriksson ET, Falkmer UG, Azavedo E, Svane G, Auer GU. Expression of the c-*erb*B-2 proto-oncogene product and nuclear DNA content in benign and malignant human breast parenchyma. *Virchows Arch A Pathol Anat Histopathol* 1992; 420:433–440.

139. Gusterson BA, Gelber RD, Goldhirsch A, et al. Prognostic importance of c-erbB-2 expression in breast cancer. International (Ludwig) Breast Cancer Study Group. *J Clin Oncol* 1992; 10:1049–1056.

140. Tandon AK, Clark GM, Chamness GC, Ullrich A, McGuire WL. HER-2/*neu* oncogene protein and prognosis in breast cancer. *J Clin Oncol* 1989; 7:1120–1128.

141. Quenel N, Wafflart J, Bonichon F, et al. The prognostic value of c-erbB2 in primary breast carcinomas: a study on 942 cases. *Breast Cancer Res Treat* 1995; 35:283–291.

142. Lee AH, Bobrow LG. Relationship of histologic grade, c-erbB-2 expression, and inflammatory infiltrate to prognosis in carcinoma of the breast. *J Clin Oncol* 1996; 14:2406–2407.

143. Soomro S, Shousha S, Taylor P, Shepard HM, Feldmann M. c-erbB-2 expression in different histological types of invasive breast carcinoma. *J Clin Pathol* 1991; 44:211–214.

144. Somerville JE, Clarke LA, Biggart JD. c-*erb*B-2 overexpression and histological type of *in situ* and invasive breast carcinoma. *J Clin Pathol* 1992; 45:16–20.

145. Diab SG, Clark GM, Osborne CK, Libby A, Allred DC, Elledge RM. Tumor characteristics and clinical outcome of tubular and mucinous breast carcinomas. *J Clin Oncol* 1999; 17:1442–1448.

146. Albanell J, Bellmunt J, Molina R, et al. Node-negative breast cancers with p53(–)/HER2-neu(–) status may identify women with very good prognosis. *Anticancer Res* 1996; 16:1027–1032.

147. O'Malley FP, Saad Z, Kerkvliet N, et al. The predictive power of semiquantitative immunohistochemical assessment of p53 and c-erb B-2 in lymph node-negative breast cancer. *Hum Pathol* 1996; 27:955–963.

148. Paterson MC, Dietrich KD, Danyluk J, et al. Correlation between c-erbB-2 amplification and risk of recurrent disease in node-negative breast cancer. *Cancer Res* 1991; 51:556–567.

149. Sauer R, Schauer A, Rauschecker HF, et al. Therapy of small breast cancer: a prospective study on 1036 patients with special emphasis on prognostic factors. *Int J Radiat Oncol Biol Phys* 1992; 23:907–914.

150. An HX, Niederacher D, Beckmann MW, et al. ERBB2 gene amplification detected by fluorescent differential polymerase chain reaction in paraffin-embedded breast carcinoma tissues. *Int J Cancer* 1995; 64:291–297.

151. Gaci Z, Bouin-Pineau MH, Gaci M, Daban A, Ingrand P, Metaye T. Prognostic impact of cathepsin D and c-erbB-2 oncoprotein in a subgroup of node-negative breast cancer patients with low histological grade tumors. *Int J Oncol* 2001; 18:793–800.

152. Allred DC, Clark GM, Tandon AK, et al. HER-2/neu in node-negative breast cancer: prognostic significance of overexpression influenced by the presence of in situ carcinoma. *J Clin Oncol* 1992; 10:599–605.

153. Baselga J, Seidman AD, Rosen PP, Norton L. HER2 overexpression and paclitaxel sensitivity in breast cancer: therapeutic implications. *Oncology (Huntingt)* 1997; 11:43–48.

154. Yu D, Hung MC. Role of erbB2 in breast cancer chemosensitivity. *Bioessays* 2000; 22:673–680.

155. Tsai CM, Chang KT, Perng RP, et al. Correlation of intrinsic chemoresistance of non-small-cell lung cancer cell lines with HER-2/neu gene expression but not with ras gene mutations. *J Natl Cancer Inst* 1993; 85:897–901.

156. O'Rourke DM, Kao GD, Singh N, et al. Conversion of a radioresistant phenotype to a more sensitive one by disabling erbB receptor signaling in human cancer cells. *Proc Natl Acad Sci USA* 1998; 95:10842–10847.

157. Yu D, Jing T, Liu B, et al. Overexpression of ErbB2 blocks Taxol-induced apoptosis by upregulation of p21Cip1, which inhibits p34Cdc2 kinase. *Mol Cell* 1998; 2:581–591.

158. Kumar R, Mandal M, Lipton A, Harvey H, Thompson CB. Overexpression of HER2 modulates bcl-2, bcl-XL, and tamoxifen-induced apoptosis in human MCF-7 breast cancer cells. *Clin Cancer Res* 1996; 2:1215–1219.

159. Zhang L, Hung MC. Sensitization of HER-2/neu-overexpressing non-small cell lung cancer cells to chemotherapeutic drugs by tyrosine kinase inhibitor emodin. *Oncogene* 1996; 12:571–576.

160. Sleijfer S, Asschert JG, Timmer Bosscha H, Mulder NH. Enhanced sensitivity to tumor necrosis factor-alpha in doxorubicin-resistant tumor cell lines due to down-regulated c-erbB2. *Int J Cancer* 1998; 77:101–106.

161. Vargas-Roig LM, Gago FE, Tello O, Martin de Civetta MT, Ciocca DR. c-erbB-2 (HER-2/neu) protein and drug resistance in breast cancer patients treated with induction chemotherapy. *Int J Cancer* 1999; 84:129–134.

162. Bacus SS, Yarden Y, Oren M, et al. Neu differentiation factor (Heregulin) activates a p53-dependent pathway in cancer cells. *Oncogene* 1996; 12:2535–2547.

163. Giani C, Casalini P, Pupa SM, et al. Increased expression of c-erbB-2 in hormone-dependent breast cancer cells inhibits cell growth and induces differentiation. *Oncogene* 1998; 17:425–432.

164. Pietras RJ, Poen JC, Gallardo D, Wongvipat PN, Lee HJ, Slamon DJ. Monoclonal antibody to HER-2/neureceptor modulates repair of radiation-induced DNA damage and enhances radiosensitivity of human breast cancer cells overxpressing this oncogene. *Cancer Res* 1999; 59:1347–1355.

165. Zhou BP, Liao Y, Xia W, Spohn B, Lee MH, Hung MC. Cytoplasmic localization of p21Cip1/WAF1 by Akt-induced phosphorylation in HER-2/neu-overexpressing cells. *Nat Cell Biol* 2001; 3:245–252.

166. Di Fiore PP, Pierce JH, Kraus MH, Segatto O, King CR, Aaronson SA. *erbB*-2 is a potent oncogene when overexpressed in NIH/3T3 cells. *Science* 1987; 237:178–182.

167. Hudziak RM, Schlessinger J, Ullrich A. Increased expression of the putative growth factor receptor p185HER2 causes transformation and tumorigenesis of NIH 3T3 cells. *Proc Natl Acad Sci USA* 1987; 84:7159–7163.

168. Klapper LN, Glathe S, Vaisman N, et al. The ErbB-2/HER2 oncoprotein of human carcinomas may function solely as a shared coreceptor for multiple stroma-derived growth factors. *Proc Natl Acad Sci USA* 1999; 96:4995–5000.

169. Graus Porta D, Beerli RR, Daly JM, Hynes NE. ErbB-2, the preferred heterodimerization partner of all ErbB receptors, is a mediator of lateral signaling. *EMBO J* 1997; 16:1647–1655.

170. Tzahar E, Waterman H, Chen X, et al. A hierarchical network of interreceptor interactions determines signal transduction by Neu differentiation factor/neuregulin and epidermal growth factor. *Mol Cell Biol* 1996; 16:5276–5287.

171. Guy PM, Platko JV, Cantley LC, Cerione RA, Carraway KL. Insect cell-expressed p180ErbB3 possesses an impaired tyrosine kinase activity. *Proc Natl Acad Sci USA* 1994; 91:8132–8136.

172. Burden S, Yarden Y. Neuregulins and their receptors: a versatile signaling module in organogenesis and oncogenesis. *Neuron* 1997; 18:847–855.

173. Pinkas-Kramarski R, Soussan L, Waterman H, et al. Diversification of Neu differentiation factor and epidermal growth factor signaling by combinatorial receptor interactions. *EMBO J* 1996; 15:2452–2467.

174. Riese DJ, II van Raaij TM, Plowman GD, Andrews GC, Stern DF. The cellular response to neuregulins is governed by complex interactions of the erbB receptor family. *Mol Cell Biol* 1995; 15:5770–5776.

175. Karunagaran D, Tzahar E, Beerli RR, et al. ErbB-2 is a common auxiliary subunit of NDF and EGF receptors: implications for breast cancer. *EMBO J* 1996; 15:254–264.

176. Alimandi M, Wang LM, Bottaro D, et al. Epidermal growth factor and betacellulin mediate signal transduction through co-expressed ErbB2 and ErbB3 receptors. *EMBO J* 1997; 16:5608–5617.

177. Pinkas-Kramarski R, Lenferink AE, Bacus SS, et al. The oncogenic ErbB-2/ErbB-3 heterodimer is a surrogate receptor of the epidermal growth factor and betacellulin. *Oncogene* 1998; 16:1249–1258.

178. Baulida J, Kraus MH, Alimandi M, Di Fiore PP, Carpenter G. All ErbB receptors other than the epidermal growth factor receptor are endocytosis impaired. *J Biol Chem* 1996; 271:5251–5257.

179. Worthylake R, Opresko LK, Wiley HS. ErbB-2 amplification inhibits down-regulation and induces constitutive activation of both ErbB-2 and epidermal growth factor receptors. *J Biol Chem* 1999; 274:8865–8874.

180. Lev S, Blechman JM, Givol D, Yarden Y. Steel factor and c-kit protooncogene: genetic lessons in signal transduction. *Crit Rev Oncog* 1994; 5:141–168.

181. Longley BJ, Reguera MJ, Ma Y. Classes of c-KIT activating mutations: proposed mechanisms of action and implications for disease classification and therapy. *Leuk Res* 2001; 25:571–576.

182. Taniguchi M, Nishida T, Hirota S, et al. Effect of c-kit mutation on prognosis of gastrointestinal stromal tumors. *Cancer Res* 1999; 59:4297–4300.

183. Hongyo T, Li T, Syaifudin M, et al. Specific c-kit mutations in sinonasal natural killer/T-cell lymphoma in China and Japan. *Cancer Res* 2000; 60:2345–2347.

184. Jhiang SM. The Ret proto-oncogene in human cancer. *Oncogene* 2000; 19:5590–5597.

185. Schuchardt A, D'Agati V, Larsson-Blomberg L, Costantini F, Pachnis V. Defects in the kidney and enteric nervous system of mice lacking the tyrosine kinase receptor Ret. *Nature* 1994; 367:380–383.

186. Klugbauer S, Rabes HM. The transcription coactivator HTIF1 and a related protein are fused to the RET receptor tyrosine kinase in childhood papillary thyroid carcinomas. *Oncogene* 1999; 18:4388–4393.

187. Durick K, Gill GN, Taylor SS. Shc and Enigma are both required for mitogenic signaling by Ret/ptc2. *Mol Cell Biol* 1998; 18:2298–2308.

188. Borrego S, Eng C, Sanchez B, Saez ME, Navarro E, Antinolo G. Molecular analysis of the ret and GDNF genes in a family with multiple endocrine neoplasia type 2A and Hirschsprung disease. *J Clin Endocrinol Metab* 1998; 83:3361–3364.

189. Murakami H, Iwashita T, Asai N, et al. Enhanced phosphatidylinositol 3-kinase activity and high phosphorylation state of its downstream signalling molecules mediated by ret with the MEN 2B mutation. *Biochem Biophys Res Commun* 1999; 262:68–75.

190. Joensuu H, Roberts PJ, Sarlomo-Rikala M, et al. Effect of the tyrosine kinase inhibitor STI571 in a patient with a metastatic gastrointestinal stromal tumor. *N Engl J Med* 2001; 344:1052–1056.

191. Slamon DJ, Leyland-Jones B, Shak S, et al. Use of chemotherapy plus a monoclonal antibody against HER2 for metastatic breast cancer that overexpresses HER2. *N Engl J Med* 2001; 344:783–792.

5

Ras-Mediated Deregulation of Gene Expression and Contribution to Oncogenesis

Gretchen A. Murphy, PhD, and Channing J. Der, PhD

CONTENTS

1. INTRODUCTION

It is now well-established that Ras proteins are critical nodal points of signal transduction. Signals initiated by diverse extracellular ligands, via stimulation of a wide spectrum of cell surface receptors, converge on and activate Ras *(1)*. Activated Ras, in turn, interacts with a multitude of downstream effector targets to initiate functionally diverse cytoplasmic signaling pathways *(1–3)*. Many of the cytoplasmic signaling components that function upstream and downstream of Ras have been identified, although more are likely to be found. While unexpected complexities, such as cross-talk of these components, as well as cell type differences in Ras signaling, have prevented our complete understanding of the details of Ras signaling, our comprehension of the details is nevertheless impressive. Similarly, it is clear that Ras signaling pathways regulate events in the cytoplasm (actin cytoskeletal organization) as well as in the nucleus (regulation of gene expression and cell cycle progression) *(3,4)*. The cross-talk between Ras and Rho family proteins has provided vital details that explain how Ras controls actin organization *(5,6)*. Links between Ras signaling and specific components of the cell cycle machinery have recently been delineated *(7–10)*. It is clear that Ras can regulate the function of a multitude of transcription factors and that their functions are essential for Ras-mediated transformation *(3)*. Ras-responsive DNA elements are common features of many promoter

From: *Oncogene-Directed Therapies*
Edited by: J. W. Rak © Humana Press Inc., Totowa, NJ

sequences. However, where our knowledge is lacking is in the identification of specific gene targets of Ras that are important for Ras-mediated oncogenesis. In this review, we summarize our knowledge of several genes whose expression is regulated by Ras and whose products may be important for oncogenic Ras function. This involves genes whose functions may control cell proliferation (transforming growth factor alpha; TGFα), cell cycle progression (cyclin D1), cell survival (COX-2), cell shape (tropomyosin), tumor cell invasion and metastases (matrix metalloproteinases; MMPs), and tumor angiogenesis (vascular endothelial growth factor; VEGF). Additionally, we summarize recent differential gene expression cloning studies *(11–16)* that have begun to shed some light on this important issue. While we are clearly in the early days of these studies, with the application and refinement of gene array expression analyses and proteomics, this area of Ras signaling is poised to explode in the coming years.

2. Ras AND ONCOGENESIS

The three human *ras* genes encode four highly related proteins, H-Ras, N-Ras, K-Ras4A, and K-Ras4B (4A and 4B differ only in their carboxyl-terminal sequences due to alternative splicing), which share approx 90% amino acid identity. To date, there is limited evidence that there are functional differences in Ras proteins. For example, isoform differences in subcellular trafficking and association with the plasma membrane and different roles in development *(17,18)*. K-*ras*, but not H-*ras* or N-*ras*, is essential for normal mouse development *(18–20)*.

Ras proteins have been the subjects of intensive research because of their important role(s) in human cancer development. Mutant forms of the three human *ras* genes are associated with the development and progression of a wide spectrum of human cancers *(4,21)*. Single amino acid substitutions (primarily at residues 12, 13, or 61) result in constitutively activated, highly oncogenic, mutant Ras proteins *(21)*. Ras mutations are found in approx 30% of all human cancers, but the frequency is not random. Some cancers show greater frequency of mutations, such as carcinomas of the pancreas (approx 90%), colon (approx 50%), lung (approx 50%), and thyroid (approx 50%), whereas *ras* mutations are infrequently observed in carcinomas of the breast, ovary, and cervix *(4,21)*. K-*ras* is the most frequently mutated *ras* gene, followed by N-*ras,* while H-*ras* mutations are less frequently observed *(22–24.)* The specific *ras* gene mutated often correlates with the tumor type *(22–24)*. For example, K-*ras* mutations are most prevalent in lung, colon, and pancreatic cancer, whereas, H-*ras* mutations are most common in bladder and kidney cancer, and N-*ras* mutations are most common in myeloid and lymphatic cancers *(21,25)*. In contrast, some cancers exhibit mutations in all three isoforms (e.g., thyroid cancers) *(21)*. Whether the activation of distinct *ras* genes in specific cancers reflects distinct oncogenic properties of the different Ras proteins is not known.

In addition to mutations in Ras itself, Ras can be activated constitutively by alterations in other signaling proteins. For example, overexpression of ErbB2/HER-2/Neu, receptor tyrosine kinase of the epidermal growth factor (EGF) receptor family, occurs in approx 30% human breast and ovarian cancers and is suggestive of a poor prognosis *(26)*. Chronic activation and/or overexpression of this or other receptor tyrosine kinases can cause persistent activation of Ras, and consequently, Ras-mediated signaling *(4,26)*. Alternatively, the loss of NF1-GAP (see Section 3.1) function in malignant schawannomas is associated with an increase in active Ras *(27)*. Thus, the involvement of Ras in oncogenesis clearly extends beyond the 30% of tumors that harbor mutated *ras* genes.

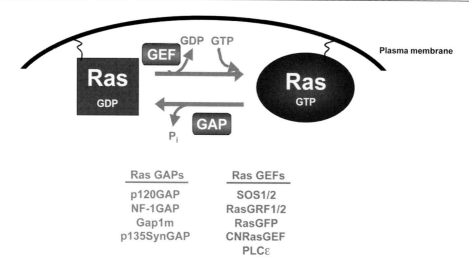

Ras GAPs	Ras GEFs
p120GAP	SOS1/2
NF-1GAP	RasGRF1/2
Gap1m	RasGFP
p135SynGAP	CNRasGEF
	PLCε

Fig. 1. The Ras molecular switch is regulated by GEFs and GAPs. Ras family proteins are membrane-bound molecular switches that bind guanine nucleotides (GTP or GDP), and catalyze both the hydrolysis of GTP to GDP and P_i and the subsequent release of bound GDP. Ras proteins are active when bound to GTP and inactive when bound to GDP. GAPs enhance GTP hydrolysis, and GEFs facilitate the release of GDP. Thus, GAPs favor the formation of inactive GTPase, and GEFs favor the formation of active GTPase. Several GAPs and GEFs have been identified that are specific for Ras, and these are indicated in the figure.

3. REGULATION OF Ras PROTEINS

3.1. Ras Molecular Switch

Ras family proteins are small GTP binding and hydrolyzing proteins (GTPases) that bind guanine nucleotides, GTP or GDP, with high affinity and exist in two functional confirmations: active when bound to GTP and inactive when bound to GDP (Fig. 1) *(23,28)*. Ras proteins transition between the two confirmations by harboring two intrinsic activities: hydrolytic release of P_1, converting bound GTP to bound GDP, and nucleotide dissociation, facilitating exchange of bound GDP for free GTP in vivo. Ras protein conformation is altered upon GDP/GTP cycling due to structural changes in two regions termed the switch I (residues 30–38) and II (residues 59–76) regions *(29–31)*. These regions, together with residues that flank the switch I region (residues 25–45), correspond to the effector domain of Ras. When Ras is bound to GTP, the effector domain displays high affinity binding to downstream effector targets such as the Raf serine/threonine kinases (see Section 4.1).

Intrinsic rates of GTP hydrolysis and nucleotide exchange by Ras proteins are slow to facilitate efficient GDP/GTP cycling in vivo, and two classes of regulatory proteins exist in the cell that enhance these activities *(23)*. Guanine nucleotide exchange factors (GEFs) enhance the release of bound nucleotide and, since the cellular amounts of GTP greatly exceed that of GDP, promote formation of active GTP-bound Ras (Fig. 1). Several GEFs have been identified that are specific for Ras family GTPases, including the CDC25 homology proteins SOS1/2, RasGRF1/2, RasGRP, CNRasGEF, and phospholipase C epsilon (PLCε) (Fig.1) *(4,32,33)*. Some Ras GEFs can also facilitate nucleotide exchange on the Ras-related proteins such as the three R-Ras proteins (R-Ras, R-Ras2/TC21, and R-Ras3/M-Ras) *(34)*. In addition to facilitating nucleotide exchange on Ras proteins, Ras GEFs are also implicated as central signaling modules that regulate and link various intracellular signaling pathways. GTPase activating proteins (GAPs) enhance the rate of GTP hydrolysis and formation of inactive, GDP-bound Ras *(35)* (Fig.1). Mutated Ras proteins (with single amino acid substitutions at residues 12, 13, or 61) are insensitive to GAPs and persist as chronically activated proteins *(23)*. Multiple Ras GAPs have been identified and include p120GAP, neurofibromin (NF-1 GAP), Gap1m, and p135SynGAP (Fig.1) *(36–40)*.

3.2. Lipid Modification and Membrane Targeting of Ras Proteins

Ras proteins are located at the inner face of the plasma membrane (Fig. 1) where they function as regulated GDP/GTP switches to relay extracellular signals to cytoplasmic signaling cascades. Ras proteins undergo a series of posttranslational modifications that mediate their association with the plasma membrane *(41)*. The carboxyl termini of all Ras proteins contain a conserved cysteine, followed by any two aliphatic amino acids, and terminating in either serine or methionine (designated the CAAX motif) *(3,42,43)*. The cysteine is covalently modified with a farnesyl isoprenoid moiety by farnesyltransferase. Subsequent to covalent lipid attachment, the AAX residues are removed by proteolytic cleavage by an intracellular membrane-bound endoprotease, RCE1 *(44)*. The cleavage event is then followed by carboxy-methylation of the now terminal, farnesylated cysteine residue. The CAAX tetrapeptide sequence is necessary and sufficient to signal these modifications and has been used as a platform for the design and development of farnesyltransferase inhibitors as possible anti-Ras drugs *(45,46)*.

The CAAX-mediated processing steps are necessary, but not sufficient, to complete the trafficking of Ras proteins to the plasma membrane *(17)*. Instead, two distinct types of "second signals" are required *(47)*. H-Ras, K-Ras4A, and N-Ras are subsequently modified by palmitoylation at one or more cysteine residues amino terminal to the CAAX motif to facilitate plasma membrane association. K-Ras4B contains a lysine-rich sequence that serves as the second signal for complete plasma membrane association. Covalent lipid attachment at the CAAX cysteine is not sufficient for plasma membrane targeting. The presence of the second signal is essential for complete localization of Ras proteins to the inner leaflet of the plasma membrane *(17)*. These posttranslational modifications have been shown to be essential for the biological activity of Ras proteins *(48)*.

4. MEDIATORS OF Ras SIGNALING AND TRANSFORMATION

To exert its effects in the cell, Ras interacts with and/or stimulates effector proteins and pathways *(1,3)*. To date, several Ras effector proteins have been discovered, and three classes have been studied extensively for their contributions to Ras-mediated transformation. Ras also utilizes other small GTPases, such as members of the Rho, Ral, and Rap families, to exert its cellular effects on growth and transformation *(49)*.

4.1. Effector Proteins of Ras Function

To date, a multitude of Ras effectors have been isolated that interact specifically with the GTP-bound, active conformation of Ras, and it is likely that Ras uses this multitude of functionally diverse effector pathways to transduce various cell signals (Fig. 2) *(1)*. The three best characterized effector families of Ras function are the Raf serine/threo-

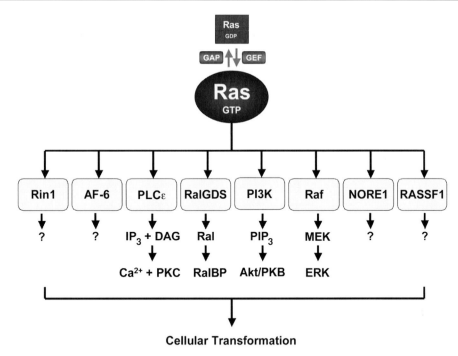

Fig. 2. Activated (GTP-bound) Ras interacts with a multitude of effector proteins that contribute to cellular transformation. Several candidate effectors of Ras signaling and transformation have been identified, including Rin1, AF-6, PLCε, RalGDS, PI3K, Raf serine/threonine kinases, NORE1, and RASSF1. Some aspects of signaling by these effectors are indicated in the figure and discussed in the text (Raf, PI3K, RalGDS). Signaling by other candidate effector proteins and their contribution to Ras-mediated transformation remain unclear.

nine kinases, Ral GEFs, and phosphatidylinositol 3-kinase (PI3K) lipid kinases. Because of the many effectors and effector pathways activated by Ras, Ras is clearly a major branch point in signal transduction. To date, it is clear that Ras-mediated oncogenesis requires activation of multiple effector signaling pathways; however, the precise role of each effector in the complex transformed phenotype is not clear.

4.1.1. Raf and Activation of the ERK MAPK Pathway

The best characterized Ras effector is the serine/threonine kinase, Raf (c-Raf-1, A-Raf, B-Raf) (Fig. 2). Activation of the Raf protein kinase occurs by Ras-mediated translocation of Raf to the plasma membrane where a complex set of other events facilitate activation of the kinase function of Raf *(50)*. Activated Raf phosphorylates the MEK1/2 dual specificity kinase, and activated MEK phosphorylates and activates ERK1/2 mitogen-activated protein kinases (MAPKs) *(51)*. ERK, in turn, activates both cytoplasmic targets, such as p90 RSK serine/threonine kinase to regulate protein synthesis *(52,53)*, and nuclear transcription factor targets, such as Elk-1 and the Ets family of transcription factors *(54,55)*, to mediate gene expression changes.

Activation of the Raf/MEK/ERK pathway alone has been shown to be necessary and sufficient to cause transformation of NIH 3T3 mouse fibroblasts *(56–63)*. However, Ras-mediated transformation also involves activation of Raf-independent pathways. For example, mutants of Ras that no longer activate Raf can still cause transformation

(64). In addition, activated Ras, but not Raf, was found to cause transformation of RIE-1 rat intestinal epithelial cells and other epithelial cell lines *(65).* These and other observations emphasize the important role of other effectors in Ras oncogenesis.

4.1.2. PHOSPHATIDYLINOSITOL 3-KINASE (PI3K)

PI3Ks were first characterized as lipid kinases that phosphorylate the 3′ position of the inositol ring of phosphatidylinositols (PI, PIP, PIP_2) (Fig. 2) *(66).* PI3Ks are composed of two subunits, a catalytic (p110) and a regulatory (p85) *(67).* Several isoforms of each subunit exist and multiple isoforms of the p110 subunit (α, β, γ, δ) have been shown to interact with GTP-bound Ras *(68).* A major function of these lipid kinases is the phosphorylation of phosphatidylinositol 4,5-bisphosphate (PIP_2) to produce phosphatidylinositol 3,4,5-triphosphate (PIP_3) *(67).* PIP_3 levels are elevated in Ras-transformed rodent fibroblasts, and dominant negative or overexpression of p85 regulatory subunit can block Ras-mediated transformation of NIH 3T3 cells *(68,69).* However, PI3K is not required for Ras-mediated transformation of RIE-1 rat intestinal epithelial cells, reflecting the cell type variation in the role of this effector in oncogenic Ras function *(70).*

Several signaling molecules have been suggested to function downstream of PI3K. One of the best characterized is the Akt/PKB serine/threonine kinase (Fig.2) *(71).* Oncogenic Ras-mediated inhibition of suspension-induced apoptosis in MDCK canine kidney epithelial cells has been attributed to PI3K-mediated activation of Akt *(72,73).* Akt can phosphorylate and alter the activity of a variety of downstream targets, including the NF-κB and forkhead transcription factors, suggesting that changes in gene expression may be an important outcome of the PI3K/Akt effector pathway *(71).*

4.1.3. RAL GUANINE NUCLEOTIDE DISSOCIATION STIMULATOR (RalGDS)

The Ral guanine nucleotide dissociation stimulator (RalGDS) family (RalGDS, RGL, RGL2/Rlf, RGL3), or GEFs, may represent a means of linking Ras family proteins to GTPases of the Ral family (Fig. 2) *(49,74,75).* Ras-mediated activation of Ral-GDS involves recruitment of RalGDS to the plasma membrane and subsequent activation of Ral *(76).* Several reports suggest that RalGDS and Ral contribute to Ras-mediated transformation. For example, co-expression of the Ras-binding domains from RGL and Rlf inhibited Ras transforming activity *(77,78).* In addition, co-expression of constitutively activated Ral-enhanced Ras focus formation; whereas, dominant negative Ral blocked Ras focus formation *(79).* Further, expression of RalGDS cooperated with activated Raf to induce synergistic focus formation *(80).* RalGEFs are also associated with up-regulation of phosphorylated (active) c-Jun *(81)* and have been shown to induce transcription of *cyclin D1*, via an NF-κB-dependent pathway, and c-fos *(82,83).* A possible mechanism by which Ras-mediated activation of RalGDS exerts its effects is by the ability of active, GTP-bound Ral to interact with a Ral effector protein, RalBP, which has GAP activity toward Rac and Cdc42 *(84).* Thus, the RalGDS effector pathway may modulate the activity of transcription factors that are regulated by Rho GTPases (see Section 3.2).

4.1.4. OTHER EFFECTOR PROTEINS

Other candidate effectors of Ras include AF-6, Rin1, Norel, RASSF1, and PLCε (Fig. 2) *(1,85,86).* To date, little is known regarding the contribution of these effectors to the oncogenic properties of Ras. AF-6 localizes to sites of cell–cell adhesion, interacts with ZO-1 adhesion molecule, and has been shown recently to disrupt epithelial junctions and cell polarity during development *(87)*. *Rin1* was isolated by screening cDNA libraries for genes that suppressed an activated RAS2 phenotype in yeast *(88)*. Early observations implicated Rin1 in growth promotion. More recent studies report that Rin1 may link the Abl tyrosine kinase to Ras function *(89)*. Currently, no function has been ascribed to Norel. RASSF1 was identified originally as a putative tumor suppressor protein *(90)*, shown subsequently to be a Ras effector, and may promote an apoptotic function of Ras *(85)*. Ras interaction with PLCε promotes its catalytic activity, which causes the production of two key second messengers (IP_3 and diacylglycerol [DAG]), which in turn cause the release of intracellular calcium and the activation of various isoforms of protein kinase C. Ras-transformed cells have been shown to exhibit elevated levels of DAG *(91)*. Interestingly, PLCε catalytic activity is also regulated by the Gα12 heterotrimeric G protein subunit and contains a separate domain that exhibits Ras GEF activity *(33)*. The role PLCε plays in Ras transformation is not known. However, since a Ras effector domain mutant (E37G) that interacts with RalGDS also retains binding to PLCε, the transforming activity of this mutant may involve activation of both RalGDS as well as PLCε *(86)*. Finally, in addition to their roles as negative regulators of Ras, effector functions have also been suggested for p120 and NF1 Ras GAPs *(92,93)*.

4.2. Linking Ras to Rho GTPases

Over the past few years, there has been growing evidence of cross-talk between Ras and Rho family GTPases, in particular, in transformation *(94,95)*. Ras-mediated transformation of fibroblasts has been shown to require the activity of several Rho family GTPases, RhoA, RhoB, Rac1, Cdc42, RhoG, and TC10 *(60,61,96–101)*. A clear example of the necessary cross-talk between Ras and Rho family GTPases is evident in the morphology of Ras-transformed cells. Ras-transformed cells adopt a mesenchymal phenotype characterized by loss of cell–cell adhesions and an increase in focal adhesions and stress fibers *(102,103)*. Ras-transformed epithelial cells show elevated levels of Rho activity *(102)*, and inhibitors of Rho partially restore the epithelial phenotype *(102)*. A recent report indicates that Ras-transformed cells have elevated levels of RhoA-GTP and that the RhoA-GTP functions to inhibit expression of p21^{CIP1}, a cell cycle inhibitor *(5,104)*. Finally, cross-talk between Ras and Rho family GTPases may converge on nuclear targets such as Ras-mediated activation of Elk-1 and Rho-mediated activation of serum response factor (SRF) to give synergistic activation of *c-fos* transcription *(95)*. In addition, it was shown that sustained ERK activation due to constitutive activation of Ras down-regulates Rho kinase and, thus, contributes to the increased motility of Ras-transformed cells *(5)*.

5. NUCLEAR TARGETS OF Ras ACTIVATION THAT CONTRIBUTE TO Ras-MEDIATED ONCOGENESIS

5.1. Complex Phenotype of Ras-Mediated Oncogenesis

Oncogenic Ras has been shown to cause and/or contribute to multiple aspects of the malignant phenotype including uncontrolled proliferation, anchorage-independent growth, survival, invasion, metastasis, and angiogenesis. Oncogenic Ras-mediated deregulation of the expression of genes whose products promote these processes have been identified. Other gene targets that facilitate the actions of oncogenic Ras remain to be identified. We first summarize the evidence that supports the importance of gene expression in Ras transformation. We then discuss the link between oncogenic Ras and specific genes whose deregulated expression may play important roles in Ras-mediated oncogenesis. Finally, we discuss the observations of several recent studies that monitor genome-wide alterations in transcription due to Ras signaling and transformation.

5.2. Nuclear Targets of Ras Activation

As described above, Ras-mediated signaling pathways can lead to the activation of a diverse spectrum of transcription factors, that include Ets-1/2, Elk-1, NF-κB, SRF, c-Fos, c-Jun, Myc, and E2F (1). Hence, it is not surprising that the promoter elements of Ras-responsive genes harbor Ets, AP-1, and NF-κB binding sites (1). Ras transforming activity has been shown to be dependent on the function of many of these transcription factors. For example, depletion of c-*myc* with specific antisense sequences (105) or expression of dominant negative mutants of Ets-1, Ets-2 (55,106,107), c-Fos (108), or c-Jun (109) can block oncogenic Ras-mediated transformation of NIH 3T3 fibroblasts. In addition, c-*Jun* null mouse embryo fibroblasts were found to be insensitive to Ras-mediated transformation (110). Further, the role of c-*fos* in Ras-mediated tumor formation was shown in c-*fos* knock-out mice carrying an H-*ras* transgene. In this mouse model, treatment with a tumor promoter induced benign tumor growth, but papillomas became hyperkeratinized and did not progress to malignancy (111). Finally, inhibition of NF-κB blocked Ras-mediated transformation and resulted in apoptosis of NIH 3T3 and Rat-1 rodent fibroblasts (112,113). When considered together, these observations indicate that changes in gene expression are critical for Ras-mediated oncogenesis.

Specific gene targets of Ras signaling have been delineated by two approaches. First, the consequences of Ras-mediated activation of the expression of specific genes whose products may contribute to transformation have been determined. Included among these are genes encoding proteins that facilitate autocrine growth factor loops (TGFα), cell cycle progression (cyclin D1), cell survival (COX-2), cell shape (tropomyosin; TM), tumor cell invasion (MMP-9), and angiogenesis (VEGF) (Fig. 3). Second, recent studies have utilized differential gene expression analyses to identify genes whose expression is altered in Ras-transformed cells. We have summarized the observations from these studies in the following sections.

5.2.1. RAS-MEDIATED UP-REGULATION OF TGFα AND AUTOCRINE GROWTH REGULATION

Oncogenic Ras-mediated transformation of a wide variety of rodent and human fibroblast and epithelial cells is associated with persistent up-regulation of the gene expression of TGFα (114–117). TGFα is a member of the EGF family of peptide growth factors and stimulates the activation of the EGF receptor. The precise details concerning how Ras stimulates TGFα gene expression remain to be determined. For at least some cell types, Ras-mediated activation of both Raf-dependent and Raf-independent effectors is required to cause up-regulation of TGFα (118).

TGFα up-regulation has been shown to be important for Ras transformation. For example, TGFα transcription and protein secretion were activated in Ras-transformed RIE-1 rat intestinal epithelial cells (118). Further, inhibition of EGF receptor function impaired the growth of Ras-transformed cells, whereas treatment of untransformed RIE-

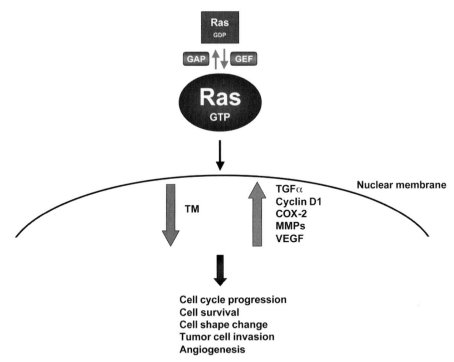

Fig. 3. Ras mediates gene expression changes that contribute to the transformed phenotype. Specific gene targets of Ras signaling and transformation have been identified. Included among these are genes encoding proteins that facilitate autocrine growth factor loops TGFα, cell cycle progression (cyclin D1), cell survival (COX-2), cell shape (TM), tumor cell invasion (MMP-9), and angiogenesis (VEGF), which, when deregulated in Ras-transformed cells, lead to the hallmarks of the transformed cell phenotype.

1 cells with exogenous TGFα alone was sufficient to cause morphological transformation and promote growth in soft agar *(118)*. Therefore, the up-regulation of TGFα is both necessary and sufficient to promote morphological and growth transformation of RIE-1 cells. Similar observations were made with Ras-transformed MCF-10A human breast epithelial cells and other cell types *(119,120)*. Finally, other EGF family ligands have also been found to be up-regulated in gene expression in Ras-transformed cells *(15)*.

5.2.2. RAS-MEDIATED UP-REGULATION OF CYCLIN D1 AND CELL CYCLE PROGRESSION

Ras signaling regulates multiple components of the cell cycle control machinery to promote hyperphosphorylation of the Rb tumor suppressor and to stimulate progression through the G1 phase of the cell cycle *(121,122)*. Cyclin D1 is the best characterized cell cycle regulatory factor target of Ras *(122)*. Cyclin D1 transcription and translation are typically elevated in mid-G1 and are associated with a second peak of Ras activation *(122)*. Maximal accumulation of cyclin D1 protein occurs closer to the G1/S boundary *(122)*. This increase in cyclin D1 promotes the formation of cyclin D1:CDK (cyclin-dependent kinases) 4/6 complexes, which in turn phosphorylate and inactivate Rb, causing activation of the E2F transcription factor, and subsequent progression of the cell cycle *(122,123)*.

Ras mediates up-regulation of cyclin D1 by transcriptional activation in a wide variety of cell types *(124–126)*. Transient induction of activated Ras expression in rodent fibroblasts and epithelial cells is accompanied by upregulation of cyclin D1 transcription and protein expression *(10,125,127)*. Serum-stimulated up-regulation of cyclin D1 expression is dependent on Ras function and constitutive expression of cyclin D1 can overcome the requirement for Ras for proliferation of NIH 3T3 cells *(128)*. Further, oncogenic Ras-mediated transformation of a variety of cell types is associated with sustained up-regulation of cyclin D1 protein *(7,10,124,126,129)*. Stimulation of cyclin D1 gene expression by oncogenic Ras requires activation of both Raf-dependent and Raf-independent effector pathways *(9,130)* and involves activation of Ets, AP-1, and NF-κB responsive motifs in the cyclin D1 promoter *(131)*.

Cyclin D1 contributes to Ras-mediated growth stimulation. For example, the treatment of Ras-transformed NIH 3T3 or IEC-18 cells with antisense cyclin D1 oligonucleotides caused an impairment in proliferation *(125,126)*. Similarly, a contribution of cyclin D1 up-regulation by Ras in tumor development was shown in a recent study where oncogenic Ras-induced tumors that developed from the cyclin D1 null cells were half the size of the tumors formed by cells heterozygous or wild-type for cyclin D1 *(121)*. However, overexpression of cyclin D1 alone is clearly not sufficient to promote Ras-mediated growth transformation *(126,130)*.

5.2.3. RAS-MEDIATED UP-REGULATION OF CYCLOOXYGENASE-2 (COX-2) AND CELL SURVIVAL

One aspect of Ras-mediated transformation involves promotion of cell survival. For example, oncogenic Ras prevents the apoptotic response that is induced when epithelial cells are deprived of matrix attachment by blocking a caspase-mediated induction of cell death *(73,132)*. Ras-mediated up-regulation of the inducible eicosanoid-producing enzyme cyclooxygenase-2 (COX-2) and COX-2-mediated production of prostaglandins (PGs; e.g., PGE$_2$) is another mechanism by which oncogenic Ras may promote cell survival. In contrast to the constitutively expressed and functionally related COX-1, COX-2 expression is transiently induced by various stimuli that include pro-inflammatory cytokines, lipopolysaccharide, mitogens, and reactive oxygen species *(133)*. COX-2 protein expression has been found to be constitutively up-regulated in a variety of Ras-transformed fibroblast and epithelial cells (e.g., Rat-1, RIE-1, MCF-10A) or in cells transformed by oncoproteins known to cause activation of Ras (e.g., Src, HER2) *(134–138)*.

To date, little is known regarding the mechanism by which Ras causes up-regulation of COX-2 gene expression. Activated Raf-expressing rat intestinal epithelial cells retain normal cell morphology and growth and display only modest up-regulation of COX-2 protein *(139)*. However, treatment of Ras-transformed cells with a MEK inhibitor caused a significant reduction in COX-2 expression that was concurrent with reversion of growth and morphologic transformation *(135)*. Thus, the Raf/ERK pathway is necessary but not sufficient to cause up-regulation of COX-2. Activation of ERK, as well as activation of Akt, were found to mediate COX-2 up-regulation in HCA-7 human colorectal carcinoma cells *(140)*. In addition, the COX-2 gene promoter sequence contains NF-κB, NFIL6, ATF/CRE, and E box regulatory sequences, and may contribute to Ras-mediated COX-2 transcriptional up-regulation *(140,141)*.

Current evidence supports a role for COX-2 and PGE$_2$ in Ras-mediated transformation. For example, DuBois and colleagues have shown that transformation of rat intestinal epithelial cells by Ras is mediated, in part, by up-regulation of COX-2 (135,139,142). Treatment of Ras-transformed cells with a COX-2 inhibitor reduced cell proliferation, inhibited colony formation and size on matrigel, and suppressed tumor formation in nude mice (142). Inhibition of COX-2 in Ras-transformed cells also decreased DNA synthesis and caused apoptosis in serum-free medium (139). Further, COX-2 overexpression in nontransformed cells caused resistance to butyrate-induced apoptosis and elevated expression of anti-apoptotic Bc12 protein (143). However, these cells maintained contact inhibition, normal morphology, and were nontumorigenic (139,143). Thus, COX-2 up-regulation alone is not sufficient to promote the transformed phenotype caused by activated Ras.

5.2.4. DOWN-REGULATION OF TROPOMYOSIN IN RAS GROWTH AND MORPHOLOGIC TRANSFORMATION

Impaired expression of high molecular weight tropomyosin (TM-1, TM-2, and TM-3), a family of cytoskeletal proteins that bind to and stabilize actin in microfilaments, has been observed in a variety of Ras-transformed fibroblasts and epithelial cells (144–148). Tropomyosins are found along stress fibers and are thought to play a role in stabilizing the organization of actin filaments, which in turn plays an important role in the maintenance of cell shape, cell motility, and cell–cell and cell–matrix interactions (149). Therefore, the loss of tropomyosin expression in transformed cells may prevent proper assembly of microfilaments, and consequently, contribute to the invasive and metastatic properties of cancer cells.

Cell type differences have been observed for the mechanism by which Ras causes down-regulation of tropomyosin gene expression. For example, in NIH 3T3 mouse fibroblasts, activation of Raf alone is sufficient to cause down-regulation (148). However, Raf-mediated down-regulation appears to be independent of ERK activation (148). In RIE-1 rat intestinal epithelial cells, both Raf-dependent and Raf-independent pathways are required for Ras to extinguish tropomyosin gene expression, in part, by promoting DNA methylation (150).

Observations from studies of Ras-transformed rodent fibroblasts support an important contribution of the loss of tropomyosin expression to Ras-mediated transformation. For example, forced re-expression of TM-1 or TM-2 in Ras-transformed NIH 3T3 fibroblasts restored anchorage-dependent growth and impaired tumorigenic growth potential (146,151). In contrast, another study showed forced re-expression of TM-2 or TM-3 in Ras-transformed fibroblasts resulted in no inhibition of growth in soft agar (146). Forced re-expression of TM-2 in Raf-transformed NRK normal rat kidney fibroblasts caused reversion of cell morphology, but did not inhibit either the growth rates of these cells or their ability to grow in soft agar (148). In contrast to fibroblast studies, we found that forced re-expression of tropomyosins did not reverse morphologic or growth transformation of RIE-1 rat intestinal epithelial cells (150). Thus, the loss of tropomyosin displays cell type differences in mediating Ras transformation.

5.2.5. RAS-MEDIATED UP-REGULATION OF MATRIX METALLOPROTEINASES (MMPS) AND TUMOR CELL INVASION

Oncogenic Ras has been shown to promote invasion and metastasis in many experimental tumor cell models (152). Invasion and metastasis are mediated in part by the ability of transformed cells to destroy the extracellular matrix (ECM) in the basement membrane (153). Ras-mediated transformation is associated with transcription of genes that encode secreted proteinases such as MMPs, cysteine proteases cathepsins, urokinase plasminogen activator, and heparanase *(152,154)*. This section will focus on up-regulation of MMPs by Ras.

MMPs are a family of divalent cation-dependent proteases whose expression is associated with advanced stages of almost all cancers following the transition of epithelial cells to a mesenchymal phenotype *(155)*. To date, more than 15 MMPs have been identified. According to domain structure and substrate specificity, the family of MMPs is subdivided into several families, including collagenases (MMP-1,-8,-13), stromelysin (MMP-3,-10,-12), gelatinases (MMP-2,-9), matrilysin (MMP-7), membrane types (MMP-14,-15,-16,-17), and others (MMP-11,-19,-20) *(156–158)*. The target substrates of this family of proteases are components of the ECM, such as collagen, a major component of basement membranes, but family members are active against most other components of basement membranes, such as laminin, entactin, and perlecan as well *(157)*.

Regulation of MMPs occurs by transcription, mRNA stability, amino-terminal proteolytic cleavage of a pro-enzyme form, and inhibition by endogenous proteins, tissue inhibitors of metalloproteinases (TIMPs) *(155)*. Transcriptional activation has been reported to occur in response to growth factors and cytokines and oncogenes *(155)*. The promoters of MMPs contain Ras-responsive DNA elements *(159,160)*. For example, the MMP-9 promoter contains Ets, AP-1, and NF-κB DNA binding motifs *(158)*. Therefore, it is not surprising that up-regulation of MMP gene expression has been reported in many Ras-transformed cells. However, the specific MMPs that are up-regulated show cell type differences. Various differential gene expression cloning strategies (*see* Subheading 5.3) have been applied to identify gene targets of Ras, and MMPs have been identified in these studies *(11)*.

The best evidence for linking Ras to up-regulation of MMPs involves MMP-9/type IV collagenase/gelatinase B *(159,161–165)*. Type IV collagen is the predominant collagen component of the basement membrane, and consequently, activation of MMP-9 may contribute significantly to invasion and metastasis *(157,158)*. Ras-mediated MMP-9 up-regulation has been shown in metastatic rodent tumor cells and human tumors. Further, Ras-transformed rat embryo fibroblasts and NIH 3T3 murine fibroblasts metastasize in nude mice, and the metastatic potential of these cells is associated with increased type IV collagenolytic activity and the secretion of MMP-9 *(166–168)*. Inhibition of metastasis by Ras-transformed cells was achieved by inhibition of MMP-9 by ribozyme targeting of the MMP-9 mRNA expression and loss of type IV collagenolytic activity *(169)*.

In addition to MMP-9, other MMPs have been shown to be up-regulated in a Ras-dependent manner *(154)*. For example, MMP-2 is implicated in regulation by Ras both in cell culture and in human tumors *(162,170)*, MMP-7 (matrilysin) expression was induced in colon tumor cells transfected with Ras *(171)*, and MMP-10 (stromelysin) expression is activated by oncogenic H-Ras *(172)*.

5.2.6. Ras-Mediated Up-Regulation of Vascular endothelial Growth Factor (VEGF) and Angiogenesis

Oncogenic Ras has been observed to be a potent stimulator of VEGF gene expression *(173–175)*. VEGF is one of a number of soluble factors that are mitogens specific for vascular endothelial cells, mediating both normal and pathological angiogenesis. Two known tyrosine kinase cell-surface receptors recognize VEGF, VEGFR-1 (flt-1), and VEGFR-2 (flk-1/KDR) *(176)*, and VEGF binding mediates its mitogenic effects on endothelial cells. Solid tumor growth beyond 1 to 2 mm in diameter requires vascularization in order to provide nutrients to sustain the metastatic growth potential. Consequently, up-regulation of VEGF may be an important for oncogenic Ras induction of this angiogenic response and promotion of malignant growth *(173,177)*.

Oncogenic Ras has been associated with the up-regulation of VEGF mRNA expression and secretion of protein in both experimental transformation cell systems and in human tumors. Transient or sustained expression of oncogenic Ras in a variety of fibroblasts, epithelial cells, and other cell types has been has been shown to cause up-regulation of VEGF transcription and protein expression *(173,175,177)*. VEGF is up-regulated in *ras* mutation positive colon carcinoma cell lines, and disruption of the mutant K-*ras* function is associated with reduction in VEGF production *(173)*. The effectors that mediate oncogenic Ras stimulation of *VEGF* gene expression exhibit significant cell type differences. For example, the Raf/ERK pathway is sufficient to promote VEGF up-regulation in rodent fibroblasts *(178,179)*. In contrast, other studies implicated PI3K in the Ras-mediated regulation of VEGF *(177,180)*. Finally, Ras has also been shown to up-regulate VEGF transcription and mRNA stability by a pathway involving Protein Kinase C ζ (PKCζ) *(181)*. Various elements in the *VEGF* promoter have been implicated in Ras-mediated stimulation and include hypoxia-inducible transcription factor 1 (HIF-1) and cAMP-responsive element (CRE) *(180)*. Furthermore, the promoter region responsible for the Raf-mediated up-regulation of *VEGF* transcription has been identified, and it has been determined that ERK activation led to an increase in binding of Sp1 and AP2 transcription factor activation and binding to GC-rich elements in the promoter region of *VEGF (179)*.

There is evidence for a functional contribution of VEGF up-regulation in oncogenic Ras-mediated transformation in some but not all cell types. For example, expression of antisense *VEGF* in the DLD-1 and HCT-116 colon carcinoma cells, which harbor an activated K-*ras* allele, caused a decrease in VEGF production and subsequent inability to form tumors in nude mice *(182)*. In contrast, while VEGF was up-regulated, Ras-induced mammary tumors were found, and this expression was dispensable for tumor formation *(183)*.

5.3. Current Techniques Used to Examine Genome-Wide Alterations in Gene Expression

During the past few years, several techniques have been developed to study genome-wide changes in gene expression. These techniques are being applied extensively to study the transcriptional changes associated with various aspects of Ras-mediated transformation. These techniques include differential display, subtractive suppression hybridization (SSH), representational difference analysis (RDA), and microchip array analyses. We have summarized the observations made from these different approaches.

Differential display was developed by Liang and Pardee as a polymerase chain reaction (PCR)-based technique to identify and isolate those genes that are differentially expressed in two different cell populations *(184)*. Recently, Liang and colleagues have applied this technique to identify genes that are deregulated in expression by oncogenic Ras transformation *(12)*. They identified 12 genes that were differentially expressed in rat embryo fibroblasts transformed by cooperation of oncogenic Ras and dominant negative p53. One gene identified encodes a small secreted protein designated Mob-1, with significant homology with the interferon-γ-inducible protein-10 proinflammatory cytokine. Mob-1 expression was constitutively up-regulated in Ras-transformed cells, and promoter analyses identified AP-1 and NF-κB motifs that may account for Ras mediated up-regulation of *Mob*-1 gene transcription. Inhibition of ERK activation abolished Mob-1 up-regulation in Ras-transformed cells, indicating that Ras stimulation of Mob-1 is dependent on the Raf/ERK effector pathway. A second gene, designated *rCop-1*, was identified as a gene whose expression was down-regulated in Ras-transformed cells *(13)*. RCop-1 encodes a protein with homology to members of the CCN cysteine-rich growth-regulatory proteins. Ectopic re-expression of rCop-1 in Ras-transformed cells caused apoptosis, supporting a negative regulatory function for this protein.

McMahon and colleagues applied the differential display technique to identify genes induced by Raf activation in NIH 3T3 cells and found that heparin-binding (HB) EGF mRNA was induced rapidly and resulted in secretion of HB-EGF *(14)*. HB-EGF secretion was also observed in Ras-transformed cells. It was determined subsequently that this autocrine mechanism contributed to Ras activation of the c-Jun N- terminal Kinase (JNK) MAPK.

SSH is a technique that is similar to RDA that was developed by Diatchenko et al. for the generation of subtracted cDNA libraries *(185)*. Baba et al. used this approach to identify differentially-expressed genes between the HCT116 human colon carcinoma cell line and a genetic variant (Hke3), in which homologous recombination in vitro was used to eliminate the mutated K-*ras* allele *(15)*. Disruption of activated K-Ras function is associated with impaired growth transformation in vitro and in vivo *(186)*. One gene identified encodes epiregulin, a member of the EGF family, and its expression was reduced in Hke3 cells. Reintroduction of a mutated K-*ras* allele into Hke3 cells resulted in up-regulation of epiregulin expression and morphologic transformation. While forced re-expression of epiregulin in Hke3 cells did not restore the ability to grow in soft agar, it did enhance tumor formation in nude mice, indicating that this gene expression change is functionally important for some aspects of K-Ras transformation.

Habets et al. *(16)* described the application of cDNA microarray analyses to identify oncogenic K-Ras-induced gene transcription. They utilized the DLD1 human colon carcinoma cell line where the endogenous mutated K-*ras* allele was removed by homologous recombination in vitro *(186)*. Loss of mutated K-*ras* has been shown to greatly impair the ability of these tumor cells to grow in soft agar and to form tumors in nude mice. Ecdysone-inducible expression of activated K-Ras was established in these cells. A strong induction of K-Ras protein was seen and corresponded with induction of ERK activation. RNA was isolated from uninduced and induced knock-out cells, as well as the parental DLD1 cell line, and hybridization was performed on 10,000 cDNA gene arrays. While the induction of known early response genes was identified *(fos, jun,* and *erg1)*, unexpectedly induction of *myc* was not detected. Previously, it was found that loss of mutated K-*ras* in DLD1 cells was associated with a 9-fold reduction in *myc* expression *(186)*. An additional unexpected observation was that induction of activated K-Ras protein expression did not induce morphologic or growth transformation. Thus, whatever gene expression changes were identified was not sufficient to promote transformation.

SSH was also employed by Schafer and colleagues to identify gene targets of oncogenic H-Ras signaling and transformation *(11)*. Overall, they determined gene expression profiles in H-Ras-transformed cells and indentified transcriptional stimulation or repression of 244 known genes, 104 expressed sequence tags (ESTs), and 45 novel sequences. Among these were some that were identified previously as genes whose expression is up-regulated (e.g., *CD44, Fra-1, Mob-1*) or down-regulated (e.g., entactin/nidogen, lysyl oxidase) by Ras. Other genes identified included up-regulation of genes involved in invasion (e.g., *MMP1, MMP3,* and *MMP-10*) and down-regulation of genes with negative roles in oncogenesis (e.g., *TIMP2, Gas-1*). Genes involved in regulation of cell proliferation and survival, stress response, cytoskeletal organization, and glycolytic energy regeneration were also identified. Overall, it was estimated that 3–8% of all expressed genes were altered in Ras-transformed cells.

Interestingly, the deregulated expression of only 16% of these gene targets were found to be dependent upon ERK activation, indicating that Raf-independent effector function is critically important for a majority of the changes in gene expression. Approximately 90% of the genes identified were also altered by mutated N-Ras and K-Ras. Thus, while it has been speculated that the different Ras isoforms may have distinct functions, this observation suggests that their roles in regulation of gene expression are quite similar. Finally, since these analyses compared Ras-transformed 208F cells with untransformed 208F cells, the observed gene expression changes may be due to activation of H-Ras or to H-Ras-induced growth transformation. However, a number of the genes were also found to be altered on transient induction of oncogenic Ras expression in 208F cells, indicating that direct targets of Ras activation were identified.

The information derived from differential gene expression analyses is immense and is certain to provide important clues for understanding the mechanism of Ras-mediated oncogenesis. However, since the level of gene expression may not accurately reflect the level of protein expression, another approach for defining the gene targets of Ras involves functional proteomics and mass spectrometry to monitor global changes in protein expression or function. For example, Ahn and colleagues applied functional proteomics to identify cellular targets of the MEK/ERK cascade *(187)*. They used selective activation and inactivation of MEK1/2 and identified 25 targets, of which only five were linked previously to this signaling pathway. Similarly, Westwick and colleagues applied functional genomics to elucidate the possible targets of farnesyltransferase inhibitors *(188)*. The application of functional genomics continues to develop, and we will certainly see greater future application of this methodology to the study of Ras "mediated" deregulation of gene and protein function.

6. CONCLUSIONS AND PERSPECTIVES

We have reviewed our current understanding of Ras signal transduction and its consequences on gene expression and function. The identification of downstream effectors of Ras continues at an impressive rate. The diversity and complexity of their functions reveal that we still have much to learn about the biological function of Ras. For example, the identification of PLCε as a Ras effector links Ras activity directly to the actions of second messengers, calcium and DAG, which in turn cause pleotropic cellular responses. How this effector may contribute to normal and oncogenic Ras function will be interesting to determine. Many of the cytoplasmic signaling events that these effectors may regulate are now well-defined, but many remain to be elucidated. What is clear is that many result in the regulation of proteins that control changes in gene expression. Some signaling events directly stimulate the activity of specific transcription factors, and the number and diversity of these factors continues to expand. Other Ras-mediated signaling events may evoke more global changes in gene expression, for example, by regulation of DNA methylation or by regulation of histone acetylation. Thus, as we continue to dissect the components and complexity of Ras signaling through the cytoplasm, elucidating the gene targets of Ras will be an important pursuit. The development of methods, such as microarray analyses and functional proteomics, to evaluate global changes in gene or protein expression is evolving rapidly. Experimental approaches to evaluate global changes in protein function, such as protein kinase activity, are also being developed. Hence, we are certain to witness great strides in this area of Ras research in the coming years. The accumulation of information has and will occur at a pace that greatly exceeds our ability to make sense of these observations. Nevertheless, our comprehension of this information will foster great advances for understanding the role of Ras in oncogenesis and for the development of therapeutic approaches to thwart that role for cancer treatment.

ACKNOWLEDGMENTS

We thank Kevin Pruitt and Aylin Ulku for helpful discussions and Misha Rand for manuscript preparation. Our studies are supported by National Institutes of Health (NIH) grants to C.J.D. (CA42978, CA55008, and CA63071). G.A.M. is supported as a Merck Fellow of the Life Science Research Foundation.

REFERENCES

1. Campbell SL, Khosravi-Far R, Rossman KL, Clark GJ, Der CJ. Increasing complexity of Ras signaling. *Oncogene* 1998; 17:1395–1413.
2. Vojtek AB, Der CJ. Increasing complexity of the Ras signaling pathway. *J. Biol Chem* 1998; 273:19925–19928.
3. Shields JM, Pruitt K, McFall A, Shaub A, Der CJ. Understanding Ras: 'it ain't over 'til it's over'. *Trends Cell Biol* 2000; 10:147–154.
4. Khosravi-Far R, Der CJ. The Ras signal transduction pathway. *Cancer Metastasis Rev* 1994; 13:67–89.
5. Sahai E, Olson MF, Marshall CJ. Cross-talk between Ras and Rho signalling pathways in transformation favours proliferation and increased motility. *EMBO J* 2001; 20:755–766.
6. Scita G, Tenca P, Frittoli E, Tocchetti A, Innocenti M, Giardina G, et al. Signaling from Ras to Rac and beyond: not just a matter of GEFs. *EMBO J* 2000; 19:2393–2398.
7. Pruitt K, Pestell RG, Der CJ. Ras inactivation of the Rb pathway by distinct mechanisms in NIH 3T3 fibroblasts and RIE-1 epithelial cells. *J Biol Chem* 2000; 275:40916–40924.
8. Takuwa N, Takuwa Y. Regulation of cell cycle molecules by the Ras effector system. *Mol Cell Endocrinol* 2001; 177:25–33.
9. Gille H, Downward J. Multiple ras effector pathways contribute to G(1) cell cycle progression. *J Biol Chem* 1999; 274:22033–22040.
10. Shao J, Sheng H, DuBois RN, Beauchamp RD. Oncogenic Ras-mediated cell growth arrest and apoptosis are associated with increased ubiquitin-dependent cyclin D1 degradation. *J Biol Chem* 2000; 275:22916–22924.
11. Zuber J, Tchernitsa OI, Hinzmann B, Schmitz AC, Grips M, Hellriegel M, et al. A genome-wide survey of RAS transformation targets. *Nat Genet* 2000; 24144–24152.
12. Liang P, Averboukh L, Zhu W, Pardee AB. Ras activation of genes: Mob-1 as a model. *Proc Natl Acad Sci USA* 1994; 91:12515–12519.
13. Zhang R, Averboukh L, Zhu W, Zhang H, Jo H, Dempsey PJ, et al. Identification of rCop-1, a new member of the CCN protein family, as a negative regulator for cell transformation. *Mol Cell Biol* 1998; 18:6131–6141.
14. McCarthy SA, Samuels ML, Pritchard CA, Abraham JA, McMahon M. Rapid induction of heparin-binding epidermal growth factor/diphtheria toxin receptor expression by Raf and Ras oncogenes. *Genes Dev* 1995; 9:1953–1964.

15. Baba I, Shirasawa S, Iwamoto R, Okumura K, Tsunoda T, Nishioka M, et al. Involvement of deregulated epiregulin expression in tumorigenesis in vivo through activated Ki-Ras signaling pathway in human colon cancer cells. *Cancer Res* 2000; 60:6886–6889.
16. Habets GG, Knepper M, Sumortin J, Choi YJ, Sasazuki T, Shirasawa S, et al. cDNA array analyses of K-ras-induced gene transcription. *Methods Enzymol* 2001; 332:245–260.
17. Choy E, Chiu VK, Silletti J, Feoktistov M, Morimoto T, Michaelson D, et al. Endomembrane trafficking of ras: the CAAX motif targets proteins to the ER and Golgi. *Cell* 1999; 98:69–80.
18. Johnson L, Greenbaum D, Cichowski K, Mercer K, Murphy E, Schmitt E, et al. K-ras is an essential gene in the mouse with partial functional overlap with N-ras. *Genes Dev* 1997; 11:2468–2481.
19. Esteban LM, Vicario-Abejon C, Fernandez-Salguero P, Fernandez-Medarde A, Swaminathan N, Yienger K, et al. Targeted genomic disruption of H-ras and N-ras, individually or in combination, reveals the dispensability of both loci for mouse growth and development. *Mol Cell Biol* 2001; 21:1444–1452.
20. Koera K, Nakamura K, Nakao K, Miyoshi J, Toyoshima K, Hatta T, et al. K-ras is essential for the development of the mouse embryo. *Oncogene* 1997; 15:1151–1159.
21. Bos JL. ras oncogenes in human cancer: a review. *Cancer Res* 1989; 49:4682–4689.
22. Bollag G, McCormick F. Regulators and effectors of ras proteins. *Annu Rev Cell Biol* 1991; 7:601–632.
23. Boguski MS, McCormick F. Proteins regulating Ras and its relatives. *Nature* 1993; 366:643–654.
24. Lowy DR, Willumsen BM. Function and regulation of ras. *Annu Rev Biochem* 1993; 62:851–891.
25. MacKenzie KL, Dolnikov A, Millington M, Shounan Y, Symonds G. Mutant N-ras induces myeloproliferative disorders and apoptosis in bone marrow repopulated mice. *Blood* 1999; 93:2043–2056.
26. Reese DM, Slamon DJ. HER-2/neu signal transduction in human breast and ovarian cancer. *Stem Cells* 1997; 15:1–8.
27. Guha A. Ras activation in astrocytomas and neurofibromas. *Can J Neurol Sci* 1998; 25:267–281.
28. Bourne HR, Sanders DA, McCormick F. The GTPase superfamily: a conserved switch for diverse cell functions. *Nature* 1990; 348:125–132.
29. Tong LA, de Vos AM, Milburn MV, Jancarik J, Noguchi S, Nishimura S, et al. Structural differences between a ras oncogene protein and the normal protein. *Nature* 1989; 337:90–93.
30. Milburn MV, Tong L, deVos AM, Brunger A, Yamaizumi Z, Nishimura S, et al. Molecular switch for signal transduction: structural differences between active and inactive forms of protooncogenic ras proteins. *Science* 1990; 247:939–945.
31. Krengel U, Schlichting L, Scherer A, Schumann R, Frech M, John J, et al. Three-dimensional structures of H-ras p21 mutants: molecular basis for their inability to function as signal switch molecules. *Cell* 1990; 62:539–548.
32. Pham N, Cheglakov I, Koch CA, de Hoog CL, Moran MF, Rotin D. The guanine nucleotide exchange factor CNrasGEF activates ras in response to cAMP and cGMP. *Curr Biol* 2000; 10:555–558.
33. Lopez I, Mak EC, Ding J, Hamm HE, Lomasney JW. A novel bifunctional phospholipase c that is regulated by Galpha 12 and stimulates the Ras/mitogen-activated protein kinase pathway. *J Biol Chem* 2001; 276:2758–2765.
34. Ohba Y, Mochizuki N, Yamashita S, Chan AM, Schrader JW, Hattori S, et al. Regulatory proteins of R-Ras, TC21/R-Ras2, and M-Ras/R-Ras3. *J Biol Chem* 2000; 275:20020–20026.
35. Wittinghofer A, Scheffzek K, Ahmadian MR. The interaction of Ras with GTPase-activating proteins. FEBS Lett 1997; 410:63–67.
36. McCormick F, Martin GA, Clark R, Bollag G, Polakis P. Regulation of ras p21 by GTPase activating proteins. *Cold Spring Harb Symp Quant Biol* 1991; 56:237–241.
37. Xu GF, O'Connell P, Viskochil D, Cawthon R, Robertson M, Culver M, et al. The neurofibromatosis type 1 gene encodes a protein related to GAP. *Cell* 1990; 62:599–608.
38. Maekawa M, Li S, Iwamatsu A, Morishita T, Yokota K, Imai Y, et al. A novel mammalian Ras GTPase-activating protein which has phospholipid-binding and Btk homology regions. *Mol Cell Biol* 1994; 14:6879–6885.
39. Kim JH, Liao D, Lau LF, Huganir RL. SynGAP: a synaptic RasGAP that associates with the PSD-95/SAP90 protein family. *Neuron* 1998; 20:683–691.
40. Xu GF, Lin B, Tanaka K, Dunn D, Wood D, Gesteland R, et al. The catalytic domain of the neurofibromatosis type 1 gene product stimulates ras GTPase and complements ira mutants of *S. cerevisiae*. *Cell* 1990; 63:835–841.
41. Seabra MC. Membrane association and targeting of prenylated Ras-like GTPases. *Cell Signal* 1998; 10:167–172.
42. Fu HW, Casey PJ. Enzymology and biology of CaaX protein prenylation. *Recent Prog Horm Res* 1999; 54:315–342.

43. Willumsen BM, Norris K, Papageorge AG, Hubbert NL, Lowy DR. Harvey murine sarcoma virus p21 ras protein: biological and biochemical significance of the cysteine nearest the carboxy terminus. *EMBO J* 1984; 3:2581–2585.
44. Kim E, Ambroziak P, Otto JC, Taylor B, Ashby M, Shannon K, et al. Disruption of the mouse Rce1 gene results in defective Ras processing and mislocalization of Ras within cells. *J Biol Chem* 1999; 274:8383–8390.
45. Cox AD, Der CJ. Farnesyltransferase inhibitors and cancer treatment: targeting simply Ras? *Biochim Biophys Acta* 1997; 1333:F51–F71.
46. Oliff A. Farnesyltransferase inhibitors: targeting the molecular basis of cancer. *Biochim Biophys Acta* 1999; 1423:C19–C30.
47. Prior IA, Hancock JF. Compartmentalization of Ras proteins. *J Cell Sci* 2001; 114:1603–1608.
48. Cox AD, Der CJ. Protein prenylation: more than just glue? *Curr Opin Cell Biol* 1992; 4:1008–1016.
49. Reuther GW, Der CJ. The Ras branch of small GTPases: Ras family members don't fall far from the tree. *Curr Opin Cell Biol* 2000; 12:157–165.
50. Morrison DK, Cutler RE. The complexity of Raf-1 regulation. *Curr Opin Cell Biol* 1997; 9:174–179.
51. Crews CM, Alessandrini A, Erikson RL. Erks: their fifteen minutes has arrived. *Cell Growth Differ* 1992; 3:135–142.
52. Blenis J. Signal transduction via the MAP kinases: proceed at your own RSK. *Proc Natl Acad Sci USA* 1993; 90:5889–5892.
53. Sturgill TW, Ray LB, Erikson E, Maller JL. Insulin-stimulated MAP-2 kinase phosphorylates and activates ribosomal protein S6 kinase II. *Nature* 1988; 334:715–718.
54. Marais R, Wynne J, Treisman R. The SRF accessory protein Elk-1 contains a growth factor-regulated transcriptional activation domain. *Cell* 1993; 73:381–393.
55. Wasylyk B, Hagman J, Gutierrez-Hartmann A. Ets transcription factors: nuclear effectors of the Ras-MAP-kinase signaling pathway. *Trends Biochem Sci* 1998; 23.
56. Kolch W, Heidecker G, Lloyd P, Rapp UR. Raf-1 protein kinase is required for growth of induced NIH/3T3 cells. *Nature* 1991; 349:426–428.
57. Schaap D, van der WJ, Howe LR, Marshall CJ, van Blitterswijk WJ. A dominant-negative mutant of raf blocks mitogen-activated protein kinase activation by growth factors and oncogenic p21ras. *J Biol Chem* 1993; 268:20232–20236.
58. Cowley S, Paterson H, Kemp P, Marshall CJ. Activation of MAP kinase kinase is necessary and sufficient for PC12 differentiation and for transformation of NIH 3T3 cells. *Cell* 1994; 77:841–852.
59. Westwick JK, Cox AD, Der CJ, Cobb MH, Hibi M, Karin M, et al. Oncogenic Ras activates c-Jun via a separate pathway from the activation of extracellular signal-regulated kinases. *Proc Natl Acad Sci USA* 1994; 91:6030–6034.
60. Qiu RG, Chen J, Kirn D, McCormick F, Symons M. An essential role for Rac in Ras transformation. *Nature* 1995; 374:457–459.
61. Khosravi-Far R, Solski PA, Clark GJ, Kinch MS, Der CJ. Activation of Rac1, RhoA, and mitogen-activated protein kinases is required for Ras transformation. *Mol Cell Biol* 1995; 15:6443–6453.
62. Mansour SJ, Matten WT, Hermann AS, Candia JM, Rong S, Fukasawa K, et al. Transformation of mammalian cells by constitutively active MAP kinase kinase. *Science* 1994; 265:966–970.
63. Leevers SJ, Paterson HF, Marshall CJ. Requirement for Ras in Raf activation is overcome by targeting Raf to the plasma membrane. *Nature* 1994; 369:411–414.
64. Khosravi-Far R, White MA, Westwick JK, Solski PA, Chrzanowska-Wodnicka M, Van Aelst L, et al. Oncogenic Ras activation of Raf/mitogen-activated protein kinase-independent pathways is sufficient to cause tumorigenic transformation. *Mol Cell Biol* 1996; 16:3923–3933.
65. Oldham SM, Clark GJ, Gangarosa LM, Coffey RJ Jr, Der CJ. Activation of the Raf-1/MAP kinase cascade is not sufficient for Ras transformation of RIE-1 epithelial cells. *Proc Natl Acad Sci USA* 1996; 93:6924–6928.
66. Carpenter CL, Cantley LC. Phosphoinositide kinases. *Curr Opin Cell Biol* 1996; 8:153–158.
67. Corvera S, Czech MP. Direct targets of phosphoinositide 3-kinase products in membrane traffic and signal transduction. *Trends Cell Biol* 1998; 8:442–446.
68. Rodriguez-Viciana P, Warne PH, Khwaja A, Marte BM, Pappin D, Das P, et al. Role of Phosphoinositide 3-OH kinase in cell transformation and control of the actin cytoskeleton by Ras. *Cell* 1997; 89:457–467.
69. Zhang QX, Davis ID, Baldwin GS. Controlled overexpression of selected domains of the P85 subunit of phosphatidylinositol 3-kinase reverts v-Ha-Ras transformation. *Biochim Biophys Acta* 1996; 1312:207–214.

70. Oldham SM, Cox AD, Reynolds ER, Sizemore NS, Coffey RJ Jr, Der CJ. Ras, but not Src, transformation of RIE-1 epithelial cells is dependent on activation of the mitogen-activated protein kinase cascade. *Oncogene* 1998; 16:2565–2573.

71. Alessi DR, Cohen P. Mechanism of activation and function of protein kinase B. *Curr Opin Genet Dev* 1998; 8:55–62.

72. Frisch SM, Francis H. Disruption of epithelial cell-matrix interactions induces apoptosis. *J Cell Biol* 1994; 124:619–626.

73. Khwaja A, Rodriguez-Viciana P, Wennstrom S, Warne PH, Downward J. Matrix adhesion and Ras transformation both activate a phosphoinositide 3-OH kinase and protein kinase B/Akt cellular survival pathway. *EMBO J* 1997; 16:2783–2793.

74. Shao H, Andres DA. A novel RalGEF-like protein, RGL3, as a candidate effector for rit and Ras. *J Biol Chem* 2000; 275:26914–26924.

75. Feig LA, Urano T, Cantor S. Evidence for a Ras/Ral signaling cascade. *Trends Biochem Sci* 1996; 21:438–441.

76. Matsubara K, Kishida S, Matsuura Y, Kitayama H, Noda M, Kikuchi A. Plasma membrane recruitment of RalGDS is critical for Ras-dependent Ral activation. *Oncogene* 1999; 18:1303–1312.

77. Okazaki M, Kishida S, Murai H, Hinoi T, Kikuchi A. Ras-interacting domain of Ral GDP dissociation stimulator like (RGL) reverses v-Ras-induced transformation and Raf-1 activation in NIH3T3 cells. *Cancer Res* 1996; 56:2387–2392.

78. Peterson SN, Trabalzini L, Brtva TR, Fischer T, Altschuler DL, Martelli P, et al. Identification of a novel RalGDS-related protein as a candidate effector for Ras and Rap1. *J Biol Chem* 1996; 271:29903–29908.

79. Urano T, Emkey R, Feig LA. Ral-GTPases mediate a distinct downstream signaling pathway from Ras that facilitates cellular transformation. *EMBO J* 1996; 15:810–816.

80. White MA, Vale T, Camonis JH, Schaefer E, Wigler MH. A role for the Ral guanine nucleotide dissociation stimulator in mediating Ras-induced transformation. *J Biol Chem* 1996; 271:16439–16442.

81. de Ruiter ND, Wolthuis RM, van Dam H, Burgering BM, Bos JL. Ras-dependent regulation of c-Jun phosphorylation is mediated by the ral guanine nucleotide exchange factor-Ral pathway. *Mol Cell Biol* 2000; 20:8480–8488.

82. Okazaki M, Kishida S, Hinoi T, Hasegawa T, Tamada M, Kataoka T, et al. Synergistic activation of c-fos promoter activity by Raf and Ral GDP dissociation stimulator. *Oncogene* 1997; 14:515–521.

83. Henry DO, Moskalenko SA, Kaur KJ, Fu M, Pestell RG, Camonis JH, et al. GTPases contribute to regulation of cyclin D1 through activation of NF-kappaB. *Mol Cell Biol* 2000; 20:8084–8092.

84. Cantor SB, Urano T, Feig LA. Identification and characterization of Ral-binding protein 1, a potential downstream target of Ral GTPases. *Mol Cell Biol* 1995; 15:4578–4584.

85. Vos MD, Ellis CA, Bell A, Birrer MJ, Clark GJ. Ras uses the novel tumor suppressor RASSF1 as an effector to mediate apoptosis. *J Biol Chem* 2000; 275:35669–35672.

86. Kelley GG, Reks SE, Ondrako JM, Smrcka AV. Phospholipase C(epsilon): a novel Ras effector. *EMBO J* 2001; 20:743–754.

87. Yamamoto T, Taya S, Kaibuchi K. Ras-induced transformation and signaling pathway. *J Biochem (Tokyo)* 1999; 126:799–803.

88. Han L, Colicelli J. A human protein selected for interference with Ras function interacts directly with Ras and competes with Raf1. *Mol Cell Biol* 1995; 15:1318–1323.

89. Han L, Wong D, Dhaka A, Afar D, White M, Xie W, et al. Protein binding and signaling properties of RINI suggest a unique effector function. *Proc Natl Acad Sci USA* 1997; 94:4954–4959.

90. Dammann R, Li C, Yoon JH, Chin PL, Bates S, Pfeifer GP. Epigenetic inactivation of a RAS association domain family protein from the lung tumour suppressor locus 3p21.3. *Nat Genet* 2000; 25:315–319.

91. Fleischman LF, Chahwala SB, Cantley L. ras-transformed cells: altered levels of phosphatidylinositol-4,5-bisphosphate and catabolites. *Science* 1986; 231:407–410.

92. Adari H, Lowy DR, Willumsen BM, Der CJ, McCormick F. Guanosine triphosphatase activating protein (GAP) interacts with the p21 ras effector binding domain. *Science* 1988; 240:518–521.

93. DeClue JE, Stone JC, Blanchard RA, Papageorge AG, Martin P, Zhang K, et al. A ras effector domain mutant which is temperature sensitive for cellular transformation: interactions with GTPase-activating protein and NF-1. *Mol Cell Biol* 1991; 11:3132–3138.

94. Kjoller L, Hall A. Signaling to Rho GTPases. *Exp Cell Res* 1999; 253:166–179.

95. Bar-Sagi D, Hall A. Ras and Rho GTPases: a family reunion. *Cell* 2000; 103:227–238.

96. Zohn IM, Campbell SL, Khosravi-Far R, Rossman KL, Der CJ. Rho family proteins and Ras transformation: the RHOad less traveled gets congested. *Oncogene* 1998; 17:1415–1438.

97. Murphy GA, Solski PA, Jillian SA, Perez de la Ossa P, D'Eustachio P, Der CJ, et al. Cellular functions of TC10, a Rho family GTPase: regulation of morphology, signal transduction and cell growth. *Oncogene* 1999; 18:3831–45.

98. Prendergast GC, Khosravi-Far R, Solski PA, Kurzawa H, Lebowitz PF, Der CJ. Critical role of Rho in cell transformation by oncogenic Ras. *Oncogene* 1995; 10:2289–2296.

99. Qiu RG, Chen J, McCormick F, Symons M. A role for Rho in Ras transformation. *Proc Natl Acad Sci USA* 1995; 92:11781–11785.

100. Roux P, Gauthier-Rouviere C, Doucet-Brutin S, Fort P. The small GTPases Cdc42Hs, Rac1 and RhoG delineate Raf-independent pathways that cooperate to transform NIH3T3 cells. *Curr Biol* 1997; 7:629–637.

101. Lebowitz PF, Du W, Prendergast GC. Prenylation of RhoB is required for its cell transforming function but not its ability to activate serum response element-dependent transcription. *J Biol Chem* 1997; 272:16093–16095.

102. Zhong C, Kinch MS, Burridge K. Rho-stimulated contractility contributes to the fibroblastic phenotype of Ras-transformed epithelial cells. *Mol Biol Cell* 1997; 8:2329–2344.

103. Zondag GC, Evers EE, ten Klooster JP, Janssen L, van der Kammen RA, Collard JG. Oncogenic Ras downregulates Rac activity, which leads to increased Rho activity and epithelial-mesenchymal transition. *J Cell Biol* 2000; 149:775–782.

104. Olson MF, Paterson HF, Marshall CJ. Signals from Ras and Rho GTPases interact to regulate expression of p21WAF1/CIP1. *Nature* 1998; 394:295–299.

105. Sklar MD, Thompson E, Welsh MJ, Liebert M, Harney J, Grossman HB, et al. Depletion of c-myc with specific antisense sequences reverses the transformed phenotype in ras oncogene-transformed NIH 3T3 cells. *Mol Cell Biol* 1991; 11:3699–3710.

106. Langer SJ, Bortner DM, Roussel MF, Sherr CJ, Ostrowski MC. Mitogenic signaling by colony-stimulating factor 1 and ras is suppressed by the ets-2 DNA-binding domain and restored by myc overexpression. *Mol Cell Biol* 1992; 12:5355–5362.

107. Wasylyk C, Maira SM, Sobieszczuk P, Wasylyk B. Reversion of Ras transformed cells by Ets transdominant mutants. *Oncogene* 1994; 9:3665–3673.

108. Wick M, Lucibello FC, Muller R. Inhibition of Fos- and Ras-induced transformation by mutant Fos proteins with structural alterations in functionally different domains. *Oncogene* 1992; 7:859–867.

109. Granger-Schnarr M, Benusiglio E, Schnarr M, Sassone-Corsi P. Transformation and transactivation suppressor activity of the c-Jun leucine zipper fused to a bacterial repressor. *Proc Natl Acad Sci USA* 1992; 89:4236–4239.

110. Johnson R, Spiegelman B, Hanahan D, Wisdom R. Cellular transformation and malignancy induced by ras require c-jun. *Mol Cell Biol* 1996; 16:4504–4511.

111. Saez E, Rutberg SE, Mueller E, Oppenheim H, Smoluk J, Yuspa SH, et al. c-fos is required for malignant progression of skin tumors. *Cell* 1995; 82:721–732.

112. Finco TS, Westwick JK, Norris JL, Beg AA, Der CJ, Baldwin AS Jr. Oncogenic Ha-Ras-induced signaling activates NF-kappaB transcriptional activity, which is required for cellular transformation. *J Biol Chem* 1997; 272:24113–24116.

113. Mayo MW, Wang CY, Cogswell PC, Rogers-Graham KS, Lowe SW, Der CJ, et al. Requirement of NF-kappaB activation to suppress p53-independent apoptosis induced by oncogenic Ras. *Science* 1997; 278:1812–1815.

114. Marshall CJ, Vousden K, Ozanne B. The involvement of activated ras genes in determining the transformed phenotype. *Proc R Soc Lond B Biol Sci* 1985; 226:99–106.

115. Ciardiello F, Kim N, Hynes N, Jaggi R, Redmond S, Liscia DS, et al. Induction of transforming growth factor alpha expression in mouse mammary epithelial cells after transformation with a point-mutated c-Ha-ras protooncogene. *Mol Endocrinol* 1988; 2:1202–1216.

116. Godwin AK, Lieberman MW. Early and late responses to induction of rasT24 expression in Rat-1 cells. *Oncogene* 1990; 5:1231–1241.

117. Glick AB, Sporn MB, Yuspa SH. Altered regulation of TGF-beta 1 and TGF-alpha in primary keratinocytes and papillomas expressing v-Ha-ras. *Mol Carcinog* 1991; 4:210–219.

118. Gangarosa LM, Sizemore N, Graves-Deal R, Oldham SM, Der CJ, Coffey RJ. A raf-independent epidermal growth factor receptor autocrine loop is necessary for Ras transformation of rat intestinal epithelial cells. *J Biol Chem* 1997; 272:18926–18931.

119. Ciardiello F, McGeady ML, Kim N, Basolo F, Hynes N, Langton BC, et al. Transforming growth factor-alpha expression is enhanced in human mammary epithelial cells transformed by an activated c-

Ha-ras protooncogene but not by the c-neu protooncogene, and overexpression of the transforming growth factor-alpha complementary DNA leads to transformation. *Cell Growth Differ* 1990; 1:407–420.

120. Basolo F, Serra C, Ciardiello F, Fiore L, Russo J, Campani D, et al. Regulation of surface-differentiation molecules by epidermal growth factor, transforming growth factor alpha, and hydrocortisone in human mammary epithelial cells transformed by an activated c-Ha-ras proto-oncogene. *Int J Cancer* 1992; 51:634–640.

121. Rodriguez-Puebla ML, Robles AI, Conti CJ. ras activity and cyclin D1 expression: an essential mechanism of mouse skin tumor development. *Mol Carcinog* 1999; 24:1–6.

122. Marshall C. How do small GTPase signal transduction pathways regulate cell cycle entry? *Curr Opin Cell Biol* 1999; 11:732–736.

123. Sherr CJ, Roberts JM. Inhibitors of mammalian G1 cyclin-dependent kinases. *Genes Dev* 1995; 9:1149–1163.

124. Arber N, Sutter T, Miyake M, Kahn SM, Venkatraj VS, Sobrino A, et al. Increased expression of cyclin D1 and the Rb tumor suppressor gene in c-K-ras transformed rat enterocytes. *Oncogene* 1996; 12:1903–1908.

125. Filmus J, Robles AI, Shi W, Wong MJ, Colombo LL, Conti CJ. Induction of cyclin D1 overexpression by activated ras. *Oncogene* 1994; 9:3627–3633.

126. Liu JJ, Chao JR, Jiang MC, Ng SY, Yen JJ, Yang-Yen HF. Ras transformation results in an elevated level of cyclin D1 and acceleration of G1 progression in NIH 3T3 cells. *Mol Cell Biol* 1995; 15:3654–3663.

127. Winston JT, Coats SR, Wang YZ, Pledger WJ. Regulation of the cell cycle machinery by oncogenic ras. *Oncogene* 1996; 12:127–134.

128. Aktas H, Cai H, Cooper GM. Ras links growth factor signaling to the cell cycle machinery via regulation of cyclin D1 and the Cdk inhibitor p27KIP1. *Mol Cell Biol* 1997; 17:3850–3857.

129. Yang N, Higuchi O, Ohashi K, Nagata K, Wada A, Kangawa K, et al. Cofilin phosphorylation by LIM-kinase 1 and its role in Rac-mediated actin reogranization. *Nature* 1998; 393:809.

130. Pruitt K, Pestell RG, Der CJ. Ras inactivation of the retinoblastoma pathway by distinct mechanisms in NIH 3T3 fibroblast and RIE-1 epithelial cells. *J Biol Chem* 2000; 275:40916–40924.

131. Albanese C, Johnson J, Watanabe G, Eklund N, Vu D, Arnold A, et al. Transforming p21ras mutants and c-Ets-2 activate the cyclin D1 promoter through distinguishable regions. *J Biol Chem* 1995; 270:23589–23597.

132. Frisch SM, Francis H. Disruption of epithelial cell-matrix interactions induces apoptosis. *J Cell Biol* 1994; 124:619–626.

133. Williams CS, Mann M, DuBois RN. The role of cyclooxygenases in inflammation, cancer, and development. *Oncogene* 1999; 18:7908–7916.

134. Vadlamudi R, Mandal M, Adam L, Steinbach G, Mendelsohn J, Kumar R. Regulation of cyclooxygenase-2 pathway by HER2 receptor. *Oncogene* 1999; 18:305–314.

135. Sheng H, Williams CS, Shao J, Liang P, DuBois RN, Beauchamp RD. Induction of cyclooxygenase-2 by activated Ha-ras oncogene in Rat-1 fibroblasts and the role of mitogen-activated protein kinase pathway. *J Biol Chem* 1998; 273:22120–22127.

136. Sheng H, Shao J, Dixon DA, Williams CS, Prescott SM, DuBois RN, et al. Transforming growth factor-beta1 enhances Ha-ras induced expression of cyclooxygenase-2 in intestinal epithelial cells via stabilization of mRNA. *J Biol Chem* 2000; 275:6628–6635.

137. Subbaramaiah K, Telang N, Bansal MB, Weksler BB, Dannenberg AJ. Cyclooxygenase-2 gene expression is upregulated in transformed mammary epithelial cells. *Ann NY Acad Sci* 1997; 833:179–185.

138. Simmons DL, Levy DB, Yannoni Y, Erikson RL. Identification of a phorbol ester-repressible v-src-inducible gene. *Proc Natl Acad Sci USA* 1989; 86:1178–1182.

139. Sheng GG, Shao J, Sheng H, Hooton EB, Isakson PC, Morrow JD, et al. A selective cyclooxygenase 2 inhibitor suppresses the growth of H-ras-transformed rat intestinal epithelial cells. *Gastroenterology* 1997; 113:1883–1891.

140. Shao J, Sheng H, Inoue H, Morrow JD, DuBois RN. Regulation of constitutive cyclooxygenase-2 expression in colon carcinoma cells. *J Biol Chem* 2000; 275:33951–33956.

141. Mestre JR, Rivadeneira DE, Mackrell PJ, Duff M, Stapleton PP, Mack-Strong V, et al. Overlapping CRE and E-box promoter elements can independently regulate COX-2 gene transcription in macrophages. *FEBS Lett* 2001; 496:147–151.

142. Sheng H, Shao J, O'Mahony CA, Lamps L, Albo D, Isakson PC, et al. Transformation of intestinal epithelial cells by chronic TGF-beta1 treatment results in downregulation of the type II TGF-beta receptor and induction of cyclooxygenase-2. *Oncogene* 1999; 18:855–867.

143. Tsujii M, DuBois RN. Alterations in cellular adhesion and apoptosis in epithelial cells overexpressing prostaglandin endoperoxide synthase 2. *Cell* 1995; 83:493–501.

144. Baum G, Suh BS, Amsterdam A, Ben Ze'ev A. Regulation of tropomyosin expression in transformed granulosa cell lines with steroidogenic ability. *Dev Biol* 1990; 142:115–128.

145. Prasad GL, Fuldner RA, Cooper HL. Expression of transduced tropomyosin 1 cDNA suppresses neoplastic growth of cells transformed by the ras oncogene. *Proc Natl Acad Sci USA* 1993; 90:7039–7043.

146. Gimona M, Kazzaz JA, Helfman DM. Forced expression of tropomyosin 2 or 3 in v-Ki-ras-transformed fibroblasts results in distinct phenotypic effects. *Proc Natl Acad Sci USA* 1996; 93:9618–9623.

147. Ljungdah1 S, Linder S, Franzen B, Binetruy B, Auer G, Shoshan MC. Down-regulation of tropomyosin-2 expression in c-Jun-transformed rat fibroblasts involves induction of a MEK1-dependent autocrine loop. *Cell Growth Differ* 1998; 9:565–573.

148. Janssen RA, Veenstra KG, Jonasch P, Jonasch E, Mier JW. Ras- and Raf-induced down-modulation of non-muscle tropomyosin are MEK-independent. *J Biol Chem* 1998; 273:32182–32186.

149. Bamburg JR, McGough A, Ono S. Putting a new twist on actin: ADF/cofilins modulate actin dynamics. *Trends Cell Biol* 1999; 9:364–370.

150. Shields, JM, Mehta H, Der CJ. DNA methylation, an opposing roles of the ERK and p38 mitogen-activated protein kinase cascades, in Ras-mediated downregulation of tropomyosin, *Mol Cell Biol* 2002; 22:2304–2317.

151. Prasad GL, Fuldner RA, Cooper HL. Expression of transduced tropomyosin 1 cDNA suppresses neoplastic growth of cells transformed by the ras oncogene. *Proc Natl Acad Sci USA* 1993; 90:7039–7043.

152. Himelstein BP, Canete-Soler R, Bernhard EJ, Dilks DW, Muschel RJ. Metalloproteinases in tumor progression: the contribution of MMP-9. *Invasion Metastasis* 1994; 14:246–258.

153. Matrisian LM. Cancer biology: extracellular proteinases in malignancy. *Curr Biol* 1999; 9:R776–R778.

154. Hernandez-Alcoceba R, del Peso L, Lacal JC. The Ras family of GTPases in cancer cell invasion. *Cell Mol Life Sci* 2000; 57:65–76.

155. MacDougall JR, Matrisian LM. Contributions of tumor and stromal matrix metalloproteinases to tumor progression, invasion and metastasis. *Cancer Metastasis Rev* 1995; 14:351–362.

156. Duffy MJ, McCarthy K. Matrix metalloproteinases in cancer: prognostic markers and targets for therapy. *Int J Oncol* 1998; 12:1343–1348.

157. Shapiro SD. Matrix metalloproteinase degradation of extracellular matrix: biological consequences. *Curr Opin Cell Biol* 1998; 10:602–608.

158. Westermarck J, Kahari VM. Regulation of matrix metalloproteinase expression in tumor invasion. *FASEB J* 1999; 13:781–792.

159. Chambers AF, Tuck AB. Ras-responsive genes and tumor metastasis. *Crit Rev Oncog* 1993; 4:95–114.

160. Bortner DM, Langer SJ, Ostrowski MC. Non-nuclear oncogenes and the regulation of gene expression in transformed cells. *Crit Rev Oncog* 1993; 4:137–160.

161. Giambernardi TA, Grant GM, Taylor GP, Hay RJ, Maher VM, McCormick JJ, et al. Overview of matrix metalloproteinase expression in cultured human cells. *Matrix Biol* 1998; 16:483–496.

162. Yanagihara K, Nii M, Tsumuraya M, Numoto M, Seito T, Seyama T. A radiation-induced murine ovarian granulosa cell tumor line: introduction of v-ras gene potentiates a high metastatic ability. *Jpn J Cancer Res* 1995; 86:347–356.

163. Ballin M, Gomez DE, Sinha CC, Thorgeirsson UP. Ras oncogene mediated induction of a 92 kDa metalloproteinase; strong correlation with the malignant phenotype. *Biochem Biophys Res Commun* 1988; 154:832–838.

164. Himelstein BP, Lee EJ, Sato H, Seiki M, Muschel RJ. Transcriptional activation of the matrix metalloproteinase-9 gene in an H-ras and v-myc transformed rat embryo cell line. *Oncogene* 1997; 14:1995–1998.

165. Bernhard EJ, Hagner B, Wong C, Lubenski I, Muschel RJ. The effect of E1A transfection on MMP-9 expression and metastatic potential. *Int J Cancer* 1995; 60:718–724.

166. Thorgeirsson UP, Turpeenniemi-Hujanen T, Williams JE, Westin EH, Heilman CA, Talmadge JE, et al. NIH/3T3 cells transfected with human tumor DNA containing activated ras oncogenes express the metastatic phenotype in nude mice. *Mol Cell Biol* 1985; 5:259–262.

167. Bernhard EJ, Muschel RJ, Hughes EN. Mr 92,000 gelatinase release correlates with the metastatic phenotype in transformed rat embryo cells. *Cancer Res* 1990; 50:3872–3877.

168. Garbisa S, Negro A, Kalebic T, Pozzatti R, Muschel R, Saffiotti U, et al. Type IV collagenolytic activity linkage with the metastatic phenotype induced by ras transfection. *Adv Exp Med Biol* 1988; 233:179–186.

169. Sehgal G, Hua J, Bernhard EJ, Sehgal I, Thompson TC, Muschel RJ. Requirement for matrix metalloproteinase-9 (gelatinase B) expression in metastasis by murine prostate carcinoma. *Am J Pathol* 1998; 152:591–596.

170. Garzetti GG, Ciavattini A, Lucarini G, Goteri G, Nictolis MD, Romanini C, et al. Ras p21 immunostaining in early stage squamous cervical carcinoma: relationship with lymph nodal involvement and 72 kDa-metalloproteinase index. *Anticancer Res* 1998; 18:609–613.

171. Yamamoto H, Itoh F, Senota A, Adachi Y, Yoshimoto M, Endoh T, et al. Expression of matrix metalloproteinase matrilysin (MMP-7) was induced by activated Ki-ras via AP-1 activation in SW1417 colon cancer cells. *J Clin Lab Anal* 1995; 9:297–301.

172. Matrisian LM, McDonnell S, Miller DB, Navre M, Seftor EA, Hendrix MJ. The role of the matrix metalloproteinase stromelysin in the progression of squamous cell carcinomas. *Am J Med Sci* 1991; 302:157–162.

173. Rak J, Mitsuhashi Y, Bayko L, Filmus J, Shirasawa S, Sasazuki T, et al. Mutant ras oncogenes upregulate VEGF/VPF expression: implications for induction and inhibition of tumor angiogenesis. *Cancer Res* 1995; 55:4575–4580.

174. Konishi T, Huang CL, Adachi M, Taki T, Inufusa H, Kodama K, et al. The K-ras gene regulates vascular endothelial growth factor gene expression in non-small cell lung cancers. *Int J Oncol* 2000; 16:501–511.

175. White FC, Benehacene A, Scheele JS, Kamps M. VEGF mRNA is stabilized by ras and tyrosine kinase oncogenes, as well as by UV radiation—evidence for divergent stabilization pathways. *Growth Factors* 1997; 14:199–212.

176. Risau W. Mechanisms of angiogenesis. *Nature* 1997; 386:671–674.

177. Arbiser JL, Moses MA, Fernandez CA, Ghiso N, Cao Y, Klauber N, et al. Oncogenic H-ras stimulates tumor angiogenesis by two distinct pathways. *Proc Natl Acad Sci USA* 1997; 94:861–866.

178. Grugel S, Finkenzeller G, Weindel K, Barleon B, Marme D. Both v-Ha-Ras and v-Raf stimulate expression of the vascular endothelial growth factor in NIH 3T3 cells. *J Biol Chem* 1995; 270:25915–25919.

179. Milanini J, Vinals F, Pouyssegur J, Pages G. p42/p44 MAP kinase module plays a key role in the transcriptional regulation of the vascular endothelial growth factor gene in fibroblasts. *J Biol Chem* 1998; 273:18165–18172.

180. Mazure NM, Chen EY, Laderoute KR, Giaccia AJ. Induction of vascular endothelial growth factor by hypoxia is modulated by a phosphatidylinositol 3-kinase/Akt signaling pathway in Ha-ras-transformed cells through a hypoxia inducible factor-1 transcriptional element. *Blood* 1997; 90:3322–3331.

181. Pal S, Datta K, Khosravi-Far R, Mukhopadhyay D. Role of PKC z in Ras-mediated transcriptional activation of vascular permeability factor/vascular endothelial growth factor expression. *J Biol Chem* 2001; 276:2395–2403.

182. Okada F, Rak JW, Croix BS, Lieubeau B, Kaya M, Roncari L, et al. Impact of oncogenes in tumor angiogenesis: mutant K-ras up-regulation of vascular endothelial growth factor/vascular permeability factor is necessary, but not sufficient for tumorigenicity of human colorectal carcinoma cells. *Proc Natl Acad Sci USA* 1998; 95:3609–3614.

183. Chin L, Tam A, Pomerantz J, Wong M, Holash J, Bardeesy N, et al. Essential role for oncogenic Ras in tumour maintenance. *Nature* 1999; 400:468–472.

184. Liang P, Pardee AB. Differential display of eukaryotic messenger RNA by means of the polymerase chain reaction. *Science* 1992; 257:967–971.

185. Diatchenko L, Lau YF, Campbell AP, Chenchik A, Moqadam F, Huang B, et al. Suppression subtractive hybridization: a method for generating differentially regulated of tissue-specific cDNA probes and libraries. *Proc Natl Acad Sci USA* 1996; 93:6025–6030.

186. Shirasawa S, Furuse M, Yokoyama N, Sasazuki T. Altered growth of human colon cancer cell lines disrupted at activated Ki-ras. *Science* 1993; 260:85–88.

187. Lewis TS, Hunt JB, Aveline LD, Jonscher KR, Louie DF, Yeh JM, et al. Identification of novel MAP kinase pathway signaling targets by functional proteomics and mass spectrometry. *Mol Cell* 2000; 6:1343–1354.

188. Alton G, Cox AD, Toussaint LG III, Westwick JK. Functional proteomics analysis of GTPase signaling networks. *Methods Enzymol* 2001; 332:300–316.

6

The Interplay Between Tumor Suppressor Genes and Oncogenes in Tumorigenesis

Eric C. Holland, MD, PhD

CONTENTS

1. INTRODUCTION

One of the great cornerstones of our understanding of cancer biology was the realization that cancer-causing genes are intrinsic to our own genome, and therefore, cancer comes from within. These genes promote cancer formation by their inappropriately elevated expression or by their failure to produce functional protein products. They encode biological pathways, and mutations of these genes results in dysregulation of these pathways. These alterations do not act alone, but cooperate to form cancer in ways that we are just beginning to understand. Hopefully, this knowledge will lead to rational mechanistic treatment strategies.

2. ONCOGENES AND TUMOR SUPPRESSORS

Throughout the early part of the 20th century, many investigators showed that some RNA viruses were capable of causing cancer in experimental animals *(1)*. Subsequently, it was demonstrated that these viruses could transform cells into a neoplastic phenotype in culture *(2)*. Encoded by these viruses were genes that, when expressed, induced neoplastic changes and, therefore, were referred to as oncogenes. A startling realization came with the recognition that src, the best-studied oncogene of the time,

From: *Oncogene-Directed Therapies*
Edited by: J. W. Rak © Humana Press Inc., Totowa, NJ

encoded by the rous sarcoma virus (RSV), had a homolog in the host's genome *(3)*. In the process of infecting the host cell, at some point earlier in evolution, RSV appeared to have stolen the src gene from the host animal and inappropriately expressed this gene in infected cells with a result of cancer formation. Following this discovery, the initial observation was extended to a more general principal when other virally encoded oncogenes were shown to be derived from cellular homolog's. These cellular genes were subsequently designated proto-oncogenes to distinguish them from their viral counterparts *(4)*. Cellularly derived proto-oncogenes frequently encode proteins that function normally to control the balance between cell proliferation and cell death. The viral oncogenes achieve their neoplastic effect by a gain of function; these genes are expressed in the wrong place at the wrong time or at inappropriate levels.

As the function of the proto-oncogenes were identified, an important clue to the underlying biology of cancer began to immerge. The protein products of these proto-oncogenes frequently function in the signal transduction cascades that cells use to transmit information between themselves during the rapid proliferation and patterning that occurs in embryonic development. In the normal developmental process, the expansion of cell populations is carefully controlled by communication between cells with growth factors and cell-to-cell contact. Secreted growth factors and membrane-bound signaling ligands bind to the extracellular portion of cell surface receptors and activate intracellular enzymatic processes. The activation progresses through many pathways of sequential cytoplasmic proteins and eventually results in the modification of transcription in the nucleus and translation in the cytoplasm. The genes that encode the members of these cascades are the proto-oncogenes, and expression of the viral forms of these genes (often mutated or constitutively active) results in the inappropriate activation of these signal transduction pathways. In essence, cells expressing these oncogenes misinterpret external environment and proliferate inappropriately. The fact that so many different cancer causing genes have been conscribed by these viruses and that the cellular homologs of these genes usually encode signal transduction pathway components emphasizes the importance of these pathways in oncogenesis.

The next intellectual breakthrough in our understanding of the biology of cancer was the realization that not only was cancer formation driven by the gain of function generated by the expression of oncogenes, but in addition, there appeared to be anti-oncogenes, or tumor suppressors, that functioned to inhibit oncogenic transformation *(5)*. The loss of these genes appeared to contribute to the formation of cancer. This phenomenon is best seen in families with predisposition to cancer and is well illustrated by the inherited predisposition to the formation of retinoblastoma. The susceptibility to form retinal tumors is inherited as a dominant trait. Classical genetic inheritance of dominant traits usually implies a gain of function of a single allele that produces an effect. At first glance, the inheritance pattern of families with predisposition to retinoblastoma might imply that they have an activation germline mutation in a proto-oncogene that is inherited as a gain of function allele. However, mapping of the gene locus responsible for this genetic predisposition identified the retinoblastoma gene (Rb), and these families pass the tumor susceptibility via disruption of one allele of the Rb locus (and therefore are heterozygous at this locus) *(6)*. These individuals develop normally due to the function of the remaining allele; however, these patients invariable develop retinoblastomas, usually bilaterally. The remaining allele is lost, and therefore, no functional Rb is produced in these cells *(7)*. The gene expression alterations appear to contribute to the formation of cancer, and the cells of the retina in humans appear exquisitely sensitive. Therefore, although loss of a tumor suppressor gene is recessive on a cell by cell basis, it is dominant on an organismal basis because of the secondary mutations that invariable occur in a few cells within a large population of susceptible cells.

Several other syndromes of familially inherited predisposition to cancer have been investigated, and their causative genes have been mapped and identified. These genes encode proteins referred to as tumor suppressors because their function suppresses tumor formation. Many of the known tumor suppressor genes encode proteins involved with G1 cell cycle arrest, such as Rb, p53, and the *INK4a-ARF* gene products p16 and p14 *(8)*. These pathways are not active during embryonic development, consistent with the rapid proliferation of cells during that time. In mice, the *INK4a-ARF* gene products p16 and p19 begin to be expressed around the time of birth with the reduction in cellular proliferation *(9)*. Dysregulation of these pathways by loss of these tumor suppressors is extremely common in malignant tumors, and in some tumor types reaches nearly 100% *(10)*.

Not all genes that function to suppress transformation act in the cell cycle arrest pathways. Some tumor suppressors function to inhibit signaling through the same signal transduction pathways that are activated by oncogene products. For example, the tumor suppressor involved with neurofibromatosis type 1 (NF-1) normally functions to inhibit the activity of Ras *(11)*. NF-1 loss elevates Ras activity and probably contributes to oncogenesis in that manner. The tumor suppressor gene PTEN is a phosphatase that inhibits the ability of PI3K to activate Akt. PTEN loss is, therefore, correlated with elevated Akt activity *(12)*. The existence of tumor suppressors that act in the signal transduction pathways further emphasize the importance of elevated activity in these signaling pathways in the formation of tumors. Still other tumor suppressor genes encode proteins involved in other biologic processes. For example, BRCA 1 is involved in chromosomal stability *(13)*, while NF-2 integrates the cellular shape and internal structure with proliferation rates *(14)*. Therefore, dysregulation of many functions can contribute to tumor formation or progression.

For unclear reasons, different tumor types tend to activate critical pathways in different ways. A particular tumor will have favorite oncogenes or tumor suppressors to achieve what appears to be the same biologic output. For example, Ras signaling is very commonly elevated in many tumor types, but the mechanism for achieving that outcome varies. In lung tumors, Ras activity is frequently elevated by the expression of a mutant constitutively active Ras *(15)*. In neurofibromas, as mentioned above, Ras activity is elevated by the loss of the RasGap NF-1 tumor suppressor, which normally inhibits Ras activity. In high-grade gliomas, while Ras is essentially never mutated, its activity is elevated by signaling from upstream tyrosine kinase receptors *(16)*. The reason for the mechanistic specificity is not clear at this time, but is undoubtedly central to the biology of these tumor types (Fig. 1). Such examples further emphasize the importance of the pathways these oncoproteins and tumor suppressors comprise.

3. MULTIPLE EVENTS COOPERATE IN THE FORMATION OF CANCER

In 1971, Knutson proposed that cancer required two distinct events to occur *(17)*. This "two hit hypothesis" originally proposed that loss of both alleles of a tumor sup-

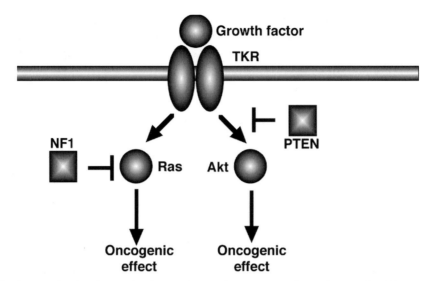

Fig. 1. Oncogenic signal transduction pathways downstream of protein tyrosine kinase receptors. EGFR platelet-derived growth factor receptor (PDGFR), insulin-like growth factor receptor (IGFR), and other tyrosine kinase receptors that recognize growth factors activate several pathways that have oncogenic effects. Illustrated here are the pathways involving Ras and Akt. Proteins with oncogenic effects, and encoded by proto-oncogenes, are illustrated as round. Proteins that inhibit the activity of these pathways and are encoded by tumor suppressor genes, are square.

pressor gene were required for tumor formation. In families with inherited loss of one allele, loss of the second allele occurs somatically, enabling transformation. This hypothesis deals with the two-stage inactivation of a single gene. However, as we now know, cancer is more complicated than the result of dysregulated output of a single gene. Since Knutson's original proposal, the two hit hypothesis has been expanded and adapted based on our ever-expanding knowledge of the oncogenic process.

In 1983, based on cell culture experiments, Weinberg and coworkers demonstrated that Ras could cooperate with either Myc or Simian Virus 40 (SV40)T antigen (blocking Rb and p53 function) to induce transformation in cultured rat fibroblasts, in which Ras or Myc alone was insufficient. Based on these experiments, he proposed that in order for transformation to occur, there needed to be a cytoplasmic and a nuclear oncogenic signal *(18)*. Binary combinations of oncogenic stimuli expressed as either nuclear vs cytoplasmic, signal transduction vs cell cycle arrest, or oncogene vs tumor suppressor, may constrain our thinking about biologic processes with artificial definitions. The important point is that multiple independent alterations seem to cooperate in the induction of transformation, and the biologic pathways that are affected by these genetic alterations appear to be causally related to the formation of the disease.

We need to remind ourselves that the ultimate effect of DNA mutations that occur is at the protein level. Although this is a well-known outcome of the central dogma, it is sometimes easy to forget that a mutation only has an effect (and is therefore is only selected for) if it changes the protein composition of the cell. Furthermore, mutations in the gene encoding a given protein are not the only way that a protein can be altered. For example, loss of expression for a protein can be caused not only by deletion of the gene, but it can also be due to methylation of a nonmutated gene resulting in the lack of its expression. Furthermore, most of these gene products are important in the biology of cancer because they have enzymatic activity, which is often regulated by upstream components of these pathways. It stands to reason that if inactivating mutations in a given gene are found in some reasonable percent of tumors analyzed, it is quite possible that this mutation frequency is an underrepresentation of the frequency that the pathway in which that protein functions is affected in the tumor population. In other words, by focusing only on DNA mutations, we may be underestimating the importance of specific pathways to cancer biology.

Whether a genetic alteration, that is found in a given percent of tumor samples, is causally related to tumor formation or simply an epiphenomenon of the tumor progression process is another matter. The observation that a given pathway is altered in a high percent of cancer specimens or cell lines does not mean that dysregulation of that pathway contributes to the etiology of the disease. For example, angiogenesis is required for a tumor of any reasonable size to form in vivo. The gene expression alterations that allow or drive the production of new blood vessels are, therefore, required for the progression of a tumor. However, simply inducing angiogenesis would not be expected to result in tumor formation. By contrast, other biologic abnormalities occurring within the tumor cells may, in fact, be necessary and sufficient to induce tumor formation in vivo. Being able to distinguish between these two possibilities is critical to identifying effective targets for therapy *(19)*.

4. COOPERATION BETWEEN ONCOGENES AND TUMOR SUPPRESSORS IN THE SAME PATHWAY

One mechanistic categorization of genetic alterations found in tumors is by the pathways in which the gene products function. Simply thinking of these genes as either oncogenes or tumor suppressors clouds the biologic processes to which these proteins contribute. The products of oncogenes and tumor suppressors that cooperate with each other can function in the same pathway and their respective gain or loss could reinforce the signaling abnormalities. Alternatively, these alterations may function in different pathways, and these pathways cooperate in tumor formation.

As pointed out previously, pathways that promote oncogenesis contain both positive and negative regulatory elements, which are frequently encoded by genes shown to be proto-oncogenes and tumor suppressors, respectively. Multiple alterations in the same pathway may either act to further activate a particular sub-branch or potentially block feedback loops that attempt to maintain homeostasis in the presence of the first mutation. For example, the signal transduction pathway initiated by tyrosine kinase receptors that proceed through PI3 kinase. PI3K is an oncogene, it is activated in the overactivity of this pathway and leads to the activation of AKT, which is also an oncogene (Fig. 1). Both PI3K and AKT are found in oncogenic viruses, and their gain of function can contribute to tumor formation *(20,21)*. The phosphatase PTEN also functions in this pathway by effectively blocking the ability for PI3K to activate AKT. PTEN's function is, therefore, counter to the two other oncogenes, and one might infer that it is a tumor suppressor. In fact, PTEN is a tumor suppressor by all criteria *(22)*. It was identified by deletion analysis in human tumors, and familial *PTEN* mutations result in Cowden's syndrome, which includes the formation of a number of cancer types *(23)*.

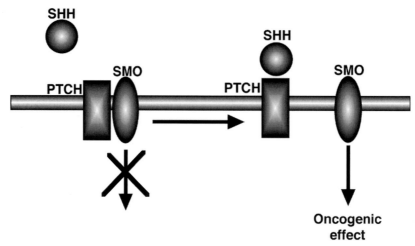

Fig. 2. Oncogenic signaling activated by SHH. The oncogenic effects of SHH are initiated by binding to PTCH, which releases a tonic inhibitory effect on SMO, resulting in activation of oncogenic signaling in some tumors, including medulloblastomas and basal cell carcinomas. SHH and SMO have oncogenic effects and are encoded by proto-oncogenes and are illustrated as round. PTCH is encoded by tumor suppressor genes and is square.

Another example of a signaling pathway, with both oncogenic and tumor suppressive components, is the signaling pathway activated by sonic hedgehog (SHH). SHH binds to its receptor patched (PTCH) and induces the floorplate during early embryonic development and also induces proliferation of cerebellar external granular cells *(24)*. Mechanistically, PTCH exerts a tonic inhibitory effect on smoothened (SMO), which is released by the binding of SHH. Therefore, SHH and SMO act as oncogenes, and PTCH is as a tumor suppressor *(25)*. Humans with inactivating germline mutations in *PTCH* (Gorlin's syndrome) develop a number of tumor types, including medulloblastomas *(26)*, and inactivating mutations in *PTCH* have been demonstrated in some sporadic medulloblastomas *(27)* (Fig. 2).

In addition, tumor suppressors and oncogenes that encode protein components of a given pathway also exist in control of cell cycle arrest. For example, the genes encoding p16 and Rb are both classical tumor suppressors. They are lost in human tumors, and the activity of their gene products inhibits tumor cell growth *(28)*. CDK4 functions in this pathway, and it is inhibited by p16 and, in turn, inactivates Rb. Because of this double negative control mechanism elevation of CDK4 activity is the equivalent of loss of p16 and Rb. In fact, CDK4 acts as an oncogene of sorts, as it is amplified in tumors (frequently the ones that do not have deletions of either p16 or Rb) *(29)* (Fig. 3).

Rather than thinking of genes as being oncogenic or tumor suppressive, it may be better to think of the pathways themselves as being oncogenic or tumor suppressive. For oncogenic pathways, mutations that activate the pathway are oncogenic, and those that inhibit the pathway are tumor suppressive. For tumor suppressive pathways the reverse is true.

Oncogenic cooperation between tumor suppressor gene products and onco-proteins, which function with a given pathway, is well documented. In these pathways, which contain oncogene and tumor suppressor gene products, such alterations may be capable of substituting for one another rather than cooperation with one another. However, the

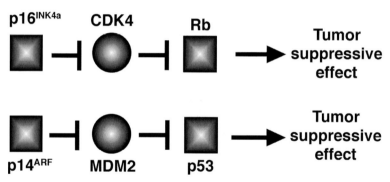

Fig. 3. Tumor suppressive signaling pathways leading to G1 cell cycle arrest. The INK4a-ARF gene encodes two tumor suppressor proteins that function to ultimately activate both p53 and Rb proteins. The control mechanisms for these pathways are a series of inhibitory functions as indicated. Proteins that activate these pathways and have tumor suppressive effects (are encoded by tumor suppressor genes) are illustrated as squares. MDM2 and CDK4, which inhibit the function of these pathways, have oncogenic effects and are illustrated as circles.

pathways are more complicated that simply being active or inactive. For example, in the transition between grade 3 and grade 4 gliomas, there are two mutations that are commonly encountered and are relative specific for grade 4 tumors. They are activating mutations and amplification of epidermal growth factor receptor (EGFR) and loss of PTEN *(30)*. One of the main functions of EGFR is to activate PI3 kinase. Loss of PTEN enhances the ability of PI3 kinase to activate Akt. Furthermore, if one analyzes the AKT activity of a series of grade 4 gliomas, one finds substantially elevated levels of Akt activity in these tumors relative to lower grade tumors *(31)*. These data do not imply that all of the AKT activity in these tumors is due to cooperation between EGFR and PTEN. Rather, AKT activity appears important for grade 4 glioma biology, and one way to achieve that goal is with cooperation between EGFR and PTEN.

5. COOPERATION BETWEEN ONCOGENES AND TUMOR SUPPRESSORS IN SEEMINGLY UNRELATED PATHWAYS

Demonstrating the oncogenic cooperation between seemingly unrelated pathways is more difficult, because there is not preexisting data leading to mechanistic hypotheses for the expected outcomes. Although it is necessary to demonstrate that two pathways are disrupted in the same tumor cells in order to validate the relevance of concurrent abnormalities to actual tumor biology, demonstration of concurrence of alterations is insufficient to prove cooperation between two pathways. It is quite possible the one or both of the pathways are an effect rather than a cause of the neoplastic phenotype. The only way to demonstrate cooperation in these circumstances is using experimental systems of tumor development.

Historically, genetic modification has been easier for cells in culture than for cells in living animals. Many experiments investigating the cooperation between oncogenes and tumor suppressors were done using transformation, the assay considered equivalent to tumor formation in vivo. Cultured cells undergoing transformation change their morphology, proliferated faster, lose contact-induced growth inhibition, and form colonies in soft agar. Although these same characteristics are found in tumor cells that have been transferred to culture, cultured tumor cells transformed cells in culture, and tumor cells in vivo have significant differences in gene expression profiles—potentially due to the different selective pressures placed on them over time. Therefore, it is not clear how many of the conclusions generated from cell culture experiments accurately reflect the molecular biology of tumor cells in a living animal. The advent of techniques that allow genetic modification of animals has allowed experiments that demonstrate cooperativity between oncogenic pathways using tumor formation as a biologic readout. Because of the relative ease of genetic manipulation and the significant numbers of genetically modified lines generated to date, the animal species used most frequently for these studies is the mouse. What follows are some vinets to illustrate the principles of interactions between apparently unrelated pathways in the formation of tumors in mice in vivo.

One of the earliest illustrations of cooperativeity in oncogenic pathways was the demonstration of the interaction between Wnt-1 and FGF3 signaling to generate mammary tumors. Initial studies using the mouse mammary tumor virus (MMTV)-generate mammary tumors showed the most common integration site for the MMTV was adjacent to the Wnt-1 gene resulting in its activation. The second most common site activated the gene encoding fibroblast growth factor 3 (FGF3). These data indicated that these pathways with no known common elements might independently contribute to the formation of these mammary tumors *(32)*. Further evidence for the importance of these pathways in mammary tumor formation was obtained with the production of two transgenic mouse lines, one expressing Wnt-1 from the MMTV promoter (with resultant expression in the mammary gland), and a second line of mice expressing FGF3 from the MMTV promoter *(33,34)*. As expected from the earlier viral studies, both lines of mice developed mammary tumors. The definitive experiment showing cooperativity between these pathways was obtained by crossing the two mouse lines to generate mice that overexpressed both Wnt-1 and FGF3 in the mammary gland. These doubly transgenic mice developed mammary tumors significantly faster than either mouse line alone *(35)*. These data indicate a synergy between these two signaling pathways in the formation of mammary tumors.

A second example of cooperation between oncogenic signaling in a signal transduction pathway and loss of a tumor suppressor controlling cell cycle arrest is the formation of melanomas in mice by concurrent activation of Ras and loss of *INK4a-ARF*. Although human melanomas frequently have deletions of the *INK4a-ARF* locus, mice with germline-targeted deletion of this locus develop sarcomas and lymphomas as adults but not melanomas. In addition, although human melanomas demonstrate elevated Ras activity, transgenic mice expressing mutant constitutively active Ras as a transgene in melanocytes only rarely form melanomas. However, when the two mouse lines are crossed, these mice develop numerous melanomas with 50% penetrance by 5.5 months of age *(36)*. Therefore, elevated Ras signaling and disruption of cell cycle arrest appears to cooperate and contribute significantly to the formation of these tumors in mice.

Demonstration of the continued cooperation between these two pathways and continued requirement for Ras signaling during melanoma development was demonstrated with an inducible oncogenic Ras transgene. A mouse line was constructed that expressed Ras in melanocytes under control of a tetracycline inducible promoter. In this mouse line, the levels of expression of the oncogenic Ras are dependent on the addition of exogenous doxicycline and, therefore, can be regulated externally. When this mouse line is crossed with the *INK4a-ARF –/–* mouse line, melanomas form in the presence of doxicycline. When doxicycline is withdrawn, resulting in loss of expression of oncogenic Ras in the preexisting melanomas, these tumors regress *(37)*.

A second illustration of the cooperative effects between signal transduction and cell cycle arrest pathways is the modeling of neurofibromas in mice with combined loss of *NF-1* and *p53*. As mentioned above, both NF-1 and p53 are tumor suppressors, NF-1 loss leads to increased Ras activity, and loss of *p53* disrupts that cell cycle arrest. Human neurofibromatosis type 1 (NF-1) is caused by germline heterozygous loss of *NF-1*. These family members develop numerous neurofibromas that demonstrate loss of the remaining *NF-1* allele *(38)*. Malignant transformation of these neurofibromas to malignant peripheral nerve sheath tumors is associated with additional mutation of *p53 (39)*. In mice, homozygous-targeted deletion of NF-1 is embryonically lethal, while in mice, heterozygous loss of NF-1 alone does not lead to the formation of neurofibromas within the life span of the mouse. In addition, mice nul for *p53*, although forming other tumor types as adults, do not develop neurofibromas. However, when these mouse lines are crossed to generate *p53–/–, NF-1+/–* mice, they show the formation of malignant peripheral nerve sheath tumors with the same histologic characteristics as their human counterparts *(40,41)*.

Another illustration of cooperativity is between subsections of signal transduction pathways initiated by growth factor receptor tyrosine kinases in the formation of glioblastomas. Human glioblastomas have elevated signaling through both the Ras and Akt pathways. Elevated Akt activity in these high-grade gliomas is due to both increased signaling through PI3 kinase and the loss of the tumor suppressor PTEN. This elevated Ras and Akt activity can be mimicked by gene transfer of oncogenic forms of Ras and Akt using somatic cell type-specific gene transfer techniques. Gene transfer of activated forms of either Ras or Akt alone to glial progenitor cells in vivo has no detectable oncogenic effect. However, gene transfer of both Ras and Akt results in combined pathway activity in these cells and gives rise to the efficient formation of glioblastomas *(30)*.

Finally, mouse modeling of skin tumors shows cooperativity between Ras signaling and disruption of cell cycle arrest pathways as well. Overexpression of oncogenic Ras in kerotinocytes as a transgene results in the formation of benign skin papillomas *(42)*. Crossing these mice into a *p53–/–* background results in the conversion of these benign tumors to malignant and undifferentiated cancer. In this case, the neoplastic transformation is not dependent on the loss of *p53*. However, the histologic grade and malignant characteristics of high-grade tumors is markedly enhanced by the loss of cell cycle control generated by *p53* mutation *(43)*. It is worth noting that loss of cell cycle control, frequently due to *p53* mutation, is a common finding in highly invasive human skin tumors *(44)*.

The above examples illustrate several general principles of oncogenesis. First, the same oncogenic pathways are altered in many of these tumor types in humans and also appear to be causally related to the equivalent experimental-induced tumors in mice. Therefore, it is likely that these pathways are causally related to many human tumors as well. Second, depending on the tumor model, the role of these pathways can be either required for tumor formation or for progression. It is possible that the cell of origin from which the experimental tumors arise may have slightly different requirements for initiation and malignant transformation, and the variable results seen in these experiments may be a reflection of that. Finally, although there are many tumor suppressors and oncogenes known, the number of pathways that contribute to oncogenesis is much more limited. These pathways are constructed from components that are the protein products of the oncogenes and tumor suppressor genes. The oncogenic role that these genes play appears directly related to the effect that the gene products have on these pathways.

6. THERAPEUTIC IMPLICATIONS

From a therapeutic standpoint, the interactions between these pathways are extremely important. The fact that the same pathways seem to cooperate with each other in many of these model systems underlines the importance of the individual pathways. In addition, these data imply that successful cancer treatment may require a combined blockade of specific pathways chosen by the interactions identified in these mouse-modeling experiments.

There are many questions that still need to be answered if we are to undertake a pathway blockade approach to the treatment of cancer. For example, in case where two or more pathways are required to form and maintain cancer, is it necessary to block all of these pathways or will blocking only one of them suffice? For any pathway that we show is capable of contributing to cancer formation experimentally, how many parallel pathways exist and do we need to block all of these parallel pathways simultaneously? Are there specific locations along these pathways that do not have multiple redundant components and act as restricted nodes or bottlenecks? If such components can be identified, could drugs be constructed to block these components and would such strategies be more effective? Finally, what is the ultimate downstream mechanism for the oncogenic effect of these pathways? Is it simply transcription, or are there alterations in mRNA translation that achieve the final neoplastic phenotype? Once we know the answers to these questions, we will be much closer to knowing whether oncogene-targeted therapies will be a viable option for cancer therapy.

ACKNOWLEDGMENTS

This work was partly supported by grants from the National Institutes of Health (NIH) and the Searle Scholars Program.

REFERENCES

1. Coffin, JM, Hughes SH, Varmus HE, eds. *Retroviruses.* CSHL, Press, NY 1997, pp1–25.
2. Temin HM, Rubin H. Characteristics of an assay for rous sarcoma virus and rous sarcoma cells. *Virology* 1958; 6:669–688.
3. Stehelin D, Varmus HE, Bishop JM, Vogt PK. DNA related to the transforming gene(s) of avain sarcoma viruses is present in normal avian DNA. *Nature* 1976; 260:170–173.
4. Varmus HE. The molecular genetics of cellular oncogenes. *Annu Rev Genet* 1984; 18:553–612.
5. Weinberg RA. Tumor suppressor genes. *Science* 1991; 254:1138–1146.
6. Gallie BL, Phillips RA. Retinoblastoma: a model of oncogenesis. *Ophthalmology* 1984; 91:666–672.
7. Cavenee WK, Hansen MF, Nordenskjold M, Kock E, Maumenee I, Squire JA, et al. Genetic origin of mutations predisposing to retinoblastoma. *Science* 1985; 228:501–503.
8. Sherr CJ. The Pezcoller lecture: cancer cell cycles revisited. *Cancer Res* 2000; 60:3689–3695.
9. Zindy F, Soares H, Herzog KH, Morgan J, Sherr CJ, Roussel MF. Expression of INK4 inhibitors of cyclin D-dependent kinases during mouse brain development. *Cell Growth Differ* 1997; 8:1139–1150.

10. Ichimura K, Schmidt EE, Goike HM, Collins VP. Human glioblastomas with no alterations of the CDKN2A (p16INK4A, MTS1) and CDK4 genes have frequent mutations of the retinoblastoma gene. *Oncogene* 1996; 13:1065–1072.

11. Xu GF, O'Connell P, Viskochil D, Cawthon R, Robertson M, Culver M, et al. The neurofibromatosis type 1 gene encodes a protein related to GAP. *Cell* 1990; 62:599–608.

12. Stambolic V, Suzuki A, de la Pompa JL, Brothers GM, Mirtsos C, Sasaki T, et al. Negative regulation of PKB/Akt-dependent cell survival by the tumor suppressor PTEN. *Cell* 1998; 95:29–39.

13. Li S, Ting NS, Zheng L, Chen PL, Ziv Y, Shiloh Y, et al. Functional link of BRCA1 and ataxia telangiectasia gene product in DNA damage response. *Nature* 2000; 406:210–215.

14. Rouleau GA, Merel P, Lutchman M, Sanson M, Zucman J, Marineau C, et al. Alteration in a new gene encoding a putative membrane-organizing protein causes neuro-fibromatosis type 2. *Nature* 1993; 363:515–521.

15. Minamoto T, Mai M, Ronai Z. K-ras mutation: early detection in molecular diagnosis and risk assessment of colorectal, pancreas, and lung cancers—a review. *Cancer Detect Prev* 2000; 24:1–12.

16. Guha A, Feldkamp MM, Lau N, Boss G, Pawson A. Proliferation of human malignant astrocytomas is dependent on Ras activation. *Oncogene* 1997; 15:2755–2765.

17. Knudson AG. Mutation and cancer: statistical study of retinoblastoma. *Proc Natl Acad Sci USA* 1971; 68:820–823.

18. Land H, Parada LF, Weinberg RA. Tumorigenic conversion of primary embryo fibroblasts requires at least two cooperating oncogenes. *Nature* 1983; 304:596–602.

19. Holland EC. Gliomagenesis: genetic alterations and mouse models. *Nat Rev Genet* 2001; 2:120–129.

20. Chang HW, Aoki M, Fruman D, Auger KR, Bellacosa A, Tsichlis PN, et al. Transformation of chicken cells by the gene encoding the catalytic subunit of PI 3-kinase. *Science* 1997; 276:1848–1850.

21. Staal SP. Molecular cloning of the akt oncogene and its human homologues AKT1 and AKT2: amplification of AKT1 in a primary human gastric adenocarcinoma. *Proc Natl Acad Sci USA* 1987; 84:5034–5037.

22. Li J, Yen C, Liaw D, Podsypanina K, Bose S, Wang SI, et al. PTEN, a putative protein tyrosine phosphatase gene mutated in human brain, breast, and prostate cancer. *Science* 1997; 275:1943–1947.

23. Liaw D, Marsh DJ, Li J, Dahia PL, Wang SI, Zheng Z, et al. Germline mutations of the PTEN gene in Cowden disease, an inherited breast and thyroid cancer syndrome. *Nat Genet* 1997; 16:64–67.

24. Jessell TM, Sanes JR. Development. The decade of the developing brain. *Curr Opin Neurobiol* 2000; 10:599–611.

25. Hahn H, Wicking C, Zaphiropoulous PG, Gailani MR, Shanley S, Chidambaram A, et al. Mutations of the human homolog of *Drosophila* patched in the nevoid basal cell carcinoma syndrome. *Cell* 1996; 85:841–851.

26. Gorlin RJ. Nevoid basal-cell carcinoma syndrome. *Medicine* 1987; 66:98–113.

27. Raffel C, Jenkins RB, Frederick L, Hebrink D, Alderete B, Fults DW, et al. Sporadic medulloblastomas contain PTCH mutations. *Cancer Res* 1997; 57:842–845.

28. Bringold F, Serrano M. Tumor suppressors and oncogenes in cellular senescence. *Exp Gerontol* 2000; 35:317–329.

29. Rasheed BK, Wiltshire RN, Bigner SH, Bigner DD. Molecular pathogenesis of malignant gliomas. *Curr Opin Oncol* 1999; 11:162–167.

30. Holland EC, Celestino J, Dai C, Schaefer L, Sawaya RE, Fuller GN. Combined activation of Ras and Akt in neural progenitors induces glioblastoma formation in mice. *Nat Genet* 2000; 25:55–57.

31. Nusse R, Varmus HE. Many tumors induced by the mouse mammary tumor virus contain a provirus integrated in the same region of the host genome. *Cell* 1982; 31:99–109.

32. Shackleford GM, MacArthur CA, Kwan HC, Varmus HE. Mouse mammary tumor virus infection accelerates mammary carcinogenesis in Wnt-1 transgenic mice by insertional activation ofint-2/Fgf-3 and hst/Fgf-4. *Proc Natl Acad Sci USA* 1993; 90:740–744.

33. Tsukamoto AS, Grosschedl R, Guzman RC, Parslow T, Varmus HE. Expression of the int-1 gene in transgenic mice is associated with mammary gland hyperplasia and adenocarcinomas in male and female mice. *Cell* 1988; 55:619–625.

34. Muller WJ, Lee FS, Dickson C, Paters G, Pattengale P, Leder P. The int-2 gene product acts as an epithelial growth factor in transgenic mice. *EMBO J* 1990; 9:907–913.

35. Kwan H, Pecenka V, Tsukamoto A, Parslow TG, Guzman R, Lin TP, et al. Transgenes expressing the Wnt-1 and int-2 proto-oncogenes cooperate during mammary carcinogenesis in doubly transgenicmice. *Mol Cell Biol* 1992; 12:147–154.

36. Chin L, Pomerantz J, Polsky D, Jacobson M, Cohen C, Cordon-Cardo C, et al. Cooperative effects of INK4a and ras in melanoma susceptibility in vivo. *Genes Dev* 1997; 11:2822–2834.

37. Chin L, Tam A, Pomerantz J, Wong M, Holash J, Bardeesy N, et al. Essential role for oncogenic Ras in tumour maintenance. *Nature* 1999; 400:468–472.

38. Colman SD, Williams CA, Wallace MR. Benign neurofibromas in type 1 neurofibromatosis (NF1) show somatic deletions of the NF1 gene. *Nat Genet* 1995; 11:90–92.

39. Legius E, Dierick H, Wu R, Hall BK, Marynen P, Cassiman JJ, et al. TP53 mutations are frequent in malignant NF1 tumors. *Genes Chromosom Cancer* 1994; 10:250–255.

40. Vogel KS, Klesse LJ, Velasco-Miguel S, Meyers K, Rushing EJ, Parada LF. Mouse tumor model for neurofibromatosis type 1. *Science* 1999; 286:2176–2179.

41. Cichowski K, Shih TS, Schmitt E, Santiago S, Reilly K, McLaughlin ME, et al. Mouse models of tumor development in neurofibromatosis type 1. *Science* 1999; 286:2172–2176.

42. Bailleul B, Surani MA, White S, Barton SC, Brown K, Blessing M, et al. Skin hyperkeratosis and papilloma formation in transgenic mice expressing a ras oncogene from a suprabasal keratin promoter. *Cell* 1990; 62:697–708.

43. Kemp CJ, Donehower LA, Bradley A, Balmain A. Reduction of p53 gene dosage does not increase initiation or promotion but enhances malignant progression of chemically induced skin tumors. *Cell* 1993; 74:813–822.

44. Moles JP, Moyret C, Guillot B, Jeanteur P, Guilhou JJ, Theillet C, et al. p53 gene mutations in human epithelial skin cancers. *Oncogene* 1993; 8:583–588.

7

Genetic Basis of Altered Responsiveness of Cancer Cells to Their Microenvironment

Amato J. Giaccia, PhD

CONTENTS

1. INTRODUCTION

1.1. Lessons Learned from the Response of Minimally Transformed Rodent Cells to Hypoxia

One insight into how oxygen deficiency may affect the aggressiveness of tumors is through the modulation of apoptosis. In experimental tumors, hypoxia can provide a selective pressure for the expansion of populations of oncogenically transformed rodent cells with reduced apoptotic sensitivity, not only to hypoxia *(1)*, but to chemotherapeutic agents as well *(2)*.

Thus, transformed cells that possess mutations in their apoptotic program due to inactivation of the *p53* tumor suppressor gene or the overexpression of anti-apoptotic genes, such as *bcl-2* will have a survival advantage under hypoxic conditions. Mixing experiments also demonstrated that small numbers of transformed cells that lack wild-type p53 possess a survival advantage over isogenic cells that lack wild-type p53 when exposed to multiple rounds of hypoxia and aerobic regrowth *(1)*. In vivo, transplanted tumors that

From: *Oncogene-Directed Therapies*
Edited by: J. W. Rak © Humana Press Inc., Totowa, NJ

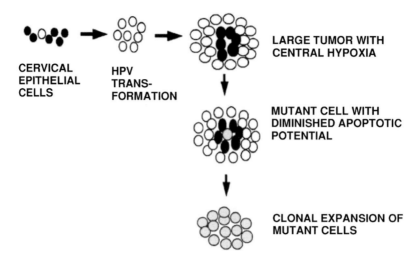

Fig. 1. The influence of HPV infection and hypoxia on the evolution of human cervical carcinomas.

possess a wild-type *p53* genotype were found to have apoptotic areas that co-localized with hypoxic areas, further supporting the hypothesis that tumor hypoxia is an important modulator of malignant progression. However, both p53 wild-type or p53 null cells can die by necrosis when exposed to hypoxia for long periods of time, indicating that this form of cell death is possible in both cell types, but does not act as a selective pressure. What genetic determinants influence a cell to die by necrosis instead of apoptosis are still unknown, but it depends, in part, on the release of cytochrome c *(3)*.

1.2. Roles of HPV E6 and E7 Viral Oncogenes in Hypoxia-Induced Apoptosis

Although the induction of apoptosis by hypoxia is strongly dependent on wild-type p53 activity, it is highly influenced by whether cells are oncogenically transformed. Since human papillomavirus (HPV) infection is strongly associated with cervical neoplasia, and tumor hypoxia has prognostic significance in human cervical carcinomas, we examined the relationship between hypoxia and apoptosis in human cervical epithelial cells expressing high risk HPV type 16 oncoproteins *(4)*. In vitro, hypoxia stimulated both p53 induction and apoptosis in primary cervical epithelial cells infected with the HPV *E6* and *E7* genes. Interestingly, cervical fibroblasts infected with *E6* and *E7* did not undergo apoptosis when exposed to hypoxia but, instead, growth arrested *(4)*. Furthermore, cell lines derived from HPV-associated human cervical squamous cell carcinomas were substantially less sensitive to apoptosis induced by hypoxia, indicating that these cell lines have acquired further genetic alterations which reduced their apoptotic sensitivity. Although the process of long term cell culturing resulted in selection for subpopulations of HPV oncoprotein expressing cervical epithelial cells with diminished apoptotic potential, exposure of cells to hypoxia greatly accelerated the selection process. These results provide evidence for the role of hypoxia-mediated selection of cells with diminished apoptotic potential in the progression of human tumors and offer an explanation of why cervical tumors, which possess low pO_2 values, are more aggressive (Fig. 1).

An elegant study by Hockel et al. investigated the relationship between hypoxia and apoptosis in spontaneous human cervical tumors *(5)*. They found that apoptotic regions were correlated with hypoxic regions in biopsy specimens of patients with squamous cell carcinoma of the cervix prior to initiation of treatment. Since 90% of cervical carcinomas possess a high risk type HPV, and at least 50% possess highly hypoxic regions, hypoxia could select for cervical epithelial cells that have lost their apoptotic ability and have a poor prognosis independent of therapy *(5,6)*.

2. APOPTOTIC SENSITIZATION TO GROWTH RESTRICTIVE CONDITIONS INDUCED BY *MYC*

Seemingly paradoxical to its role in proliferation and oncogenic transformation is the fact that overexpression of *myc* primes cells for apoptotic cell death under growth restrictive conditions generated by nutrient deprivation or low oxygen conditions *(1,7,8)*. It is this paradox that has set forth the hypothesis that *myc* deregulation results in a cellular state in which increased proliferation or apoptotic death are both equally possible depending on the cellular microenvironment and the activity of certain crucial genetic determinants, such as the p53 tumor suppressor gene. Evidence has accumulated that oncogenes such as *myc* and the adenovirus E1A gene increase p53 protein stabilization and sensitize cells to killing by growth restrictive conditions *(1,7–11)*. Loss of p53 through mutation or functional inactivation severely attenuates the sensitivity of these same oncogene-expressing cells to stress-induced apoptosis *(10–13)*. Analysis of p19^{ARF}-deficient cells indicates that *myc* can signal to p53 by two different mechanisms *(14)*. One mechanism is through p19^{ARF} cyclin-cdk inhibitor and also involves E2F-1. The second mechanism seems to involve direct activation of p53 by a yet unknown mechanism. Loss of p19^{ARF} also attenuates the sensitivity of *myc* expressing cells to apoptosis even in the presence of wild-type p53 *(14)*. Furthermore, genetic analysis of tumor cells indicates that they possess either p53 mutations or p19^{ARF} mutations, but rarely both mutations *(15,16)*. Implicit in this hypothesis is that *myc* deregulation favors proliferation and that a growth restrictive state such as lack of nutrients or oxygen starvation is needed to substantially tip the cellular balance to favor apoptotic cell death. Therefore, increased sensitivity to growth-restrictive conditions that induce apoptotic cell death will result in a selective pressure for the loss or inactivation of p19^{ARF}, p53, or other components of this stress-induced pathway.

During the malignant progression of a tumor in which *myc* deregulation is an early event, changes in tumor oxygenation could act to induce apoptosis and apply a selective pressure on these cells for the loss of their apoptotic sensitivity to this stress inducing microenvironment *(1,17,18)*. Recently, studies have demonstrated that nongenotoxic stresses found in the tumor microenvironment such as hypoxia, growth factor deprivation, and cell detachment all lead to apoptosis in transformed cells in which *myc* is deregulated and possesses functional apaf-1 and caspase 9, and adaptor and signaling molecules involved in initiating the activation of enzymatic effectors of the apoptotic process *(19,20)*. If apaf-1 or caspase 9 activity are lost through mutation, these same *myc* deregulated cells will become highly refractory to killing by these stresses *(3,21)*. Thus, loss of apaf-1 or caspase 9 activity is equivalent to the loss of the p53 tumor suppressor gene, suggesting that these apoptotic regulators could also be tumor suppressor genes and work epistatically in the same pathway.

Myc and *bcl-2* cooperate in lymphomagenesis in vivo, suggesting that overcoming apoptosis may be an important step in the progression of tumors stimulated by *myc* *(22)*. In addition to the p53 pathway, *myc* may also receive signals from Fas and tumor necrosis factor (TNF) receptors to signal cell death *(23,24)*. Although preliminary data suggest that p53 may also be involved in this pathway, further experiments will be needed to understand the direct and indirect interactions between these signaling molecules. With so many different stimuli proposed to signal cell death in *myc*-activated cells, it is not surprising that most solid tumor cells derived from human specimens possess diminished apoptotic programs in response to radiotherapy or chemotherapy, as they have already acquired genetic alterations that render them refractory to this form of cell death by the time they are diagnosed.

Finally, the question of what function or functions of *myc* are necessary to induce apoptotic cell death have recently been addressed using a transactivation deficient *myc* allele *(25)*. Surprisingly, this mutant *myc* allele, which was unable to induce transcriptional activation from E-box elements, was still able to stimulate proliferation and induce apoptosis. These provocative results will require further investigation as they do not eliminate the possibility that the crucial effectors for *myc*-induced apoptosis do not contain E-box elements or require transcriptional activation. In addition, they also do not rule out the possibility that both transcriptionally dependent and independent mechanisms exist in the signaling of the cell death by *myc*. For example, direct activation of p53 by *myc* could explain cell death induced by this transactivation defective *myc*.

Myc expression and activity is modulated by a variety of mechanisms at different levels. *Myc* transcription is autoregulated at transcription by cellular *myc* protein levels. *Myc* is also regulated posttranscriptionally by phosphorylation, although the critical phospho-residues have not fully been elucidated. The transcriptional activity of *myc* and *max* dimers is opposed by the transcriptional repressive activity of *max* and *mad* dimers. Cells with deregulated *myc* expression will promote proliferation or cell death by responding to external signals from their microenvironment. Apoptosis in cells with activated *myc* is influenced by the coordinate and complex interaction of death receptors at the cell surface, tumor suppressor gene sensors, and caspase effectors. Mutations or inactivation of any of these inputs to *myc* or outputs from *myc* will antagonize *myc's* ability to signal apoptosis. Deregulated *myc* antagonizes the function of key negative regulators of the cell cycle to promote cell proliferation. Overexpression of these negative regulators inhibits *myc's* ability to stimulate proliferation.

The importance of *myc* mutations in tumor progression has not been fully appreciated. Studies in rodent cells gave insights into the immortalizing ability of *myc* and its cooperativity with other oncogenes in transforming cells. We now have a much clearer insight into the mechanisms by which *myc* performs both functions. Immortalization by *myc* is, in part, do to deregulation of the cell cycle and, in part, do to reactivation of telomerase in cells in which it had been turned off. The relative contributions of each still need to be determined. The cooperativity of *myc* and other oncogenes in promoting transformation results from the combination of individual effects of each oncogene on critical cellular targets, as well as interaction between the oncogenes themselves. Lastly, deregulated *myc* activity and the tumor microenvironment act synergistically to select for transformed cells to lose their ability to commit suicide by apoptosis. The consequence of this selective pressure is the expansion of cell populations with diminished apoptotic programs that will possess increased resilience to the fluctuations of oxygen and nutrients in their microenvironment which constantly occur during tumor development. In addition, solid tumors that have evolved through this selection will now be more refractory to cell killing induced by the therapeutic modalities, such as radiotherapy and chemotherapy, that are used to shrink the tumor.

Now that many of the signals that feed into and out of *myc* have been identified, the challenge of the field will be to understand the genetic, biochemical, and cellular context that lead to the paradoxical effects attributed to deregulated *myc* activity. In particular, the regulation of *myc* protein domains and dimerization partners will be a critical step in understanding the biological consequences of *myc* in nontransformed and transformed cells.

3. DIVERGENCE OF THE Ras PATHWAY IN SIGNALING TO NF-κB AND HIF-1 TRANSCRIPTION FACTORS

NF-κB is a transcription factor that is composed of proteins that are related to the rel family of proteins. The regulation of NF-κB involves the interaction of two rel family subunits and an inhibitory subunit designated Ikb. Modulation of this trimeric complex is both unique and complex and has been reported to involve a myriad of signal transduction pathways *(26)*. Previous studies suggest that tyrosine phosphorylation of IκBα by hypoxia is necessary to dissociate it from the p65 subunit of NF-κB in the cytoplasm and to permit NF-κB nuclear translocation *(27–30)*. Previous studies have indicated that inhibition of IκBα phosphorylation inhibits NF-κB activity under hypoxic conditions *(27)*. In contrast, TNF and phorbol 12-myristate-13-acetate (PMA) treatment also signal for the dissociation of IκBα, but the accumulation of phosphotyrosine residues on IκBα occurs as a result of either of these stresses *(26)*. It has also been proposed that oxidative stresses that induce phosphorylation of IκBα do so in an unknown matter that does not require degradation of the protein *(26)*. The link between phosphorylation and degradation may be so rapid for these latter stresses that the phosphorylated form of IκBα cannot be detected even if it occurs, or that each stress induces multiple kinases that signal for the dissociation of IκBα. This latter hypothesis is very attractive, as it could explain many conflicting reports about the role of phosphorylation in IκBα degradation.

The early events in the pathway for the inactivation of IκBα by hypoxia possess slower kinetics than UV, TNF, and PMA *(27)*. Although the latter three stresses signal for the inactivation of IκBα, presumably through a free radical mechanism that is inhibited by radical scavengers *(26)*, unpublished data suggests that hypoxic inactivation of IκBα or increased NF-κB binding is not inhibited by these scavengers (E.Y. Chen, A.C. Koong, and A.J. Giaccia, unpublished results). It is also noteworthy that hypoxia, UV, TNF, and PMA signal for the inactivation of IκBα through *Ras* and *Raf-1* kinases *(31–33)* and that *Raf-1* kinase may activate divergent downstream kinases such as MEK and IκBα kinase, depending on the stress. Therefore, it seems that many pathways involved in the activation of NF-κB are regulated by *Raf-1* kinase, making it a worthy target for cancer therapy *(34)*.

In contrast to the NF-κB pathway, oncogenic Ras predominately uses the phosphatidylinositol 3-kinase [PI(3) kinase] pathway in signaling the hypoxia inducible transcription factor HIF-1, heterodimeric factor composed of a constitutive expressed subunit, and an oxygen sensitive subunit *(35)* for a recent review. Previous studies have demonstrated a direct role for a Ras signaling pathway in HIF induction by hypoxia *(36,37)*. A mutant form of Ha-*ras* (RasN17; Asn-17) *(38)*, which inhibits Ras activity, also blocked vascular endothelial growth factor (VEGF) induction in both transformed and untransformed NIH 3T3 cells. Studies have shown that Ras, in the active GTP-bound conformation, interacts with PI(3) kinase *(39–41)*, and hypoxia also increases PI(3) kinase activity *(37,42)*. Thus, inhibitors of PI(3) kinase, such as LY294002 (or derivatives), can be added on the list with farnesyltransferase inhibitors *(43,44)* as having a potent antitumor effect by inhibiting hypoxia inducible gene expression *(42,45–47)*. Recent preclinical and phase I clinical studies have suggested that farnesyltransferase inhibitors may impart exert their antitumor effects by reducing tumor hypoxia *(48,49)*. While the underlying mechanism responsible for the reduction of tumor hypoxia is still under investigation, the combination of farnesyltransferase inhibitors and radiotherapy holds great promise for many solid tumors in that it acts to eliminate the age-old problem of tumor hypoxia. When more efficient vectors are developed for use in gene therapy, then other modulators of PI(3) kinase pathway, such as the PTEN suppressor gene, could also be used to inhibit tumor growth by impeding hypoxia inducible gene induction *(50)*.

4. HYPOXIA, Akt AND HIF-1 ACTIVITY

The study of how hypoxia modulates cell signaling is the focus of much research interest. Recently, the identification of the transcription factor HIF-1 has advanced the understanding of hypoxia-induced intracellular signaling pathways *(35,51)*. Studies of HIF-1 knock-out embryos indicate that HIF-1 is necessary for proper embryonic development, presumably through the transcriptional activation of genes involved in angiogenesis, glycolysis, and tissue remodeling *(52–55)*. As regulation of HIF-1 appears to be a result of posttranslational modifications of the HIF-1α subunit through hydroxylation *(56–58)* and phosphorylation *(59–65)*, which results in its stabilization, the list of proteins that may bind or somehow modify HIF-1 specifically under a hypoxic microenvironment is rapidly expanding, thereby providing possible targets for intervention in treatment of cancer, stroke, coronary artery disease, and peripheral vascular disease.

In some cell types, hypoxia-induced PI(3) kinase/Akt/HIF-1 pathway leads to increased stabilization of HIF-1α and increased transcriptional activity of HIF-1 effector genes, such as VEGF. These studies suggested that Akt or protein kinase B (PKB) is one of the protein kinases that lies downstream of the phospholipid products of PI(3) kinase and transduces the signal induced by hypoxia that results in HIF-1α stabilization. Recently, it was shown that 3′-phosphorylated phosphoinositides (PI 3-Ps) target Akt to the plasma membrane, which is an event that leads to the phosphorylation of Akt at two residues, Thr308 and Ser473, by phosphatidylinositol $(3,4,5)P_3$-dependent protein kinases (PDK) *(66–69)*. Phosphorylation of these critical residues in turn releases Akt from an inhibited conformation, thereby activating its kinase function. The downstream targets of Akt, which regulate its metabolic functions such as glycogen synthesis, glucose uptake, and glycolysis, include glycogen synthase kinase-3 (GSK-3) *(70,71)*, glucose transporter 4 (GLUT4) *(72,73)*, and 6-phosphofructose 2-kinase (PFK2) *(74)*. The substrates of Akt, which are involved with its anti-apoptotic function, include CED-3, c-Myc, Fas, NF-κB, and p53 *(75–79)*.

Several signaling molecules in addition to PI(3) kinase (Src, Ras, MAPK) have been shown to be modulated by hypoxia and to be involved with HIF-1 activation, but how these molecules are initially activated by hypoxia is currently unknown *(37,80–82)*. Since

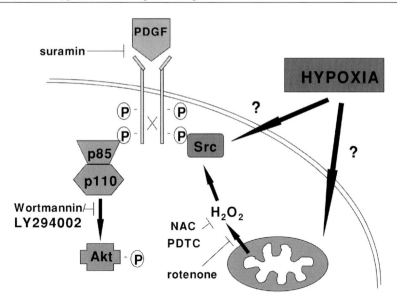

Fig. 2. Speculative growth factor receptor activation and proximal signaling events under hypoxic conditions. Hypoxia can induce growth factor activation through modulation of src kinase or through the generation of free radicals by the mitochondria. Growth factor activation can then lead to the activation of the PI(3) kinase pathway and the activation of the Akt. Growth factor activation by hypoxia can be disrupted by free radical scavengers, the growth receptor poison suramin, or the PI(3) kinase inhibitors wortmannin or LY294002. It should be noted that dysregulation of this pathway often occurs in human tumors, as many of the key signaling components are considered proto-oncogenes.

many of these signaling molecules are also activated by or associated with growth factors, we hypothesized that hypoxia may induce the activation of growth factor receptors. The general scheme of growth factor receptor activation proceeds through a series of well-studied events. First, the growth factor binds to the extracellular domain of a heterodimeric receptor. The binding of the ligand results in dimerization of the receptor, which leads to autophosphorylation of the receptor at specific residues in the intracellular domain of the receptor. Several Src homology 2 (SH2)-containing signaling molecules then bind to these phosphorylated tyrosines and activate several signal transduction pathways, the most studied of which are the MAPK pathway and the PI(3) kinase pathway.

Activation of growth factor receptors by UV irradiation, osmotic stress, and heat shock has been previously reported to proceed through a ligand-independent mechanism *(83–85)*. Rosette and Karin showed that UV light and osmotic stress cause aggregation of growth factor receptors, which results in the activation of the JNK signaling pathway *(83)*. They hypothesized that physical stress could cause changes in the cell membrane, resulting in clustering and activation of growth factor receptors and downstream signaling cascades. Huang et al. showed that UV treatment causes an accumulation of reactive oxygen species (ROS), which then activate several growth factor receptors, most notably the epidermal growth factor receptor (EGFR) *(86)*. Interestingly, recent publications have proposed that hypoxia induces a mitochondria-dependent accumulation of ROS, suggesting the necessity of mitochondrial function in hypoxia-induced activation of the growth factor receptor signaling pathway *(87–89)*. However, the mechanism of activation of growth factor receptors in a ligand-independent manner and the role of ROS in hypoxia signaling remain unclear and controversial (Fig. 2).

A recent study by Chen et al. reported that within an hour of hypoxia treatment, platelet-derived growth factor receptor (PDGFR)β and EGFR are tyrosine-phosphory-lated, indicating that hypoxia initiates growth factor receptor signaling pathways in a ligand-independent manner *(42)*. The activation of Akt by hypoxia was inhibited by wortmannin, suggesting its dependence upon PI(3) kinase activity. However, suramin did not inhibit Akt activation by hypoxia, suggesting that this pathway was not acti-vated by either autocrine or paracrine release of growth factors or other extracellular ligands. Additionally, evidence that hypoxia-induced activation of Akt/PKB is depen-dent upon mitochondrial function was indicated by cells treated with rotenone, a mito-chondrial inhibitor, or cells depleted of mitochondrial DNA that exhibited substantially decreased Akt phosphorylation by hypoxia. Hypoxia also resulted in the phosphoryla-tion and, hence, inactivation of GSK-3, a downstream target of Akt/PKB *(42)*. Taken together, these data suggest that hypoxia initiates a PI(3) kinase/Akt/GSK-3 signaling cascade through ligand-independent activation of growth factor receptors.

Since the PI(3) kinase pathway is important for the regulation of the HIF-1 tran-scription factors and angiogenesis, the tumor suppressor gene PTEN would serve to check the hypoxia-induced stimulation of the PI(3) kinase-HIF-VEGF pathway. PTEN inhibits the hypoxia-induced activation of the PI(3) kinase downstream effector Akt *(46,50)*. In fact, PTEN inhibits endogenous VEGF induction by hypoxia to the same extent as wortmannin, which is a potent PI(3) kinase inhibitor. In cotransfection exper-iments, PTEN inhibits the activation of VEGF by inhibiting the activation of HIF-1 by PI(3) kinase. Interestingly. PTEN inhibited the hypoxia-stimulated accumulation of HIF-1α, although not through direct phosphorylation or interaction with the protein. This observation suggests that tumor cells deficient in PTEN will have dysregulated HIF-1 activity under hypoxic conditions. Thus, PTEN is an important modulator of the cellular response to hypoxia, oncogenic mutations, and growth factors by regulating VEGF and HIF activity

5. MODULATION OF HIF-1 EXPRESSION UNDER AEROBIC AND HYPOXIC CONDITIONS: THE ROLE OF THE VHL TUMOR SUPPRESSOR GENE

One consequence of cellular exposure to hypoxia is inhibition of oxidative phospho-rylation and increased glycolysis. This adaptation of cells to an anaerobic environment is achieved by the transcriptional induction of genes that encode glycolytic enzymes *(90)*. In addition, hypoxia has also been shown to increase the transcriptional activity of genes that increase tumor oxygenation through promoting angiogenesis *(91)* and tis-sue remodeling *(92)*, regulating vascular tone *(93)*, blood pressure *(94)*, and stimulat-ing hematopoiesis *(95,96)*. Perhaps, the earliest insight into the transcriptional regulation of gene expression by hypoxia came from studies on erythropoietin (EPO) gene regulation. Several groups have shown that the hypoxia inducibility of the EPO gene was due in large part to a hypoxia responsive element (HRE) localized in its 3′ untranslated region (UTR) *(97,98)*. The transcription factor that bound this HRE was designated HIF-1. Purification and characterization of HIF-1 revealed that it was com-posed of two subunits, an oxygen-sensitive HIF-1α subunit and a constitutively expressed HIF-1β subunit *(99)*. This heterodimeric complex recognizes a core consensus sequence 5'-TACGTG-3' based on gel mobility shift analysis and DNA methylation interference assays. The HIF-1β subunit was identified as the ARNT gene *(99)*, and it plays an important role in directing an activated AH receptor to enhancer elements to increase gene transcription in response to dioxin signaling *(100)*. Three important points should be noted about the structure of the HIF-1β/ARNT gene. First, HIF-1α/ARNT contains an Helix Loop Helix (HLH) domain and a Per Arnt Sim (PAS) domain. In general, HLH domains are involved in protein dimerization and aid in positioning protein contact with target sequences such as HREs in the major groves of DNA. Second, PAS domains act as a surface for interactions with other PAS-containing proteins and with cellular chaperones such as hsp90. Third, the transactivation domain is located in the carboxyl terminus of the protein. Recently, two additional family members of ARNT, designated ARNT2 *(101,102)* and MOP3 *(103–105)*, have been identified. In vitro experiments have demonstrated that ARNT2 and MOP3 are able to form complexes with AHR or HIF-1β family members and activate reporter genes containing dioxin or hypoxia responsive elements *(106,107)*. Although ARNT2 shares only 57% overall sequence identity with ARNT, it exhibits 81% conservation in its bHLH-PAS domains *(101,102)*.

In contrast to the constitutively expressed HIF-β/ARNT subunit, HIF-1α is an oxygen labile protein that becomes stabilized in response to hypoxia, iron chelators, and divalent cations. As all three inducers of HIF-1α have some direct or indirect relationship with heme, it has been postulated that the cellular oxygen sensor is a heme-associated protein *(96,108)*. To date, there has been no as yet definitive identification of such a protein. Under hypoxic conditions, HIF-1α mRNA levels do not change, but HIF-1α protein levels increase *(109,110)*. Although multiple signaling pathways involving MAP kinase *(81)*, PKC *(59,60)*, and PI(3)kinase *(37,42,45–47,50)* have been shown to affect the accumulation of HIF-1α, the details on how these pathways modulate HIF-1α are still unclear. HIF-1α, like ARNT, also possesses an HLH and PAS domain *(111)*. However, the most critical point for this review concerning the labile nature of HIF-1α under oxic conditions is that it can be transferred to other proteins *(112,113)*. In fact, fusion of different HIF-1α domains to gal4 identified two separable hypoxia responsive domains. One domain is localized between residues 531–575 and is important in modulating HIF-1α protein stability *(112,114)*. The second domain is localized between residues 786–826 and is involved in modulating transcriptional activation of HIF-1α under hypoxic conditions. The finding that transfer of residues 531–575 to a heterologous protein can confer oxygen instability, suggests that the oxygen sensor itself does not have to be directly associated with HIF-1. Interestingly, two additional members of the HIF-1α family, designated HIF-2α (also called EPAS1 or MOP2) *(103,115–117)* and HIF-3α have been identified *(118)*. HIF-2α is highly similar to HIF-1α in both structure and function, but exhibits more restricted tissue-specific expression. In contrast to HIF-2α, HIF-3α also exhibits conservation with HIF-1α and HIF-2α in the HLH and PAS domains, but does not possess a similar hypoxia-inducible transactivation domain *(118)*.

So how does hypoxia signal HIF-1α stabilization? Hypoxia regulates HIF-1α at the level of protein stability by inhibiting its ubiquitin-mediated degradation *(119–121)*. This concept is highly supported by studies on cell lines derived from tumors that have lost the Von Hippel Lindau (VHL) tumor suppressor gene that display aerobic HIF-1α protein expression *(122,123)*. Tumors such as renal cell carcinomas, which possess

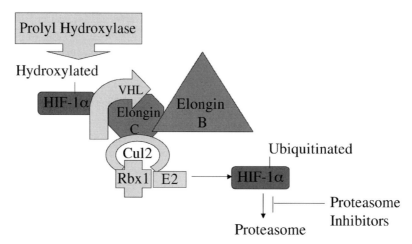

Fig. 3. Model for HIF-1α stabilization under hypoxia. The key points in this model are the hydroxylation of HIF-1α by a prolyl hydroxylase in its oxygen degradation domain. Hydroxylated HIF-1α binds to a VHL complex that results in its ubiquitination and degradation by the proteasome. Mutations in the prolyl hydroxylase and VHL will result in stabilization of HIF-1α under aerobic conditions.

mutations in VHL, exhibit high aerobic expression of HIF-1 regulated genes, whereas reintroduction of wild-type VHL substantially reduces the aerobic expression of HIF-1α to levels found in nontransformed or transformed cells that express wild-type VHL. Recent studies have directly linked changes in oxygen sensing, HIF-1α modification, and VHL (Fig. 3). In the current model, under normoxic conditions, HIF-1α is hydroxylated in its oxygen degradation domain by a prolyl hydroxylase, and this modification results in its ubiquitin-mediated degradation through VHL-"binding" *(56–58)*. As extracellular oxygen levels fall, the activity of the HIF-1α prolyl hydroxylase decreases, resulting in decreased hydroxylation of the oxygen degradation domain of HIF-1α and its increased stabilization under hypoxic conditions. Protein stability of HIF-1α is separable from its heterodimerization with ARNT as ARNT-deficient cells still exhibit HIF-1α stabilization *(124)*.

6. PROTEIN TRANSDUCTION OF ODD REGULATED PROTEIN EXPRESSION AS A NEW FORM OF ANTICANCER THERAPEUTICS

A fundamental problem for any form of cancer gene or protein therapy is the ability to derive tumor-specific activity. While novel approaches to overcome the problems of tumor-specific delivery and activity are currently being undertaken through the use of stealth liposomes and genetically modified anaerobic bacteria, the need for therapeutics that can be readily used by researchers that are not skilled in such technically burdensome strategies still exists. For example, the use of obligate anaerobic bacteria such as *Clostridium oncolyticum* as a gene therapy vector holds great promise in delivering tumor-specific production of enzymes that can activate chemically modified pro-drug chemotherapeutic agents *(125,126)*. However, manipulation of *C. oncolyticum* requires specialized equipment and experience that make it difficult to be used except in a few specialized laboratories throughout the world.

One powerful means of transducing proteins into cells is to link them to protein transduction domains (PTDs) derived from *Drosophila* or viral genes *(127)*. Three very robust PTDs have been derived from the human immunodeficiency virus type 1 (HIV-1) TAT protein *(128,129)*, the antennapedia homeotic transcription factor *(130,131)* and the herpes-simplex virus, VP22 *(132)*. Although the mechanisms of how these three PTDs aid in the transduction of heterologous proteins is still unknown, they all share in common large stretches of basic amino acids, which permit the entry of peptides in a receptor or endocytosis independent mechanism *(127)*. In fact, oligomers of basic amino acids, such as arginine, seem to be sufficient to enhance protein transduction *(133,134)*. At present, protein transduction strategies are increasing in number, but still possess several limitations. First, the choice of PTD needs to be addressed. While PTDs are derived from the HIV-1 TAT protein, the antennapedia homeotic transcription factor and the herpes-simplex virus VP22 all possess the ability to transduce fusion proteins; there are limitations with each. Peptides derived from the antennapedia homeotic transcription factor will only efficiently transduce proteins that are 100 residues or less *(135)*, thereby limiting the choice of proteins based on size. The use of VP22 to transduce proteins is cumbersome, in that the VP22 fusion construct is introduced into cells as DNA, and the cellular machinery is then used to make protein that has to exit the original transfected cells and enter surrounding cells *(132,136)*. Clearly, this is not a technique that will allow direct transduction and will have limited uses. In fact, VP22 is not that significant an improvement over viral transduction systems that rely on the bystander effect to increase cell killing. Of the three PTDs described above, peptides derived from the HIV TAT protein are the most efficient and direct means of introducing proteins of any size by transduction *(137,138)*. However, this transduction domain is derived from a virus and could potentially stimulate an immune response in patients. In the present application, this is not a concern, as we are using it in immune-deficient mice and are confident that synthetic nonimmunogenic PTDs will be developed in the near future. Interestingly, experimental data indicates that denatured protein transduces more efficiently than nondenatured proteins *(137,138)*, almost counterintuitive to conventional thinking. The higher efficiency of transduction of denatured proteins raises a second issue, in that, for a transduced protein to function properly, it must be able to be renatured after transduction. Surprisingly, most mammalian proteins that have been tested in this system do renature after transduction and, more importantly, exhibit biological activity. However, while proteins transduce rapidly across the cell membrane, restoration of their activity exhibits slower kinetics *(138)*. Whether proteins renature with the same efficiency and with the same kinetics in hypoxic cells as in oxic cells will need to be investigated. A second point that requires examination is the stability of the protein in hypoxic cells. While proteins of up to 120 kDa transduce efficiently within 10–20 min after application to culture *(137,138)*, the lifespan of these proteins may vary under hypoxic conditions. Therefore the half-life of transduced proteins under oxic and hypoxic conditions will also be examined.

A second hurdle to overcome in the use of protein transduction is specificity for tumor cells. Studies indicate that both transformed and nontransformed cells exhibit similar protein transduction efficiencies. In this situation, the efficiency of protein transduction in both types of cells will decrease therapeutic benefit. Therefore, the combination of TAT-mediated transduction and oxygen degradation domain (ODD)-modified proteins would provide a novel approach to specifically attack tumor cells and

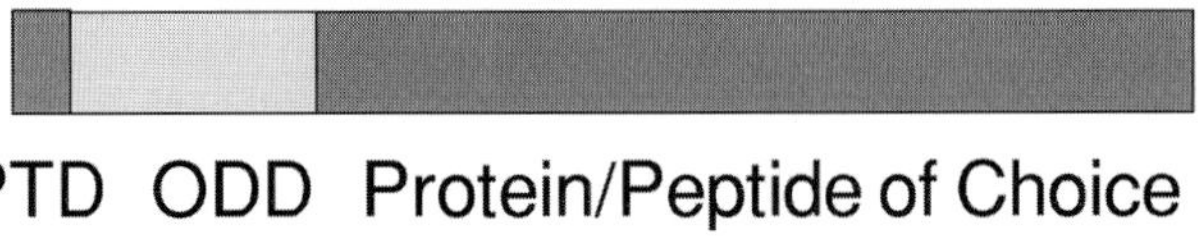

PTD ODD Protein/Peptide of Choice

Fig. 4. Hypoxia-regulated protein delivery system. This hybrid molecule is depicted as having a PTD at the amino terminus and an ODD fused to the protein or peptide of choice. However, this schema can be altered to maximize protein transduction efficiency and destabilization under aerobic conditions.

spare normal tissue toxicity (Fig. 4). In addition, such an approach would be targeting the very cells that represent a therapeutic impediment *(139)*. While there are clearly problems associated with this approach, the high levels of transduction achieved by using PTDs are the most feasible means to use in delivering oxygen-regulated proteins in vivo.

ACKNOWLEDGMENT

This work was supported in part by National Institutes of Health (NIH) Grant Nos. PO1 CA67166 and RO1-CA88480. I would also like to thank Sharon Clarke for assistance in manuscript preparation.

REFERENCES

1. Graeber TG, Osmanian C, Jacks T, et al. Hypoxia mediated selection of cells with diminished apoptotic potential in solid tumors. *Nature* 1996; 379:88–91.
2. Lowe SW, Bodis S, McClatchey A, et al. p53 status and the efficacy of cancer therapy in vivo. *Science* 1994; 266:807–810.
3. Alarcon RM, Denko NC, Giaccia AJ. Genetic determinants that influence hypoxia-induced apoptosis. In. The Tumour Microenvironment: Causes and Consequences of Hypoxia and Acidity. Goode, J. A. and Chadwick, D.J. (eds), John Wiley & Sons, Ltd., Chichester, United Kingdom, pp115-132, 2001.
4. Kim CY, Tsai MH, Osmanian C, et al. Selection of human cervical epithelial cells that possess reduced apoptotic potential to low-oxygen conditions. *Cancer Res* 1997; 57:4200–4204.
5. Hockel M, Schlenger K, Hockel S, Vaupel P. Hypoxic cervical cancers with low apoptotic index are highly aggressive. *Cancer Res* 1999; 59:4525–4528.
6. Hockel M, Vaupel P. Biological consequences of tumor hypoxia. *Semin Oncol* 2001; 28:36–41.
7. Evan GI, Wyllie AH, Gilbert CS, et al. Induction of apoptosis in fibroblasts by c-myc protein. *Cell* 1992; 69:119–128.
8. Hermeking H, Eick D. Mediation of c-Myc-induced apoptosis by p53. *Science* 1994; 265:2091–2093.
9. Lowe SW, Ruley HE. Stabilization of the p53 tumor suppressor is induced by adenovirus 5 E1A and accompanies apoptosis. *Genes Dev* 1993; 7:535–545.
10. Lowe SW, Ruley HE, Jacks T, Housman DE. p53-dependent apoptosis modulates the cytotoxicity of anticancer agents. *Cell* 1993; 74:957–967.
11. Wagner AJ, Kokontis JM, Hay N. Myc-mediated apoptosis requires wild-type p53 in a manner independent of cell-cycle arrest and the ability of p53 to induce p21waf-1/cip1. *Genes Dev* 1994; 8:2817–2830.
12. Debbas M, White E. Wild-type p53 mediates apoptosis by E1A, which is inhibited by E1B. *Genes Dev* 1993; 7:546–554.
13. Lowe SW, Jacks T, Housman DE, Ruley HE. Abrogation of oncogene-associated apoptosis allows transformation of p53-deficient cells. *Proc Natl Acad Sci USA* 1994; 91:2026–2030.
14. Zindy F, Quelle DE, Roussel MF, Sherr CJ. Expression of the p16INK4a tumor suppressor versus other INK4 family members during mouse development and aging. *Oncogene* 1997; 15:203–211.
15. Kamijo T, Zindy F, Roussel MF, et al. Tumor suppression at the mouse INK4a locus mediated by the alternative reading frame product p19[ARF]. *Cell* 1997; 91:649–659.
16. Zindy F, Eischen CM, Randle DH, et al. Myc signaling via the ARF tumor suppressor regulates p53-dependent apoptosis and immortalization. *Genes Dev* 1998; 12:2424–2433.

17. Alarcon RM, Rupnow BA, Graeber TG, Knox SJ, Giaccia AJ. Modulation of c-Myc activity and apoptosis in vivo. *Cancer Res* 1996; 56:4315–4319.
18. Shim H, Chun Y, Lewis B, Dang CV. A unique glucose-dependent apoptotic pathway induced by c-Myc. *Proc Natl Acad Sci USA* 1998; 95:1511–1516.
19. Srinivasula SM, Ahmad M, Fernandes-Alnemri T, Alnemri ES. Autoactivation of procaspase-9 by Apaf-1-mediated oligomerization. *Mol Cell* 1998; 1:949–957.
20. Zou H, Henzel WJ, Liu X, Lutschg A, Wang X. Apaf-1, a human protein homologous to *C. elegans* CED-4, participates in cytochrome c-dependent activation of caspase-3. *Cell* 1997; 90:405–413.
21. Soengas MS, Alarcon RM, Yoshida H, et al. Apaf-1 and caspase-9 in p53-dependent apoptosis and tumor inhibition. *Science* 1999; 284:156–159.
22. Schmitt CA, Rosenthal CT, Lowe SW. Genetic analysis of chemoresistance in primary murine lymphomas. *Nat Med* 2000; 6:1029–1035.
23. Hueber A-O, Zornig M, Lyon D, Suda T, Nagata S, Evan GI. Requirement for the CD95 receptor-ligand pathway in c-myc induced apoptosis. *Science* 1997; 278:1305–1309.
24. Klefstrom J, Arighi E, Littlewood T, et al. Induction of TNF-sensitive cellular phenotype by c-myc involves p53 and impaired NF-κB activation. *EMBO J* 1997; 24:7382–7392.
25. Xiao Q, Claassen G, Shi J, Adachi S, Sedivy J, Hann SR. Transactivation-defective c-MycS retains the ability to regulate proliferation and apoptosis. *Genes Dev* 1998; 12:3803–3808.
26. Janssen-Heininger YM, Poynter ME, Baeuerle PA. Recent advances towards understanding redox mechanisms in the activation of nuclear factor kappaB. *Free Radic Biol Med* 2000; 28:1317–1327.
27. Koong AC, Chen EY, Giaccia AJ. Hypoxia causes the activation of nuclear factor-κB through the phosphorylation of IκBα on tyrosine residues. *Cancer Res* 1994; 54:1425–1430.
28. Beraud C, Henzel WJ, Baeuerle PA. Involvement of regulatory and catalytic subunits of phosphoinositide 3-kinase in NF-kappaB activation. *Proc Natl Acad Sci USA* 1999; 96:429–434.
29. Digicaylioglu M, Lipton SA. Erythropoietin-mediated neuroprotection involves cross-talk between Jak2 and NF-kappaB signalling cascades. *Nature* 2001; 412:641–647.
30. Siebenlist U. Signal transduction. Barriers come down. *Nature* 2001; 412:601–602.
31. Finco TS, Baldwin AS, Jr. Kappa B site-dependent induction of gene expression by diverse inducers of nuclear factor kappa B requires Raf-1. *J Biol Chem* 1993; 268:17676–17679.
32. Finco TS, Westwick JK, Norris JL, Beg AA, Der CJ, Baldwin AS Jr. Oncogenic Ha-Ras-induced signaling activates NF-kappaB transcriptional activity, which is required for cellular transformation. *J Biol Chem* 1997; 272:24113–24116.
33. Koong AC, Chen EY, Mivechi NF, Denko NC, Stambrook P, Giaccia AJ. Hypoxic activation of nuclear factor-kB is mediated by a Ras and Raf signaling pathway and does not involve MAP kinase (ERK1 or ERK2). *Cancer Res* 1994; 54:5273–5279.
34. Mayo MW, Baldwin AS. The transcription factor NF-kappaB: control of oncogenesis and cancer therapy resistance. *Biochim Biophys Acta* 2000; 1470:M55-M62.
35. Semenza GL. HIF-1 and mechanisms of hypoxia sensing. *Curr Opin Cell Biol* 2001; 13:167–171.
36. Mazure NM, Chen EY, Yeh P, Laderoute KR, Giaccia AJ. Oncogenic transformation and hypoxia synergistically act to modulate vascular endothelial growth factor expression. *Cancer Res* 1996; 56:3436–3440.
37. Mazure NM, Chen EY, Laderoute KR, Giaccia AJ. Induction of vascular endothelial growth factor by hypoxia is modulated by a phosphatidylinositol 3-kinase/Akt signaling pathway in Ha-ras-transformed cells through a hypoxia inducible factor-1 transcriptional element. *Blood* 1997; 90:3322–3331.
38. Stacey DW, Feig LA, Gibbs JB. Dominant inhibitory Ras mutants selectively inhibit the activity of either cellular or oncogenic Ras. *Mol Cell Biol* 1991; 11:4053–4064.
39. Rodriguez-Viciana P, Warne PH, Dhand R, et al. Phosphatidylinositol-3-OH kinase as a direct target of Ras. *Nature* 1994; 370:527–532.
40. Rodriguez-Viciana P, Vanhaesebroeck B, Waterfield MD, Downward J. Activation of phosphoinositide 3-kinase by interaction with Ras and by point mutation. *EMBO J* 1996; 15:2442–2451.
41. Franke TF, Yang S-I, Chan TO, et al. The protein kinase encoded by the *Akt* proto-oncogene is a target of the PDGF-activated phosphatidylinositol 3-kinase. *Cell* 1995; 81:727–736.
42. Chen EY, Mazure NM, Cooper JA, Giaccia AJ. Hypoxia activates a platelet-derived growth factor receptor/phosphatidylinositol 3-kinase/Akt pathway that results in glycogen synthase kinase-3 inactivation. *Cancer Res* 2001; 61:2429–2433.
43. Gibbs JB, Oliff A, Kohl NE. Farnesyltransferase inhibitors: Ras research yields a potential cancer therapeutic. *Cell* 1994; 77:175–178.

44. Rak J, Mitsuhashi Y, Bayko L, et al. Mutant ras oncogenes upregulate VEGF/VPF expression: implications for induction and inhibition of tumor angiogenesis. *Cancer Res* 1995; 55:4575–4580.

45. Chen C, Pore N, Behrooz A, Ismail-Beigi F, Maity A. Regulation of glut1 mRNA by hypoxia-inducible factor-1. Interaction between H-ras and hypoxia. *J Biol Chem* 2001; 276:9519–9525.

46. Jiang BH, Jiang G, Zheng JZ, Lu Z, Hunter T, Vogt PK. Phosphatidylinositol 3-kinase signaling controls levels of hypoxia-inducible factor 1. *Cell Growth Differ* 2001; 12:363–369.

47. Blancher C, Moore JW, Robertson N, Harris AL. Effects of ras and von Hippel-Lindau (VHL) gene mutations on hypoxia-inducible factor (HIF)-1alpha, HIF-2alpha, and vascular endothelial growth factor expression and their regulation by the phosphatidylinositol 3′-kinase/Akt signaling pathway. *Cancer Res* 2001; 61:7349–7355.

48. Cohen-Jonathan E, Evans SM, Koch CJ, et al. The farnesyltransferase inhibitor L744,832 reduces hypoxia in tumors expressing activated H-ras. *Cancer Res* 2001; 61:2289–2293.

49. Brown JM. Therapeutic targets in radiotherapy. *Int J Radiant Oncol Biol Phys* 2001; 49:319–326.

50. Zundel W, Schindler C, Haas-Kogan D, et al. Loss of PTEN facilitates HIF-1-mediated gene expression. *Genes Dev* 2000; 14:391–396.

51. Semenza GL. Hif-1, o(2), and the 3 phds. how animal cells signal hypoxia to the nucleus. *Cell* 2001; 107:1–3.

52. Iyer NV, Kotch LE, Agani F, et al. Cellular and developmental control of O2 homeostasis by hypoxia-inducible factor 1 alpha. *Genes Dev* 1998; 12:149–162.

53. Ryan HE, Lo J, Johnson RS. HIF-1 alpha is required for solid tumor formation and embryonic vascularization. *EMBO J* 1998; 17:3005–3015.

54. Kozak KR, Abbott B, Hankinson O. ARNT-deficient mice and placental differentiation. *Dev Biol* 1997; 191:297–305.

55. Maltepe E, Schmidt JV, Baunoch D, Bradfield CA, Simon MC. Abnormal angiogenesis and responses to glucose and oxygen deprivation in mice lacking the protein ARNT. *Nature* 1997; 386:403–407.

56. Ivan M, Kondo K, Yang H, et al. HIFalpha targeted for VHL-mediated destruction by proline hydroxylation: implications for O2 sensing. *Science* 2001; 292:464–468.

57. Jaakkola P, Mole DR, Tian YM, et al. Targeting of HIF-alpha to the von Hippel-Lindau ubiquitylation complex by O2-regulated prolyl hydroxylation. *Science* 2001; 292:468–472.

58. Yu F, White SB, Zhao Q, Lee FS. HIF-1alpha binding to VHL is regulated by stimulus-sensitive proline hydroxylation. *Proc Natl Acad Sci USA* 2001; 98:9630–9635.

59. Wang GL, Jiang BH, Semenza GL. Effect of protein kinase and phosphatase inhibitors on expression of hypoxia-inducible factor 1. *Biochem Biophys Res Commun* 1995; 216:669–675.

60. Salceda S, Beck I, Srinivas V, Caro J. Complex role of protein phosphorylation in gene activation by hypoxia. *Kidney Int* 1997; 51:556–559.

61. Minet E, Arnould T, Michel G, et al. ERK activation upon hypoxia: involvement in HIF-1 activation. *FEBS Lett* 2000; 468:53–58.

62. Sodhi A, Montaner S, Miyazaki H, Gutkind JS. MAPK and Akt act cooperatively but independently on hypoxia inducible factor-1alpha in ras V12 upregulation of VEGF. *Biochem Biophys Res Commun* 2001; 287:292–300.

63. Minet E, Michel G, Mottet D, Raes M, Michiels C. Transduction pathways involved in hypoxia-inducible factor-1 phosphorylation and activation. *Free Radic Biol Med* 2001; 31:847–855.

64. Hofer T, Desbaillets I, Hopfl G, Gassmann M, Wenger RH. Dissecting hypoxia-dependent and hypoxia-independent steps in the HIF-1α activation cascade: implications for HIF-1α gene therapy. *FASEB J* 2001; 15:2715–2717.

65. Czyzyk-Krzeska MF. Molecular aspects of oxygen sensing in physiological adaptation to hypoxia. *Respir Physiol* 1997; 110:99–111.

66. Coffer PJ, Jin J, Woodgett JR. Protein kinase B (c-Akt): a multifunctional mediator of phosphatidylinositol 3-kinase activation. *Biochem J* 1998; 335:1–13.

67. Alessi DR, Deak M, Casamayor A, et al. 3-Phosphoinositide-dependent protein kinase-1 (PDK1): structural and functional homology with the *Drosophila* DSTPK61 kinase. *Curr Biol* 1997; 7:776–789.

68. Klippel A, Kavanaugh WM, Pot D, Williams LT. A specific product of phosphatidylinositol 3-kinase directly activates the protein kinase Akt through its pleckstrin homology domain. *Mol Cell Biol* 1997; 17:338–344.

69. Stokoe D, Macdonald SG, Cadwallader K, Symons M, Hancock JF. Activation of Raf as a result of recruitment to the plasma membrane. *Science* 1994; 264:1463–1467.

70. van Weeren PC, de Bruyn KM, de Vries-Smits AM, van Lint J, Burgering BM. Essential role for protein kinase B (PKB) in insulin-induced glycogen synthase kinase 3 inactivation. Characterization of dominant-negative mutant of PKB. *J Biol Chem* 1998; 273:13150–13156.

71. Cross DA, Alessi DR, Cohen P, Andjelkovich M, Hemmings BA. Inhibition of glycogen synthase kinase-3 by insulin mediated by protein kinase B. *Nature* 1995; 378:785–789.

72. Wang Q, Somwar R, Bilan PJ, et al. Protein kinase B/Akt participates in GLUT4 translocation by insulin in L6 myoblasts. *Mol Cell Biol* 1999; 19:4008–4018.

73. Tanti JF, Grillo S, Gremeaux T, Coffer PJ, Van Obberghen E, Le Marchand-Brustel Y. Potential role of protein kinase B in glucose transporter 4 translocation in adipocytes. *Endocrinology* 1997; 138:2005–2010.

74. Deprez J, Vertommen D, Alessi DR, Hue L, Rider MH. Phosphorylation and activation of heart 6-phosphofructo-2-kinase by protein kinase B and other protein kinases of the insulin signaling cascades. *J Biol Chem* 1997; 272:17269–17275.

75. Kennedy SG, Wagner AJ, Conzen SD, et al. The PI 3-kinase/Akt signaling pathway delivers an anti-apoptotic signal. *Genes Dev* 1997; 11:701–713.

76. Kauffmann-Zeh A, Rodriguez-Viciana P, Ulrich E, et al. Suppression of c-Myc-induced apoptosis by Ras signaling through PI(3)K and PKB. *Nature* 1997; 385:544–548.

77. Peli J, Schroter M, Rudaz C, et al. Oncogenic Ras inhibits Fas ligand-mediated apoptosis by down-regulating the expression of Fas. *EMBO J* 1999; 18:1824–1831.

78. Romashkova JA, Makarov SS. NF-kappaB is a target of AKT in anti-apoptotic PDGF signalling. *Nature* 1999; 401:86–90.

79. Sabbatini P, McCormick F. Phosphoinositide β-OH kinase (PI3K) and PKB/Akt delay the onset of p53-mediated, transcriptionally dependent apoptosis. *J Biol Chem* 1999; 274:24263–24269.

80. Jiang BH, Agani F, Passaniti A, Semenza GL. V-SRC induces expression of hypoxia-inducible factor 1 (HIF-1) and transcription of genes encoding vascular endothelial growth factor and enolase 1: involvement of HIF-1 in tumor progression. *Cancer Res* 1997; 57:5328–5335.

81. Richard DE, Berra E, Gothie E, Roux D, Pouyssegur J. p42/p44 mitogen-activated protein kinases phosphorylate hypoxia-inducible factor 1alpha (HIF-1alpha) and enhance the transcriptional activity of HIF-1. *J Biol Chem* 1999; 274:32631–32637.

82. Gleadle JM, Ratcliffe PJ. Induction of hypoxia-inducible factor-1, erythropoietin, vascular endothelial growth factor, and glucose transporter-1 by hypoxia: evidence against a regulatory role for Src kinase. *Blood* 1997; 89:503–509.

83. Rosette C, Karin M. Ultraviolet light and osmotic stress: activation of the JNK cascade through multiple growth factor and cytokine receptors. *Science* 1996; 274:1194–1197.

84. Lin RZ, Hu ZW, Chin JH, Hoffman BB. Heat shock activates c-Src tyrosine kinases and phosphatidylinositol 3-kinase in NIH3T3 fibroblasts. *J Biol Chem* 1997; 272:31196–31202.

85. Coffer PJ, Burgering BM, Peppelenbosch MP, Bos JL, Kruijer W. UV activation of receptor tyrosine kinase activity. *Oncogene* 1995; 11:561–569.

86. Huang RP, Wu JX, Fan Y, Adamson ED. UV activates growth factor receptors via reactive oxygen intermediates. *J Cell Biol* 1996; 133:211–220.

87. Vanden Hoek TL, Becker LB, Shao Z, Li C, Schumacker PT. Reactive oxygen species released from mitochondria during brief hypoxia induce preconditioning in cardiomyocytes. *J Biol Chem* 1998; 273:18092–18098.

88. Chandel NS, Maltepe E, Goldwasser E, Mathieu CE, Simon MC, Schumacker PT. Mitochondrial reactive oxygen species trigger hypoxia-induced transcription. *Proc Natl Acad Sci USA* 1998; 95:11715–11720.

89. Duranteau J, Chandel NS, Kulisz A, Shao Z, Schumacker PT. Intracellular signaling by reactive oxygen species during hypoxia in cardiomyocytes. *J Biol Chem* 1998; 273:11619–11624.

90. Semenza GL, Roth PH, Fang H-M, Wang GL. Transcriptional regulation of genes encoding glycolytic enzymes by hypoxia-inducible factor 1. *J Biol Chem* 1994; 269:23757–23767.

91. Shweiki D, Itin A, Soffer D, Keshet E. Vascular endothelial growth factor induced by hypoxia may mediate hypoxia-initiated angiogenesis. *Nature* 1992; 359:843–845.

92. Graham CH, Fitzpatrick TE, McCrae KR. Hypoxia stimulates urokinase receptor expression through a heme-dependent pathway. *Blood* 1998; 91:3300–3307.

93. Bodi I, Bishopric NH, Discher DJ, Wu X, Webster KA. Cell-specificity and signaling pathway of endothelin-1 gene regulation by hypoxia. *Cardiovas Res* 1995; 30:975–984.

94. Czyzyk-Krzeska MF, Furnari BA, Lawson EE, Millhorn DE. Hypoxia increases rate of transcription and stability of tyrosine hydroxylase mRNA in pheochromocytoma (PC12) cells. *J Biol Chem* 1994; 269:760–764.

95. Goldberg MA, Glass GA, Cunningham JM, Bunn HF. The regulated expression of erythropoietin by two human hepatoma cell lines. *Proc Natl Acad Sci USA* 1987; 84:7972–7976.

96. Goldberg MA, Dunning SP, Bunn HF. Regulation of the erythropoietin gene: evidence that the oxygen sensor is a heme protein. *Science* 1988; 242:1412–1415.

97. Semenza GL, Nejfelt MK, Chi SM, Antonarakis SE. Hypoxia-inducible nuclear factors bind to an enhancer element located 3′ to the erythropoietin gene. *Proc Natl Acad Sci USA* 1991; 88:5680–5684.

98. Imagawa S, Goldberg MA, Doweiko J, Bunn HF. Regulatory elements of the erythropoietin gene. *Blood* 1991; 77:278–285.

99. Wang GL, Semenza GL. Purification and characterization of hypoxia-inducible factor 1. *J Biol Chem* 1995; 270:1230–1237.

100. Hoffman EC, Reyes H, Chu FF, et al. Cloning of a factor required for activity of the Ah (dioxin) receptor. *Science* 1991; 252:954–958.

101. Hirose K, Morita M, Ema M, et al. cDNA cloning and tissue-specific expression of a novel basic helix-loop-helix/PAS factor (Arnt2) with close sequence similarity to the aryl hydrocarbon receptor nuclear translocator (Arnt). *Mol Cell Biol* 1996; 16:1706–1713.

102. Drutel G, Kathmann M, Heron A, Schwartz JC, Arrang JM. Cloning and selective expression in brain and kidney of ARNT2 homologous to the Ah receptor nuclear translocator (ARNT). *Biochem Biophys Res Commun* 1996; 225:333–339.

103. Hogenesch JB, Chan WK, Jackiw VH, et al. Characterization of a subset of the basic-helix-loop-helix-PAS superfamily that interacts with components of the dioxin signaling pathway. *J Biol Chem* 1997; 272:8581–8593.

104. Ikeda M, Nomura M. cDNA cloning and tissue-specific expression of a novel basic helix-loop-helix/PAS protein (BMAL1) and identication of alternatively spliced variants with alternative translation initiation site usage. *Biochem Biophys Res Commun* 1997; 233:258–264.

105. Takahata S, Sogawa K, Kobayashi A, et al. Transcriptionally active heterodimer formation of an Arnt-like PAS protein, Arnt3, with HIF-1a, HLF, and clock. *Biochem Biophys Res Commun* 1998; 248:789–794.

106. Hogenesch JB, Gu YZ, Jain S, Bradfield CA. The basic-helix-loop-helix-PAS orphan MOP3 forms transcriptionally active complexes with circadian and hypoxia factors. *Proc Natl Acad Sci USA* 1998; 95:5474–5479.

107. Gu YZ, Hogenesch JB, Bradfield CA. The PAS superfamily: sensors of environmental and developmental signals. *Annu Rev Pharmacol Toxicol* 2000; 40:519–561.

108. Goldberg MA, Schneider TJ. Similarities between the oxygen-sensing mechanisms regulating the expression of vascular endothelial growth factor and erythropoietin. *J Biol Chem* 1994; 269:4355–4359.

109. Wenger RH, Kvietikova I, Rolfs A, Gassmann M, Marti HH. Hypoxia-inducible factor-1 alpha is regulated at the post-mRNA level. *Kidney Int* 1997; 51:560–563.

110. Huang LE, Arany Z, Livingston DM, Bunn HF. Activation of hypoxia-inducible transcription factor depends primarily upon redox-sensitive stabilization of its alpha subunit. *J Biol Chem* 1996; 271:32253–32259.

111. Jiang BH, Rue E, Wang GL, Roe R, Semenza GL. Dimerization, DNA binding, and transactivation properties of hypoxia-inducible factor 1. *J Biol Chem* 1996; 271:17771–17778.

112. Pugh CW, O'Rourke JF, Nagao M, Gleadle JM, Ratcliffe PJ. Activation of hypoxia-inducible factor-1; definition of regulatory domains within the alpha subunit. *J Biol Chem* 1997; 272:11205–11214.

113. Srinivas V, Zhang LP, Zhu XH, Caro J. Characterization of an oxygen/redox-dependent degradation domain of hypoxia-inducible factor alpha (HIF-alpha) proteins. *Biochem Biophys Res Commun* 1999; 260:557–561.

114. Jiang BH, Zheng JZ, Leung SW, Roe R, Semenza GL. Transactivation and inhibitory domains of hypoxia-inducible factor 1alpha. Modulation of transcriptional activity by oxygen tension. *J Biol Chem* 1997; 272:19253–19260.

115. Ema M, Taya S, Yokotani N, Sogawa K, Matsuda Y, Fujii-Kuriyama Y. A novel bHLH-PAS factor with close sequence similarity to hypoxia-inducible factor 1alpha regulates the VEGF expression and is potentially involved in lung and vascular development. *Proc Natl Acad Sci USA* 1997; 94:4273–4278.

116. Tian H, McKnight SL, Russell DW. Endothelial PAS domain protein 1 (EPAS1), a transcription factor selectively expressed in endothelial cells. *Genes Dev* 1997; 11:72–82.

117. Flamme I, Frohlich T, von Reutern M, Kappel A, Damert A, Risau W. HRF,a putative basic helix-loop-helix-PAS-domain transcription factor is closely related to hypoxia-inducible factor-1 alpha and developmentally expressed in blood vessels. *Mech Dev* 1997; 63:51–60.

118. Gu YZ, Moran SM, Hogenesch JB, Wartman L, Bradfield CA. Molecular characterization and chromosomal localization of a third alpha-class hypoxia inducible factor subunit, HIF3alpha. *Gene Expr* 1998; 7:205–213.

119. Salceda S, Caro J. Hypoxia-inducible factor 1alpha (HIF-1alpha) protein is rapidly degraded by the ubiquitin-proteasome system under normoxic conditions. Its stabilization by hypoxia depends on redox-induced changes. *J Biol Chem* 1997; 272:22642–22647.

120. Huang LE, Gu J, Schau M, Bunn HF. Regulation of hypoxia-inducible factor 1alpha is mediated by an O2-dependent degradation domain via the ubiquitin-proteasome pathway. *Proc Natl Acad Sci USA* 1998; 95:7987–7992.

121. Wiesener MS, Turley H, Allen WE, et al. Induction of endothelial PAS domain protein-1 by hypoxia: characterization and comparison with hypoxia-inducible factor-1alpha. *Blood* 1998; 92:2260–2268.

122. Maxwell PH, Wiesener MS, Chang GW, et al. The tumour suppressor protein VHL targets hypoxia-inducible factors for oxygen-dependent proteolysis [see comments]. *Nature* 1999; 399:271–275.

123. Ohh M, Park CW, Ivan M, et al. Ubiquitination of hypoxia-inducible factor requires direct binding to the beta-domain of the von Hippel-Lindau protein [see comments]. *Nat Cell Biol* 2000; 2:423–427.

124. Gassmann M, Chilov D, Wenger RH. Regulation of the hypoxia-inducible factor-1 alpha. ARNT is not necessary for hypoxic induction of HIF-1 alpha in the nucleus [in process citation]. *Adv Exp Med Biol* 2000; 475:87–99.

125. Fox ME, Lemmon MJ, Mauchline ML, et al. Anaerobic bacteria as a delivery system for cancer gene therapy: in vitro activation of 5-fluorocytosine by genetically engineered clostridia [published erratum appears in Gene Ther 1996 Aug;3(8):741]. *Gene Ther* 1996; 3:173–178.

126. Lemmon MJ, van Zijl P, Fox ME, et al. Anaerobic bacteria as a gene delivery system that is controlled by the tumor microenvironment. *Gene Ther* 1997; 4:791–796.

127. Schwarze SR, Hruska KA, Dowdy SF. Protein transduction: unrestricted delivery into all cells? *Trends Cell Biol* 2000; 10:290–295.

128. Frankel AD, Pabo CO. Cellular uptake of the tat protein from human immunodeficiency virus. *Cell* 1988; 55:1189–1193.

129. Green M, Loewenstein PM. Autonomous functional domains of chemically synthesized human immunodeficiency virus tat trans-activator protein. *Cell* 1988; 55:1179–1188.

130. Derossi D, Joliot AH, Chassaing G, Prochiantz A. The third helix of the Antennapedia homeodomain translocates through biological membranes.*J Biol Chem* 1994; 269:10444–10450.

131. Derossi D, Calvet S, Trembleau A, Brunissen A, Chassaing G, Prochiantz A. Cell internalization of the third helix of the Antennapedia homeodomain is receptor-independent. *J Biol Chem* 1996; 271:18188–18193.

132. Elliott G, O'Hare P. Intercellular trafficking and protein delivery by a herpesvirus structural protein. *Cell* 1997; 88:223–233.

133. Wender PA, Mitchell DJ, Pattabiraman K, Pelkey ET, Steinman L, Rothbard JB. The design, synthesis, and evaluation of molecules that enable or enhance cellular uptake: peptoid molecular transporters. *Proc Natl Acad Sci USA* 2000; 97:13003–13008.

134. Rothbard JB, Garlington S, Lin Q, et al. Conjugation of arginine oligomers to cyclosporin A facilitates topical delivery and inhibition of inflammation. *Nat Med* 2000; 6:1253–1257.

135. Derossi D, Chassaing G, Prochiantz A. Trojan peptides: the penetratin system for intracellular delivery. *Trends Cell Biol* 1998; 8:84–87.

136. Elliott G, O'Hare P. Intercellular trafficking of VP22-GFP fusion proteins. *Gene Ther* 1999; 6:149–151.

137. Nagahara H, Vocero-Akbani AM, Snyder EL, et al. Transduction of full-length TAT fusion proteins into mammalian cells: TAT-p27Kip1 induces cell migration. *Nat Med* 1998; 4:1449–1452.

138. Schwarze SR, Ho A, Vocero-Akbani A, Dowdy SF. In vivo protein transduction: delivery of a biologically active protein into the mouse. *Science* 1999; 285:1569–1572.

139. Brown JM, Giaccia AJ. The unique physiology of solid tumors: opportunities (and problems) for cancer therapy. *Cancer Res* 1998; 58:1408–1416.

II THE FUNCTIONAL IMPACT OF ONCOGENE EXPRESSION ON CANCER CELLS—THERAPEUTIC IMPLICATIONS

8

Deregulation of Cell Cycle Progression by Oncogenic Transformation

Marcelo L. Rodriguez-Puebla, PhD,
Adrian M. Senderowicz, MD,
and Claudio J. Conti, DVM, PhD, MD

Contents

1. INTRODUCTION

The regulation of cell cycle and proliferation has been extensively studied in the last few years and a consensus paradigm of cell cycle regulation has been developed *(1)*. According to this paradigm, the master switch of the cell cycle is the Rb family of proteins. Proliferation is turned on by phosphorylation of these proteins by cyclin-dependent kinases (CDKs) (Fig. 1) *(2)*. These kinases are activated by D-type cyclins (D1, D2, and D3) and cyclin E, and inhibited by two families of CDK inhibitors (CKIs), the Ink (p16^{Ink4a}, p15^{Ink4b}, p18^{Ink4c}, and p19^{Ink4d}) and Cip/Kip families (p21^{Cip1}, p27^{Kip1}, and p57^{Kip2}) *(3,4)*.

pRb proteins are pocket proteins that sequester E2F transcription factors preventing them from activating critical genes in cell proliferation. In addition, Rb/E2F binds to histone deacetylase to form complexes that act as transcriptional repressors *(5)*. After Rb phosphorlation by CDK4 and/or CDK6 complexes during G1 phase and CDK2 at G1/S interphase, E2F proteins are released and promote the transcription of genes essential for the transition to S phase of cell cycle (Fig. 1B) *(1,6)*. CDK4,6/D-type cyclins, therefore, execute their critical functions during mid-to-late G1 phase, as cells cross a G1 restriction point and become independent of mitogens for completion of the division cycle. These features suggest that the fundamental role of these complexes is to integrate extracellular signals with the cell cycle machinery *(7)*.

From: *Oncogene-Directed Therapies*
Edited by: J. W. Rak © Humana Press Inc., Totowa, NJ

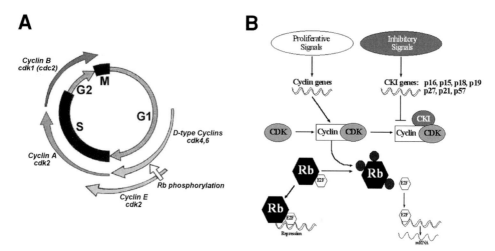

Fig. 1. Regulation of cell cycle in mammalian cells. (**A**) Specific CDKs participate in the regulation of each phase of the cell cycle by phosphorylating some substrates. In G1 phase, phosphorylation of *retinoblastoma* (Rb) is essential for G1/S phase transition. (**B**) Rb phosphorylation is performed in sequential manner by CDK4 and CDK2. After Rb phosphorylation, E2F transcription factor is release from Rb complex and participates in the transcription of important genes for S phase progression. On the other hand, CKIs are regulated by extracellular inhibitor signals and bind and inactivate the CDK–cyclin complex.

Although this paradigm of cell cycle regulation is a useful framework for under-standing the basis of cell homeostasis, it has become clear that it is also an oversimpli-fication of a much more complex phenomenon. Not only are the interactions between the different components of the cell cycle more intricate than anticipated, but cross-talk between cell cycle regulatory pathways and pathways regulating apoptosis and differ-entiation have become evident.

In addition to binary and ternary complexes with D-type cyclins and CKIs, CDK4 was also found associated with other proteins. For example, CDK4 association with $p50^{Cdc37}$, a protein subunit of the chaperone heat shock protein 90, was recently described (8,9). Also, CDK4 interaction with survivin (a member of the inhibitor of apoptosis [IAP] family) was recently established as part of the caspase 3 apoptotic pathway (10). The expression of survivin is cell cycle regulated and strong expression is observed in G2/M phase. Also, association of survivin with microtubules suggests that this protein participates in a cytoskeleton protective pathway that has an important role in the G2 checkpoint (11). Thus, it was suggested that CDK4 might also partici-pate in the G2 checkpoint by interacting with survivin (11).

Other important points of regulation have been described in G2 and mitosis. In these phases, also, the specific expression of certain regulators is essential to control the cor-rect sequence of events that lead to cell division. Basically, the cyclins B1, B2, and its partner cdc2 (CDK1), together with other kinases and phosphatases (wee1, cdc25), regulated the final phases of the cell cycle (Fig. 1A).

In the last decade, several proteins that participate in the tight control of cell division have been found to be mutated, deleted, amplified, or overexpressed in human and experimental tumors. In the first part of this chapter, we want summarize the principal points of deregulation found in human and experimental tumors. Furthermore, we will point to specific proteins whose importance in tumor development is now evident. In this regard, we will focus only on the regulators that play an important role in the modulation of the cell cycle machinery per se, and minimal details will be given to retinoblastoma mutations, which have been described in other chapters.

2. CELL CYCLE ALTERATIONS IN NEOPLASIA

In the last few years, work from our own, as well as other laboratories, has shown that cyclins, CDK complexes, and other cell cycle regulators are mechanistically involved in the development of chemically induced epidermal tumors (12–16). This is consistent with a large body of literature showing the importance of inactivation of the pRb pathway in tumor development (1,17,18). The inactivation of pRb is produced by direct mutation of the Rb protein, but this is a relatively rare event occurring in retinoblastomas, osteosarcomas, and a minority of breast and some other tumors (1,17,18). More frequent alterations of this pathway occur by functional inactivation of Rb by hyperphosphorylation. This is normally the result of elevated CDK activities caused by overexpression of cyclins, CDKs, or loss of function of CKIs, being the most commonly deleted p16[Ink4a] (Fig. 1B).

For example, several laboratories have reported that some tumors show loss of pRb or, alternatively, overexpression of cyclin D1 (19–21). Similarly, in other tumors, loss of p16[Ink4a] and pRb are mutually exclusive (22–24). This observation led to the hypothesis that inactivation of the cyclin D/CDK/p16/pRb pathway can promote tumor development and that either loss of the suppressor activity of pRb or p16[Ink4a], or overexpression of cyclin D1 can override this checkpoint (1,25). However, these alterations may not all have the same impact on the pathway. While functional inactivation of pRb itself would completely eliminate the checkpoint, alterations in p16[Ink4a] and cyclin D1, which operate upstream of pRb, might cooperate to provide an additional growth advantage. This point of view is supported by experiments showing that, in normal cells, the decision to enter S phase depends on the balance between functional cyclin D1 and p16[Ink4a] and that several human tumor cell lines have both cyclin D1 and p16[Ink4a] abnormalities (26). Therefore, the ultimate result of these changes is loss of proliferative control and loss of balance between proliferation, apoptosis, and differentiation. Several reports have implicated D-type cyclins in the neoplastic development, although limited information is available on the participation of its partner, CDK4, in these events. The involvement of CDK4 in the neoplastic process was suggested by the fact that CDK4 amplification and/or overexpression were detected in human glioblastomas, but, in these tumors, overexpression and/or amplification of D-type cyclins were not detected (27–29). In addition, CDK4 mutations were identified in patients with familial melanoma (30,31), and recently, amplification and overexpression of CDK4 were also detected in sporadic breast carcinomas (32) and sarcomas (33).

3. G1 CYCLINS AND CDKS IN CARCINOGENESIS

The mechanisms that link growth factor signaling to the activation of the cell cycle progression in G1 are the key to understanding how cells decide whether or not to undergo the division process. Major emphasis is being placed on the identification of components that are activated in mid to late G1. In this sense, D-type cyclins are major downstream targets of extracellular signaling pathways and, together with cyclin E, regulate the G1/S phase transition. Transcriptional induction of D-type cyclins occurs in response to a wide variety of mitogenic stimuli, including the Ras signaling cascade *(34)* and the adenomatous polyposis coli (APC)/β-catenin/Tcf-Lef pathway *(35)*. These data have led to the idea that D-type cyclins act as growth factor sensors. A prediction from this would be that deregulated expressions of D-type cyclins contribute to tumorigenesis by making cells less dependent on growth factors. Both D-type cyclins/CDK4,6 and cyclin E/CDK2 complexes phosphorylate sequentially the product of the tumor suppressor gene Rb. Thus, it was not unexpected that D-type cyclins and cyclin E were found amplified, rearranged, or overexpressed in several kinds of experimental and human tumors. In fact, cyclin D1 was first identified on 11q13 as a chromosomal breakpoint region rearranged with the parathyroid hormone gene in a subset of parathyroid adenomas (PRAD1 gene) *(36,37)*, and rearrangement of that region on chromosome 11q13 also appears to be highly characteristic of centrocytic lymphoma (BCL1, B-cell lymphoma 1) *(36–39)*. At present, amplification and overexpression of cyclin D1 have also been reported in the pathogenesis of other types of cancer, including carcinomas of human breast, upper aerodigestive tract, and head and neck squamous cell carcinomas *(20,40–42)*. Among them, cyclin D1 plays an important role in deregulating proliferation of breast cancer. The cyclin D1 gene is amplified in approx 20% of mammary carcinomas, and the protein is overexpressed in approx 50% of cases *(43,44)*. The relevance of cyclin D1 overexpression in breast cancer is further emphasized by the finding that transgenic expression of cyclin D1 in mice results in mammary hyperplasia and adenocarcinoma *(45)*. The prominent role of cyclin D1 in growth of breast epithelium was also supported by the fact that cyclin D1 knock-out mice show a marked defect in breast epithelium development during pregnancy *(46,47)*. In addition, Yu et al. have recently reported that cyclin D1-deficient mice are resistant to breast cancer induced by the neu and ras oncogenes, although, these animals remain fully sensitive to other oncogenic pathways, such as those driven by c-myc or wnt-1 *(48)*. CDK-independent activities of cyclin D1 also appear to be involved in the development of mammary carcinomas *(49)*. Two recent studies indicate that expression of cyclin D1 leads to hormone-independent activation of estrogen receptor (ER) *(50,51)*. Estrogens are major determinants of proliferation of breast epithelial cells, where activation of ER leads to increased cyclin D1 transcription. Indeed, an estrogen-responsive element has been found in the cyclin D1 promoter *(52)*. Interestingly, whereas only 50–60% of human breast cancers express a functional ER, cyclin D1 overexpression is seen preferentially in ER-positive breast cancers *(53,54)*. Surprisingly, the effect of cyclin D1 on ER does not require CDK binding. In fact, the cyclin D1/CDK4 complex is unable to activate the ER, supporting the notion that cyclin D1 acts on ER in a CDK-independent fashion. Other experiments showed that cyclin D1 forms a direct physical complex with ER *(50,51)*. Altogether, these results suggest the existence in breast cancers of an autostimulatory loop, in which activation of ER by hormone leads to transcriptional induction of cyclin D1, and furthermore, the newly synthesized cyclin D1 protein can bind ER to cause ER activation and stimulate breast cancer growth. Another role of D-type cyclins described, independent of CDK, has been that of forming a complex with the androgen receptor and inhibiting its transcriptional transactivation ability *(55)*. These findings may explain the low frequency of cyclin D1 amplification in prostatic adenocarcinomas.

Several lines of evidence have shown that the cell-cycle machinery, specifically the circuit cyclin D1/CDK4,6-p16-pRb, lies downstream of oncogenic ras. In fact, increased expression of cyclin D1 by activated ras was observed in epithelial cells from rat intestine and mammary gland (56,57) and in fibroblast cell lines (58). This increased expression of cyclin D1 was apparently mediated through the MAP kinase cascade and involves activation of the cyclin D1 promoter by AP1 sequences (59,60). Furthermore, recent studies have indicated that ras may independently coordinate the up-regulation of cyclin D1 and down-regulation of p27[Kip1] expression by the respective activation of MAP kinase and RhoA pathways (61,62). Cyclin D1 up-regulation and p27[Kip1] down-regulation may depend on temporally distinct roles of ras throughout the G1 phase (61–63). Consistent with the main role of cyclin D1 in ras-dependent tumorigenesis, cyclin D1-deficient mice show a reduced level of mouse skin tumor development when the two-stage carcinogenesis model was used. In this model, mutation and activation of the Ha-ras gene is induced by topical treatment with the genotoxic carcinogen 7,12-dimethylbenz(a)-anthracene (DMBA) (64). The link between cyclin D1 and p27[Kip1] has been studied by using knock-out mice, and a clear difference has been observed between normal and neoplastic proliferation. For instance, the development of double knock-out mice has shown genetic evidence for the interaction of cyclin D1 and p27[Kip1]. Two different groups have shown that deletion of the p27[Kip1] gene restores normal development in cyclin D1-deficient mice and corrects the p27-null to wild-type phenotypes (65,66). However, the unique role of cyclin D1 in tumorigenesis has been demonstrated by the fact that the cyclin D1/p27[Kip1] double-null mice did not show compensation in mouse skin tumor development (Rodriguez-Puebla et al., unpublished results). Altogether, these results demonstrate that down-regulation of p27[Kip1] can compensate for the lack of cyclin D1 in normal but not in neoplastic proliferation. The development of transgenic mice also has shown that cyclin D1 overexpression behaves as an oncogene in some tissue, such as mammary gland (45), but not in other tissue such as skin (67). In fact, overexpression of cyclin D1 increases CDK activity and cell proliferation but does not affect skin tumor development (67,68).

Several other signaling pathways participate in activation of the cyclin D1 gene and further deregulation of its expression in tumorigenesis. However, the more relevant finding in the last few years has been that the cyclin D1 gene is a target of the β-catenin/LEF pathway (69). β-catenin plays a dual role in the cells; one in cell–cell contact and an additional role in signaling together with the transcription factor LEF-1. In this regard, elevated β-catenin levels in colorectal cancer, caused by mutation in β-catenin, result in increased transcriptional activation of its target genes. Thus, although the cyclin D1 gene is not amplified in human colon cancer, the expression of cyclin D1 is elevated in about 30% of human adenocarcinomas (70,71).

Cyclin D2 overexpression or amplification was also described in several tumors. In fact, cyclin D2 accumulation in the cytoplasm of gastric carcinoma cells appears to play a role in cancer progression (72). Also, the overexpression of cyclin D2 in carcinoma in situ identified it as a candidate gene in male germ cell malignancies (73,74). Cyclin D2 is also overexpressed in chronic B-cell malignancies (75). In addition, recent studies have shown increased levels of expression of cyclin D2 in human ovarian granulose cell tumors (76). Apart from high cyclin D2 levels, granulose cell tumors expressed very little cyclin D1 and cyclin D3. Moreover, overexpression of cyclin D2 was demonstrated in cell lines derived from human testicular germ cell tumors (76). These data are consistent with the phenotype observed in female cyclin D2-null mice, in which the ovarian granulose cells showed an inability to proliferate normally in response to hormone follicle stimulating hormone (FSH), whereas males display hypoplastic testes *(76)*. Cyclin D2 appears to play a specific role in other tissue, as demonstrated in transgenic mice. In this case, development of thymic hyperplasia was observed in the cyclin D2 and cyclin D1 transgenic mice, whereas on the other end of the spectrum, the cyclin D3 mice did not develop thymic hyperplasia *(68,77)*. Although, fewer reports suggest that cyclin D3 plays a role in tumorigenesis, cyclin D3 overexpression was associated with increased expression of p27[Kip1] in a subset of aggressive B-cell lymphomas *(78)*. In addition, coordinated elevation of cyclin D3 and cyclin D1 was observed in the breast cell line MCF-7 *(79)*.

Cyclin E is another G1 cyclin, which has been implicated in cancer development. In fact, overexpression and/or amplification of cyclin E has been described in several human cancers such as breast, invasive bladder, non-small cell lung, ovarian, and gastric cancer *(80–91)*. Also, forced expression of human cyclin E in the mammary gland of transgenic mice led to develop of hyperplasia and carcinomas *(92)*. However, the role of cyclin E in proliferation and cancer development appears to be much more complicated that D-type cyclins. In this sense, while cells lacking a functional Rb molecule apparently no longer require the activity of D-type cyclin/CDK complexes *(93,94)*, cyclin E/CDK2 activity remains indispensable *(95)*. In addition, in the last few years a second isoform of cyclin E called cyclin E2 was described *(96)*, and other splice variants of cyclin E were also observed in breast cancer, although, specific roles for these variants have not yet been established *(97,98)*. Also, interactions of cyclin E with different proteins have been reported, and the more important of those appear to be the cyclin E association with components of the pre-mRNA splicing machinery *(99)* and the stimulation of DNA polymerase by CDK2/cyclin E phosphorylated Rb protein *(100)*. These activities could be important in the regulation of the cell cycle engine and the interaction with the DNA replication and repair systems during tumor development. In fact, phosphorylation of mammalian cdc6, a component of the prereplication complex by CDK2, was described a few years ago *(101)*.

Not only the regulatory subunits, such us D-type cyclins and cyclin E, have been implicated in the tumorigenesis process, but the catalytic subunit of D-type cyclins, CDK4, was found amplified or overexpressed in several human cancers. In fact, an early description of co-amplification of CDK4 with other putative oncogenes such as MDM2 and GLI was reported in human sarcomas *(102)*. As was mentioned above, CDK4 mutations were also identified in patients with familial melanoma *(30,31)*. This missense mutation results in a mutant CDK4 protein, which loses its affinity for the CDK-inhibitor p16[Ink4a] without affecting its ability to bind D-type cyclins *(30,31)*. However, the more relevant finding was that CDK4 amplification or overexpression is an alternative mechanism to p16[Ink4a] or pRb mutation in human gliomas *(27,29,103–105)*. Serrano et al. demonstrated that p16[Ink4a] acts as a negative regulator of cell proliferation, through its binding to CDK4, by preventing it from forming an active complex with cyclin D *(106)*. The finding that amplification of the CDK4 gene occurs in glioblastomas without abnormalities in the p16[Ink4a] region suggests that aberrations of the cell cycle are critical for the development of these tumors. In fact, when aberrations of these genes are included, 85% of the glioblastomas show abnormalities *(27)*. Another important finding was that cyclin D1, which is also part of this cell cycle regulatory mechanism, was not amplified or overexpressed in these tumors *(27,29)*. These results, suggest that CDK4 amplification can act in a different way than its catalytic activity phosphorylating pRb family of proteins. The generation of CDK4 transgenic mice has shown that overexpression of CDK4 in epidermis results in strong hyperplasia and hyperproliferative phenotype without overexpression of D-type cyclins *(107)*. In the last few years, a noncatalytic function of CDK4 has been suggested by sequestering the CDK2-inhibitor p27[Kip1], resulting in further activation of CDK2 (107–109). However, the actual role of the noncatalytic function of CDK4 in human and experimental tumors has not been clearly established. In this sense, overexpression of CDK4 in mouse skin result in increased susceptibility to chemically induced squamous cell carcinoma development (Miliani de Marval and Rodriguez-Puebla, in preparation). On the other hand, abrogation of CDK4 expression in CDK4-deficient mice showed minimal phenotype alterations; mainly a defect in β-islet cell proliferation *(110,111)*, although complete inhibition of chemically induced skin tumors was observed in these mice (Rodriguez-Puebla and Conti, in preparation). Another interesting possibility is that CDK4 could participate in the c-myc induced tumorigenesis. C-myc is a transcription factor that has been implicated in a variety of human and experimental tumors, and recently, CDK4 was identified as a target of c-myc, opening the possibility of cooperation between CDK4 and c-myc in carcinogenesis *(112,113)*. At present, we have limited information about the participation of other CDKs in the tumorigenesis process, although, CDK6 has been involved in the development of NK/T-cell lymphomas, glioblastomas multiform and breast cancer *(114–116)*.

Among the negative regulators of the cell cycle that have been described as tumor suppressor genes, we can mention p16[Ink4a] and pRb. As was mentioned above, not only the deregulation of factors involved in Rb phosphorylation have been observed in human and experimental tumors, but also mutations in the Rb gene have been detected in some human tumors, mainly in retinoblastomas and osteosarcomas, although functional inactivation of Rb appears to be more frequent. p16[Ink4a] is a negative regulator that binds and inhibits the activity of the complexes CK4,6/D-type cyclins and, hence, avoids the inhibition of Rb protein. However, the fact that the p16[Ink4a] locus also encodes other important tumor suppressor genes (p19[Arf] in mouse and p14[Arf] in human) in an alternative reading frame has lead to the question of the actual role of p16[Ink4a] in carcinogenesis.

4. CELL CYCLE PROTEOLISIS AND TUMORIGENESIS

In the last few years, intense efforts have been made to elucidate the machinery responsible for the degradation of proteins involved in the control of the G1 phase. The ubiquitin-proteasome proteolityc pathway mediates the degradation of short-lived regulatory proteins, including cyclins and other cell cycle regulators *(117,118)*. The ubiquitin-mediated pathway comprises two discrete steps: the covalent attachment of multiple ubiquitin molecules to the protein substrate and degradation of the polyubiquitylated protein by the 26S proteasome complex (Fig. 2) *(118)*. The ubiquitin attachment system consists of at least three enzymes: a ubiquitin-activating enzyme (E1), a ubiquitin-conjugative enzyme (E2), and a ubiquitin ligase (E3). The E3 components are thought to be primarily responsible for substrate recognition. Two major types of E3 enzymes are thought to regulate cell cycle progression: the anaphase-promoting complex or cyclosome (APC/C), and the SCF complex, which promote the degradation of G1 phase regulators *(118)*. The SCF complexes consist of the invariable components Skp1, Cull, and

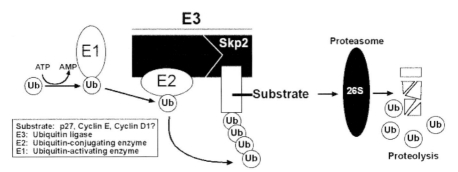

Fig. 2. Proteolysis mediated by the ubiquitination pathway. The activation of ubiquitin by E1 enzyme is followed by transfer to an E2 enzyme. The E2 enzyme transfers the ubiquitin molecule to an E3, which ligates the ubiquitin to the substrate protein via an isopeptide bond. The marked substrate is targeted to the 26S proteosome for degradation and ubiquitin is recycled.

ROC1, as well as a variable component, known as an F-box protein, that binds to Skp1 through its F-box motif and is responsible for substrate recognition *(119–121)*. Mammals likely posses several hundred F-box proteins, providing the basis for multiple substrate-specific ubiquitination pathways. Skp2, which contains an F-box domain, was identified originally as a protein that interacts with CDK2-cyclinA complex. This protein is responsible for the recognition of the cell cycle regulators cyclin E, cyclin D1, and p27^{Kip1} (Fig. 2) *(122,123)*. Skp2 is required for the G1-S transition in both transformed cells and diploid fibroblasts, and Skp2 overexpression induces quiescent fibroblasts to replicate their DNA in low serum *(124)*. Skp2 only binds to and allows the ubiquitination of p27^{Kip1}, when the latter is phosphorylated in Thr-187 by CDK2 *(122)*. In quiescent cells levels of p27^{Kip1} are high, but in response to mitogenic stimuli, levels of cyclin E, cyclin A, and Skp2 increase, resulting in the Thr-187 phosphorylation of p27^{Kip1} and its subsequent ubiquitin-mediated degradation. Interestingly, p27^{Kip1} degradation is enhanced in many aggressive human tumors *(125)*. Skp2 also is required for the ubiquitination of cyclin E, but only in its free non-CDK2 bound form, whereas cyclin E complex formation with CDK2 is not affected by Skp2 *(126)*. Thus, given the role of Skp2 in inducing S-phase entry, it has been hypothesized that Skp2 can be deregulated in tumors. In fact, ubiquitin-mediated proteolysis has been involved in several human diseases such as Parkinson disease, Liddle syndrome, Angelman syndrome, cervical cancer, and Von Hippel Lindau syndrome *(127)*. The role of Skp2 in oncogenesis has recently been described in human and experimental tumors. A possible causative role of a increased level of Skp2 and decreased level of p27^{Kip1} was observed in colorectal carcinomas *(128)*. In addition, analysis of different stages of malignant oral cancer progression has also shown that an increased Skp2 level is associated with a reduced level of p27^{Kip1} *(129)*. Gstaiger et al. have also demonstrated that Skp2 has oncogenic potential and cooperates with Ha-ras to transform primary rodent fibroblasts *(129)*. Supporting these results, the generation of a transgenic mouse, in which Skp2 was targeted to the T-lymphoid lineage (130), showed a strong cooperative effect between overexpression of Skp2 and N-ras (double transgenic mice), which induce T-cell lymphomas *(130)*. However, recent analysis of Skp2 knock-out mice has revealed that the loss of Skp2 also may contribute to tumorigenesis. In fact, these mutant mice contain markedly enlarged nuclei with polyploidy and multiple centrosomes *(126)*. The results with transgenic and knock-out mice are consistent with the role of Skp2 regulating the proteolysis of positive (cyclin E and likely cyclin D1) and negative (p27^{Kip1}) regulators of cell cycle *(122,123)*. Finally, the chromosome mapping of Skp2 and Skp1 have shown that these loci are associated with karyotipic alterations, known amplifications or suspected tumor suppressor genes *(131)*.

5. THERAPEUTICS IMPLICATIONS

5.1. Therapeutic Approaches for the Manipulation of the Cell Cycle Machinery

Several strategies could be considered to modulate CDK activity. These strategies are divided into direct effects on the catalytic CDK subunit or indirect modulation of regulatory pathways that govern CDK activity *(132,133)*. The small molecular endogenous CDK inhibitors (SCDKI) are compounds that directly target the catalytic CDK subunit. Most of these compounds modulate CDK activity by interacting specifically with the ATP binding site of CDKs *(132–136)*. The second class of CDK inhibitors are compounds that inhibit CDK activity by targeting the regulatory "upstream pathways" that modulate the activity of CDKs: by altering the expression and synthesis of the CDK/cyclin subunits or the CDK inhibitory proteins; by modulating the phosphorylation of CDKs; by targeting CDK-activating kinase, cdc25, and wee1/myt1 or by manipulating the proteolytic machinery that regulates the catabolism of CDK/cyclin complexes or their regulators *(132,133)*.

5.2. Small Molecule CDK Modulators

5.2.1. PURINE DERIVATIVES: OLOMUCINE, ROSCOVITINE, AND DERIVATIVES

The first CDK inhibitor discovered was dimethylaminopurine *(137)*. This compound demonstrated clear evidence of inhibition of mitosis in sea urchin embryos without evidence of protein synthesis inhibition, due to inhibition of CDK1 (cdc2) activity (IC$_{50}$, 120 µM) *(134)*. Subsequent studies demonstrated that this molecule is relatively non-specific. Isopentenyladenine, a derivative of this compound, was somewhat more potent and specific for the CDKs (IC$_{50}$, 55 µM) *(138)*, although not a very potent antiproliferative agent. Subsequent screening efforts yielded more specific and potent inhibitors. Olomucine (Fig. 3) displayed potent ability to inhibit CDK1 (cdc2) and CDK2 (IC$_{50}$, 7 µM) *(134,138)*. Roscovitine (Fig. 3), an even more potent CDK inhibitor (IC$_{50}$s for CDK1/CDK2 of 0.7 µM), was derived from the olomucine structure *(139)*, showing more potent effects on cellular proliferation assays in the 60-cell line anticancer screen panel. The crystal structure of CDK2 in complex with isopentenyladenine, olomucine, or roscovitine was resolved, confirming that that all three inhibitors can bind to the ATP site *(136)*. Another novel purine analogue, CVT-313 (a potent CDK2 inhibitor), was obtained using a combinatorial library strategy and the knowledge of the crystal structure of CDK2 bound to chemical CDK inhibitors. Similar to the previous analogs, CVT-313 (Fig. 3) was specific for CDK1 (cdc2) and CDK2 with an IC$_{50}$ of 4.2 and 1.5 µM, respectively *(140)*. Not only CVT-313 showed expected cell cycle arrest, but also demonstrated potent inhibition in neointima revascularization after balloon angioplasty in in vivo preclinical models *(140)*. Although there are no clear plans to start clinical trials with these compounds, they clearly serve as important tools to dissect cellular effects due to CDK action.

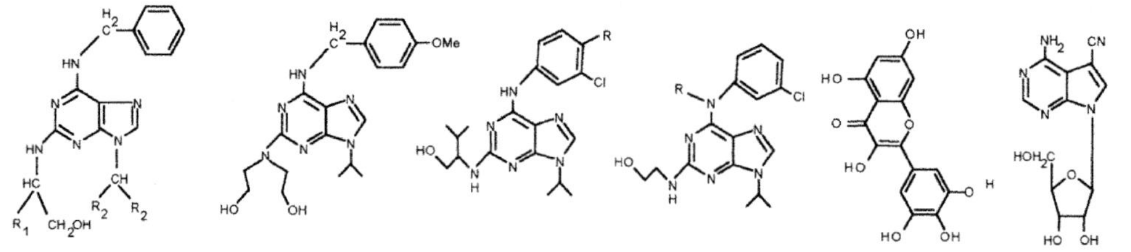

Olomucine (R_1=H, R_2=H) Roscovitine(R_1=C_2H_5, R_2=CH_3) | CVT - 313 | Purvalanol A (R=H) Purvalanol B (R=CO_2H) | Compound 52 (R=H) Compound 52Me (R=CH_3) | Myrecetin | Toyocamycin

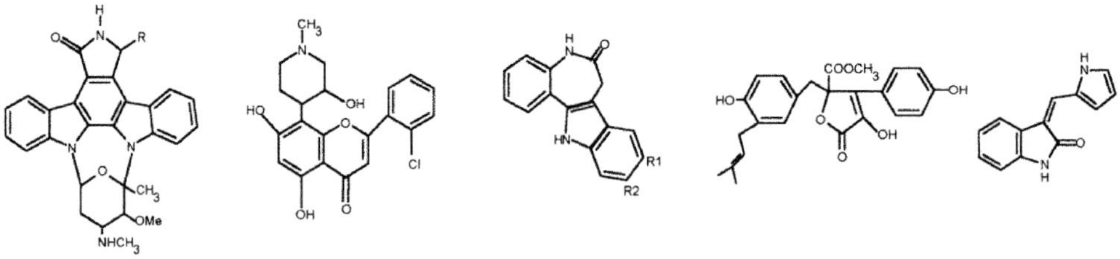

Staurosporine (R=H) UCN-01 (R=OH) | Flavopiridol | Kenpaullone (R_1=Br) 10-Br paullone (R_2=Br) | Butyrolactone I | Oxindole I

Fig. 3. Chemical structures of small molecular CDIs.

Based on the knowledge of the binding properties of olomucine to the ATP binding site of CDK2, a combinatorial approach to modifying the purine scaffold revealed several compounds with very potent and specific inhibitory properties against CDK1 (cdc2) and CDK2. Four novel compounds, purvalanol A, purvalanol B, compound 52, and compound 52E were characterized in a battery of in vitro kinase experiments (Fig. 3) *(141)*. Crystal structure studies of purvalanol B and CDK2 showed that this compound fits into the ATP-binding pocket, resembling the binding of olomucine to CDK2. Moreover, cell cycle studies with a more permeable membrane, purvalanol A, in exposed human fibroblasts revealed a clear arrest in G1/S and G2/M, compatible with the putative inhibitory properties in CDK2 and CDK1 (cdc2), respectively *(141)*.

5.2.2. Paullones

Using flavopiridol's antiproliferative in vitro profile in the National Cancer Institute (NCI) anticancer drug screen, several compounds display similar antiproliferative pattern to flavopiridol. Kenpaullone (NSC 664704, Fig. 3) displayed potent inhibitory properties against CDK1/cyclin B (IC_{50}, 0.4 μM), CDK2/cyclin A (IC_{50}, 0.68 μM), CDK2/cyclin E (IC_{50}, 7.5 μM), and CDK5/p25 (IC_{50}, 0.4 μM) with much less effect on other kinases *(135)*. Unfortunately, kenpaullone was not a very potent antiproliferative agent with GI_{50}s approx 42 μM. Kenpaullone behaves as a competitor with respect to ATP with an apparent Ki of approx 2.5 μM. Molecular modeling studies demonstrated that Kenpaullone may bind in the ATP binding site with residue contacts similar to other CDK2 inhibitors *(135)*. When kenpaullone was tested in serum-starved synchronized MCF10A breast epithelial cells, loss in S progression was observed in the presence of 30 μM kenpaullone. Thus, the G1/S arrest observed underscores the cellular effects of kenpaullone on the activity of G1 CDKs and cell cycle progression. Alsterpaullone (9-nitro-paullone-9NP) is an analogue of kenpaullone with more potent CDK inhibitory activity and lower GI_{50}s for tumor growth *(142,143)*. Further preclinical studies with these compounds and novel analogues are being undertaken.

5.2.3. OTHER CDK INHIBITORS

Kent et al. *(144)* discovered several new small molecule CDK inhibitors by high-throughput screening of small molecule compound libraries. They were able to discover 4 distinct CDK inhibitors, oxindole I (Fig. 3), urea I, urea II, and benzoic acid *(144)*. Interestingly, the last 3 compounds show some selectivity against CDK4/cyclin D1 with IC_{50}s approx 1.2–6.7 μM *(144)*. In contrast, oxindole I, showed nonselective inhibitory activity against CDK4/cyclin D1, CDK2/cyclin E, and CDK1(cdc2)/cyclin B1 (4.9, 10, and 10.2 μM, respectively). The effects and specificity of these compounds with respect to other kinases are not known *(144)*. When these 4 compounds were tested against 3 different tumor cell lines, only the less potent, albeit nonselective, compound oxindole I was able to promote antiproliferative effects, suggesting that in order to have potent antiproliferative activity in vitro, small molecule CDK inhibitors need to target more than one CDK *(144)*. Interestingly, flavopiridol, also a nonspecific CDK inhibitor, has more potent in vitro antiproliferative activity compared with more selective ones such as olomucine and roscovitine. This potent antiproliferative property, again, may reflect the nonspecific inhibitory nature of flavopiridol with respect to different CDKs.

A novel flavonoid, Myrecetin (Fig. 3), was recently discovered by Walker *(145)*. Preliminary studies demonstrated that this compound is a less potent CDK2 inhibitor (IC_{50}, approx 10 μM). Also, preliminary crystal structural efforts demonstrated that myrecetin binds in the ATP binding pocket of CDK2 in reverse orientation as compared to flavopiridol *(145)*. However, the specificity of this compound with respect to CDKs or the effects of this compound in cellular systems are not known.

5.3. Cellular Effects of Loss in CDK Activity

Several possible approaches to assess the role of CDKs in cellular models may involve the use of dominant negative (dn) forms of CDKs, heterologous expression of CKIs such as p16[INK4a] or p27[kip1], use of chemical CDK inhibitors or the use of CKI peptidomimetics *(132,133)*.

Several models could be studied in order to assess the functional role of CDKs in cellular physiology. Initial studies in yeast cells were possible because only one CDK (cdc2) is responsible for the cell cycle progression. However, human cells are more complex: several CDKs govern cell cycle progression, and their inhibition leads to either cell cycle arrest at different periods and/or apoptosis (programmed cell death).

5.3.1. CELL CYCLE ARREST

Initial studies by Van den Heuvel et al. *(146)* demonstrated that forced expression of CDK1(cdc2) (dn) alleles was able to block cell cycle progression of U2OS osteosarcoma cell lines at the G2/M boundary. In contrast, expression of either CDK2- or CDK3-dn prevented S phase progression *(146)*. Thus, this seminal observation helped to determine the role of most CDKs in human cell cycle progression. Forced expression of CKIs, such as p16[Ink4a], p21[Cip1], or p27[Kip1], or peptidomimetics derived from p21[Cip1], p16[Ink4a], or E2F1 *(132,133)*, clearly demonstrates G1/S cell cycle arrest. Furthermore, several small molecular CDK inhibitors including roscovitine, olomucine, purvalanol, and flavopiridol arrest cells at either the G1/S or G2/M boundaries

(134,140,141,147–149). It is unclear why these agents provoke a G1/S arrest phenotype in some cells and a G2/M or combined arrest in others; as mentioned later, in the case of flavopiridol, the arrest is independent of functional p53 or Rb *(148,150).* Interestingly, in some experimental models, the antiproliferative effect was accompanied, in the case of olomucine, flavopiridol, and roscovitine, by the induction of apoptosis *(134,151,152).*

5.3.2. APOPTOSIS

As mentioned earlier, these small molecular CDK inhibitors may induce apoptosis in some preclinical models. In one example, susceptibility to apoptosis by chemical CDK inhibitors (flavopiridol and olomucine) varied depending on the growth state of the cells. Thus, postmitotic nondividing PC-12 cells were protected from apoptosis, induced by nerve growth factor (NGF) deprivation, by the presence of flavopiridol or olomucine; on the other hand, cycling PC-12 cells were not protected from NGF withdrawal, but actually were induced to undergo apoptosis after exposure to flavopiridol *(153).* In a similar model of apoptosis, only CDK4- and CDK6-dn, but not CDK2- or CDK3-dn, protected neurons against NGF deprivation *(154).* Further evidence of the role of CDKs in apoptosis is based on the protective role of DN-cdc2, CDK2 or CDK3 in the apoptosis in HeLa cells is induced by staurosporine and TNFα. Finally, it has become clear that certain apoptotic stimuli provoke the induction of cleavage in CKIs (p21^{cip1}/p27^{kip1}) or CDK inhibitory proteins (wee1 and cdc27) by caspases leading to activation of CDKs *(155–157).* Clearly, the final outcome of loss of CDK activity to promote cell cycle arrest/apoptosis depends on several factors, including the mechanism of inhibition, cell type, and proliferation status. Thus, some cell types cannot tolerate loss of CDK activity and/or cell cycle arrest leading to cell death.

5.3.3. DIFFERENTIATION

It became clear recently that cells become differentiated when exit of the cell cycle (GO) and loss of CDK2 activity occurs. Based on this information, Lee and coworkers tested flavopiridol and roscovitine, both known CDK2 inhibitors, to determine if they induce a differentiated phenotype. For this purpose, NCI-H358 lung carcinoma cell lines were exposed to CDK2 antisense construct, flavopiridol, or roscovitine. Clear evidence of mucinous differentiation along with loss in CDK2 activity was observed. However, each CDK2-antagonist therapy had different cell cycle regulatory expression despite a similar differentiated phenotype *(158).*

In another effort to study the differentiating effects of aminopurvalanol, U937 myelomonocytic leukemia cell lines were treated with this compound. These cells acquired a phenotype characteristic of differentiated macrophages. Moreover, this potent CDK1 and CDK2 inhibitor displayed evidence of G2/M arrest with subsequent apoptosis *(159).* Thus, it is possible for a cell to become differentiated with 4N DNA content as observed in experiments where ectopic expression of p21^{cip1} or p27^{kip1} results in a differentiated phenotype as cells arrest in G1/S or G2/M phases *(160).*

5.3.4. TRANSCRIPTIONAL EFFECTS

To compare the effects of several CDK inhibitors on mRNA expression from yeast cells, Gray et al. exposed *Saccharomyces cerevisae* to compound 52 and flavopiridol (25 µM) for 2 h and quantified mRNA by oligonucleotide array methods *(141).* It became clear that 2–3% of a total of 6200 yeast genes showed significant (greater than twofold) changes in transcript level when treated with these agents. Interestingly, almost 50% of affected transcripts were shared by compound 52 and flavopiridol. These genes belong to genes that regulate the progression of cell cycle, phosphate and cellular energy metabolism, and GTP or ATP binding proteins. However, more than 40% of mRNA changes are not concordant between flavopiridol and compound 52. These discrepant behaviors could be explained by the universal CDK inhibitory activity of flavopiridol compared with the selective CDK2/CDK1 (cdc2) effects of compound 52, by the different intracellular concentrations achieved of these inhibitors, their distinctive molecular structures, or from their putative effects on other cellular targets. When the compound 52E (inactive analogue to compound 52) or a yeast strain (cdc28p) that is mutant for the putative target for both flavopiridol and compound 52 were studied, very few mRNA alterations were noted with 52E, implying that the net effect of these agents is due to the inhibition of CDKs and not due to chemical structural motifs of the compound. Moreover, the mutant cdc28p revealed some overlapping effects with compound 52 and flavopiridol *(141)*. Modulation in transcription (cyclin D1 and vascular endothelial growth factor [VEGF]) was also observed in human cells.

6. SUMMARY

The results accumulated in the last few years have demonstrated that deregulation of cell cycle proteins have a deep impact on tumor development. At present, we know that deregulation of cell proliferation is achieved by deregulated transcription, translation, or modulation of protein stability through the ubiquitin-mediated pathway.

Based on the frequent aberration in cell cycle regulatory pathways in human cancer by "CDK activation", novel ATP competitive CDK inhibitors are being developed. The first two tested in clinical trials, flavopiridol and UCN-01, showed promising results with evidence of antitumor activity and plasma concentrations sufficient to inhibit CDK-related functions. The best schedule to be administered, the combination with standard chemotherapeutic agents, and a demonstration of CDK modulation from tumor samples from patients in these trials are important issues that need to be answered in order to advance these agents to the clinic.

REFERENCES

1. Sherr CJ. Cancer cell cycles. *Science* 1996; 274:1672–1677.
2. Sherr CJ. G1 phase progression: cyclin on cue. *Cell* 1994; 79:551–555.
3. Sherr CJ, Roberts JM. Inhibitors of mammalian G1 cyclin-dependent kinases. *Genes Dev* 1995; 9:1149–1163.
4. Xiong Y. Why are there so many CDK inhibitors? *Biochim Biophys Acta* 1996; 1288:1–5.
5. Zhang HS, Gavin M, Dahiya A, Postigo AA, Ma D, Luo RX, et al. Exit from G1 and S phase of the cell cycle is regulated by repressor complexes containing HDAC-Rb-hSWI/SNF and Rb-hSWI/SNF. *Cell* 2000; 101:79–89.
6. Nevins JR. E2F: a link between the Rb tumor suppressor protein and viral oncoproteins. *Science* 1992; 258:424–429.
7. Sherr CJ. D-type cyclins. *Trends Biochem Sci* 1995; 20:187–190.
8. Dai K, Kobayashi R, Beach D. Physical interaction of mammalian CDC37 with CDK4. *J Biol Chem* 1996; 271:22030–22034.
9. Stepanova L, Leng X, Parker S, Harper J. Mammalian p50CDC37 is a protein kinase targeting subunit of Hsp90 that binds and stabilizes Cdk4. *Genes Dev* 1999; 10:1491–1502.
10. Suzuki A, Hayashida M, Ito T, Kawano H, Nakano T, Miura M, et al. Survivin intiates cell cycle entry by the competitive interactions with CDK4/p16Ink4a and CDK2/cyclin E complex activation. *Oncogene* 2000; 19:3225–3234.

11. Li F, Ambrosini G, Chu E, Plescia J, Tognin S, Marchisio P, et al. Control of apoptosis and mitotic spindle checkpoint by survivin. *Nature* 1998; 396:580–584.

12. Rodriguez-Puebla ML, LaCava M, Gimenez-Conti IB, Jonhson DG, Conti CJ. Deregulated expression of cell-cycle proteins during premalignant progression in SENCAR mouse skin. *Oncogene* 1998; 17:2251–2258.

13. Rodriguez-Puebla M, LaCava M, Bolontrade M, Rusell J, Conti C. Increased expression of mutated Ha-ras during premalignant progression in SENCAR mouse skin. *Mol Carcinog* 1999; 26:150–156.

14. Weinberg R. The molecular basis of carcinogenesis: understanding the cell cycle clock. *Cytokines Mol Ther* 1996; 2:105–110.

15. Motokura T, Arnold A. Cyclins and oncogenesis. *Biochim Biophys Acta* 1993; 1155:63–78.

16. Jacks T, Weinberg R. The expanding role of Cell cycle regulators. *Science* 1998; 280:1035–1036.

17. Hunter T, Pines J. Cyclins and cancer. II: cyclin D and CDK inhibitors come of age [see comments]. *Cell* 1994; 79:573–582.

18. Bianchi AB, Fischer SM, Robles AI, Rinchik EM, Conti CJ. Overexpression of cyclin D1 in mouse skin carcinogenesis. *Oncogene* 1993; 8:1127–1133.

19. Bartkova J, Lukas J, Strauss M, Bartek J. The PRAD1/cyclin D1 oncogene product accumulate aberrantly in a subset of colorectal carcinomas. *Int J Cancer* 1994; 58:568–573.

20. Jiang W, Zhang Y, Kahn S, Hollstein M, Santella R, Lu S, et al. Altered expression of the cyclin D1 and retinoblastoma genes in human esophageal cancer. *Proc Natl Acad Sci USA* 1993; 90:9026–9030.

21. Schauer IE, Siriwardana S, Langan TA, Sclafani RA. Cyclin D1 overexpression vs. retinoblastoma inactivation: implications for growth control evasion in non-small cell and small cell lung cancer. *Proc Natl Acad Sci USA* 1994; 91:7827–7831.

22. Aagaard L, Lukas J, Bartkova J, Kjerulff A, Strauss M, Bartek J. Aberrations of p16Ink4 and retinoblastoma tumour-suppressor genes occur in distinct sub-sets of human cancer cell lines. *Int J Cancer* 1995; 61:115–120.

23. Otterson GA, Kratze RA, Coxon A, Kim YW, Kaye FJ. Absence of p16Ink4 protein is restricted to a subset of lung cancer cell lines that retains wildtype RB. *Oncogene* 1994; 9:3375–3378.

24. Shapiro G, Edwards C, Kobzik L, Godleski J, Richards W, Sugarbaker D, et al. Reciprocal Rb inactivation and p16INK4 expression in primary lung cancers and cell lines. *Cancer Res* 1995; 55:505–509.

25. Weinberg RA. The retinoblastoma protein and cell cycle control. *Cell* 1995; 81:323–330.

26. Lukas J, Aagaard L, Strauss M, Bartek J. Oncogenic aberrations of p16INK4/CDKN2 and cyclin D1 cooperate to deregulate G1 control. *Cancer Res* 1995; 55:4818–4823.

27. Schmit E, Ichimura K, Reifenberger G. CdkN2 (p16/MTST1) gene deletion or Cdk4 amplification occurs in the majority of glioblastomas. *Cancer Res* 1994; 54:6321–6324.

28. Sonoda Y, Yoshimoto T, Sekiya T. Homozygous deletion of the MTS1/p16 and MTS2/p15 genes and amplification of the CDK4 gene in glioma. *Oncogene* 1995; 11:2145–2149.

29. He J, Allen JR, Collins VP, Allalunis-Turner MJ, Godbout R, Day RS, et al. CDK4 amplification is an alternative mechanism to p16 homozygous deletion in glioma cell lines. *Cancer Res* 1994; 54:5804–5807.

30. Zuo L. Germline mutation in the p16Ink4a binding domain of cdk4 in familial melanoma. *Nat Genet* 1996; 12:97–99.

31. Wölfel T, Hauer M, Schneider J, Serrano M, Wölfel C, Klehmann-Hieb E, et al. A p16INK4a-insensitive CDK4 mutant targeted by cytolytic T lymphocytes in a human melanoma. *Science* 1995; 269:1281–1284.

32. An H, Beckmann MW, Reifenger G, Bender HG, Niederacher D. Gene amplification and overexpression of CDK4 in sporadic breast carcinomas is associated with high tumor cell proliferation. *Am J Pathol* 1999; 154:113–118.

33. Kanoe H, Nakayama T, Murakami H, Hosaka T, Yamamoto H, Nakashima Y, et al. Amplification of CDK4 gene in sarcomas: tumor specificity and relationship with the Rb mutation. *Anticancer Res* 1998; 18:2317–2321.

34. Peeper DS, Upton TM, Ladha MH, Neuman E, Zaldive J, et al. Ras signalling linked to the cell-cycle machinery by the retinoblastome protein. *Nature* 1997; 386:177–181.

35. Testu O, McCormick F. Beta-catenin regulates expression of cyclin D1 in colon carcinoma cells. *Nature* 1999; 398:422–426.

36. Arnold A, Kim H, Gaz R, Eddy R, Fukushima Y, Byers M, et al. Molecular cloning and chromosomal mapping of DNA rearranged with the parathyroid hormona gene in a parathyroid adenoma. *J Clin Invest* 1989; 83:2034–2040.

37. Rosenberg CL, Wong E, Petty E, Bale A, Tsujimoto Y, Harris N, et al. PRAD1, a candidate BCL1 oncogene: mapping and expression in centrocytic lymphoma. *Proc Natl Acad Sci USA* 1991; 88:9638–9642.

38. Motokura T, Bloom T, Goo-Kim H, Junpper H, Rudermann J, Kronenberg H, et al. A novel cyclin encoded by a bcl1-linked candidate oncogene. *Nature* 1991; 350:512–515.

39. Arnold A. The cyclin D1/PRAD1 oncogene in human neoplasia. *J Investig Med* 1995; 43:543–549.

40. Bartkova J, Lukas J, Strauss M, Bartek J. Cyclin D1 oncoprotein aberrantly accumulates in malignancies of diverse histogenesis. *Oncogene* 1995; 10:775–778.

41. Lammie G, Fantl V, Smith R, Schuuring E, Brookes S, Michalides R, et al. D11S287, a putative oncogene on chromosome 11q13, is amplified and expressed in squamous cell and mammary carcinomas and linked to BCL-1. *Oncogene* 1991; 6:439–444.

42. Weinstat-Saslow D, Merino M, Manrow R, Lawrence J, Bluth R, Wittenbel K, et al. Overexpression of cyclin D mRNA distinguishes invasive and in situ breast carcinomas from non-malignant lesions [see comments]. *Nat Med* 1995; 1:1257–1260.

43. Barnes D. Cyclin D1 in mammary carcinoma. *J Pathol* 1997; 181:267–269.

44. Barnes D, Gillet C. Cyclin D1 in breast cancer. *Breast Cancer Res Treat* 1998; 52:1–15.

45. Wang T, Cardiff R, Zukerberg L, Lees E, Arnold A, Schmidt E. Mammary hyperplasia and carcinoma in MMTV-cyclin D1 transgenic mice. *Nature* 1994; 369:669–671.

46. Sicinski P, Donaher J, Parker S, Li T, Fazeli A, Gardener H, et al. Cyclin D1 provides a link between development and oncogenesis in the retina and breast. *Cell* 1995; 82:621–630.

47. Fantl V, Stamp G, Andrews A, Rosewell I, Dickson C. Mice lacking cyclin D1 are small and show defects in eye and mammary gland development. *Genes Dev* 1995; 9:2364–2372.

48. Yu Q, Geng Y, Sicinski P. Specific protection against breast cancers by cyclin D1 ablation. *Nature* 2001; 411:1017–1021.

49. Bernards R. CDK-independent activities of D type cyclins. *Biochim Biophys Acta* 1999; 1424:M17–M22.

50. Zwijsen R, Wientjens E, Klompmaker R, van der Sman J, Bernards R, Michalides R. CDK-independent activation of estrogen receptor by cyclin D1. *Cell* 1997; 88:405–415.

51. Neuman E, Ladha M, Lin N, Upton T, Miller S, DiRenzo J, et al. Cyclin D1 stimulation of estrogen receptor transcriptional activity independent of cdk4. *Mol Cell Biol* 1997; 17:5338–5347.

52. Altucci L, Addeo R, Cicatiello L, Dauvois S, Parker M, Truss M, et al. 17beta-Estradiol induces cyclin D1 gene transcription, p36D1-p34cdk4 complex activation and p105Rb phosphorylation during mitogenic stimulation of G(1)-arrested human breast cancer cells. *Oncogene* 1996; 12:2315–2324.

53. van Diest PJ, Michalides RJ, Jannink L, van der Valk P, Peterse H, de Jong JS, et al. Cyclin D1 expression in invasive breast cancer. Correlations and prognostic value. *Am J Pathol* 1997; 150:705–711.

54. Gillett C, Smith P, Gregory W, Richards M, Millis R, Peters G, et al. Cyclin D1 and prognosis in human breast cancer. *Int J Cancer* 1996; 69:92–99.

55. Knudsen KE, Cavenee WK, Arden KC. D-type cyclins complex with androgen receptor and inhibits its transcriptional transactivation ability. *Cancer Res* 1999; 59:2297–2301.

56. Arber N, Sutter T, Miyake M, Kahn SM, Venkatraj VS, Sobrino A, et al. Increased expression of cyclin D1 and the RB tumor suppressor gene in c-K-ras transformed rat enterocytes. *Oncogene* 1996; 12:1903–1908.

57. Filmus J, Robles AI, Shi W, Wong MJ, Colombo LL, Conti CJ. Induction of cyclin D1 overexpression by activated ras. *Oncogene* 1994; 9:3627–3633.

58. Liu JJ, Chao JR, Jiang MC, Ng SY, Yen JJ, Yang YH. Ras transformation results in an elevated level of cyclin D1 and acceleration of G1 progression in NIH3T3 cells. *Mol Cell Biol* 1995; 15:3654–3663.

59. Albanese C, Johnson J, Watanabe G, Eklund N, Vu D, Arnold A, et al. Transforming p21ras mutants and c-Ets-2 activated the cyclin D1 promoter through distinguishable regions. *J Biol Chem* 1995; 270:23589–23597.

60. Mechta F, Lalleman D, Pfarr CM, Yaniv M. Transformation by ras modifies AP1 composition and activity. *Oncogene* 1997; 14:837–847.

61. Weber JD, Hu W, Jefcoat SC, Raben DM, Baldassare JJ. Ras-stimulated extracellular signal-related kinase 1 and RhoA activities coordinate platelet-derived growth factor-induced G1 progression through the independent regulation of cyclin D1 and p27Kip1. *J Biol Chem* 1997; 272:32966–32971.

62. Aktas H, Cai H, Cooper G. Ras links growth factor signaling to the cell cycle machinery via regulation of cyclin D1 and the cdk inhibitor p27Kip1. *Mol Cell Biol* 1997; 17:3850–3857.

63. Takuwa N, Takuwa Y. Ras activity in G1 phase required for p27 downregulation, passage through the restriction point, and entry into S phase in growth factor-stimulated NIH3T3 fibroblasts. *Mol Cell Biol* 1997; 17:5348–5358.

64. Robles A, Rodriguez-Puebla M, Glick A, Trempus C, Hansen L, Sicinski P, et al. Reduced skin tumor development in cyclin D1 deficient mice highlights the oncogenic ras pathway in vivo. *Genes Dev* 1998; 12:2469–2474.

65. Tong W, Pollard JW. Genetic evidence for the interactions of cyclin D1 and p27Kip1 in Mice. *Mol Cell Biol* 2001; 21:1319–1328.

66. Geng Y, Yu Q, Sicinska E, Das M, Bronson RT, Sicinski P. Deletion of the p27Kip1 gene restores normal development in cyclin D1-deficient mice. *Proc Natl Acad Sci USA* 2001; 98:194–199.

67. Rodriguez-Puebla ML, LaCava M, Conti C. Cyclin D1 overexpression in mouse epidermis increases cyclin-dependent kinase activity and cell proliferation in vivo but does not affect skin tumor development. *Cell Growth Diff* 1999; 10:467–472.

68. Robles AI, Larcher F, Whalin RB, Murillas R, Richie E, Gimenez-Conti IB, et al. Expression of cyclin D1 in epithelial tissues of transgenic mice results in epidermal hyperproliferation and severe thymic hyperplasia. *Proc Natl Acad Sci USA* 1996; 93:7634–7638.

69. Shtutman M, Zhurinsky J, Simcha I, Albanese C, D'Amico M, Pestell R, et al. The cyclin D1 gene is a target of the B-catenin/LEF-1 pathway. *Proc Natl Acad Sci USA* 1999; 96:5522–5527.

70. Bartkova J, Lukas J, Strauss M, Bartek J. The PRAD-1/cyclin D1 oncogene product accumulates aberrantly in a subset of colorectal carcinomas. *Int J Cancer* 1994; 58:568–573.

71. Arber N, Hibshoosh H, Moss S, Sutter T, Zhang Y, Begg M, et al. Increased expression of cyclin D1 is an early event in multistage colorectal carcinogenesis. *Gastroenterology* 1996; 110:669–674.

72. Yasogawa Y, Takamo Y, Okayasu I, Kakita A. The 5D4 abtibody (anti-cyclin D1/D2) related antigen: cytoplasmic staining is correlated to the progression of gastric cancer. *Pathol Int* 1998; 48:717–722.

73. Murty V, Chaganti R. A genetic perspective of male germ cell tumors. *Semin Oncol* 1998; 25:133–144.

74. Houldsworth J, Reuter V, Bosl G, Chaganti R. Aberrant expression of cyclin D2 in an early event in human male germ cell tumorigenesis. *Cell Growth Differ* 1997; 8:292–299.

75. Delmer A, Ajchenbaum-Cymbalista F, Tang R, Ramond S, Faussat A, Marie J, et al. Overexpression of cyclin D2 in chronic B-cell malignancies. *Blood* 1995; 85:2870–2876.

76. Sicinski P, Donaher J, Geneg Y, Parker S, Garder H, Park M, et al. Cyclin D2 is an FSH-responsive gene involved in gonadal cell proliferation and oncogenesis. *Nature* 1996; 384:470–474.

77. Rodriguez-Puebla ML, LaCava M, Miliani de Marval PL, Jorcano JL, Richie E, Conti CJ. Cyclin D2 overexpression in transgenic mice induces thymic and epidermal hyperplasia where as cyclin D3 expression results only in epidermal hyperplasia. *Am J Pathol* 2000; 157:1039–1050.

78. Sanchez-Beato M, Camacho F, Martinez-Montero J, Saez A, Villuendas R, Sanchez-Verde L, et al. Anomalous high p27/Kip1 expression in a subset of aggressive B-cell lymphomas is associated with cyclin D3 overexpression. p27/Kip1-cyclin D3 colocalization in tumor cells. *Blood* 1999; 94:765–772.

79. Russell A, Thompson M, Hendley J, True L, Armes J, Germain D. Cyclin d1 and D3 associate with the SCF complex and are coordinately elevated in breast cancer. *Oncogene* 1999; 18:1983–1991.

80. Juan G, Cordon-Cardo C. Intranuclear compartmentalization of cyclin E during the cell cycle: disruption of the nucleoplasm-nucleolar shuttling of cyclin E in bladder cancer. *Cancer Res* 2001; 61:1220–1226.

81. Muller-Tidow C, Kigler M, Diederichs S, Idos G, Thomas M, Dockhorn-Dworniczak B, et al. Cyclin E is the only cdk2-associated cyclin that predicts metastasis and survival in early stage non-small cell lung cancer. *Cancer Res* 2001; 61:647–653.

82. Hirata F, Naiki H, Hitomi S, Wada H. Prognosis significance of cyclin E overexpression in resected non-small cell lung cancer. *Cancer Res* 2000; 60:242–244.

83. Takano Y, Kato Y, van Diest P, Masuda M, Mitomi H, Okayasu I. Cyclin D2 overexpression and lack of p27 correlate positively and cyclin E inversely with a poor prognosis in gastric cancer cases. *Am J Pathol* 2000; 156:585–594.

84. Nielsen N, Emdin S, Cajander J, Landberg G. Deregulation of cyclin E and D1 in breast cancer is associated with inactivation of the retinoblastoma protein. *Oncogene* 1997; 14:295–304.

85. Nielsen N, Arnerlov C, Cajander S, Landberg G. Cyclin E expression and proliferation in breast cancer. *Anal Cell Pathol* 1998; 17:177–188.

86. Jang S, Park Y, Park M, Lee J, Lee Y, Jung T, et al. Expression of cell-cycle regulators, cyclin E and p21 Wak1/Cip1, a potential prognosis markers for gastric cancer. *Eur J Surg Oncol* 1999; 25:157–163.

87. Keyomarsi K, Herliczek T. The role of cyclin E in cell proliferation, development and cancer. *Prog Cell Cycle Res* 1997; 3:171–191.

88. Keyomarsi K, Conte DJ, Toyofuku W, Fox M. Deregulation of cyclin E in breast cancer. *Oncogene* 1995; 11:941–950.

89. Keyomarsi K, O'Leary N, Molnar G, Lees E, Fingert H, Pardee A. Cyclin E, a potential prognostic marker for breast cancer. *Cancer Res* 1994; 54:380–385.

90. Gray-Bablin J, Zalvide J, Fox M, Knickerbocker C, DeCaprio J, Keyomarsi K. Cyclin E, a redundant cyclin in breast cancer. *Proc Natl Acad Sci USA* 1996; 93:15215–15220.

91. Marone M, Scambia G, Giannitelli C, Ferrandina G, Masciullo V, Bellacosa A, et al. Analysis of cyclin E and CDK2 in overian cancer: gene amplification and RNA overexpression. *Int J Cancer* 1998; 75:34–39.

92. Bortner D, Rosenberg M. Induction of mammary gland hyperplasia and carcinomas in transgenic mice expressing human cyclin E. *Mol Cell Biol* 1997; 17:453–459.

93. Lukas J, Bartkova J, Rohde M, Strauss M, Bartek J. Cyclin D1 is dispensable for G1 control in retinoblastoma gene-deficient cells independently of cdk4 activity. *Mol Cell Biol* 1995; 15:2600–2611.

94. Tam S, Theodoras J, Shay G, Draetta F, Pagano M. Differential expression and regulation of cyclin D1 protein in normal and tumor human cells: association with Cdk4 is required for cyclin D1 function in G1 progression. *Oncogene* 1994; 9:2663–2674.

95. Ohtsubo M, Theodoras A, Schumacher J, Roberts J, Pagano M. Human cyclin E, a nuclear protein essential for the G1-toS phase transition. *Mol Cell Biol* 1995; 15:1559–1571.

96. Lauper N, Beck A, Cariou S, Richman L, Hofmann K, Reith W, et al. Cyclin E2: a novel CDK2 partner in the late G1 and S phase of the mammalian cell cycle. *Oncogene* 1998; 17:2637–2643.

97. Porter DC, Keyomarsi K. Novel splice variants of cyclin E with altered substrate specificity. *Nucleic Acid Res* 2000; 28:1–8.

98. Harwell RM, Porter DC, Danes C, Keyomarsi K. Processing of cyclin E differs between normal and tumor breast cells. *Cancer Res* 2000; 60:481–489.

99. Seghezzi W, Chua K, Shanahan F, Gozani O, Reed R, Lees E. Cyclin E associates with components of the pre-mRNA splicing machinery in mammalian cells. *Mol Cell Biol* 1998; 18:4526–4536.

100. Takemura M, Yamamoto T, Kitagawa M, Taya Y, Akiyama T, Asahara H, et al. Stimulation of DNA polymerase a activity by Cdk2-Phosphorylated Rb protein. *Biochem Biophys Res Commun* 2001; 282:984–990.

101. Otzen Petersen B, Lukas J, Storgaard Sorensen C, Bartek J, Helin K. Phosphorylation of mammalian CDC6 by Cyclin A/CDK2 regulates its subcellular localization. *EMBO J* 1999; 18:396–410.

102. Khatib Z, Matsushime H, Valentine M. Coamplification of the Cdk4 gene with MDM2 and GL1 in human sarcomas. *Cancer Res* 1993; 53:5535–5541.

103. Ichimura K, Schmidt EE, Goike HM, Collins VP. Human glioblastomas with no alterations of the CDKN2A and CDK4 genes have frequent mutations of the retinoblastoma gene. *Oncogene* 1996; 13:1065–1072.

104. He J, Olson J, James C. Lack of p16 or retinoblastoma protein (pRb), or amplification-associated overexpression of cdk4 is observed in distinct subsets of malignant glial tumors and cell lines. *Cancer Res* 1995; 55:4833–4836.

105. Holland EC, Hively WP, Gallo V, Varmus HE. Modeling mutations in the G1 arrest pathway in human gliomas: overexpression of CDK4 but not loss of INK4a-ARF induces hyperploidy in cultured mouse astrocytes. *Genes Dev* 1998; 12:3644–3649.

106. Serrano M, Hannon GJ, Beach D. A new regulatory motif in cell-cycle control causing specific inhibition of cyclin S/cdk4. *Nature* 1993; 366:704–707.

107. Miliani de Marval P, Gimenez-Conti I, LaCava M, Martinez L, Conti C, Rodriguez-Puebla M. Transgenic Expression of CDK4 results in epidermal hyperplasia and severe dermal fibrosis. *Am J Pathol* 2001; 159:369–379.

108. Parry D, Mahony D, Wills K, Lees E. Cyclin-CDK subunit arrangement is dependent on the availability of competing INK4 and p21 class inhibitors. *Mol Cell Biol* 1999; 19:1775–1783.

109. McConnell B, Gregory F, Stott F, Hara E, Peters G. Induced expression of p16Ink4a inhibits both CDK4- and CDK2-associated kinase activity by reassorment of cyclin-CDK-inhibitor complexes. *Mol Cell Biol* 1999; 19:1981–1989.

110. Rane SG, Dubus P, Mettus RV, Galbreath EJ, Boden G, Premkumar Reddy E, et al. Loss of Cdk4 expression causes insulin-deficient diabetes and Cdk4 activation results in B-islet cell hyperplasia. *Nat Genet* 1999; 22:44–52.

111. Tsutsui T, Hesabi B, Moons DS, Pandolfi P, Hansel K, Koff A, et al. Targeted disruption of CDK4 delays cell cycle entry with enhanced p27Kip1 activity. *Mol Cell Biol* 1999; 19:7011–7019.

112. Hermeking H, Rago C, Schuhmacher M, Li Q, Barret J, Obaya A, et al. Identification of CDK4 as a target of c-Myc. *Proc Natl Acad Sci USA* 2000; 97:2229–2234.

113. Haas K, Staller P, Geisen C, Bartek J, Eilers M, Moroy T. Mutual requirement of CDK4 and Myc in malignant transformation: evidence for cyclin D1/CDK4 and p16INK4A as upstream regulators of Myc. *Oncogene* 1997; 15:179–192.

114. Lapointe J, Lachance Y, Labrie Y, Labrie C. A p18 mutant defective in CDK6 binding in human breast cancer cells. *Cancer Res* 1996; 56:4586–4589.

115. Lam P, Di Tomaso E, Ng H, Pang J, Roussel M, Hjelm N. Expression of p19INK4d, CDK4, CDK6 in glioblastoma multiforme. *Br J Neurosurg* 2000; 14:28–32.

116. Huang-Chun L, Chun-Wu L, Pei-Hsin H, Min-Lee C, Su-Ming H. Expression of cyclin-dependent kinase 6 (cdk6) and frequent loss of CD44 in nasal-nasopharyngeal NKT/T-Cell lymphomas: comparison with CD56-negative peripheral T-cell lymphomas. *Lab Invest* 2000; 80:893–900.

117. Peters J-M, Harris J, Finley D. *Ubiquitin and Biology of the Cell*. Plenum Press, New York, 1998.

118. Hershko A, Ciechanover A. The ubiquitin system. *Annu Rev Biochem* 1998; 67:425–479.

119. Elledge S, Harper J. The role of protein stability in the cell cycle and cancer. *Biochim Biophys Acta* 1998; 1377:M61–M70.

120. Patton E, Willems A, Tyers M. Combinatorial control in ubiquitin-dependent proteolysis: don't Skp the F-box hypothesis. *Trends Genet* 1998; 14:236–243.

121. Deshaies R. SCF and cullin/ring H2-based ubiquitin ligases. *Annu Rev Cell Dev Biol* 1999; 15:435–467.

122. Nakayama K-I, Hatakeyama S, Nakayama K. Regulation of the cell cycle at the G1-S transition by proteolysis of cyclin E and p27Kip1. *Biochem Biophys Res Commun* 2001; 282:853–860.

123. Ganiatsas S, Dow R, Thompson A, Schulman B, Germain D. A splice variant of Skp2 is retained in the cytoplasm and fails to direct cyclin D1 ubiquitination in the uterine cancer cell line SK-UT. *Oncogene* 2001; 20:3641–3650.

124. Zhang H, Kobayashi R, Galatinonov K, Beach D. p19Skp1 and p45Skp2 are essential elements of the cyclin A-cdk2 S phase kinase. *Cell* 1995; 82:915–925.

125. Slingerland JM, Pagano M. Regulation of the cdk inhibitor p27 and its deregulation in cancer. *J Cell Physiol* 2000; 183:10–17.

126. Nakayama K, Nagahama H, Minamishima Y, Matsumoto M, Nakamichi I, Kitagawa K, et al. Targeted disruption of Skp2 results in accumulation of cyclin E and p27Kip1, polyploidy and centrosome overeduplication. *EMBO J* 2000; 19:2069–2081.

127. Vu P, Sakamoto K. Ubiquitin-mediated proteolysis and human disease. *Mol Genet Metab* 2000; 71:261–266.

128. Hershko D, Bornstein G, Ben-Izhak O, Carrasco A, Pagano M, Krauss M, et al. Inverse relation between levels of p27Kip1 and of its ubiquitin ligase subunit Skp2 in colorectal carcinomas. *Cancer* 2001; 91:745–751.

129. Gstaiger M, Jordan R, Lim M, Catzavelos C, Mestan J, Slingerland JM, et al. Skp2 is oncogenic and overexpressed in human cancers. *Proc Natl Acad Sci USA* 2001; 98:5043–5048.

130. Latres E, Chiarle R, Schulman B, Pavletich N, Pellicer A, Inghirami G, et al. Role of the F-box protein Skp2 in lymphomagenesis. *Proc Natl Acad Sci USA* 2001; 98:2515–2520.

131. Demetrick D, Zhang H, Beach D. Chromosomal mapping of the genes for the human CDK2/cyclin A-associated proteins p19(SKP1A and SKP1B) and p45 (SKP2). *Cytogenet Cell Genet* 1996; 73:104–107.

132. Senderowicz AM. Small molecule modulators of cyclin-dependent kinases for cancer therapy. *Oncogene* 2000; 19:6600–6606.

133. Senderowicz AM, Sausville EA. Preclinical and clinical development of cyclin-dependent kinase modulators. *J Natl Cancer Inst* 2000; 92:376–387.

134. Meijer L, Kim S. Chemical inhibitors of cyclin-dependent kinase. *Methods Enzymol* 1997; 283:113–128.

135. Zaharevitz D, Gussio R, Leost M, Senderowicz A, Lahusen T, Kunicj C, et al. Discovery and initial characterization of the paullones, a novel class of small-molecule inhibitors of cyclin-dependent kinases. *Cancer Res* 1999; 59:2566–2569.

136. De Azevedo W, Leclerc S, Meijer L, Havlicek L, Strnad M, Kim S. Inhibition of cyclin-dependent kinases by purine analogues: crystal structure of human cdk2 complexed with roscovitine. *Eur J Biochem* 1997; 243:518–526.

137. Meijer L, Ondaven P. Cyclic activation of histone H1 kinase during sea urchin egg mitotic divisions. *Exp Cell Res* 1988; 174:116–129.

138. Rialet V, Meijer L. A new screening test for antimitotic compounds using the universal M phase-specific protein kinase, p34cdc2/cyclin Bcdc13, affinity-immobilized on p13suc1-coated microtitration plates. *Anticancer Res* 1991; 11:1581–1590.

139. Meijer L, Borgne A, Mulner O, Chong J, Blow J, Inagaki N, et al. Biochemical and cellular effects of roscovitine, a potent and selective inhibitor of cyclin-dependent kinase cdk2, cdc2 and cdk5. *Eur J Biochem* 1997; 243:527–536.

140. Brooks E, Gray N, Joly A, Kerwar S, Lum R, Mackman R, et al. CVT-313, a specific and potent inhibitor of CDK2 that prevents neointimal proliferation. *J Biol Chem* 1997; 272:207–229.

141. Gray N, Wodicka L, Thunnissen A, Norman T, Kwon S, Espinoza F, et al. Exploiting chemical libraries, structure, and genomics in the search for kinase inhibitors. *Science* 1998; 281:533–538.

142. Lahusen J, Loaiza-Perez A, Sausville EA, Senderowicz AM. Flavopiridol-induced apoptosis is associated with p38 and MEK activation and is prevented by caspase and MAPK inhibitors. *Proc Annu Meet Am Assoc Cancer Res* 2000.

143. Schultz R, Patel V, Worzalla J, Shih C. Role of thymidylate synthase in the antitumor activity of the multitargeted antifolate, LY231514. *Anticancer Res* 1999; 19:437–443.

144. Kent L, Hull-Campbell N, Lau T, Wu J, Thompson S, Nori M. Characterization of novel inhibitors of cyclin-dependent kinases. *Biochem Biophys Res Commun* 1999; 260:768–774.

145. Walker D. Small-molecule inhibitors of cyclin-dependent kinases: molecular tools and potential therapeutics. *Curr Top Microbiol Immunol* 1998; 227:149–165.

146. van den Heuvel S, Harlow E. Distinct roles for cyclin-dependent kinases in cell cycle control. *Science* 1993; 262:2050–2054.

147. Carlson B, Pearlstein R, Naik R, Sedlacek H, Sausville EA, Worland P. Inhibition of CDK2, CDK4 and CDK7 by flavopiridol and structural analogs. *Proc Am Assoc Cancer Res* 1996.

148. Carlson B, Dubay M, Sausville E, Brizuela L, Worland P. Flavopiridol induces G1 arrest with inhibition of cyclin-dependent kinase (CDK) 2 and CDK4 in human breast carcinoma cells. *Cancer Res* 1996; 56:2973–2978.

149. Buquet-Fagot C, Lalleman F, Montagne M, Mester J. Effects of olomucine, a selective inhibitor of cyclin-dependent kinases, on cell cycle progression in human cancer cell lines. *Anticancer Drugs* 1997; 8:2425–2432.

150. Chien M, Astumian M, Liebowitz D, Rinker-Schaeffer C, Stadler W. In vitro evaluation of flavopiridol, a novel cell cycle inhibitor, in bladder cancer. *Cancer Chemother Pharmacol* 1999; 44:81–87.

151. Park S, Cheon J, Lee Y, Park Y, Lee K, Lee C, et al. A specific inhibitor of cyclin-dependent protein kinase. *Mol Cell* 1996; 6:679–683.

152. Parker B, Nieves-Neira W, Taimi M, Kolhagen G, Shimizu T, Pommier Y, et al. Early induction of apoptosis in hematopoietic cell lines after exposure to flavopiridol. *Blood* 1998; 91:458–465.

153. Park D, Farinelli S, Greene L. Inhibitors of cyclin-dependent kinases promote survival of post-mitotic neuronally differentiated PC12 cells and sympathetic neurons. *J Biol Chem* 1996; 271:8161–8169.

154. Park S, Kang S, Lee D, Kang M, Kim S, Koh G. Temporal expression of cyclins and cyclin-dependent kinases during renal development and compensatory growth. *Kidney* 1997; 51:762–769.

155. Gervais JL, Seth P, Zhang H. Cleavage of CDK inhibitor p21(Cip1/Waf1) by caspases is an early event during DNA damage-induced apoptosis. *J Biol Chem* 1998; 273:19207–19212.

156. Levkau B, Koyama H, Raines E, Clurman B, Herren B, Orth K, et al. Cleavge of p21Cip1/Waf1 and p27Kip1 mediates apoptosis in endothelial cells through activation of Cdk2: role os a caspase cascade. *Mol Cell* 1998; 1:553–563.

157. Zhou B, Li H, Yuan J, Kirscher M. Caspase-depandent activation of cyclin-dependent kinases during Fas- induced apoptosis in Jurkat cells. *Proc Natl Acad Sci USA* 1991; 95:6785–6790.

158. Lee H, Chang T, Tebalt M, Senderowicz A, Szabo E. Induction of differentiation accompanies inhibition of cdk2 in a non-small cell lung cancer cell line. *Int J Cancer* 1999; 15:161–166.

159. Rosania G, Merlie J, Gray N, Chang Y, Schult P, Heald R. A cyclin-dependent kinase inhibitor inducing cancer cell differentiation: biochemical identification using *Xenopus* egg extracts. *Proc Natl Acad Sci USA* 1999; 96:4797–4802.

160. Liu M, Subramanyam Y. Preparation and analysis of cDNA from a small number of hematopoietic cells. *Methods Enzymol* 1999; 303:45–55.

9 Oncogenes as Regulators of Cell Survival

The Role of Oncogenes and Tumor Suppressor Genes in the Induction of Resistance to Anoikis and Hypoxia

Kirill Rosen, PhD, and Jorge Filmus, PhD

CONTENTS

1. INTRODUCTION

During the past few years, it has become obvious that resistance to programmed cell death, or apoptosis, plays a major role in the process of malignant transformation and subsequent tumor progression. Molecular mechanisms of such resistance induced by the activation of various proto-oncogenes and the loss of activity of tumor suppressor genes have begun to emerge. In parallel, our knowledge of the principles governing the functioning of the intrinsic cell death machinery has expanded considerably.

During solid tumor progression, malignant cells are forced to grow in the absence of contact with a properly formed basement membrane and in hypoxic conditions. These changes create a highly hostile environment that can potentially induce apoptosis in the malignant cells. We will discuss here how cell death is triggered by such a "tumor specific environment" and the molecular mechanisms by which oncogenes and tumor suppressor genes induce resistance to these potentially lethal conditions in the context of solid tumor progression.

From: *Oncogene-Directed Therapies*
Edited by: J. W. Rak © Humana Press Inc., Totowa, NJ

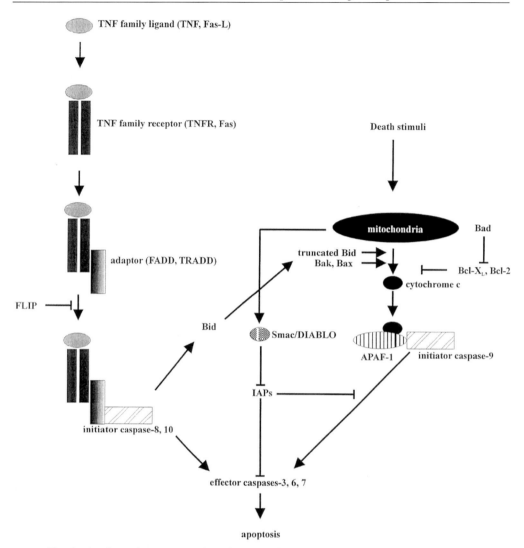

Fig. 1. A schematic representation of current views on basic mechanisms of apoptosis.

1.1. Molecular Mechanisms of Apoptosis

The current knowledge of the molecular mechanisms governing apoptosis has been recently reviewed by several investigators *(1–3)*.

In brief, two major apoptotic pathways in mammalian cells are presently known (Fig. 1). One of them, the mitochondria pathway, is induced by various stimuli and involves the release of cytochrome c from this organelle into the cytoplasm and subsequent cytochrome c-dependent activation of the caspases *(4–6)*. Caspases are serine proteases that cleave a set of critical cellular targets and ultimately cause death *(7–9)*. They are organized in a hierarchical manner, with some caspases, such as caspase 9, acting upstream in the apoptotic pathway. Upon activation, these upstream caspases trigger the activity of the downstream caspases (i.e., caspase 3), which act as the executioners in the degradation of the cellular targets. The release of cytochrome c from the mitochondria is both positively and negatively regulated by pro- and anti-apoptotic members of the Bcl-2 protein family. Bcl-2, Bcl-X_L, and Mcl-1 are some of the anti-apoptotic members of this family, whereas Bax, Bak, and Bad are examples of the pro-apoptotic group *(10,11)*. Caspase activity can also be controlled by members of a separate family of proteins known as inhibitors of apoptosis (IAPs), which regulate activity of some caspases by directly binding to them *(12–15)*. IAPs, in turn, can be sequestered and inactivated by the pro-apoptotic factor Smac/DIABLO, which is released from the mitochondria in response to various death signals *(16,17)*.

The second major apoptotic pathway is triggered by the engagement of members of the tumor necrosis factor (TNF) receptor family, such as TNF receptor and Fas, which in turn results in activation of caspases *(18,19)*. In some specific cell types, the death receptor pathway also requires the involvement of the mitochondrial pathway to fully activate the death process *(20)* (Fig. 1).

1.2. Oncogenes and Tumor Suppressor Genes as Activators of Anti-Apoptotic Signaling Pathways

Numerous studies have demonstrated that activation of many proto-oncogenes, as well as inactivation of tumor suppressor genes, results in the induction of resistance to apoptosis *(21,22)*. Survival signals triggered by oncogenic Ras represent one of the best-studied examples. Ras is a GTPase normally activated by receptor tyrosine kinases and other extracellular stimuli *(23,24)*. Once activated, Ras is capable of acting on several effectors, including Raf and phosphatidyl inositol 3-kinase (PI 3-kinase). Raf, in turn, activates a cascade of mitogen-activated kinases (MAP-kinases), whereas PI 3-kinase stimulates the activity of protein kinase B (PKB) *(25,26)*. Both Ras-induced pathways have a direct impact on the activity of various components of apoptotic machinery *(27)*. One of these components is Bad, a pro-apoptotic member of the Bcl-2 family of proteins. Bad can bind to Bcl-X_L and block its pro-survival function *(28)*. This activity of Bad is inhibited by phosphorylation at various serine residues. One of such serines, Ser 136, represents a target of PKB *(29)*. Another serine located at position 112 is phosphorylated by MAP kinases *(30)*. Both phosphorylations were shown to block apopotosis in several cell types *(31)*. In addition to Bad, PI 3-kinase and PKB can induce the phosphorylation of other targets, including FKHRL1, one of the members of the forkhead family of transcription factors *(32)*. This factor appears to be required for the expression of Fas ligand, a well-known inducer of apoptosis. FKHRL1 phosphorylation leads to inactivation and, consequently, to the inhibition of transcription from the Fas ligand promoter *(32)*. It has also been reported that the PI 3-kinase/PKB signaling pathway stimulates the expression of Mcl-1, which is an anti-apoptotic member of Bcl-2 family *(33)*. Another component of the apoptotic machinery that is affected by activated Ras is Bak, a pro-apoptotic member of the Bcl-2 family. It has been shown that Bak expression is significantly down-regulated by this oncogene *(34)*.

In addition to *ras*, other oncogenes have been reported to act on the apoptotic machinery. For example, oncogenic Src has been shown to trigger the expression of Bcl-X_L, an anti-apoptotic member of the Bcl-2 family *(35,36)*.

The loss of tumor suppressor genes can also induce resistance to apoptosis. For instance, p53 is a well known inducer of cell death that is frequently mutated in cancer *(37)*. p53 is a transcription factor that regulates the expression of several components of the apoptotic machinery, including Bax, a pro-apoptotic member of the Bcl-2 family *(38)*.

PTEN is another example of a tumor suppressor gene that can affect the apoptotic machinery. PTEN is a phosphatase capable of removing phosphate groups from phosphoinositols and inhibits, therefore, PI 3 kinase-induced activation of PKB *(39)*. Thus, tumors that have mutated PTEN display an activation of this anti-apoptotic pathway *(40,41)*.

Although the effect of oncogenes and tumor suppressor genes on the expression of many components of the apototic machinery was originally described in cultured cells, it is now established that the expression of many of these molecules is also altered in human tumors in a similar fashion. For example, Bak expression is reduced in a high proportion of colorectal cancers, while the expression of Bcl-X_L is frequently elevated in tumors derived from colon, ovary, and other tissues *(42–44)*.

The data described above regarding the resistance of malignant cells to apoptosis are in an apparent contradiction with the observation that many human solid tumors display a high apoptotic index *(45)*. How can this paradox be explained?

In vivo, normal epithelial cells grow as monolayers attached to a mesh of extracellular matrix (ECM) proteins usually called basement membrane (BM). Detachment of epithelial cells from the BM results in apoptosis. Such form of programmed cell death has been named anoikis (which means "homeless" in Greek) *(46)*. Unlike normal cells, malignant cells exist as multicellular aggregates in which they are forced to survive in the absence of contact with a properly assembled BM. In addition, a large proportion of cells within the tumor mass is often deprived of oxygen *(47)*. Even though many types of carcinomas are highly angiogenic, the vasculature in such tumors is usually disorganized, and, as a consequence, a large fraction of cells within the tumor is hypoxic *(48)*. Similarly to detachment from the ECM, hypoxia is known to induce apoptosis *(49)*. Thus, the lack of attachment to the ECM and the insufficient supply of oxygen constitute a highly hostile environment for cancer cells. In view of this, the fact that a proportion of these cells dies in the course of tumor progression is not surprising. Many cancer cells, however, are obviously capable of withstanding both types of pro-apoptotic challenges and give rise to a viable clinically relevant cellular population capable of invasion and metastasis. Therefore, resistance to cell death triggered by detachment from the BM, and hypoxia, likely represents one of the most critical features of the malignant phenotype. Specific oncogene- and tumor suppressor gene-triggered mechanisms of inhibition of anoikis and hypoxia-induced apoptosis and the role of such mechanisms in the progression of solid tumors are discussed below.

2. ROLE OF ANOIKIS RESISTANCE IN ONCOGENE-INDUCED TRANSFORMATION

2.1. Mechanisms of Anoikis

Anoikis is thought to be critical for the maintenance of proper tissue architecture, since it precludes growth of epithelial cells at ectopic locations *(50,51)*. In addition, this form of apoptosis is thought to play a major role in several physiologically important processes, such as mammary gland involution and developmental morphogenesis *(52,53)*.

Which molecular mechanisms are responsible for the induction of anoikis? Adhesion of epithelial cells to the ECM is controlled by specialized receptors called integrins

(50,54). Different proteins composing the ECM represent specific ligands for various integrins *(55)*. Upon engagement by these ECM proteins, integrins trigger various signaling pathways that contribute to cell survival and proliferation *(56,57)*. Thus, it has been proposed that in detached cells, integrins are unable to trigger such pathways *(58,59)*.

Another potentially important regulator of anoikis is the cytoskeleton. Upon detachment from the ECM, cells round up, which results in a dramatic change of the cytoskeletal organization. Experiments with endothelial cells (which, similarly to epithelial cells, are prone to anoikis) have demonstrated that distortion of the cell shape and, consequently, of the cytoskeleton, is *per se* sufficient for the induction of apoptosis *(60)*. Therefore, it has been proposed that efficient integrin-induced signaling requires a properly organized cytoskeleton *(61)*.

What are the mechanisms by which integrins and/or cytoskeleton could regulate anoikis? Several studies indicate that the ability of growth factor receptors to support survival and proliferation signals requires attachment of cells to the ECM *(58,59,62–65)*. For example, it has been shown that ligand-induced activation of the epidermal growth factor receptor (EGFR) in NIH 3T3 fibroblasts is strongly reduced upon cell detachment. This requirement for cell–ECM interactions was abrogated in the presence of activating antibodies against β1 integrin subunit. In addition, EGFR and β1 integrin were demonstrated to form a complex in monolayer, but not in suspension culture, suggesting that this particular integrin is capable of triggering EGFR activity. Such activity was presumably required for cell survival, as detachment or treatment of cells with a pharmacological inhibitor of EGFR resulted in apoptosis. The authors of this study report that activation of the receptor by the integrin occurred in the absence of EGFR ligands, but the precise mechanism of such ligand-independent EGFR activation remains unknown *(63)*. The inability of EGFR to support anti-apoptotic signals in the absence of cell–ECM interactions has also been demonstrated in case of dog kidney epithelial cells (MDCK) *(66)*.

Inhibition of the EGFR caused by cell detachment results in the reduction of the activity of MAP kinases MEK, Erk-1, and Erk-2, which are well known stimulators of cell survival *(67–69)*. This phenomenon has been observed in NIH 3T3 and MDCK cells. The significance of such reduction for anoikis has been made evident by the fact that overexpression of Raf, an activator of the MAP kinase cascade, prevented detachment-induced down-regulation of MAP kinase activity and subsequent death of MDCK cells *(70)*. PKB is another kinase relevant for anoikis and can also be stimulated by EGF. The capacity of EGF to induce PKB was shown to be strongly reduced upon detachment of MDCK cells *(66)*. In addition, apoptosis caused by detachment was completely abrogated in cells expressing activated mutants of PI 3 kinase and PKB *(66)*.

The receptors for insulin and insulin-like growth factor 1(IGF-1) are two other examples of survival-inducing signaling molecules, whose activity requires adhesion to the ECM *(65)*. The ability of both insulin and IGF-1 to rescue primary mouse mammary epithelial cells from apoptosis strongly depends on the attachment of these cells to the ECM. Similarly to what was observed for EGFR, the anti-anoikis activity of these growth factors was mediated by PI 3 kinase and, presumably, PKB *(65)*.

Focal adhesion kinase (FAK) is another molecule that plays a critical role in integrin signaling. This kinase is activated by integrin engagement, and it is thought to transduce integrin-generated signals by binding to multiple cellular proteins such as c-Src, Grb2, and PI 3-kinase, as well as by activating Ras *(71)*. The activity of FAK is known to be reduced upon detachment of several types of cells, including MDCK cells *(72)*. Constitutively active FAK mutants rescue MDCK cells as well as normal immortalized human keratinocytes HaCat from anoikis *(72)*.

A recent report has suggested that at least some integrins can actively trigger pro-apoptotic signals when they are not engaged by the respective ECM ligands *(73)*. Using human pancreatic carcinoma cells Capan-1, as well as normal epithelial cells MDCK, it was shown that these cells become more prone to anoikis when transfected with the cell cycle inhibitor p16$^{INK4a.}$ Expression of this protein resulted in a strong increase in the levels of the α5 subunit of α5β1 integrin. The causal role of this integrin in anoikis was made evident by the fact that addition of fibronectin, which acts as an α5β1 ligand, completely abolished anoikis. The same result was achieved by ectopic expression of antisense α5 cDNA. Whether the effect of p16 on the levels of the α5 subunit is related to the ability of this cell cycle inhibitor to regulate cell proliferation is unknown. Likewise, the mechanisms of nonengaged α5β1 integrin-induced anoikis remain to be identified.

How do cell–ECM interactions and subsequent activation of specific signaling pathways affect the cell death machinery? One important clue to answer this question has been provided by studying anoikis in normal human neonatal keratinocytes, as well as immortalized normal rat intestinal epithelial cells IEC-18 *(74,75)*. Detachment of these cells from the ECM results in the down-regulation of the anti-apoptotic effector Bcl-X$_L$ *(74,75)*. Such down-regulation is required for the induction of cell death, and ectopic expression of Bcl-X$_L$ in IEC-18 cells partially prevents anoikis *(75)*. Expression of Bcl-X$_L$ in adherent cells is known to require constitutive EGFR activity. In attached cells, inhibition of EGFR function with drugs or monoclonal antibodies down-regulates Bcl-X$_L$ *(75)*. Given the fact that EGFR activity requires attachment to the ECM, it is tempting to speculate that down-regulation of Bcl-X$_L$ in response to cell detachment is caused by the preceding inhibition of the EGFR. However, a direct experimental evidence supporting this hypothesis remains to be obtained.

Another component of apoptotic machinery involved in anoikis is Bax. This protein is normally cytoplasmic and triggers cell death through integration into the mitochondrial membrane and subsequent stimulation of cytochrome c release into the cytoplasm *(10,76)*. The pro-apoptotic function of Bax requires the presence of its BH3 domain. Detachment of mouse mammary FSK-7 cells, another anoikis-sensitive cell line, results in a conformational change in Bax, such that its BH3 domain becomes exposed *(77)*. This, presumably, allows for the insertion of Bax into the mitochondrial membrane and triggers subsequent cytochrome c release and anoikis. Ectopic expression of dominant-negative FAK in FSK-7 cells causes a similar conformational change in Bax accompanied by apoptosis. These events could be prevented by co-expression of activated PI 3-kinase and Src, indicating that these two kinases can regulate Bax conformation, and pro-apoptotic activity caused by cell detachment.

One major pathway known to induce apoptosis is initiated by the engagement of the "death" receptors, such as Fas and the TNF receptor (TNFR). Once activated, these receptors trigger initiator caspases-8 and -10 through the adapter molecule Fas-associated death domain (FADD) *(18,19)*. Initiator caspases, in turn, either directly activate downstream caspases outside of the mitochondria or cause the cleavage of a pro-apoptotic Bcl-2 family member Bid. The truncated form of Bid is thought to facilitate the insertion of Bax into the mitochondria, and the subsequent release of cytochrome c and cytochrome c-dependent activation of the effector caspases *(20)*.

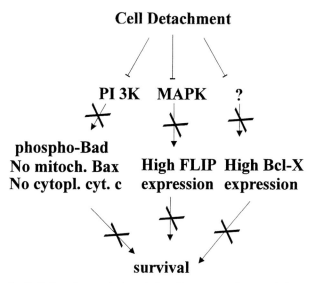

Fig. 2. Cell detachment-induced signaling events that result in anoikis.

Expression of dominant-negative FADD in MDCK, HaCat, and human endothelial HUVEC cells strongly inhibits their susceptibility to apoptosis upon detachment, indicating that anoikis could be mediated by the death receptor-dependent pathway *(78–80)*. However, the mechanism by which this pathway is involved seems to be cell type-specific, since in the case of MDCK and HaCat cells, anoikis appears to occur in a death receptor ligand-independent manner *(79)*, but in HUVEC cells, it is triggered by the interaction of Fas with its ligand *(80)*. In addition, detachment of HUVEC cells induces the expression of Fas and the down-regulation of c-Flip, a known inhibitor of caspase-8 and caspase-10 *(80)*. In the case of epithelial cells on the other hand, the mechanism by which the death receptor pathway is activated by detachment remains unknown. Cell detachment induced signaling events that result in anoikis are shown in Fig. 2.

2.2. Oncogenes as Inhibitors of Anoikis

The ability to grow in an anchorage-independent manner is one of the most typical in vitro features of solid tumor-derived and oncogene-transformed cells. This ability has frequently been assessed by growing the cells in agar. To explain the lack of anchorage-independent growth of nonmalignant cells, it was initially argued that detachment from the ECM causes an arrest in the G1 phase of the cell cycle. This, indeed, is true for many fibroblastic cell lines, especially in the presence of high concentrations of serum *(54,81,82)*. However, in the case of normal epithelial cells, the lack of anchorage-independent growth is mostly due to apoptotic death—anoikis *(46,83)*. In view of this, the fact that oncogenes are capable to inhibit anoikis is not surprising.

Ras oncogenes are present in a large proportion of human cancers *(84,85)*, and their ability to inhibit anoikis has been clearly established *(46,83)*. For example, it has been shown that *ras*-transformed MDCK and IEC-18 cells are, unlike their parental counterparts, highly resistant to this form of cell death *(46,83)*. In the case of MDCK cells, the anti-anoikis effect of activated *ras* seems to be entirely dependent on PI 3-kinase and

PKB, since activated mutants of PI 3-kinase and PKB rescue cells from anoikis to the same extent as oncogenic *ras(66)*. Similarly to what has been shown for mammary epithelial cells *(77)*, detachment of MDCK cells from the ECM resulted in the integration of Bax into the mitochondrial membrane, and in the release of cytochrome c into the cytoplasm *(70)*. Activated Ras and PKB mutants were capable to prevent both of these pro-apoptotic events.

Additional mechanisms through which *ras* could inhibit anoikis have been described for human and rat intestinal epithelial cells. In this case, the anti-anoikis effect was shown to be due in part to the ability of activated Ras to down-regulate the expression of the pro-apoptotic Bcl-2 family member Bak *(34)*. The reduction in Bak expression could be reversed by a pharmacological inhibitor of PI 3-kinase, supporting the role of this enzyme in detachment-induced apoptosis. However, re-expression of Bak or inhibition of PI 3-kinase in *ras*-transformed intestinal epithelial cells prevented the inhibitory effect of this oncogene on anoikis only partially, suggesting the existence of another, PI 3-kinase-independent ras-induced anti-anoikis pathway. Indeed, it turned out that in addition to its effect on Bak expression, activated *ras* is capable of preventing down-regulation of Bcl-X$_L$ expression caused by detachment of intestinal epithelial cells from the ECM. This property of activated *ras* is essential for anoikis resistance, as abrogation of Bcl-X$_L$ expression in the *ras*-transformed cells through an antisense RNA approach partially blocked the anti-anoikis effect of this oncogene *(75)*. The impact of activated *ras* on Bcl-X$_L$ expression was PI 3-kinase-independent and MAP-kinase-independent, suggesting that other *ras* effectors are involved.

It is important to note that *ras*-transformed cells transfected with Bak or deprived of Bcl-X$_L$ remained completely viable when attached to the ECM. Apoptosis observed in response to these changes occurred only when cells were forced to detach, suggesting that, in addition to the ras-induced changes in Bak and Bcl-X$_L$, other pro-anoikis alterations occur in the *ras*-transformed IEC cells upon detachment. These changes, however, resulted in apoptosis only when complemented by overexpression of Bak or down-regulation of Bcl-X$_L$.

Another oncogene capable of inhibiting anoikis in MDCK cells is v-Src *(46,66)*. The mechanisms of the anti-anoikis effect of this oncogene are presently unknown. v-Src activates Bcl-X$_L$ expression in fibroblasts *(35)*. Given the well documented role of Bcl-X$_L$ in anoikis *(75)*, it is tempting to speculate that the ability of v-Src to prevent detachment-induced cell death is, at least in part, due to the effect of this oncogene on Bcl-X$_L$ expression.

Resistance to anoikis by cancer cells could also result from the inactivation of tumor suppressor genes. In the case of PTEN, for example, reintroduction of this gene into human glioma (U251) and breast cancer (BT549) cell lines, which do not express functional PTEN, notably increases susceptibility of these cells to anoikis *(86,87)*. In both cases, reexpression of PTEN results in the inhibition of PKB and Bad phosphorylation, suggesting that inactivation of the PI 3-kinase-PKB-Bad signaling pathway is the cause of increased anoikis in these cells.

Another tumor suppressor gene that has been implicated in anoikis is the adenomatous polyposis coli (APC). APC inhibits transformation of normal epithelial cells by binding to β-catenin and inducing its degradation. This prevents β-catenin-mediated activation of Tcf-Lef family of transcription factors. Constitutive activation of the APC-β-catenin signaling pathway in cancer can be achieved either through inactivating mutations in APC or through activating mutations in β-catenin *(88,89)*. Expression of the transforming mutants of β-catenin in MDCK, as well as RK3E rat kidney epithelial cells, induces anchorage-independent growth, and suppression of anoikis *(90,91)*. The molecular mechanisms of such inhibition are currently unknown.

2.3. Role of Anoikis Resistance in Cancer Progression

As discussed above, cancer cells derived from solid tumors, as well as oncogene-transformed epithelial cells are able to survive in tissue culture in the absence of attachment to the ECM. Several studies indicate that this property of cancer cells is highly relevant for the progression of solid tumors in vivo and does not represent just a tissue culture artifact.

Disruption of the BM is one of the first events that can be observed at the cellular level during progression of most cancers of epithelial origin. This disruption is required for invasion of the surrounding stroma by the malignant cells. Histological studies of invasive cancer clearly show that the invading cells survive and grow without the attachment to a properly formed basement membrane. Thus, the ability of tumor cells to survive in the absence of such attachment likely represents a critical prerequisite for cancer progression. If this were correct, inhibition of susceptibility to anoikis in normal epithelial cells would be expected to render them tumorigenic. On the other hand, inhibition of anoikis resistance in cancer cells should reduce their tumorigenicity. This, indeed, is the case. MDCK cells expressing activated FAK, a genuine regulator of integrin-mediated signaling and anoikis, become tumorigenic in nude mice *(72)*. In addition, variants of IEC-18 cells, selected for the ability to resist anoikis by intermittent culturing in suspension, were also demonstrated to acquire tumorigenic potential *(83,92)*. On the other hand, the capacity of *ras*-transformed IEC-18 cells to form subcutaneous tumors in nude mice is strongly inhibited by ectopic Bak expression *(34)*. The same phenomena have been demonstrated for IEC-*ras* and human ovarian carcinoma HEY cells deprived of Bcl-X_L *(75,93)*. In the case of the ovarian cancer cells, it is important to note that they are characterized by the ability to grow in the intraperitoneal cavity, especially at the late stage of the disease. This growth condition can be considered an in vivo suspension culture. Importantly, reduction of Bcl-X_L expression in HEY cells severely inhibits their tumorigenicity when injected in the peritoneum *(93)*. Taken together, these observations indicate that acquisition of resistance to anoikis represents a critical step in the progression of carcinomas.

3. ROLE OF RESISTANCE TO HYPOXIA IN SOLID TUMOR PROGRESSION

3.1. Metabolic Mechanisms of Adaptation to Hypoxia in Cancer Cells

Solid tumors are known to contain a significant proportion of microregions that are chronically or transiently hypoxic. A strong reduction in oxygen concentration has been observed in tumor cells located at least 100–200 μm away from a functional supply of blood *(94)*. Hypoxia is thought to be one of the main factors resulting in the formation of a core of dead cells within solid tumors. For some time, the lack of oxygen was believed to result in necrosis of cancer cells *(95)*. However, recent studies indicate that hypoxia can lead to apoptotic death *(96,97)*. The fact that tumors are capable to grow and metastasize despite this highly unfavorable environment suggests that at least a proportion of cancer cells is resistant to hypoxia.

Tumor cells are thought to ensure a continuous supply of oxygen through angiogenesis. However, new microvessels are usually limited in quantity and disorganized (47). One mechanism of tumor adaptation to hypoxia is the induction of a high rate of aerobic glycolysis by tumor cells. This allows for the production of ATP levels compatible with survival, even in a low-oxygen environment. This phenomenon has been observed in the majority of human and experimental animal tumors and is called the Warburg effect (98). This effect is thought to be achieved through the increase in the expression of genes encoding several proteins involved in the intracellular transport of glucose and its conversion into ATP. A critical regulator of the expression of such genes in normal cells is the hypoxia inducible transcription factor HIF-1 (99,100). For example, HIF-1 induces the expression of several glycolytic enzymes such as phosphofructokinase L, aldolase A, phosphoglycerate kinase-1, pyruvate kinase M, enolase-1, and lactate dehydrogenase A (LDH-A). In addition, HIF-1 can stimulate the expression of vascular endothelial growth factor (VEGF), a very potent angiogenic factor (47). HIF-1 consists of two subunits, HIF-1α, and HIF-1β, also known as arylhydrocarbon-receptor nuclear translocator (ARNT) (101). ARNT is a nuclear protein whose expression is hypoxia-independent (48). Cellular levels of HIF-1α, on the other hand, are known to strongly increase under hypoxic conditions (102). In normoxia, HIF-1α is degraded by the proteasome pathway. When concentration of oxygen is low, the protein is stabilized and translocates from the cytoplasm to the nucleus where it heterodimerizes with ARNT into a transcriptionally active complex (101,102). The mechanisms of HIF-1α stabilization in response to hypoxia are not well understood.

HIF-1 has attracted a great deal of interest in the field of cancer research due to the fact that its levels, as well as the expression of its target genes involved in the Warburg effect and angiogenesis, are frequently increased in response to activation of several oncogenes. For example, cells transformed with activated v-Src display higher levels of HIF-1 and its targets enolase-1 and VEGF, as well as an increased rate of aerobic glycolisis (103).

Activated Ras, in turn, has been shown to trigger VEGF expression by a mechanism that requires the presence of a HIF-1 binding site in the VEGF promoter, suggesting that this oncogene is capable of triggering glycolitic pathways. In agreement with this, the consumption of glucose by the *ras*-transformed cells is also known to be increased (104).

myc, another oncogene frequently implicated in human cancer, has been shown to trigger overexpression of LDH-A in Rat-1 fibroblasts (105). LDH-A is one of the components of the glycolitic pathway, whose levels are known to be increased in response to hypoxia in an HIF-1-dependent way (106,107). In addition, transgenic mice that overexpress Myc in the liver display increased glycolisis in this organ (108). Also, both Myc and LDH-A were shown to trigger glycolisis when overexpressed in rodent fibroblasts (109).

Inactivation of tumor suppressor genes represents another mechanism through which tumor cells can adapt to low levels of oxygen. It has been demonstrated that reexpression of the von Hippel-Lindau (pVHL) tumor suppressor gene in renal carcinoma cells results in reduced expression of hypoxia-dependent proteins such as the glucose transporter GLUT-1 and VEGF (110).

Another tumor suppressor gene capable of suppressing hypoxia-induced stabilization of HIF-1α, as well as the expression of its target genes, is PTEN (111). Reintroduction of wild-type PTEN into the PTEN-deficient glioblastoma cell line U373 has been shown to completely suppress stabilization of HIF-1α. This effect of PTEN has been demonstrated to occur via the activation of PKB *(112)*. In addition, wild-type PTEN and a pharmacological inhibitor of PI 3-kinase were found to inhibit the expression of hypoxia-inducible genes such as VEGF, COX-1, PGK-1, and PFK. In this case, however, PTEN failed to alter the sensitivity of U373 cells to hypoxia-triggered apoptosis, suggesting that this cell line acquired additional mutations sufficient for the protection against the lack of oxygen.

3.2. Mechanisms of Hypoxia-Induced Apoptosis

Although tumor cells develop various mechanisms of resistance to hypoxic conditions, a significant proportion of these cells still die as a result of such conditions *(47)*. Recent studies have demonstrated that one of the likely reasons of tumor cell death in response to oxygen deprivation is, paradoxically, hypoxia-induced glycolisis.

One major product of glycolisis is lactic acid. Since hypoxia and oncogenes can both independently activate glycolisis, lactic acid production in hypoxic tumor cells is usually much higher than in hypoxic normal cells *(113)*. Acidosis resulting from overproduction of lactic acid is thought to be a powerful inducer of apoptosis. It has been shown that normal rat embryo fibroblasts (REF) undergo growth arrest under hypoxic conditions. In contrast, similar treatment of their Myc/Ras transformed counterparts as well as of E1a/Ras transformed mouse embryo fibroblasts (MEF) resulted in a noticeable acidosis and strong apoptosis *(113)*. Acidification was demonstrated to be the cause of cell death, as increasing the buffer capacity of the conditioned medium strongly protected these cells from apoptosis. On the other hand, the same cells became apoptotic when they were exposed to acidic medium, even under normoxic conditions *(113)*.

Another consequence of increased glycolysis in cancer cells is the high rate of glucose consumption. Glucose, therefore, can no longer serve as the only source of carbon for normal aerobic respiration. An alternative source of carbon for tumor cells exposed to reduced amounts of oxygen is glutamine. This aminoacid is known to have the ability to enter the abnormal truncated Krebs cycle. Oxidative metabolism of glutamine generate reactive oxygen species (ROS), which can in certain circumstances cause apoptosis. For example, L929 fibrosarcoma cells undergo death in response to TNF-α only when grown in the presence of glutamine. Depletion of glutamine, but not glucose, from the growth medium was shown to protect these cells from a TNF-α-induced apoptosis *(114)*.

An important regulator of hypoxia-induced cell death, whose elevated expression may be the consequence of both increased glycolisis and acidosis, is the p53 tumor suppressor protein. p53 levels increase in response to hypoxia in several cellular systems *(115,116)*. One study indicated that the accumulation of this tumor suppressor protein under hypoxic conditions results from acidosis, since inhibition of culture medium acidification abrogated the accumulation of p53 in transformed hypoxic cells *(113)*. Another study, however, suggested that this accumulation is the consequence of hypoxia-induced increase in HIF-1α expression and the subsequent direct or indirect interaction of HIF-1α with p53. This interaction was shown to prevent proteasome-mediated p53 degradation, triggering apoptosis *(116)*.

In addition to being able to generate acidosis, HIF-1α appears to have the capacity to directly induce the expression of pro-apototic components of the cell death machinery *(117)*. For example, hypoxic conditions elevate the levels of pro-apoptotic bcl-2 family members such as NIP 3 and Nix in Chinese hamster ovary cells (CHO) *(117)*. The inductive effect of hypoxia on Nip 3 expression has also been observed in several other types of cells. In addition, both hypoxia and HIF-1α were shown to activate the NIP 3 promoter, suggesting that this pro-apoptotic protein represents a direct target of HIF-1α *(117)*.

3.3. Mechanisms of Resistance to Hypoxia in Cancer Cells

Even though relatively little is known about the mechanisms of resistance to hypoxia-induced cell death in cancer, several direct and indirect regulators of apoptosis have been implicated in this process.

One way tumor cells can resist hypoxia-induced apotosis is through the inactivation of p53. p53-negative E1a/Ras-transformed MEFs are significantly more resistant to the hypoxia-induced apoptosis in tissue culture than their p53-positive counterparts *(115,118)*. Examination of tumors formed by such cells upon injection into immuno-compromised mice revealed that cells located in regions poorly supplied with blood undergo a p53-dependent apoptosis. On the other hand, cells in which active p53 was lost were demonstrated to acquire a survival advantage over cells with wild-type p53 *(115,118)*.

Another mechanism through which cancer cells could potentially acquire resistance to apoptosis triggered by the lack of oxygen involves the up-regulation of anti-apop-totic Bcl-2 family members, such as Bcl-2 and Bcl-X_L. For example, Bcl-2 has been shown to protect *myc*-transformed Rat-1 fibroblasts from hypoxia-induced cell death. A similar effect of Bcl-2 has been demonstrated in the rat hepatoma cell line 7316A and the rat pheochromocytoma cells PC 12 *(49)*. An even more potent protection from hypoxia-induced apoptosis of PC 12 cells has been observed in response to overexpres-sion of Bcl-X_L *(49)*. Since both Bcl-2 and Bcl-X_L are frequently overexpressed in many types of cancers *(42–44)*, it is reasonable to speculate that oncogenes that can induce the expression of these proteins will confer resistance to hypoxia-triggered death. A direct poof of this hypothesis, however, has not yet been reported. Signaling events that are triggered by activation of oncogenes and loss of tumor suppressor genes in cancer cells under the normoxic and hypoxic conditions are shown in Fig. 3.

4. CONCLUSIONS

Recent observations strongly suggest that acquisition of resistance to anoikis and hypoxia-induced apoptosis represent two important mechanisms of progression of can-cers originated from epithelial cells. The role of oncogenes and tumor suppressor genes in the generation of such resistance is now clearly established. Moreover, the results discussed above indicate that certain oncogenes or tumor suppressor genes could be involved in the simultaneous induction of resistance to both anoikis and hypoxia-induced apoptosis.

This means that therapies aimed at the reversal of the activation or inactivation of such oncogenes and tumor suppressor genes, respectively, may be able to sensitize tumor cells to both anoikis and hypoxia. Since normal epithelial cells in vivo are attached to the BM and are generally not exposed to hypoxic conditions, at least some of such therapeutic approaches would be expected to preferentially attack tumor cells.

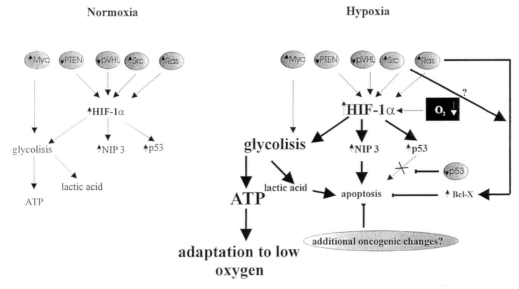

Fig. 3. Signaling events that are triggered by activation of oncogenes and loss of tumor suppressor genes in cancer cells under the normoxic and hypoxic conditions.

REFERENCES

1. Hengartner H. The biochemistry of apoptosis. *Nature* 2000; 407:770–776.
2. Reed JC. Mechanisms of apoptosis. *Am J Pathol* 2000; 157:1415–1430.
3. Li H, Yuan J. Deciphering the pathways of life and death. *Curr Opin Cell Biol* 1999; 11:261–266.
4. Desagher S, Martinou JC. Mitochondria as the central control point in apoptosis. *Trends Cell Biol* 2000; 10:369–377.
5. Loeffler M, Kroemer G. The mitochondrion in cell death control: certainties and incognita. *Exp Cell Res* 2000; 256:19–26.
6. Kroemer G, Reed JC. Mitochondrial control of cell death. *Nat Med* 2000; 6:513–519.
7. Wang J, Lenardo MJ. Roles of caspases in apoptosis, development, and cytokine maturation revealed by homozygous gene deficiencies. *J Cell Sci* 2000; 113:753–757.
8. Budihardjo I, Oliver H, Lutter M, Luo X, Wang X. Biochemical pathways of caspase activation during apoptosis. *Annu Rev Cell Dev Biol* 1999; 15:269–290.
9. Salvesen GS, Dixit VM. Caspase activation: the induced-proximity model. *Proc Natl Acad Sci USA* 1999; 96:10964–10967.
10. Antonsson B, Martinou JC. The Bcl-2 protein family. *Exp Cell Res* 2000; 256:50–57.
11. Gross A, McDonnell JM, Korsmeyer SJ. BCL-2 family members and the mitochondria in apoptosis. *Genes Dev* 1999; 13:1899–1911.
12. Green DR. Apoptotic pathways: paper wraps stone blunts scissors. *Cell* 2000; 102:1–4.
13. Deveraux QL, Reed JC. IAP family proteins—suppressors of apoptosis. *Genes Dev* 1999; 239–252.
14. LaCasse EC, Baird S, Korneluk RG, Mackenzie AE. The inhibitors of apoptosis (IAPs) and their emerging role in cancer. *Oncogene* 1998; 17:3247–3259.
15. Nicholson DW. Baiting death inhibitors. *Nature* 2001; 410:33–34.
16. Chai J, Du C, Wu JW, Kyin S, Wang X, Shi Y. Structural and biochemical basis of apoptotic activation by Smac/Diablo. *Nature* 2000; 406:855–862.
17. Ekert PG, Silke J, Hawkins CJ, Verhagen AM, Vaux DL. DIABLO promotes apoptosis by removing MIHA/XIAP from processed caspase 9. *J Cell Biol* 2001; 152:483–490.
18. Locksley RM, Killeen N, Lenardo MJ. The TNF and TNF receptor superfamilies: integrating mammalian biology. *Cell* 2001; 104:487–501.
19. Walczak H, Krammer PH. The CD95(APO-1/Fas) and the TRAIL (APO-2L) apoptosis systems. *Exp Cell Res* 2000; 256:58–66.

20. Nagata S. Biddable death. *Nat Cell Biol* 1999; 1:E143–E145.
21. Lowe SW, Lin AW. Apoptosis in cancer. *Carcinogenesis* 2000; 21:485–495.
22. Kaufmann SH, Gores GJ. Apoptosis in cancer: cause and cure. *Bioessays* 2000; 22:1007–1017.
23. Shields JM, Pruitt K, McFall A, Shaub A, Der CJ. Understanding Ras: 'it ain't over 'til it's over'. *Trends Cell Biol* 2000; 10:147–154.
24. McCormick F. How receptors turn ras on. *Nature* 1993; 363:15–16.
25. Katz ME, McCormick F. Signal transduction from multiple Ras effectors. *Curr Opin Genet Dev* 1997; 7:75–79.
26. Vojtek AB, Der CJ. Increasing complexity of the ras signaling pathway. *J Biol Chem* 1998; 273:19925–19928.
27. Downward J. Ras signaling and apoptosis. *Curr Opin Genet Dev* 1998; 8:49–54.
28. Sy MS, Guo YJ, Stamenkovic I. Distinct effects of two CD44 isoforms on tumor growth in vivo. *J Exp Med* 1991; 174:859–866.
29. Datta SR, Dudek H, Tao X, Masters S, Fu H, Gotoh Y, et al. Akt phosphorylation of BAD couples survival signals to the cell-intrinsic death machinery. *Cell* 1997; 91:231–241.
30. Scheid MP, Schubert KM, Duronio V. Regulation of Bad phosphorylation and association with Bcl-X_L by the MAPK/Erk kinase. *J Biol Chem* 1999; 274:31108–31113.
31. Downward J. How BAD phosphorylation is good for survival. *Nat Cell Biol* 1999; 1:E33–E35.
32. Brunet A, Bonni A, Zigmond MJ, Lin MZ, Juo P, Hu LS, et al. Akt promotes cell survival by phosphorylating and inhibiting a forkhead transcription factor. *Cell* 1999; 96:857–868.
33. Wang JM, Chao JR, Chen W, Kuo ML, Yen JJY, Yen HFY. The antiapoptotic gene *mcl-1* is up-regulated by the phosphatidylinositol 3-kinase/Akt signaling pathway through a transcription fator complex containing CREB. *Mol Cell Biol* 1999; 19:6195–6206.
34. Rosen K, Rak J, Jin J, Kerbel RS, Newman MJ, Filmus J. Downregulation of the pro-apoptotic protein Bak is required for the ras-induced transformation of intestinal epithelial cells. *Curr Biol* 1998; 8:1331–1334.
35. Karni R, Jove R, Levitzki A. Inhibition of pp60^{c-src} reduces Bcl-X_L expression and reverses the transformed phenotype of cells overexpressing EGF and HER-2 receptors. *Oncogene* 1999; 18:4654–4662.
36. Bromberg JF, Wrzeszczynska MH, Devgan G, Zhao Y, Pestell RG, Albanese C, et al. STAT3 as an oncogene. *Cell* 1999; 98:295–303.
37. Vogelstein B, Kinzler KW. p53 function and disfunction. *Cell* 1992; 70:523–526.
38. Miyashita T, Reed JC. Tumor suppressor p53 is a direct transcriptional activator of the human bax gene. *Cell* 1995; 80:293–299.
39. Stambolic V, Suzuki A, de la Pompa JL, Brothers GM, Mirtsos C, Sasaki T, et al. Negative regulation of PKB/Akt-dependent cell survival by the tumor suppressor PTEN. *Cell* 1998; 95:29–39.
40. Cantley L, Neel BG. New insights into tumor suppression: PTEN suppresses tumor formation by restraining the phosphoinositide 3-kinase/AKT pathway. *Proc Natl Acad Sci USA* 1999; 96:4240–4245.
41. Di Cristofano A, Pandolfi PP. The multiple roles of PTEN in tumor suppression. *Cell* 2000; 100:387–390.
42. Krajewska M, Moss SF, Krajewski S, Song K, Holt PR, Reed JC. Elevated expression of Bcl-X and reduced Bak in primary colorectal adenocarcinomas. *Cancer Res* 1996; 56:2422–2427.
43. Liu JR, Fletcher B, Page C, Hu C, Nunez G, Baker V. Bcl-xL is expressed in ovarian carcinoma and modulates chemotherapy-induced apoptosis. *Gynecol Oncol* 1998; 70:398–403.
44. Marone M, Scambia G, Mozzetti S, Ferrandina G, Iacovella S, De Pasqua A, et al. bcl-2, bax, bcl-XL, and bcl-XS expression in normal and neoplastic ovarian tissues. *Clin Cancer Res* 1998; 4:517–524.
45. Soini Y, Paakko P, Lehto VP. Histopathological evaluation of apoptosis in cancer. *Am J Pathol* 1998; 153:1041–1053.
46. Frisch SM, Francis H. Disruption of epithelial cell-matrix interactions induces apoptosis. *J Cell Biol* 1994; 124:619–626.
47. Dang CV, Semenza GL. Oncogenic alterations of metabolism. *Trends Biochem Sci* 1999; 24:68–72.
48. Eguchi H, Ikuta T, Tachibana T, Yoneda Y, Kawajiri K. A nuclear localization signal of human aryl hydrocarbon receptor nuclear translocator/hypoxia-inducible factor 1 beta is a novel bipartite type recognized by the two components of nuclear pore-targeting complex. *J Biol Chem* 1997; 272:17640–17647.
49. Shimizu S, Eguchi Y, Kosaka H, Kamiike W, Matsuda H, Tsujimoto Y. Prevention of hypoxia-induced cell death by Bcl-2 and Bcl-xL. *Nature* 1995; 374:811–813.

50. Frisch SM, Ruoslahti E. Integrins and anoikis. *Curr Opin Cell Biol* 1997; 9:701–706.

51. Meredith JE, Fazeli B, Schwartz MA. The extracellular matrix as a cell survival factor. *Mol Biol Cell* 1993; 4:953–961.

52. Wiesen J, Werb Z. Proteinases, cell cycle regulation, and apoptosis during mammary gland involution. *Mol Reprod Dev* 2000; 56:534–540.

53. Jacobson MD, Weil M, Raff MC. Programmed cell death in animal development. *Cell* 1997; 88:347–354.

54. Meredith JE, Schwartz MA. Integrins, adhesion and apoptosis. *Trends Cell Biol* 1997; 7:147–150.

55. Giancotti FG, Ruoslahti E. Integrin signaling. *Science* 1999; 285:1028–1032.

56. Howe A, Aplin AE, Alahari SK, Juliano RL. Integrin signaling and cell growth control. *Curr Opin Cell Biol* 1998; 10:220–231.

57. Giancotti F. Integrin signaling: specificity and control of cell survival and cell cycle progression. *Curr Opin Cell Biol* 1997; 9:691–700.

58. Aplin AE, Juliano RL. Integrin and cytoskeletal regulation of growth factor signaling to the MAP kinase pathway. *J Cell Sci* 1999; 112:695–706.

59. Renshaw MW, Price LS, Schwartz MA. Focal adhesion kinase mediates the integrin signaling requirement for growth factor activation of MAPK kinase. *J Cell Biol* 1999; 147:611–618.

60. Chen CS, Mrksich M, Huang S, Whitesides GM, Ingber DE. Geometric control of cell life and death. *Science* 1997; 276:1425–1428.

61. Huang S, Ingber DE. The structural and mechanical complexity of cell-growth control. *Nat Cell Biol* 1999; 1:E131–E138

62. Renshaw MW, Ren XD, Schwartz MA. Growth factor activation of MAP kinase requires cell adhesion. *EMBO J* 1997; 16:5592–5599.

63. Moro L, Venturino M, Bozzo C, Silengo L, Altruda F, Beguinot L, et al. Integrins induce activation of EGF receptor: role in MAP kinase induction and adhesion-dependent cell survival. *EMBO J* 1998; 17:6622–6632.

64 Miyamoto S, Teramoto H, Gutkind JS, Yamada KM. Integrins can collaborate with growth factors for phosphorylation of receptor tyrosine kinases and MAP kinase activation: roles of integrin aggregation and occupancy of receptors. *J Cell Biol* 1996; 135:1633–1642.

65. Farrelly N, Lee YJ, Oliver J, Dive C, Streuli CH. Extracellular matrix regulates apoptosis in mammary epithelium through a control on insulin signaling. *J Cell Biol* 1999; 144:1337–1347.

66. Khwaja A, Rodriguez-Viciana P, Wennstrom S, Warne PH, Downward J. Matrix adhesion and ras transformation both activate a phosphoinositide 3-OH kinase and protein kinase B/Akt cellular survival pathway. *EMBO J* 1997; 16:2783–2793.

67. Xia Z, Dickens J, Raingeaud J, Davis RJ, Greenberg ME. Opposing effects of ERK and JNK-p38 MAP kinases on apoptosis. *Science* 1995; 270:1326–1331.

68. Bonni A, Brunet A, West AE, Datta SR, Takasu MA, Greenberg ME. Cell survival promoted by the Ras-MAPK signaling pathway by transcription-dependent and -independent mechanisms. *Science* 1999; 286:1358–1362.

69. Gire V, Marshall C, Wynford-Thomas D. PI-3-kinase is an essential anti-apoptotic effector in the proliferative response of primary human epithelial cells to mutant RAS. *Oncogene* 2000; 19:2269–2276.

70. Rytomaa M, Lehman K, Downward J. Matrix detachment induces caspase-dependent cytocrome c release from mitochondria: inhibition by PKB/Akt but not Raf signalling. *Oncogene* 2000; 19:4461–4468.

71. Schlaepfer DD. Hunter T. Integrin signalling and tyrosine phosphorylation: just the FAKs? *Trends Cell Biol* 1998; 8:151–157.

72. Frisch SM, Vuori K, Ruoslahti E, Chan-Hui PY. Control of adhesion-dependent cell survival by focal adhesion kinase. *J Cell Biol* 1996; 134:793–799.

73. Plath T, Detjen K, Welzel M, von Marschall Z, Murphy D, Schirner M, et al. A novel function for the tumor suppressor p16INK4a: induction of anoikis via upregulation of the $\alpha_5\beta_1$ fibronectin receptor. *J Cell Biol* 2000; 150:1467–1477.

74. Rodeck U, Jost M, DuHadaway J, Kari C, Jensen PJ, Risse B, et al. Regulation of Bcl-x$_L$ expression in human keratinocytes by cell-substratum adhesion and the epidermal growth factor receptor. *Proc Natl Acad Sci USA* 1997; 94:5067–5072.

75. Rosen K, Rak J, Leung T, Dean NM, Kerbel RS, Filmus J. Activated ras prevents downregulation of Bcl-X$_L$ triggered by detachment from the extracellular matrix: a mechanism of *ras*-induced resistance to anoikis in intestinal epithelial cells. *J Cell Biol* 2001; 149:447–455.

76. Adams JM, Cory S. The Bcl-2 protein family: arbiters of cell survival. *Science* 1998; 281:1322–1326.

77. Gilmore AP, Metcalfe AD, Romer LH, Streuli CH. Integrin-mediated survival signals regulate the apoptotic function of Bax through its conformation and subcellular localization. *J Cell Biol* 2000; 149:431–445.

78. Frisch SM. Evidence for a function of death-receptor-related, death-domain-containing proteins in anoikis. *Curr Biol* 1999; 9:1047–1049.

79. Rytomaa M, Martins LM, Downward J. Involvement of FADD and caspase-8 signaling in detachment-induced apoptosis. *Curr Biol* 1999; 9:1043–1046.

80. Aoudjit F, Vuori K. Matrix attachment regulates Fas-induced apoptosis in endothelial cells: a role for c-flip and implications for anoikis. *J Cell Biol* 2001; 152:633–643.

81. Guadagno TM, Ohtsubo M, Roberts JM, Assoian RK. A link between cyclin A expression and adhesion-dependent cell cycle progression. *Science* 1993; 262:1572–1575.

82. Fang F, Orend G, Watanabe N, Hunter T, Ruoslahti E. Dependence of cyclin E-CDK2 kinase activity on cell anchorage. *Science* 1996; 271:499–502.

83. Rak J, Mitsuhashi Y, Erdos V, Huang S-N, Filmus J, Kerbel RS. Massive programmed cell death in intestinal epithelial cells induced by three-dimensional growth conditions: suppression by mutant C-H-*ras*oncogene. J Cell Biol 1995; 131:1587–1598.

84. Bos JL, Fearon ER, Hamilton SR, Verlaan-de Vries M, van Boom JH, van der Eb AJ, et al. Prevalence of ras gene mutations in human colorectal cancers. *Nature* 1987; 327:293–297.

85. Barbacid M. ras Genes. *Annu Rev Biochem* 1987; 56:779–827.

86. Davies MA, Lu Y, Sano T, Fang X, Tang P, Lapushin R, et al. Adenoviral transgene expression of MMAC/PTEN in human glioma cells inhibits Akt activation and induces anoikis. *Cancer Res* 1998; 58:5285–5290.

87. Lu Y, Lin YZ, LaPushi R, Cuevas B, Fang X, Yu SX, et al. The PTEN/MMAC1/TEP tumor suppressor gene decreases cell growth and induces apoptosis and anoikis in breast cancer cells. *Oncogene* 1999; 18:7034–7045.

88. Polakis P. Wnt signaling and cancer. *Genes Dev* 2000; 14:1837–1851.

89. van Es JH, Giles RH, Clevers HC. The many faces of the tumor suppressor gene APC. *Exp Cell Res* 2001; 264:126–134.

90. Orford K, Orford CC, Byers SW. Exogenous expression of β-catenin regulates contact inhibition, anchorage-independent growth, anoikis, and radiation-induced cell cycle arrest. *J Cell Biol* 1999; 146:855–867.

91. Kolligs FT, Kolligs B, Hajra KM, Hu G, Tani M, Cho KR, et al. γ-catenin is regulated by the APC tumor suppressor and its oncogenic activity is distinct from the β-catenin. *Genes Dev* 2000; 14:1319–1331.

92. Rak J, Mitsuhashi Y, Sheehan C, Krestow JK, Florenes VA, Filmus J, et al. Collateral expression of proangiogenic and tumorigenic properties in intestinal epithelial cell variants selected for resistance to anoikis. *Neoplasia* 1999; 1:23–30.

93. Frankel AD, Rosen K, Filmus J, Kerbel RS. Induction of anoikis and suppression of human ovarian tumor growth in vivo by downregulation of Bcl-XL. *Cancer Res* 2001, in 61:4837–4841.

94. Helmlinger G, Yuan F, Dellian M, Jain RK. Interstitial pH and pO$_2$ gradients in solid tumors in vivo: high-resolution measurements reveal a lack of correlation. *Nat Med* 1997; 3:177–182.

95. Jozsa L, Reffy A, Demel S, Szilagyi I. Ultrastructural changes in human liver cells due to reversible acute hypoxia. *Hepatogastroenterology* 1981; 28:23–26.

96. Muschel RJ, Bernhard EJ, Garza L, McKenna WG, Koch CJ. Induction of apoptosis at different oxygen tensions: evidence that oxygen radicals do not mediate apoptotic signaling. *Cancer Res* 1995; 55:995–998.

97. Tanaka M, Ito H, Adachi S, Akimoto H, Nishikawa T, Kasajima T, et al. Hypoxia induces apoptosis with enhanced expression of Fas antigen messenger RNA in cultured neonatal rat cardiomyocytes. *Circ Res* 1994; 75:426–433.

98. Warburg O. *The Metabolism of Tumors.* Constable, London, England, 1930.

99. Wang GL, Semenza GL. General involvement of hypoxia-inducible factor 1 in transcriptional response to hypoxia. *Proc Natl Acad Sci USA* 1993; 90:4304–4308.

100. Wang GL, Semenza GL. Characterization of hypoxia-inducible factor 1 and regulation of DNA binding activity by hypoxia. *J Biol Chem* 1993; 268:21513–21518.

101. Wang GL, Jiang BH, Rue EA, Semenza GL. Hypoxia-inducible factor 1 is a basic-helix-loop-helix-PAS heterodimer regulated by cellular O$_2$ tension. *Proc Natl Acad Sci USA* 1995; 92:5510–5514.

102. Salceda S, Caro J. Hypoxia-inducible factor 1alpha (HIF-1alpha) protein is rapidly degraded by the ubiquitin-proteasome system under normoxic conditions. Its stabilization by hypoxia depends on redox-induced changes. *J Biol Chem* 1997; 272:22642–22647.

103. Jiang BH, Agani F, Passaniti A, Semenza GL. V-SRC induces expression of hypoxia-inducible factor 1 (HIF-1) and transcription of genes encoding vascular endothelial growth factor and enolase 1: involvement of HIF-1 in tumor progression. *Cancer Res* 1997; 57:5328–5335.

104. Mazure NM, Chen EY, Yeh P, Laderoute KR, Giaccia AJ. Oncogenic transformation and hypoxia synergistically act to modulate vascular endothelial growth factor expression. *Cancer Res* 1996; 56:3436–3440.

105. Lewis BC, Shim H, Li Q, Wu CS, Lee LA, Maity A, et al. Identification of putative c-Myc-responsive genes: characterization of rcl, a novel growth-related gene. *Mol Cell Biol* 1997; 17:4967–4978.

106. Firth JD, Ebert BL, Ratcliffe PJ. Hypoxic regulation of lactate dehydrogenase A. Interaction between hypoxia-inducible factor 1 and cAMP response elements. *J Biol Chem* 1995; 270:21021–21027.

107. Semenza GL, Jiang BH, Leung SW, Passantino R, Concordet JP, Maire P, et al. Hypoxia response elements in the alsolase A, enolase 1, and lactate dehydrogenase A gene promoters contain essential binding sites for hypoxia-inducible factor 1. *J Biol Chem* 1996; 271:32529–32537.

108. Valera A, Pujol A, Gregori X, Riu E, Visa J, Bosch F. Evidence from transgenic mice that myc regulates hepatic glycolysis. *FASEB J* 1995; 9:1067–1078.

109. Shim H, Dolde C, Lewis BC, Wu CS, Dang G, Jungmann RA, et al. c-Myc transactivation of LDH-A: implications for tumor metabolism and growth. *Proc Natl Acad Sci USA* 1997; 94:6658–6663.

110. Gnarra JR, Zhou S, Merrill MJ, Wagner JR, Krumm A, Papavassiliou E, et al. Post-transcriptional regulational of vascular endothelial growth factor mRNA by the product of the VHL tumor suppressor gene. *Proc Natl Acad Sci USA* 1996; 93:10589–10594.

111. Zundel W, Schindler C, Haas-Kogan D, Koong A, Kaper F, Chen E, et al. Loss of PTEN facilitates HIF-1-mediated gene expression. *Genes Dev* 2000; 14:391–396.

112. Willecke K, Schafer R. Human oncogenes. *Hum Genet* 1984; 66:132–142.

113. Schmaltz C, Hardenbergh PH, Wells A, Fisher DE. Regulation of proliferation-survival decisions during tumor cell hypoxia. *Mol Cell Biol* 1998; 18:2845–2854.

114. Goossens V, Grooten J, Fiers W. The oxidative metabolism of glutamine. A modulator of reactive oxygen intermediate-mediated cytotoxicity of tumor necrosis factor in L929 fibrosarcoma cells. *J Biol Chem* 1996; 271:192–196.

115. Graeber TG, Peterson JF, Tsai M, Monica K, Fornace AJ, Giaccia AJ. Hypoxia induces accumulation of p53 protein, but activation of a G1-phase checkpoint by low-oxygen conditions is independent of p53 status. *Mol Cell Biol* 1994; 14:6264–6277.

116. An WG, Kanekal M, Simon MC, Maltepe E, Blagosklonny MV, Neckers LM. Stabilization of wild-type p53 by hypoxia-inducible factor 1 alpha. *Nature* 1998; 392:405–408.

117. Bruick RK. Expression of the gene encoding the proapoptotic Nip3 protein is induced by hypoxia. *Proc Natl Acad Sci USA* 2000; 97:9082–9087.

118. Kinzler KW, Vogelstein B. Life (and death) in a malignant tumour. *Nature* 1996; 379:19–20.

10 Oncogenes and Tumor Angiogenesis

Janusz Rak, MD, PhD
and Robert S. Kerbel, PhD

CONTENTS

1. INTRODUCTION

A reductionist viewpoint, which assumes that all important properties of cancer are ultimately encoded in a cancer cell, has provided an important stimulus for studies on oncogenes *(1)*. Although this approach proved to be very powerful in establishing the genetic causes of cancer, it was in itself insufficient to properly interpret the resulting complexity of the unfolding pathological process *(2)*. Indeed, cancer as a disease involves a multitude of interactions between heterotypic cellular and matrix components, of which cancer cells are the central, but by no means the only relevant element *(2)*. In this sense, the intimate interrelationship and interdependence between cancer cells and the adjacent host vasculature are indispensable aspects of tumor very growth

From: *Oncogene-Directed Therapies*
Edited by: J. W. Rak © Humana Press Inc., Totowa, NJ

and dissemination *(3)*. Based on this premise, Folkman proposed that tumor vasculature can be an attractive and universal target for anticancer therapy *(3)*. This chapter is intended as a discussion of the linkage between formation of the tumor vasculature (tumor angiogenesis) and the causal disease-triggering effects of cancer-associated genetic alternations, particularly expression of activated oncogenes. Here, it is argued that there are multiple ways by which oncogenes can impinge upon the course, the outcome, and the consequences of the tumor angiogenesis process. More importantly, oncogene-directed therapies (signal transduction inhibitors) can interfere with various aspects of tumor neovascularization and possibly synergize with other blood vessel-targeting and cancer cell-targeting agents.

2. TUMOR ANGIOGENESIS

Progressive spatially unrestricted 3-dimensional cellular growth is a hallmark of cancer *(4,5)*. It is now evident that this abnormal growth pattern or topology is not solely a function of various intrinsic properties of *individual* cancer cells (e.g., anchorage-independence, increased mitogenesis, survival under unfavorable conditions, invasiveness, morphological transformation), but also involves *collective* multicellular properties of cancer *(6)* resulting in recruitment and maintenance of host-derived tumor-associated blood vessels *(3)*.

2.1. Dependence of Tumor Growth and Progression on the Vasculature

Development of the tumor-associated blood vessel network plays a pivotal role in cancer progression. In simple terms, the absolute necessity for tumor neovascularization stems from the fact that diffusion of essential metabolites, growth factors, and oxygen between blood and tumor parenchyma can only occur at relatively short distances *(7)*. Therefore, the distances between tumor cells and their nearest capillaries are viewed as ultimate determinants of sustained metabolic activity of tumor cells, their proliferation, and very survival. In this sense, 3-dimensional tumor expansion beyond the reach of the diffusion from the preexisting established vascular bed in a given organ is conditional upon new blood vessel recruitment *(3)*. This is best exemplified by the observation that in the absence of angiogenesis, (avascular) tumor growth is limited to the size of only 1 to 2 mm in diameter *(3,7)* and is often held in a steady state of dormancy until new capillaries can be attracted *(3,8)*. During the state of dormancy the increase in cancer cell numbers in areas of sufficient perfusion is usually (out)balanced by induction of mitotic arrest and apoptotic cell death in more ischemic regions of the tumor cell nodule (at a distance from capillaries). This explains the lack of net increase in tumor volume despite sometimes fairly rapid tumor cell turnover *(9,10)*.

Although tumor cells may remain in the state of dormancy for extended periods of time *(9)*, the ingrowth of new blood vessel may eventually take place leading to cessation of this silent phase of the disease and to the exponential tumor expansion *(10)*. At this time, blood *(10)* and lymphatic *(11–13)* vessel networks develop in and around the tumor, ultimately allowing the release of tumor cells into the circulation and their local, regional, and distant metastatic dissemination *(14)*. Thus, the onset of angiogenesis (angiogenic) switch is belived to be a precondition for macroscopic, clinically apparent manifestation of cancer, as well as its eventual morbidity and mortality *(3)*.

Tissue perfusion is not the only relevant consequence of tumor angiogenesis *(15)*. It is believed that tumor-associated endothelial cells acquire unique properties *(16)*, and may become capable of releasing a plethora of growth factors, cytokines, small molecular weight mediators (e.g., nitric oxide, reactive oxygen species) proteases, and extracellular matrix (ECM) proteins *(15)*. These various biologically active entities could, in turn, stimulate in a paracrine manner tumor cell growth *(17)*, survival *(18)*, migration *(19)*, invasion *(20,21)* and metastasis *(22)*. Some of these vascular influences simply promote these various cancer-associated processes, while others may participate in selection of distinct phenotypic tumor cell variants, usually of increased malignancy *(23)*. This paracrine supportive/selective role of the tumor vasculature may be particularly relevant in hematopoietic malignancies (leukemias, lymphomas), where, with possible exception of the bone marrow and/or lymphoid organs sites, tumor cell access to blood is not restricted by anatomical barriers *(24,25)*.

The notion that cancer growth and dissemination is angiogenesis-dependent carries fundamentally important therapeutic implications *(3)*. In particular, Folkman first realized that inhibition (anti-angiogenic therapy) of tumor blood vessel formation or their selective destruction (anti-vascular therapy) could constitute an effective strategy to treat cancer *(3)*. Indeed, the accuracy of this prediction is supported by ample preclinical evidence *(3,10,26–28)*. Morever, a large group of anti-angiogenics is curretly in various phases of clinical testing as prospective anti-cancer agents (http://cancertrials.nci.nih.go and www.angio.org). While the early results in many cases appear promising, in that the drugs are usually devoid of severe toxicity associated with traditional cytoreductive anti-cancer agents, their efficacy under specific clinical circumstances remains to be firmly established, optimized, and their role in mono-or combination therapy protocols more precisely defined *(29)*. Further progress in this area will likely require a more refined mechanistic understanding of cellular and molecular interactions that constitute the process of tumor angiogenesis in its many inducer, organ-, and tumor-specific forms.

2.2. Processes Leading to Tumor Blood Vessel Formation

Several distinct cellular processes can participate in the development of tumor vasculature *(30–33)*. It is believed that, for the most part, tumor-associated vascular structures originate by direct branching and extension of preexisting host capillaries or postcapillary venules *(31)*. At the center of this process (termed sprouting angiogenesis) is the directional deployment of endothelial cell cohorts (vascular sprouts) from the wall of the existing vessel toward the source of the inducing stimulus. Formation of new capillaries usually involves a cascade of distinct sequential events including: dissociation (drop-out) of supporting mural cells (pericytes, smooth muscle cells) from their underlying inner endothelial tube and resulting local vessel destabilization. This is followed by proteolytic dissolution of the endothelial basement membrane, endothelial cell invasion into the surrounding ECM, and their subsequent migration, proliferation, and alignment into a solid cellular cord *(31)*. Further steps involve lumen formation and anastomosis with analogous neighboring vascular sprouts, all of which brings about the establishement of blood circulation in the newly formed capillary loop *(31)*.

While the above generic sequence is relatively well described, alternative processes also do exist. For instance, new capillary loops may be formed by formation, first of a larger thin walled mother vessel, which is then subdivided into smaller endothelial channels (daughter vessels) *(34)*. This transition is accomplished, either by external pressure of surrounding tissue pillars (intussusceptive angiogenesis) *(35)* or by aberrant intraluminal bridges formed by activated endothelial cells (splitting angiogenesis) *(31)*. Some of the preformed vascular structures might also merge through a process of microvacular fusion to form larger vessels *(36)*. Tumor vasculature may, to some degree, expand through incorporation into the vessel wall of circulating bone marrow-derived endothelial progenitor cells (EPCs) *(37,38)*, a process often referred to as postnatal vasculogenesis *(30)*. It has also been proposed, that, at least some vascular segments of uveal melanoma, are composed of tumor cells, which are said to adopt endothelial-like functions and phenotype (i.e., undergo vasculogenic mimicry) *(39)*. While the existence and extent of this form of tumor neovascularization remains controversial in itself *(40)*, it is important to point out that even blood channels with incomplete or absent endothelial lining must, by definition, maintain anatomical and functional continuity with, and dependence on, the remaining fully endothelialized vasculature, present both within and outside of the tumor. To a degree, tumor vascularization may also occur via invasion and engulfment *(41)*, or cooption *(42)* by growing tumor masses of preexisting autochtonous tissue blood vessels. In some circumstances this process, rather than bona fide vessel recruitment through angiogenesis, is thought to accompany early stages of tumor expansion *(42)*. To one degree or another, all these forms of tumor vascularization may be present within, support, and be induced by various types of cancers. As such, these various processes, often collectively referred to as tumor angiogenesis can be viewed as implicitly linked to expression of cancer-causing genes including activated oncogenes.

Intratumoral vascular networks are often described as caricatures of their normal orthotopic counterparts. Physiologically, angiogenesis occurrs infrequently and is mainly restricted to such processes as embryo development, corpus luteum formation, growth of the exercising skeletal muscle, accumulation of the fatty tissue, regeneration of organs, and granulation tissue formation. In all such instances, the outcome is a well-organized tree-like (arborized) quasifractal vascular structure, the geometry of which is well adapted to the topology and perfusion needs of a particular site, organ, and tissue. The general feature of such normal vasculature is the gradual decrease in vessel caliber and regular branching towards the organ's periphery *(7)*. In contrast, tumor blood vessels display a wide array of morphological and functional abnormalities including: lack or proper branching and arborization, aberrant and inconsistent vessel size distribution (dilatations, pseudostenosis), as well as bizarre tortuosities, loops, and corkscrew structures *(7)*. Tumor blood vessels are thought to lack functional innervation and are often immature, i.e., display poor and discontinuous coverage of endothelial channels with pericytes and smooth muscle cells *(41,43,44)*. The functionality of such abnormal vessel networks is severely compromised as indicated by sluggish blood flow, shunting, and leakage of plasma proteins into the extravascular milleau *(7)*.

In contrast to largely quiescent endothelium of normal blood vessels, the mitotic indices of tumor-associated endothelial cells is often remarkably high *(45)*. This is accompanied by elevated expression of various molecular markers of endothelial cell activation including: adhesion molecules (including "αv" intergrins), growth factor receptor tyrosine kinases (e.g., vascular endothelial growth factor receptors VEGFR-1, and -2) *(46)*, tie-1*(47)*, and tie-2*(48–50)*, proteases *(20)*, and induction of pro-coagulant properties (e.g., overexpression of tissue factor) *(51)*. Indeed, application of genomic technologies, such as sequential analysis of gene expression (SAGE), has revealed that endothelial cells associated with human colorectal carcinoma display a distinct gene expression profile (including the so called tumor endothelial markers [TEMs], which can be qualitatively distinguished from endothelium lining blood vessels of normal or even inflammatory gut mucosa, as well as that from cultured endothelial cells *(16)*.

2.3. Effector Molecules of Angiogenesis

Formation of vascular structures is orchestrated by a complex series of cellular interactions, the molecular intricacies of which continue to be unveiled *(31)*. Nevertheless, VEGF and its receptors (VEGFR-1/flt-1, VEGFR2/flk-1/KDR, VEGFR3/flt-4, and neuropilin-1/NP1) are believed to be cornerstones of this regulatory network *(31,52)*. Six members of the VEGF family have been identified thus far (designated VEGF-A,-B, -C,-D,-E, and placenta growth factor, PlGF) along with functionally similar but unrelated endocrine gland VEGF (EG-VEGF), of which the main ligand (VEGF-A) is expressed in at least five different protein isoforms: $VEGF_{121}$, $VEGD_{145}$, $VEGF_{165}$, $VEGF_{189}$, and $VEGF_{209}$, due to alternative splicing of the single VEGF mRNA *(52,53)*. Gene knockout studies have demonstrated an absolute requirement for diploid expression of VEGF-A *(54–56)* and for the intact isoform profile *(57)*, during embryonal and postnatal vascular development, respectively. Multiplicity of pro-angiogenic effects elicited by VEGF-A includes: endothelial mitogenesis, motility and invasiveness, endothelial cell survival and longevity, vascular permeability, vascular fusion, induction of endothelial cell-associated procoagulant activity, up-regulation of endothelial proteases and adhesion molecules, and many other, but less clearly defined, changes *(36,53,58)*. For the most part, these various biological activities have been traced to activation of the major signaling VEGF receptor known as VEGFR-2/KDR/flk-1, but there is also an increasing interest in several modulating effects of other VEGFRs, such as VEGFR-1/flt-1 and neuropilins (e.g., NP-1). For example, VEGFR-1 may act as a decoy or molecular sink for VEGF *(59)*, or, in its soluble form, as a natural VEGF antagonist *(52)*. This receptor also serves as the high affinity binding site for PlGF *(60)*, a recently recognized important coregulator of VEGF-induced vascular permeability *(61)*. It is noteworthy that engagement of VEGFRs and resulting formation of signaling complexes is conditional upon simultaneous ligation of endothelial cell adhesion molecules such as VE-cadherin and αv integrins *(62,63)*.

Endothelial cell-specific signaling queues are also received through tie-1 and tie-2 receptor tyrosine kinases (RTKs) *(33)*. While the former remains an orphan receptor, the latter interacts with several different ligands of the angiopoietin family (Ang-1 to Ang-4) *(33)*. Ang-1, the natural tie-2/tek agonist is thought to be responsible for interaction between endothelial cells and pericytes, vascular maturation, vascular remodeling, and endothelial cells survival, particularly in the absence of VEGF *(33,64–66)*. Up-regulation of Ang-2 by endothelial or perivascular cells antagonizes the action of Ang-1 and leads to vessel destabilization, a necessary precondition for VEGF-induced angiogenesis. In the absence of VEGF, Ang-2 triggers regression of unstable vessels *(33,66)*. In addition, arterial or venous identity is imposed upon developing endothelial cells by expression of the membrane-bound ligand, Ephrin B2, or its receptor, EPH-B4, respectively *(33,67)*. Moreover, angiogenic growth factors may also regulate endothelial cell function in an organ-specific manner. This is exemplified by endocrine gland vascular endothelial growth factor (EG-VEGF), a polypeptide growth factor, which,

Table 1
Direct Impact of Oncogenes on the Angiogenic Phenotype of Cancer Cells[a]

Oncogene	Angiogenic activities affected	References
K-ras, H-ras	VEGF up-regulation, TSP-1 down-regulation.	89,90,92,161
v-src	VEGF up-regulation, TSP-1 down-regulation.	89,170,191,284
c-myb	TSP-2 down-regulation.	285
N-myc	Down-regulation of angiogenesis inhibitors (activin A).	286–290
c-myc	Complex angiogenic properties in epidermis.	291
HER-2	VEGF up-regulation.	104,239,292
EGFR	VEGF, bFGF, IL-8 up-regulation.	104,272,274,275
bcl-2	Hypoxic induction of VEGF.	293
PyMT	TSP-1 down-regulation.	294
c-fos	VEGF expression.	295
trkB	Down-regulation of angiogenic factors.	296,297
HPV-16	Secretion of VEGF and IFN-a.	298,299
MDM-2	VEGF up-regulation.	300
v-P3k	VEGF production and angiogenesis.	165
ODC	Novel angiogenic factor.	301
PTTG1	VEGF and bFGF up-regulation.	302
E2a-Pbx1	Induction of mouse angiogenin-3 and VEGF.	153,303
v-Abl	VEGF up-regulation.	153
v-sis	VEGF up-regulation.	153
PML-RARa	VEGF up-regulation.	209
RhoC	VEGF and cytokine upregulation.	140
HHV8	VEGF up-regulation.	304,305
eIF-4E	VEGF up-regulation (translation).	127
NOX-1	VEGF up-regulation.	316

[a] Nomenclature: *EGFR*, epidermal growth factor receptor; *HER-2/ErbB-2/neu*, homologue of EGFR; *HPV-16*, human papilloma virus; *PyMT*, polyoma middle T antigen; *ODC*, ornithine decarboxylase; *v-p3K*, oncogenic PI3K p110; *PTTG1*, pituitary tumor transforming gene 1; *E2a-Pbx1*, chimeric leukemia oncogene.

through activation of an unknown receptor interacts with endothelial cells in steroidogenic organs *(317)*. All the aforementioned endothelial-specific ligand–receptor systems constitute the core of known molecular regulatory networks, which integrate various endothelial cell activities involved in blood vessel formation, maturation, maintenance, and remodeling *(33)*. However, endothelial cells are also able to respond to other cues, including a wide range of growth factors, cytokines, ECM components, polypeptides, lipids, and other mediators. Collectively, all these influences can be broadly classified as either angiogenesis stimulators or inhibitors, depending on the global outcome of their respective interactions with the vasculature under specific biological circumstances *(68)*.

In normal mature tissues angiogenesis inhibitors are in excess, while stimulators are either not expressed or otherwise biologically unavailable *(69)*. In tumors, the onset of angiogenesis (angiogenic switch) is believed to be triggered by a reversal of this negative balance *(69,70)*. For example, tumor cells themselves are known to overexpress and/or liberate multiple pro-angiogenic growth factors and cytokines including: VEGF, basic fibroblast growth factor (bFGF), hepatocyte growth factor (HGF), or inter leukin

(IL)-8, as well as down-regulate angiogenesis inhibitors such as interferons (IFNs), or thrombospondins (TSPs) *(70)*. Alternatively, the effects of the latter, could also be bypassed in tumors by recently uncovered elaborate escape mechanisms *(71)*.

It will be discussed later in this article, how various endogenous pro-angiogenic tumor cell properties may be induced by expression of transforming oncoproteins (Table 1). In addition, angiogenic activities could also be produced by inflammatory cells and tumor stroma present within and around the tumor mass *(72,73)*. It is noteworthy, that besides this local control, tumor angiogenesis is also regulated at the systemic level by either tumor-derived circulating angiogenesis inhibitors (e.g., angiostatin) *(68)* or by preexisting state of constitutive angiogenic susceptibility linked to the genetic background of the host *(74–76)*. All these various levels of regulation contribute to the onset, pathway, and magnitude of the angiogenic response elicited in a given tumor.

3. ONCONGENES AS INDUCERS OF TUMOR ANGIOGENESIS

The source of virtually all clinical manifestations of cancer can ultimately be traced to one or more of genetic hits sustained by tumor cells during the course of the disease progression *(5)*. Such transforming genetic lesions result in either a gain of function or a loss of function events resulting in activation of dominant oncogenes or inactivation of tumor suppressor genes, respectively *(1,5)*. An overt malignant phenotype usually includes both types of changes accumulated sequentially over many years and often preceding the clinical manifestation of the disease *(5)*.

There are over 100 known genes that, under certain conditions, can act as transforming oncogenes *(1)*. In this regard, relatively well described Ras oncoproteins can serve as a paradigm for the functional linkage between molecular mechanisms of malignant transformation, 3-dimensional tumor growth, and tumor angiogenesis. Thus, three existing *ras* genes (*H-ras, N-ras,* or *K-ras*) encoding four protein isoforms (H-, N-, K-rasA, and K-rasB, respectively) are known to be frequently activated in human cancer *(77)*. In colorectal adenoma, activating *K-ras* mutations are found at relatively early stages of tumor progression *(5)*, around the time when onset of angiogenesis would be expected to take place *(69)* (i.e., prior to expansion of early adenoma to intermediate adenoma). Interestingly, the incidence of such mutations is 3- to 4-fold greater in the type of colonic (polypoid) adenomas, which *a priori* assume 3-dimensional growth pattern as compared to the so called "flat" or "superficial" adenoma lesions, which are characterized by horizontal tumor expansion within the colonic mucosa *(78,79)*. Again, polypoid growth of colorectal adenomas would likely require extensive and rapid rearrangements and expansion of the local vasculature, whereas superficial tumors could rely on more modest vascular response and preexisting mucosal microcirculation. The correlation of 3-dimensional tumor growth, angiogenesis, and high frequency of *K-ras* mutations is, therefore, thought provoking.

Indeed, in many instances, the continued expression of Ras oncoproteins has been formally shown to be indispensable for sustained 3-dimensional growth of ras-dependent tumors *in vivo (80–82)*. Furthermore, even in the absence of an overt *ras* mutation, the biochemical activity of wild-type, normal Ras proteins is often chronically elevated in cancer, and thus it can contribute to induction and maintenance of exponential tumor expansion *(83)*. Such permanent increases in Ras activity are thought to result from up-regulation, constitutive activation, or mutation of upstream acting oncogenic proteins

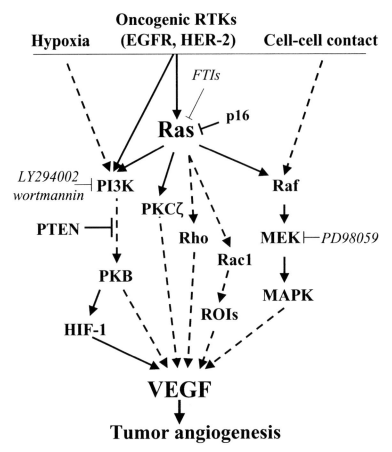

Fig. 1. Genetic and epigenetic control of VEGF expression in cancer cells. Several signal transduction pathways are involved in expression of VEGF and regulation of the angiogenic phenotype of cancer cells. In many instances the impact of activated oncogenes can be modulated by the expression status of certain tumor suppressor genes (e.g., p16 or PTEN) and by epigenetic influences such as hypoxia and cell–cell contact. These various stimuli activate intracellular signaling pathways, often in a synergistic manner. Synergy between epigenetic and oncogene-dependent induction of tumor angiogenesis is an attractive target for oncogene-targeting signal transduction inhibitors (*see* text for details).

such as members of the epidermal growth factor receptor (EGFR) or platelet-derived growth factor receptor (PDGFR) families *(83,84)*. In all these various scenarios, Ras-activation leads to triggering several crucial intracellular signaling cascades *(77)* and alterations in expression of a large numbers of *ras*-responsive genes *(85–87)*, many of which could be relevant for tumor angiogenesis *(see Fig. 1 and Table 2)*.

3.1. Up-Regulation of VEGF by Mutant ras: A Paradigm for a Direct Linkage Between Oncogenes and Tumor Angiogenesis

Constitutive expression of mutant *H-ras* oncogene in immortalized but nontumorigenic IEC-18 rat intestinal epithelial cell line leads, in one apparent step, to the overt tumorigenic conversion of these quasi normal cells *(88,89)*. Because tumors induced by injection of mutant *ras*-expressing IEC-18 cell variants exponentially reach large

Table 2
Ras-Responsive Angiogenesis Regulators

Factor[a]	Angiogeic activity	Impact of ras	Reference
VEGF	stimulator	up-regulation	89,92
bFGF	stimulator	up-regulation	306
aFGF	stimulator	up-regulation	307
TGF-α	stimulator	up-regulation	308
TGF-β	stimulator	up-regulation	309
TNF-α	stimulator (at low concentration)	up-regulation	310
G-CSF	stimulator	up-regulation	311
IGF-1	stimulator	up-regulation	312
PDGF	stimulator	up-regulation	313
OPN	stimulator	up-regulation	314
TSP-1	inhibitor	down-regulation	161
TIMP	inhibitor	down-regulation	85
PAI-1,2	modulator	down-regulation	315
PGE	stimulator	up-regulation	308

[a] Abbreviations: VEGF, vascular endothelial growth factor; bFGF, basic fibroblast growth factor; TGF-α, transforming growth factor alpha; TGF-β, transforming growth factor beta; TNF-α, tumor necrosis factor alpha; G-CSF, granulocyte colony-stimulating factor; IGF-1, insulin like growth factor 1; PDGF, platelet-derived growth factor; OPN, osteopontin; TSP-1, thrombospondin 1; PAI-1 and PAI-2, plasminogen activator inhibitors 1 and 2; TIMP, tissue inhibitor of metalloproteinases; PGE, prostaglandin E.

sizes (≥ 10mm) not achievable in the absence of new blood vessel ingrowth, we surmised that *ras* expression itself must somehow trigger the angiogenic switch in these *a priori* non-angiogenic epithelial cells *(89)*. Indeed, in contrast to parental IEC-18 cells, conditioned medium from their *ras*-transformed malignant counterparts was found to contain an activity capable of supporting growth and survival of growth factor-deprived human umbilical vein endothelial cells (HUVEC) *(89)*. Upon closer analysis, this effect was attributed to copious amounts of VEGF present in this material *(89,90)*. Moreover, expression of mutant *H-ras* in IEC-18 cells under control of various constitutive (simian virus 40SV40), or conditional (heavy metal, inducible; tetracyclin, repressible) promoters was strictly paralleled by massive up-regulation of VEGF mRNA and by the onset of the VEGF reporter activity (unpublished observations), which not only confirmed but also suggested a transcriptional nature of these stimulatory influences *(Fig.2) (89–91)*. Conversely, blockade of *H-ras*-dependent transformation in the case of two independent IEC-18-derived clones (RAS-3 and RAS-4) by treatment with a farnesyl transferase inhibitor (L-739, 749) efficiently abrogated their elevated VEGF expression *(89)*. Similar conclusions were reported by Grugel et al., who documented VEGF up-regulation in *H-ras*-and *v-Raf*-transformed NIN3T3 fibroblasts *(92)* and these observations were later confirmed by a large number of independent studies reviewed elsewhere *(93)*.

Initial analyses of VEGF production by rodent cells expressing oncogenic *H-ras,* while intriguing, differ from human pathology in two important aspects. First, *H-ras*-transfected cell lines usually express multiple copies of the oncogene, which is in sharp contrast to a single point mutation that is believed to play a transforming role in human cancers. Second, the oncogenic *H-ras* isoform used in many experimental studies is far less prevalent in major human cancers (i.e., that of colon, pancreas, and lung) than its mutant *K-ras* counterpart *(94)*. To address these concerns, we employed two human colorectal cancer cell lines (HCT-116, DLD-1), each harboring a single mutant *K-ras* allele and their respective variants (Dks-8, Hkh-2), in which the mutant (but not the wild-type) *K-ras* gene had been disrupted by homologous recombination by Shirasawa, Sasazuki and colleagues *(80)*. The results of these *ras*-knock-out experiments matched what was previously observed with IEC-18 cells (i.e., *ras*-knock-in approach). Thus, parental cells (DLD-1 and HCT116) were found to express high levels of VEGF protein and mRNA, while in their mutant *K-ras*-knock-out derivatives (Dks-8, Hkh-2, respectively) production of this angiogenic factor was reduced by at least 4- to 5-fold *(89)*, a property that coincided with near complete loss of the tumor forming capacity of the latter cell lines *(80,89)*. We have also observed a dramatic increase in VEGF expression in rat kidney epithelial (RK-3E) cells transformed with the mutant *K-ras* oncogene (Rak, Fearon, Kerbel, unpublished observation). Taken together, these results demonstrate that both *H-* and *K-ras* isoforms are capable of up-regulating VEGF, even if only a single copy of the oncogene is expressed. Furthermore, since VEGF production consistently co-segregated with the onset of the tumor forming capacity in various *ras*-transformed cell lines, it was postulated that VEGF-dependent angiogenesis may play an essential role in supporting the aggressive growth of such cells as tumors in vivo *(89)*.

3.2. VEGF as a Mediator of Oncogene-Dependent Tumor Angiogenesis

Endogenous production of VEGF by cancer cells is, at least in some instances, absolutely required for tumor growth and angiogenesis. This notion is supported by several lines of experimental and histopathological evidence including: *(i)* frequent up-regulation of VEGF in human cancers *(95)* and under the influence of many different transforming oncogenes (Table 1); *(ii)* suppression of tumorigenic properties of various cancer cells engineered to down-regulate their VEGF production by antisense *(96–102)* or gene knock-out *(54,103)* approaches; *(iii)* synchronous inhibition of both VEGF expression and tumor growth by certain oncogene-targeting agents *(6,104)*; and *(iv)* considerable preclinical anticancer efficacy of anti-VEGF antibodies *(53,105,106)*, soluble VEGF receptors *(53,107–109)*, and VEGF receptor inhibitors *(53,110–114)*.

In this context, it was reasonable to ask whether VEGF is also indispensable for tumorigenesis driven, specifically, by mutant *ras* oncogene. An affirmative answer to this question would strengthen the rationale for using VEGF/VEGFR inhibitors in treatment of cancers, in which *ras* oncogenes are likely to play a major transforming role (e.g., pancreatic carcinoma, colorectal cancer). In order to explore this possibility, two independent human colorectal carcinoma cell lines (DLD-1 and HCT-116), in which, as we have shown previously, *K-ras* oncogene drives overexpression of VEGF were transfected with expression vectors encoding $VEGF_{121}$ antisense cDNA *(115)*. In the resulting successful transfectants, VEGF production dropped to levels similar to those achieved by disruption of the mutant *K-ras* allele (i.e., 3- to 4-fold) *(89,115)*. Remarkably, even such incomplete VEGF down-regulation significantly diminished the tumor forming potential of all VEGF-suppressed clones analyzed *(115)*. These results, along with subsequent independent studies *(103,116,117)*, suggest that VEGF-overexpression is, at least in some cases, absolutely necessary for full expression of the tumor forming properties attributed to the influence of mutant *ras* (Table 3), but is clearly not

Table 3
The Role of Tumor Cell-Derived VEGF in Mutant ras-Dependent Tumor Formation

Approach	Observation	Reference
Experimental systems, in which VEGF up-regulation IS essential for ras-dependent tumor formation		
VEGF antisense transfection	Enforced down-regulation of VEGF expression abrogated K-ras-dependent tumorigenicity of human colorectal cancer cells.	*115*
VEGF gene knock-out	Transfection of VEGF –/– ES cells with mutant ras did not rescue the tumorigenic phenotype.	*116*
VEGF gene knock-out	v-H-ras transformed VEGF –/– mouse embryo fibroblasts are deficient in tumor forming ability.	*103,117*
Experimental systems in which VEGF up-regulation is NOT essential for ras-dependent tumor formation		
VEGF gene knock-out	H-ras-transformed VEGF–/– adult mouse fibroblasts (528ras1) form angiogenic tumors in SCID mice.	*198*
Inducible ras expression	Cessation of mutant H-ras expression leads to regression of spontaneous melanoma in transgenic mice regardless of residual VEGF expression.	*81*

sufficient *(81,115)*. This is evident from experiments involving enforced expression of $VEGF_{121}$ in *K-ras*-disrupted variants of both DLD-1 and HCT-116 cell lines *(115)*. These VEGF-proficient, but *K-ras*-negative cell lines, despite producing copious amounts of the angiogenic activity, fail to recapitulate the aggressive in vivo growth of their parental (*K-ras*-positive) counterparts *(115)*. This is not surprising as angiogenic competence is one of many cellular characteristics that must cooperate for tumor take *(118,119)* or tumor maintenance *(81)* to be fully realized.

3.3. Signaling Pathways Involved in ras-Dependent VEGF Up-Regulation

The notion that overexpression of VEGF may significantly contribute to *ras*-dependent tumor formation naturally leads to the idea that signal transduction inhibitors, able to block this effect, may act as indirect anti-angiogenic agents *(27,89)*. In support of this view, pharmacological inhibitors targeting protein farnesyl transferase (Ftase), or geranylgeranyl transferase I (GGTase-I), enzymes involved in essential posttranslational processing steps of Ras proteins have been shown not only to abrogate many features of cellular transformation *(120)*, but also to markedly suppress VEGF production in certain cancer cells (compare Table 4). Moreover, given the central role of Ras in cellular regulatory pathways, some of the elements involved in the Ras-to-VEGF signaling could, at least in theory, be utilized by a wide variety of oncogenic, hypoxic, paracrine, or inflammatory stimuli. Therfore, understanding how activated/mutant Ras triggers VEGF production could potentially have attractive as well as broad biological and therapeutic implications.

Table 4
Anti-Angiogenic Effects of Oncogene-Targeting Agents

Inhibitor	Target	Anti-angiogenic effect	Reference
FTIs (L-739, 749;L-744-832; A-170634; RPR 115 135; AFC)	Ras, Rho	VEGF down-regulation, direct inhibition of endothelial cells	*89,143–145, 153*
Herceptin (trastuzumab)	HER-2	VEGF down-regulation changes in Aug1 and TSP-1	*104*
IMC-C225 (cetuximab)	EGFR	VEGF, FGF, IL-8 down-regulation	*104,273,274*
Iressa (ZD1839)	EGFR	VEGF, bFGF and TGFa down-regulation	*277*
Tarceva (OSI-774)	EGFR	?*	*NT***
PKI-166	EGFR	VEGF and IL-8 down-regulation, apoptosis of endothelial cells	*278*
Gleevec (STI571)	Bcr-abl	?	*NT*
ATRA	PML-RARa	VEGF down-regulation	*209*

*? = unknown; **NT = not tested.

The principal difficulty in establishing the exact mode of VEGF up-regulation by mutant *ras* lies with the molecular complexity on both sides of this interaction. Thus, regulation of VEGF expression and activity can be influenced at multiple levels *(53)*, including regulation of the gene transcription *(121,122)*, mRNA stability *(122–125)*, mRNA splicing *(126)*, as well as the rate of translation *(127,128)* or posttranslational protein modifications *(129)*. Each of these regulatory levels could, in principle, be affected by the oncogenic *ras* (Fig. 2).

A large number of intracellular signaling modules can be triggered by activated GTP-bound Ras, all of which could be considered as plausible VEGF regulators *(77)* (Fig. 1). Furthermore, some of the phenotypic changes attributed to *ras* transformation are induced indirectly, namely through activation of autocrine growth factor feedback loops driven, for example, by members of the transforming growth factor-α (TGF-α) family, principal ligands of the EGFR protooncogene *(130,131)*. Finally, *ras*-induced cellular transformation, can be modulated by a variety of accompanying genetic and epigenetic influences *(6)*, a circumstance that may affect apparent magnitude of VEGF production in different experimental (as well as clinical) settings.

In the case of IEC-18 cells, up-regulation of VEGF by mutant *ras* appears to be controlled by a direct intracellular signal transduction mechanism rather than being secondary to *ras*-induced autocrine growth factor circuitry *(90)*. The evidence for this is twofold. First, addition of the conditioned medium of *ras*-transformed IEC-18 cells (RAS-3) did not induce VEGF mRNA expression in their nontransformed parental counterparts *(90)*. Second, *ras*-dependent increase in VEGF expression remained undiminished in the presence of the tyrosine kinase inhibitor, genistein, or neutralizing antibodies directed against TGF-α or EGFR *(90)*.

Several direct effectors of Ras were implicated in up-regulation of VEGF. In NIH3T3 and CCL39 fibroblasts, the expression of constitutively activated forms of Raf *(90)* or MEK-1 *(90,132)* was sufficient to up-regulate VEGF to a level comparable to that of cells harboring mutant *v-H-ras* oncogene itself *(90,92,132–134)*. In addition,

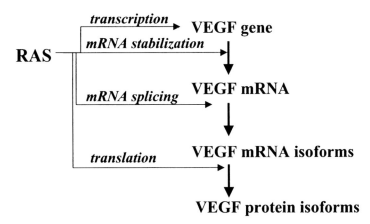

Fig. 2. Multiple levels of VEGF regulation that can be affected by expression of the activated/mutant ras oncogene. Complex regulatory mechanisms that control VEGF expression and activity under various physiological conditions could be altered in cancer cells as a result oncogene expression (see text).

treatment of *ras*-transformed fibroblasts with the MEK-1 inhibitor (PD98059) normalized (lowered) their VEGF expression *(90,132)*. This inhibitor was also effective in lowering high levels of VEGF expressed by the rat liver epithelial cell line (RLE) expressing mutant *v-H-ras* oncogene *(35)*. These observations could be interpreted as an indication that Raf/MEK/MAPK pathway is the main and universal mediator of VEGF up-regulation under the influence of mutant *H-ras (134)*. However, such a generalization is inconsistent with the fact that in *H-ras*-transformed epithelial, i.e., IEC-18 cells (RAS-3), treatment with PD98059 exhibited only a marginal decrease in VEGF production. Moreover, expression of the constitutively activated MEK-1 mutant in parental IEC-18 cells was insufficient to substitute for oncogenic *ras* in terms of both VEGF overexpression and cellular transformation in general *(90)*. The reasons why these cells are resistant to transforming effects of the activated MEK-1 are unclear, but a negative feedback mechanism mediated through MAP kinase phosphatases (e.g., MKP-1 and 2) or other similarly acting circuitry cannot be ruled out *(136)*. Nevertheless, unlike in fibroblasts, Ras-induced increase in VEGF mRNA and protein expression could be profoundly suppressed by exposure of the transformed intestinal epithelial cells (IEC-18/RAS3) to the phosphatidyl inositol 3′-OH kinase (PI3K) inhibitor (LY294002) *(90)*. Combination of both MEK-1 and PI3K inhibitors was of even greater potency bringing VEGF production to nearly normal (i.e., barely detectable) levels *(90)*. The latter observation suggests that, while PI3K activity appears to be crucial for VEGF up-regulation in RAS-3 epithelial cells, MEK/MAPK pathway can potentiate this effect *(90)*.

   A distinct pathway, that only recently has been implicated in mutant *ras*-dependent VEGF up-regulation involves activation of protein kinase C czeta (PKCZ) (137). PKCZ is one of the professional *ras* effectors and, as such, can substitute for, and enhance the impact of mutant *ras* on VEGF expression. This is, at least in part, executed by the ability of PKCZ to phosphorylate and activate the SP-1 transcription factor *(137)* known to regulate both baseline and growth factor stimulated activity of the VEGF promoter *(137,138)*.

   In addition to classical Ras-activated pathways such as MEK/MAPK or PI3K/Akt, up-regulation of VEGF could, at least in part, be influenced by other, less studied mediators of *ras* transformation such as Rho/rac/cdc42 cascade, or reactive oxygen interme-diates (ROIs) *(77)* (Fig. 1). In this regard, preliminary evidence suggests that activated Rho GTPases can, in some cases, substitute for Ras activation in causing up-regulation of VEGF *(139)*. In particular, one member of this family, RhoC, has recently been found to be overexpressed at very high frequency (90%) in inflammatory breast cancer (IBC), a disease in which profuse production of VEGF occurs with no apparent muta-tion of *ras* proto-oncogenes *(140)*. The causative role RhoC in triggering angiogenic properties of IBC cells is strongly suggested by the fact that enforced expression of this small GTPase in human mammary epithelial cells (HME) stimulates production of VEGF along with bFGF, IL-8, and IL-6 *(140)*. Another member of the Rho family, RhoB, has recently elicited a great deal of interest, owing to the notion that this puta-tive mediator of Ras-induced cellular transformation may (instead of activated Ras itself) represent the primary target for farnesyltransferase inhibitors (FTIs) *(141,142)*. It cannot be ruled out at this time, that also the FTI-mediated reversal of VEGF up-reg-ulation in cells harboring activated Ras *(89,143–145)* is due to inhibition of RhoB *(142)*. It is interesting that the Rho/rac/cdc42 cascade, in addition to mediating some of the intracellular signals emanating from the activated Ras, is strongly linked to the con-trol of the physical interface between cancer cells and their exterior *(146)*. For exam-ple, the activity of Rho-like proteins is linked to cytoskeletal organization, membrane ruffling, and cellular motility *(146)*. The type of physical forces involved in these inter-action (sheer stress, contact, stretching, pressure, solid stress) are known to be associ-ated with signaling events and changes in gene expression *(147,148)*. It is possible that VEGF overexpression in cancer cells may also be a function of the interplay between these mechanical signals, activation of Ras, and action of Rho-like GTPases.

Rac1 is another small GTPase, which is viewed as a mediator of Ras-dependent cel-lular transformation *(146,149)*. In addition to its possible role in cell–cell interactions and cell motility *(146,150)*, Rac1 is also a component of the multimolecular enzymatic complex (NADPH oxydase) implicated in generating reactive oxygen intermediates (ROIs) in neutrophils *(151)*. Expression of mutant *ras* in fibroblasts also triggers ROI generation, an event that results in changes in gene transcription and triggers cellular mitogenesis, possibly through the action of Racl *(151)*. This is of interest, because ROIs can up-regulate VEGF mRNA expression, whereas antioxidants and ROI scav-engers, such as N-acetyl-cysteine (NAC), down-regulate it, at least in retinal pigment epithelial cells *(152)*. These circumstances may point to ROIs and the Rac/NADPH pathway as *ras*-responsive elements regulating VEGF gene expression in cancer cells. Although, this possibility cannot be definitively ruled in or ruled out, elevated VEGF mRNA expression in IEC-18 cells harboring mutant *ras* oncogene (e.g., RAS-3) remains unchanged in the presence of NAC *(90)*. However, endogenous ROIs may par-ticipate in other, still poorly defined, posttranscriptional event(s) required for efficient syntesis/secretion of the VEGF polypeptide. This can be inferred from the observation that NAC treatment can reduce the levels of immunodetectable VEGF protein (but not mRNA) produced by various types of VEGF overexpressing cells, including those transformed with oncogenic *ras* or *v-src (90)*.

At least in some experimental settings, posttranscriptional VEGF regulation may become a major target for transforming oncogenes (Fig. 1). This is exemplified by increased VEGF protein production in cultures of transformed fibroblasts overexpress-ing the translation factor eIF-4e *(127)*. Increase in VEGF mRNA stability is also enhanced in the presence of several oncogenes including *H-ras, v-src, v-abl, neu,* or *v-sis (153),* albeit not in all model systems *(90).* Expression of the *H-ras* oncogenic transgene in FVB/N mice has also been linked to changes in VEGF mRNA splicing *(126)* (Fig. 2).

Much remains to be learned about how activated Ras controls VEGF production, particularly so, because the emerging picture does not appear to be simple, linear or universally applicable (see Figs. 1 and 2). Instead, cell type-specific and -complex pathways/networks seem to be involved in Ras-induced VEGF production in various experimental settings *(90,132,153,154).* Therefore, development of signal transduction inhibitors to block the intermediate steps involved in expression of the oncogene-dependent angiogenic phenotype may need to be tailored to specific biochemical properties of the given type of cancer cells and genetic alterations they carry.

3.4. Interplay Between Genetic and Epigenetic Factors in VEGF Up-Regulation by Cancer Cells

VEGF production by cancer cells may change dramatically in response to various external conditions. Also in this regard, *ras*-mediated cellular transformation can provide an informative example as to how genetic and epigenetic factors co-operate during tumor angiogenesis. While multiple epigenetic influences may have their bearing on angiogenic profiles of various types of cancers, we will illustrate this point by discussing mainly the effects of hypoxia and cell–cell contact.

3.4.1. Oncogenes, Tumor Angiogenesis, and Hypoxia

Hypoxia represents a primordial stimulus leading to VEGF up-regulation and angiogenesis in various physiological conditions, but also in pathology, including cancer *(155).* It is, therefore, of considerable interest to understand the relationship between hypoxic and oncogene-dependent aspects of tumor angiogenesis regulation. Significant progress has been recently made in this area *(156).* For example, studies conducted with NIH3T3 fibroblasts demonstrated that stimulation of the VEGF promoter activity and gene transcription by hypoxia is dramatically amplified in the presence of the oncogenic *H-ras (157).* In other words, cells expressing the mutant oncogene became hypersensitive to hypoxic conditions, at least, insofar as their level of VEGF transcription was concerned *(157,158).* A similar effect was also observed in NIH3T3 cells engineered to overexpress certain oncogenic tyrosine kinases, such as mutant *neu/HER-2 (104).*

Several distinct signaling events have been implicated in the cross-talk between oncogenes and hypoxia (Fig. 2). In this regard, studies of Mazure et al. indicated that in NIH3T3 fibroblasts, the synergistic activation of the VEGF gene transcription by combined action of mutant *ras* and oxygen withdrawal is executed in a PI3K-dependent and MEK/MAPK-independent manner *(158).* In this case, the burst of VEGF expression was mediated, primarily, by activation of the hypoxia inducible factor-1 (HIF-1), a dimeric transcription factor that binds to and activates the hypoxia responsive element (HRE) present in the VEGF gene promoter *(156).* HIF-1 is a target of PI3K, which is, in turn, activated by mutant *H-ras (158).* The convergence of hypoxia- and *ras*-activated pathways on PI3K is consistent with the earlier observation that the PI3K inhibitor, wortmannin, can suppress VEGF production stimulated in murine endothelioma cell line by the combined effects of *ras*-transformation and low oxygen conditions *(154)*. Further evidence of this interrelationship has also recently come to light. For example, in human glioblastoma cells, otherwise known for their high constitutive levels of Ras activity *(83)*, the expression of lipid phosphatase and tension homologue on chromosome 10 (PTEN) was found to effectively block the burst of VEGF synthesis under hypoxic conditions *(159)*. It is noteworthy, that PTEN may also block tumor angiogenesis through increased expression of thrombospondin-1 *(160)*, a potent endogenous angiogenesis inhibitor and a subject of mutant *ras* induced *(90,161)*, as well as hypoxia-induced *(162)*, down-regulation. PTEN acts as a negative regulator of PI3K activity and as a potent tumor suppressor *(163,164)*, a property that could likely entail blocking the aforementioned pro-angiogenic synergy between activated Ras and hypoxia. Conversely, the enforced expression of various constitutively active and oncogenic forms of p110a, the catalytic PI3K subunit (e.g., Myr-P3k or v-p3k) led in chick embryo fibroblasts and endothelial cells, to marked constitutive VEGF up-regulation, as did constitutively active forms of Akt/PKB (Myr-Akt), a downstream target/effector of PI3K *(165)*. Moreover, activation of the pathway involving PI3K, Akt, and their further downstream kinase known as FKBP-rapamycin associated protein (FRAP) was recently found to have an essential role in mRNA translation and efficient expression of HIF-1α (the oxygen/growth signal regulated HIF-1 subunit) *(156,166)*. This (posttranscriptional) regulation of HIF-lα could be an important, rate limiting step in HIF-1 mediated transcription of hypoxia-responsive genes, including VEGF *(166)*. Interestingly, this mode of HIF-lα up-regulation is involved in stimulation of VEGF production by both, heregulin and oncogenic HER-2/neu receptor kinase, even in normoxia *(166)*. Hypoxic conditions could further cooperate with these known VEGF inducers by inhibition of the ubiquitin-mediated HIF-1 degradation *(156,166)*.

The MAPK pathway has recently been implicated in certain stages of hypoxic VEGF regulation *(134,167,168)*. Despite the apparent dissociation of the MEK/MAPK module from the synergistic interaction between mutant *ras* and hypoxia in NIH3T3 fibroblasts *(158)*, MAP kinases, namely Erk1/2, may in some experimental settings (e.g., in CCL39 hamster lung fibroblasts) directly phosphorylate HIF-lα, and thereby potentiate HIF-1/HRE-dependent VEGF transcription *(168)*. MAPK inhibition was shown to interfere with hypoxia/Ras-induced VEGF up-regulation in human astrocytoma cell lines *(167)*. The generality and the relative significance of these respective modes of VEGF regulation *in vivo* remain to be established.

While in some experimental systems transforming oncogenes induce a state of apparent hypoxia hypersensitivity, in others their effects could be described as hypoxia mimicry. The latter scenario is often manifested by a constitutive up-regulation of hypoxia-resposive genes (e.g., VEGF, Glut-1) in cancer cells harboring certain activated oncogenes, even under normoxic conditions *(169,170)*. For example, cellular transformation with oncogenic *v-src*, can stimulate HIF-1 activity and thereby up-regulate VEGF expression, regardless of the actual oxygen levels *(170)*. Interestingly, several cellular proto-oncogenes such as c-src, Ras, and Raf were implicated as mediators of various aspects of normal cellular response to hypoxia, including activation of transcription factors (e.g., HIF-1, NFκB) known to directly regulate expression of VEGF *(156,170–172)*. Our recent observations suggest that in certain human colorectal cancer cell lines, mutant *K-ras* expression may mimic, rather than synergize with, hypoxia *(115)*. For example, treatment of HCT116 cells with cobalt chloride (a hypoxia mimetic and inducer of HIF-1-dependent transcription) *(173)* was associated with minimal and variable up-regulation of already high VEGF levels, a result that would be expected if hypoxia response was *a priori* constitutively activated *(6,115,174)*. Indeed, abnormal HIF-1 levels and aberrant hypoxia responses are common in cancer *(156)*. Taken together, these various observations exemplify how the angiogenic phenotype of cancer cells might be turned on as a result of the distortion of hypoxia response mechanisms by the transforming action of activated oncogenes (e.g., *ras, src*) and/or loss of tumor suppressor genes *(VHL, p53, PTEN) (156,157,162,175–177)*.

3.4.2. Oncogenes and Cell–Cell Contact as Co-Regulators of the Angiogenic Phenotype of Cancer Cells

The impact of the oncogenic transformation on expression of VEGF can be significantly modulated by cell–cell contact. In various types of cancer cells cultured under confluent conditions, VEGF was found to be dramatically up-regulated as compared to cultures where the close cell–cell contact was prevented *(90,178–180)*. Malignant transformation appears to be a prerequisite for such communal VEGF stimulation, as parental nontransformed IEC-18 cells do not up-regulate VEGF even in very dense monolayer cultures, whereas such up-regulation occurs readily in confluent cultures of their *ras*-transformed (RAS-3) counterparts *(90)*. Interestingly, RAS-3 cells grown at high density become relatively less responsive to VEGF suppression by the PI3K inhibitor LY294002 *(90)*. This observation suggests that cell–cell contact may cause not only changes in the magnitude of VEGF expression, but may also re-route some of the *ras*-dependent VEGF-stimulating signals *(90)*.

It is not clear what is the molecular sensor that elicits VEGF up-regulating signals under conditions of high cell density. In this regard, homotypic adhesion molecules such as members of the cadherin family and their associated β-catenin/GSK-3/LEF signaling modules could be viewed as conceivable candidates *(181)*. Moderate up-regulation of the constitutive VEGF production was, indeed, detected in rat kidney epithelial (RK-3E) cells *(182)* engineered to express transforming mutants of β-catenin (Rak, Fearon and Kerbel, unpublished observation). However, in IEC-18 cells, the expression of E-cadherin is virtually undetectable upon transfection with mutant *H-Ras (183)*, and hence a different mechanism of VEGF up-regulation by cell–cell contact should be sought in this case. In relation to this, it noteworthy that transformed IEC-18 sublines engineered to overexpress the integrin linked kinase (ILK) secrete markedly elevated levels of VEGF protein (our unpublished observation). Further indication that membrane-associated adhesion complexes may play a pivotal role in regulation of VEGF production by cancer cells comes from the recent work by Sheta et al *(180)*. In this study transfection of the dominant negative mutant of focal adhesion kinase (FAK), as well as analogous mutants of key signaling partners of FAK (i.e., c-src, Rap-1, Raf, MEK, but not Ras) prevented density-dependent up-regulation of VEGF in prostatic cancer cells *(180)*.

It is not unreasonable to assume that, in addition to the effects of hypoxia and cell–cell contact, the oncogene-driven tumor angiogenesis could also be augmented by other epigenetic influences such as paracrine growth factors, inflammatory cytokines, hemostatic proteases, and hormones. A corollary to this point is that, even if tumor neovascularization appears to be triggered by the presence of an evident microenvironmental pro-angiogenic stimulus (e.g., severe hypoxia or inflammation), targeting oncogenes could still exert a significant anti-angiogenic effect by eliminating an important element of the underlying genetic-epigenetic synergy *(6)*.

4. REGULATION OF THE ANGIOGENIC PHENOTYPE BY INTERACTIONS BETWEEN ONCOGENES AND TUMOR SUPPRESSOR GENES

Cell transformation by a given activated oncogene is usually conditional upon pre-existing genetic alterations *(184)*. For example, while mutant *ras* can readily transform immortalized fibroblastic cell lines, expression of this oncogene in primary cultures leads to growth arrest and cellular senescence, mainly due to up-regulation of p16/INK4a cyclin-dependent kinase inhibitor and tumor suppressor *(185)*. Hence, loss of p16/INK4a expression is thought to be a prerequisite for oncogene-dependent transformation of various cell types including primary murine fibroblasts *(185)*, astrocytes *(186)*, and melanocytes *(81)*. Moreover, recent studies implicated losses of other tumor suppressors such as *PML* and *p53* as additional requirements for effective *ras*-dependent cellular transformation *(187)*. Likewise, it would be expected that the ability of the activated Ras (and other oncoproteins, as well) to drive the angiogenic phenotype of cancer cells will be realized only in a permissive (i.e., *p16/PML/p53* tumor suppressor-negative) genetic context.

In high grade astrocytoma, many features of malignant transformation, including dramatic up-regulation of VEGF, have been linked to constitutive activation of the Ras signaling pathway *(167,186)*, a property that is almost always concomitant with the loss of p16/INK4a *(186)*. Interestingly, at least two independent studies demonstrated that the abundant production of VEGF in several human glioma/astrocytoma cell lines could be abrogated when the expression p16/INK4a was genetically restored *(6,188)*. Similar suppression of VEGF was recently observed in cell lines engineered to re-express p130/Rb2 tumor suppressor gene *(189)*. Both p16/INK4a and p130/Rb2 were originally thought to suppress tumorigenesis solely by regulation of cell cycle checkpoints. It is, therefore, intriguing that the cell autonomous role of such *bona fide* cell cycle regulators appears to be tightly coupled with their ability to control the expression of angiogenesis-related genes, a property that, at least from a teleological standpoint, would be essential for full realization of the mitotic capacity of cancer cells *in vivo*.

Several tumor suppressor genes *(p53, APC, PTEN, DPC4/Smad4, or VHL)* are known to control the expression of molecular mediators of angiogenesis (both stimulators and inhibitors) *(70,177,190)*. Again, in many such cases tumor suppressors manifest their anti-angiogenic activities primarily in the context of activated oncogenes. In this regard Mukhopadhyay et al. have originally observed that *v-src*-dependent activation of the VEGF promoter can be suppressed by co-transfection of the cDNA encoding wild-type *p53* tumor suppressor gene *(191)*. Other mitigating effects of p53 on VEGF production have been described as well *(192)*. Volpert et al. have recently demonstrated a complementation between mutant *p53* and oncogenic *ras* in triggering tumor angiogenesis *(193)*. Thus, in fibroblasts derived from patients with the Li-Fraumeni syndrome (germline p53+/–), spontaneous loss of the remaining *p53* allele was accompanied by a dramatic decrease in expression of TSP-1, slight up-regulation of VEGF, and a mild pro-angiogenic phenotype *(193)*. Subsequent expression of mutant *ras* in those cells led to a dramatic increase in VEGF production and to an overt angiogenic switch *(193)*. Observations such as this, point to a parallel between the sequential genetic hits that cancer cells sustain during the natural history of the disease and progressively pro-angiogenic properties they express *in vivo*, a process we termed "angiogenesis progression" *(15)* (Fig. 3). Recent studies by Bergers et al. point to the

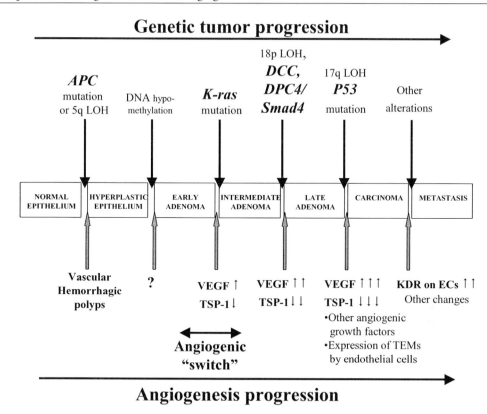

Fig. 3. Angiogenesis progression in tumors. Evolution of cancer as a disease and accompanying changes in expression of oncogenes and tumor suppressor genes are likely to leave their signatures on angiogenic pathways cancer cells utilize. Therefore, the nature and the treatment sensitivity of the vascular compartment in progressively growing tumors is likely to undergo a gradual change.

practical importance of this evolutionary process by demonstrating that successful inhibition of tumor angiogenesis may require therapeutic approaches specific for different stages of the disease progression *(194)*.

5. VEGF-DEPENDENT AND -INDEPENDENT ANGIOGENIC PHENOTYPES IN DIFFERENT TYPES OF TUMORS

Tumor growth is often, but not always, dependent on VEGF endogenously produced by cancer cells themselves. For instance, copious expression of VEGF is clearly required for experimental tumor formation by such cell types as: certain mutant *K-ras*-positive human colorectal carcinoma cells (DLD-1 and HCT116) *(115)*, wild-type embryonic stem (ES) cells *(195)*, their *H-ras* transfected derivatives *(116)*, and *H-ras*-transformed mouse embryo fibroblasts (MEFs) *(103,117)*. However, alternative (VEGF-independent) scenarios have also been described *(81,196,197)* (Table 3).

In order to better understand the nature of such diversity, we compared the impact of VEGF gene inactivation on tumor forming capacity in a series of clonally-related cell lines, which represent different states of cellular ontogenesis (ES cells vs mature fibroblasts) and different corresponding tumor histotypes (teratoma vs ras-induced fibrosarcoma). The R1 strain of totipotential ES cells was previously engineered to inactivate VEGF gene *(55)* and along with its VEGF–/– derivatives was used to generate a series of adult fibroblastic VEGF–/– cell lines, either nontransformed or transformed with mutant *ras* or *neu* oncogenes. In order to generate such cell lines, chimeric (VEGF–/– plus VEGF+/+) mice were created from wild-type (VEGF+/+) blastocysts by aggregating them with VEGF–/– R1 ES cells *(55)*. Skin explants were removed from these chimeric mice when they reached the age of maturity (approx 4 mo) in order to isolate VEGF-deficient dermal fibroblasts, which were then established in culture as spontaneously immortalized nontransformed polyclonal cell line (MDF528). These nontumorigenic MDF528 cells were subsequently transfected with an expression vector encoding mutant *v-H-ras* oncogene to yield 528ras fibrosarcoma-like cell line *(198)*.

Wild-type ES cells (R1-VEGF+/+), VEGF-defficient ES cells (R1-VEGF–/–,) VEGF-deficient nontransformed fibroblasts (MDF528) and their *ras*-transformed derivatives (528ras) were then injected subcutaneously into immune deficient (SCID) mice for assessment of their respective tumor forming and angiogenic competence. As expected, based on earlier studies *(195)*, parental VEGF-positive R1/ES cells formed highly vascular rapidly growing teratomas, while their VEGF-inactivated variants were devoid of such capacity. Because of this and other results obtained with various VEGF-negative murine embryonal cell lines *(103,116,117)*, VEGF-negative 528ras cells were also expected to be non/poorly-tumorigenic. Contrary to this prediction, and despite their inability to elaborate VEGF, 528ras cells (derived from adult mouse fibroblasts) formed aggressive angiogenic fibrosarcoma-like tumors in SCID mice *(198)*. Clearly in this case, the tumorigenic and pro-angiogenic effects of the *ras* oncogene were executed via alternative mechanisms independent on the endogenous production of VEGF by tumor cells themselves.

This observation reinforces the notion that mutant *ras* can trigger production of other than VEGF and possibly redundant angiogenic growth factors (Table 2). The presence and identity of such factors in the 528ras system remains to be established, but it is of interest that formation of subcutaneous 528ras fibrosarcomas in SCID mice was accompanied by considerable recruitment of fibroblastic host (VEGF+/+) stromal cells. It is possible, therefore, that in this particular case, *ras*-transformation bypassed the requirement for endogenous tumor cell VEGF expression by triggering production of growth factors/chemoattractants for intratumoral host cells. Arrival of such stromal and inflammatory cells could, in turn, deliver a threshold quantity of VEGF (and other angiogenesis stimulators as well) to the tumor site and promote angiogenesis in a host-VEGF-dependent manner *(73,196)*. Down-regulation of angiogenesis inhibitor-TSP-1, observed in 528ras cells could also, to some degree, compensate for their VEGF deficiency *(198)*. Thus, tumor angiogenesis may be driven by oncogenes in several direct, as well as indirect ways, and by utilizing, in a manner that still needs to be understood, such host components as stromal fibroblasts, inflammatory cells, and/or the elements of the hemostatic system (Fig. 4). Whatever the specific mechanism, the comparison of VEGF-deficient (nontumorigenic) ES cells with their VEGF-deficient, but *H-ras*-transformed (tumorigenic), direct clonal descendants (528ras cells) revealed that the very requirement for endogenous VEGF production for inducing and maintaining tumor growth and angiogenesis may be dependent on the intrinsic properties of tumor cells, their ontogenesis, and differentiation status *(198)*.

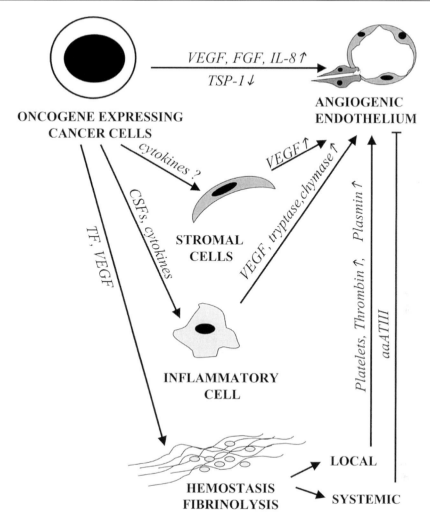

Fig. 4. Direct and indirect influences of oncogenes on tumor angiogenesis. Expression of activated oncogenes in cancer cells may not only alter their expression of angiogenesis stimulators (e.g., VEGF, bFGF) or inhibitors (e.g., TSP-1), but also influence recruitment and activation of stromal cells and inflammatory cells, both of which can serve as a source of pro-angiogenic stimuli. In addition, changes in pro-coagulant properties of cancer cells are likely a function of their genetic profile. The hemostatic alterations in cancer are intimately linked to angiogenesis (*see* text).

The role of the tumor cell-derived VEGF in inducing angiogenesis may change not only with tumor type, but also with the disease progression *(197,199)*. For example, the human T-47D breast cancer cell line, engineered to express VEGF in an inducible/repressible manner, was employed to demonstrate that VEGF withdrawal in incipient tumors inhibits their further growth, but is inconsequential when the tumors are larger and more established *(197)*. Finally, in a model of murine melanoma, in which tumor growth was triggered by tissue specific and inducible expression of the oncogenic *H-ras* transgene (in a p16INK4a –/– background), the onset of VEGF production could be temporally and functionally separated from the impact of this oncogene on the overall tumor maintenance *(81)*. In view of these results, it is clear that the role of endogenous VEGF production as a driving force of tumor angiogenesis may vary depending upon specific pathological circumstances (tumor type and stage of progression), i.e., is hardly universal for all tumors. This should be taken into account when assessing clinical trial results with such drugs as VEGF neutralizing antibodies or VEGFR inhibitors (patients who do not respond fully to such treatments may have cancers, the angiogenesis of which is not driven by VEGF).

Indeed, even in the same cellular background various transforming genetic alterations elicit different forms of angiogenic competence. Thus, in IEC-18 cells oncogene-specific angiogenic phenotypes can be induced by expression of either mutant *H-ras* or *v-src (90)*. In the former case, transformed cells simultaneously up-regulate VEGF and down-regulate TSP-1, whereas *v-src* (IEC-18) transformants up-regulate VEGF, but retain their wild-type TSP-1 expression *(90)*. Such a genetic determination of tumor angiogenesis pathways has also been documented in an elegant recent study where transgenic expression of distinct transforming genetic lesions (e.g., *neu* oncogene, BRCAI anisense, mutant p53) was directed to the murine mammary gland (under control of the mouse mammary tumor virus [MMTV] promoter). Interestingly, the resulting tumors not only displayed different profiles of angiogenesis regulators, but also different types of vascular patterning and different responses to anti-angiogenic treatment regimens *(Iruela-Arispe, personal communication)*. Again, this observation reinforces the notion that different tumors or tumor sites may be associated with distinct types of angiogenic response, which may be a function of such variables as organ site, cellular background, tumor microenvironment, the stage of tumor progression, and the transforming genetic events involved (Table 1).

6. ONCOGENES, ANGIOGENESIS, AND CANCER COAGULOPATHY

Dvorak et al. proposed that tumor angiogenesis is, to a significant degree, driven by the pathologic consequences of the increased vascular permeability *(200)*. This effect, as mentioned earlier, is largely attributed to the action of VEGF, which for this reason is also known as vascular permeability factor (VPF) *(200)*. It was argued that the VEGF/VPF-dependent leakage of plasma proteins from hyperpermeable tumor-associated capillaries leads to activation of the extravascular clotting and formation of a pro-angiogenic fibrin matrix (or gel) within the tumor mass *(200)*. In fact, activation of the hemostatic system (as well as fibrinolysis) often is not limited to the tumor site, but rather spills-over to the general circulation causing systemic thrombotic abnormalities described under a collective term of cancer coagulopathy or paraneoplastic syndrome *(201)*. In this regard, two obvious questions need to be raised. First, what is the relationship between cancer-inducing oncogenic lesions and cancer-induced abnormalities in blood coagulation? Second, what, if any, is the contribution of hemostatic/fibrinolytic events and processed occurring in tumor bearing hosts (animals and humans) to the outcome of oncogene-dependent tumor growth and angiogenesis?

Some of the links between cancer coagulopathy and oncogene-driven tumor angiogenesis are quite apparent *(202)*. Because of the causative role of oncogenes (including mutant *ras*) in up-regulation of VEGF in tumors, it can be argued that, through VEGF (or otherwise), oncogenic transformation could be an important (albeit indirect) trigger of plasma protein leakage, intratumoral fibrin formation, and activation of various proteolytic cascades that control hemostasis and fibrinolysis, both locally and systemically

(202). In addition, VEGF is known to induce procoagulant properties in endothelial cells, mainly through up-regulating their surface expression of tissue factor (TF) *(203,204)*. TF, in its own right, is an important regulator of angiogenesis *(205)*. On the other hand, frequent overexpression of this inducer of the extrinsic coagulation pathway (and cellular signaling receptor) by the cells of tumor parenchyma *(204)* is thought to potentiate their production of VEGF and angiogenic properties in general *(206)*. This is likely executed through proteolytic action of coagulation factors VIIa, Xa, and thrombin, and resulting stimulation of their respective protease activated receptors (PARs) *(207)*. It is of interest that, as we observed recently, TF expression appears to positively correlate with the presence of mutant *K-ras* oncogene and, to a lesser extent, also with the absence of *p53* tumor suppressor gene in human colorectal cancer cell lines in culture (J. Rak, unpublished observations). This observation suggests that oncogenic transformation may directly and simultaneously impact both procoagulant and pro-angiogenic properties of tumor cells *(202)* (Fig. 4).

Another case for the linkage between deregulated hemostasis (i.e., disseminated intravascular coagulation DIC) and transforming genetic events (i.e., expression of *PML-RARa* oncogene) could be made in acute promyelocytic leukemia (APL) *(208)*. In this disease, administration of all trans retinoic acid (ATRA) and resulting inhibition of *PML-RARa* transforming activity invariably leads to a reversal of cancer coagulopathy *(208)*, suggesting a causal role of the oncogene in the latter syndrome *(202)*. At the same time, ATRA also inhibits VEGF production and angiogenic competence of APL cells *(209)* (Table 4). The linkage between these respective events is under investigation.

An activated hemostatic system in cancer is also a potential source of powerful angiogenesis inhibitors *(210)*. The list of endogenous angiogenesis inhibitors is continuously expanding and currently includes, besides the two anti-angiogenic members of the thrombospondin family (TSP-1 and TSP-2) *(211)*, also certain ADAMTS proteins (Meth-1 and Meth-2) *(212)*, pigment epithelium-derived factor (PEDF) *(213)*, glioma-derived angiogenesis inhibitory factor (GD-AIF) *(214)*, vascular endothelial growth inhibitor (VEGI) *(215)*, murine EGF fragment (33–42) *(216)*, brain-specific angiogenesis inhibitor 1 (BAII) *(217)*, maspin *(218)*, endostatin *(219)*, PEX domain *(220)*, kininostatin *(221)*, 16 KD a prolactin fragment *(222)*, fibronectin fragment *(223)*, restin *(224)*, arresten *(225)*, canstatin *(226)*, tumstatin *(227)*, vasostatin *(228)*, angiostatin *(229)*, and the antiangiogenic form of antithrombin III (aaATIII) *(230)*. As mentioned earlier, many of these inhibitors can act not only at the tumor site, but also/rather are released into the circulation, whereby they could impose a state of angiogenic anergy on tumor micrometastases in distant organs *(219,229,230)*. With very few exceptions, including some known targets of tumor suppressor genes (e.g., TSP-1, BAII, GDAIF) *(70)*, the role of cancer-associated genetic lesions (particularly oncogenes) in regulation of angiogenesis inhibitors remains poorly understood *(202)*. This is particularly obvious in the case of circulating inhibitors, the relationship of which to oncogenic changes in cancer cells is unknown and requires formal experimental investigation *(202)*.

A study on aaATIII could be used as an informative, if unintended, example to illustrate the possible connection between genetic cancer cell heterogeneity, tumor progression, and the tumor-specific release of circulating angiogenesis inhibitors, in this case, through proteolytic cleavage of plasma proteins *(230)*. In this study, NCI-H69 human lung carcinoma cells were injected into immunodeficient mice in two distant subcutaneous sites. Upon tumor take, it was noticed that the larger tumors were often able to suppress the growth of their smaller contralateral counterparts *(230)*. This effect was chiefly mediated by a then novel systemic angiogenesis inhibitor, a cleaved form of antithrombin III (aaATIII), which was elaborated at the tumor site and released into the circulation *(230)*. Although, the native plasma-derived antiprotease (serpin)-ATIII, is a crucial regulator of hemostasis and a potent heparin-dependent antagonist of thrombin, aaATIII does not express such properties *(230)*. This suggests that the anti-angiogenic activity of aaATIII is unrelated to the anticoagulant action of its ATIII precursor.

Interestingly, various random clones of NCI-H69 cells were found to differ in their ability to trigger aaATIII production *in vivo (230)*. In particular, while parental NCI-H69 cells or, even more so, their H69i variant were efficient aaATIII producers, the subline designated H69ni was devoid of such capacity or, for that matter, the ability to suppress tumor growth and angiogenesis at distant organ sites *(230)*. Although the molecular basis for this heterogeneity in aaATIII generation amongst H69 cell lines is unknown, its very existence raises a number of interesting questions. For example, could activated oncogenes (or inactivated tumor suppressor genes) be responsible for the ability of cancer cells to elaborate aaATIII and other systemically acting anti-angiogenic polypeptides *(202)*? How would such a regulation be executed (directly or indirectly)? Could such genetic control (suppression) of angiogenesis inhibitor production/responsiveness explain fulminant progression and accelerated metastasis at late stages of certain malignancies, such as melanoma or breast carcinoma?

Whether oncogenes can regulate or influence the levels of systemic angiogenesis inhibition is also potentially important for a number of practical reasons. First, oncogene-responsive circulating angiogenesis inhibitors could perhaps be used as indicators (surrogate markers) to monitor the efficacy of oncogene-directed therapies. Second, the overall profile of local and circulating angiogenesis inhibitors (as well as stimulators) could be important for predicting the efficacy of various exogenously administered direct anti-angiogenic treatment strategies. This is because the action of the latter would always be projected on the background or the preexisting angiogenic balance, of which endogenous inhibitors are an important component. For example, it could be argued that tumors that retain expression of at least some inhibitors (e.g., still produce aaATIII or endostatin) could be considerably more sensitive to anti-angiogenic therapies than their inhibitor-negative counterparts, because, in the latter cases, the therapy would encounter less resistance in tripping the angiogenic switch to the off position. Finally, it would be expected that oncogene antagonists (i.e., oncogene-targeted signal transduction inhibitors) should, at least in part, restore the levels of angiogenesis inhibitors that were down-regulated by their respective targets (e.g., mutant *ras*). It follows that, oncogene-directed therapies may, therefore, be ideal synergistic partners for combination treatments involving direct acting angiogenesis inhibitors.

7. ROLE OF ONCOGENES IN SELECTION OF THE ANGIOGENIC PHENOTYPE IN TUMOR CELL POPULATIONS: A HYPOTHESIS

It would seem reasonable to propose that an overt angiogenic switch in the growing tumor could take place only if there was a critical mass of angiogenically competent tumor cells. In this sense, the angiogenic phenotype could be viewed as collective or multicellular in nature, rather than unicellular, or cell autonomous. Hence, the formation of a cluster of angiogenic cells (or an angiogenic unit) *(231)* within the incipient tumor would be required for both the development of a sufficient concentration/gradient of stimulatory growth factors, as well as for a meaningful local reduction in expression of angiogenesis inhibitors. Especially with respect to the latter effect, even a dramatic decrease in inhibitor expression at the single-cell level would not be expected to relieve the overall angiogenesis suppression and permit tumor angiogenesis to be set in motion. For these reasons, a significant enrichment in the fraction of tumor cells equipped with the overt angiogenic capacity would be required to actually initiate the process of tumor blood vessel formation *(6)*.

It is unclear exactly, how the enrichment in such angiogenically competent tumor cells could be realized. Most of the malignant characteristics of cancer cells are believed to emerge as a result of the clonal evolution *(232)* or clonal dominance *(233)* processes, whereby specific heritable traits are selectively amplified in the tumor cell population due to competitive growth and survival advantage they bestow on individual tumor cells and their clones vis-a-vis the remaining nonexpressors *(232)*. In this setting, the pro-angiogenic phenotype, on its own, would not be expected to be associated with a particularly strong selective advantage *(234,235)*. Quite simply, it is difficult to imagine how the presence of a blood vessel capillary within a given tumor microdomain would favor growth of one specific cancer cell (clone) over a neighboring cell, particularly as a function of the difference in their respective angiogenic capacities *(235)*. Instead, it seems likely that blood vessels would be "altruistically" shared among heterogenous tumor cells present in their immediate proximity. In contrast, a selective growth advantage could clearly be conferred upon individual tumor cells, if they expressed certain "selfish" properties such as intrinsically higher mitotic activity, reduced growth factor requirements, higher apoptotic threshold, or increased resistance to metabolic stress.

The actual coexistence in tumors of various selfish (e.g., apoptosis-resistant) or altruistic (e.g., angiogenic-competent) cancer cell characteristics is somewhat paradoxical, as it is not obvious how the latter would be maintained in such a competitive tumor cell population. A possible, albeit hypothetical, explanation is that the altruistic features emerge because they are tightly linked to more selectable traits by virtue of having a common molecular/genetic cause or regulation, e.g., by being concomitantly triggered by activation of a cellular oncogene. In this regard, some clues as to the feasibility of such co-selection, could be drawn form our earlier analysis of the relationship between the tumorigenic phenotype of various sublines of IEC-18 cells and their susceptibility to anoikis which is a programmed cell death that can be induced in normal epithelial cells when they are forced to grow under tumor-like 3-dimensional conditions, i.e., without a proper attachment to the ECM *(236,237)*. In such 3-dimensional (spheroid) cultures, parental, nontumorigenic IEC-18 cells invariably succumbed to massive programmed cell death, whereas their tumorigenic *H-ras* or *v-src* transformed variants remained viable and mitotically active, i.e., displayed oncogene-induced anoikis-resistant (AR) phenotype *(236,237)*. Naturally, such oncogene-expressing IEC-18/RAS (or SRC) cells also exhibited a variety of other properties typically associated with malignant trasformation, such as changes in cell shape, deregulated mitogenesis, and pro-angiogenic phenotype, all of which could contribute to their apparent tumorigenic competence *in vivo (6)*.

In order to establish whether acquisition of anoikis resistance could, in its own right, confer any degree of tumorigenic competence upon IEC-18 cells, the parental anoikis-sensitive cells were subjected to a lengthy *in vitro* selection (in spheroid culture) in order to obtain cellular variants specifically enriched for cells with exclusively increased anchorage-independent survival capacity, and not with other features of malignancy *(237)*. This was the intent, but not the outcome. AR IEC-18 variants (called AR1.10 and AR2.10) were, indeed, generated after 5–10 selection cycles, and shown competent to survive in spheriod culture *(237)*. Furthermore, upon subcutaneous injection, the variant cell lines formed slow growing tumors in nude mice *(237)*. This could have been taken as evidence for the critical and sufficient role of anoikis resistance in initiation of tumor formation, if not for the fact that, unexpectedly, tumor expansion did not stop at the size thought to constitute the limit for the avascular tumor growth (i.e., 1 to 2 mm in thickness) *(3)*. Instead, growth of AR1.10 and AR2.10 cells as tumors continued in an apparently angiogenesis-dependent manner (tumors reached relatively large sizes of 500–1500 mg and were vascularized) *(237)*. It was established *a posteriori,* that selection in vitro of the AR IEC-18 variants was paralleled by, and inseparable from, a marked constitutive up-regulation of VEGF in these cells *(237)*.

Thus, selection of IEC-18 cells for survival under bona fide angiogenesis-independent growth conditions *(in vitro)* resulted in expression of pro-angiogenic properties, even though such properties would be of no apparent biological significance in this particular biological *in vitro* context *(237)*. The pleiotrophic (i.e., apoptosis-resistant, angiogenic, and tumorigenic) phenotype of AR variants, although the specific cause of its expression is unknown, bears a striking resemblance to changes induced in IEC-18 cells by enforced expression of mutant *ras, src,* and other transforming oncogenes *(238)*. In both cases, the angiogenic phenotype is tightly linked to highly selectable intrinsic cellular traits, such as apoptosis resistance, especially under 3-dimensional conditions. It remains to be established, whether in naturally occurring human tumors the angiogenic phenotype propagates throughout the cell population by virtue of being coupled with other more selectable traits encoded by common genetic lisions (e.g., activated oncogenes) *(237)*. It is also possible that in addition to clonal selection, other mechanisms such as horizontal DNA transfer may be involved in the enrichment of tumors in both oncogene-expressing and angiogenically competent cancer cells *(239)*. In most of these circumstances, oncogenes would nevertheless act as carriers of tumor cell associated pro-angiogenic properties.

8. ONCOGENES AND THE VASCULAR DEPENDENCE OF CANCER CELLS

Although tumors may induce a vigorous angiogenic response, the resulting vasculature is often insufficient to uniformly perfuse the tumor mass and sustain optimal cancer cell growth and viability *(7)*. Instead, it is often the case that tumor cells thrive in the immediate vicinity of functional blood vessels, but undergo growth arrest and ischemic cell death with increasing distances from capillaries *(9)*. This manifestation of the vascular dependence principle can sometimes be directly observed histologically as so called perivascular cuffing i.e., formation of multilayered cylinders of viable tumor cells surrounding the central capillary and separated from other cuffs by areas of tissue necrosis. Indeed, the very distance between the central capillary and the rim of apoptotic tumor cells at the periphery of the vascular cuff defines the ultimate limit of tumor cell tolerance for ischemia and growth factor deprivation (Fig 5).

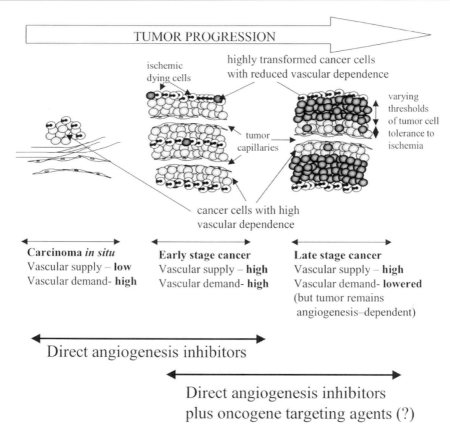

Fig. 5. Changing relationships between tumor cells and the vasculature during cancer progression. Cancer cells posses an intrinsic limit of tolerance to ischemia (i.e., defined vascular dependence), which is a function of their genetic make-up, including expression of activated oncogenes. With tumor progression cancer cell populations become heterogenous with respect to their vascular dependence. Less malignant (more vascular dependent) cellular variants (left side panel) can survive only at relatively short distances from their adjacent capillaries (or at high blood vessel density), while their more malignant counterparts (less vascular dependent) can be found throughout the tumor including its hypoxic regions (right side panel). The ability of the latter cells to survive at greater distances from the capillaries and at lower blood vessel density could be a target for signal transduction inhibitors (*see [15,240,244]* and the text for details).

In theory, two parameters could influence this distance, i.e., the thickness of the perivascular cuff: *(i)* the effective perivascular diffusion rate of critical growth factors, gasses, and metabolites *(7,32);* and *(ii)* the individual tolerance to growth factor/oxygen/metabolite deprivation exhibited by a particular type of cancer cells *(240)*. It is noteworthy, that the latter property of cancer cells (i.e., their relative vascular dependence) would likely vary as a function of tumor progression, as thresholds for growth arrest and apoptosis become increasingly higher with increasing levels of tumor malignancy *(240)*. Bedi et al demonstrated directly that the intrinsic susceptibility of colorectal cancer cells to undergo apoptotic cell death *ex vivo* negatively correlates with the stage of the disease progression *(241)*. This is not surprising, as colorectal cancer progression is associated with multiple genetic alterations (involving such genes as *APC, ras,* or *p53,* many of which are now known for their pro-survival effects and interference with various intracellular apoptosis-regulating pathways *(242)*. Among factors that participate in progressive natural selection of increasingly apoptosis-resistant tumor cell variants, chronic or intermitted hypoxia, growth factor deprivation, and metabolic stress are likely to play a major role.

There are some illuminating examples of the relationship between genetic cancer progression and tumor cell resistance to hypoxia-induced apoptosis. For instance, cells lacking the *p53* tumor suppressor gene were found to be protected from pro-apoptotic effects of hypoxia, and thereby capable of outcompeting their *p53+/+* counterparts in an oxygen deprived microenvironment *(175)*. Loss of p53 expression is often associated with late stages of colorectal carcinoma progression *(5)* (among other tumor types), where large tumor sizes, necrotic regions, and overall poor tumor perfusion, i.e., conditions detrimental for p53 expressing cells, clearly exist. Moreover, studies involving certain strains of ES cells, in which the HIF-1a gene has been inactivated, and, thereby, the main pathway of hypoxia-response has been disabled *(243)*, indicate that the rate of growth arrest and apoptosis normally (i.e., in HIF-1α +/+ cells) elicited by low oxygen tension were largely attenuated, along with expression of hypoxia-inducible genes, such as VEGF *(175)*. Notwithstanding the latter effect, HIF-1α-deficient ES cells formed large (albeit hypovascular) tumors upon subcutaneous injection into mice, suggesting that their increased apoptotic threshold could, to some degree, compensate for their relatively deficient angiogenic activity and hence, scarece perfusion of the tumor mass *(175)*.

We have previously hypothesized that with genetic disease progression (including expression of activated oncogenes) the responsiveness of cancer cells to hypoxia and growth factor deprivation would, in all probability, gradually diminish, leading to reduction in the relative vascular dependence of such increasingly malignant tumor cells *(240)*. It could, therefore, be predicted that tumor cells, which remain sensitive to hypoxia/ischemia conditions, would preferentially home to areas immediately adjacent to functional capillaries, whereas their more malignant (and ischemia-resistant) cellular variants could propagate throughout the tumor (including in its most hypoxic regions) *(5,240)*. To examine more directly whether this is the case, mixtures of wild-type, i.e., HIF-1α-positive ES, cells and their HIF-1α-negative (HIF-lα –/–) hypoxia-resistant counterparts were injected into SCID mice, and the tumors were allowed to develop to a palpable size *(244)*. Tumor-bearing mice were then injected intravenously with the DNA binding nontoxic fluorescent dye (Hoechst 33342), which, after a short circulation in blood, is known to diffuse spontaneously out of the capillaries to form perivascular concentration gradients *(245)*. Because, tumor cells incorporate the dye proportionately to its local concentration, their fluorescence intensity could be used as a marker of their position relative to the nearest perfused capillary, both *in situ* and after extraction of such cells from the tumor *(15,245)*. This technique was successfully used for isolation (by fluorescence-activated cell sorter-FACS) and analysis of tumor cells in areas either immediately adjacent to tumor capillaries (bright fluorescence), or from more hypoxic tumor periphery, i.e., areas distant from the vasculature (dim fluorescence) *(15)*. In the case of mixed teratomas containing HIF-la+/+ and HIF-la–/– ES cells, the Hoechst 33342-based sorting revealed, as expected, that the former (hypoxia-sensitive) cell type resided almost exclusively in the close proximity to blood vessels (bright fluorescence), whereas the HIF-la–/– ES cells (hypoxia-resistant) populated all areas of the tumor including the most hypoxic regions (both bright and dim fluorescence) *(244)*. This result suggests that indeed, impaired hypoxia response (i.e., HIF-1α-null-like properties) can endow tumor cells with a selective growth advantage in the heterogenous cell population and extend the distance from blood vessels, at which such cells can remain viable and mitotically active (Fig. 5).

The intratumoral cell segregation is, by no means, a peculiarity of ES cells only. A more clinically relevant tumor model, namely WM239 human malignant melanoma, was subjected to several rounds of vascular selection *in vivo* (as xenografts in nude mice), during which cell subpopulations preferentially colonizing perivascular regions of the tumor (bright fluorescence) were separated by FACS from the cells homing to areas distant from the vasculature (dim fluorescence). After a short expansion in culture, both subpopulations were reinjected into separate mice, and the enrichment cycle was repeated for up to 4× *(244)*. Finally, both subsets of WM239 tumor cells (i.e., the subpopulation enriched for proximal or distal tumor cells relative to blood vessels) were again reinjected into nude mice, and the tumors were analyzed with respect to their growth rate and vascularity *(244)*. Interestingly, both the distal WM239 subpopulation and the parental WM239 cells formed rapidly growing tumors, while their proximal (perivascular) WM239 counterparts displayed a reduced aggressiveness and slower growth rate *(244)*.

What was even more surprising (but, in retrospect, is not) was the fact that the slow growing tumors, composed of proximal WM239 cells, exhibited markedly increased microvascular density (MVD), relative to more aggressive distal WM239 subpopulation *(244)*.

This high blood vessel density associated with slow growing tumors, composed of purely perivascular (proximal) WM239 cell variants, was not due to their more angiogenic properties, i.e., it was not associated with an increase in *supply* of angiogenic blood vessels or their inducing growth factors, at least as indicated by the endothelial cell proliferation and VEGF ELISA assays with the respective conditioned medium *(244)*. Instead, this paradoxical hypervascularity of poorly tumorigenic proximal WM239 variants likely represents an increase in *demand* for blood vessels (or heightened vascular dependence), an interpretation consistent with the fact that these cells originated from the immediate proximity of the capillaries *(244)*. Thus, it seems likely that proximal WM239 cells may cease/slow-down their proliferation or undergo apoptosis at relatively closer distances to their supplying capillary, as compared to distal variants of WM239 cells. The proximal cells would then resume their growth only after a new (extra) capillary had been recruited to their immediate vicinity *(244)*. The increase in MVD would be a natural consequence of such a process *(244)*.

At this point it should be noted that, while in certain early and intermediate stage tumors (e.g., node negative breast cancer), increase in MVD is a marker of unfavourable prognosis *(246)*, in other cases, e.g., in advanced colorectal carcinoma, MVD appears to actually decrease at the late stages of disease progression *(247)*. It could be speculated that the former trend is a manifestation of the increasing angiogenic activity (*supply*) of the tumor, whereas the latter heralds decreasing vascular dependence (demand), each occuring at certain distinct stages during the disease progression (Fig. 5).

It is unclear what molecular mechanisms are responsible for the heterogenous vascular dependence of WM239 melanoma cells and whether oncogenic changes are involved. However, similar apparent perivascular selection of tumor cells was also detected in our earlier study describing two tumorigenic clones of IEC-18 cells expressing either high (RAS-7) or low (RAS-3) levels of the H-Ras oncoprotein *(15)*. The impetus for this study originally came from our observation that RAS-3 cells express a lower grade of cellular transformation and greater susceptibility to a variety of growth inhibitory and pro-apoptotic stimuli, as compared to their RAS-7 counterparts *(15,248)*. Also in this case, Hoechst 33342 injection and cell sorting revealed that, in mixed tumors containing both RAS-3 and RAS-7 cell subpopulations, the former (less malignant) cells were restricted to areas immediately adjacent to the tumor vasculature, while the clonogenic RAS-7 cells could be found throughout the tumor including its most hypoxic (distal) regions *(15)*. Thus, in three independent experimental systems (HIF-1α–/– ES cells, WM239 melanoma, IEC-18/RAS cells), of which at least one (IEC-18/RAS) involves a defined activated oncogene (H-ras), increasingly malignant properties of tumor cells brought about a relative decrease in their vascular dependence. In the context of this article, the latter example is not insignificant, as it demonstrates the possible contribution of oncogenes to changes in vascular dependence.

An important aspect of the genetically driven reduction in vascular dependence of cancer cells is the possible impact of such changes on the outcome of the antiangiogenic therapy (319,320). Since genetic tumor progression (including expression of activated oncogenes) results in tumor cells being increasingly angiogenesis proficient, but, at the same time, decreasingly vascular dependent, it follows that, at least transiently, a vascular reserve or excess of blood vessels relative to what is actually required may develop within the tumor. This reserve could, in theory, soften or mitigate the impact of even very effective anti-angiogenic agents. Tumor growth could simply continue, despite changes in vascularity and blood flow, until the functional vasculature is reduced below a certain threshold, which might be tumor-specific. A corollary to this point is that, even partial pharmacological reversal of cellular transformation, for example, by using oncogene-targeted drugs, might sensitize tumors to various direct angiogenesis antagonists (e.g., peptide inhibitors *(10)*, metronomic chemotherapy *(27,249,250)*, at last in part, by restoring higher levels of their vascular dependence *(6)*.

9. ONCOGENES AND ANGIOGENESIS IN HEMATOPOIETIC MALIGNANCIES

There are reasons to believe that, despite their liquid nature, various hematopoietic malignancies are also angiogenesis/vascular-dependent *(24)*. This contention is supported by the observation that bone marrow of leukemic patients often becomes hypervascular *(25,251)* and that leukemic cells produce VEGF, FGF, and possibly other angiogenic growth factors *(209,252–255)*. More importantly, anti-angiogenic treatments can inhibit development of experimental leukemias in mice *(249,256)*. An explanation for this, somewhat counterintuitive relationship between blood-borne malignancies and blood vessels, may lie with the fact that leukemic cells are likely responsive to paracrine growth and colony-stimulating factors released by adjacent activated endothelial cells present in the bone marrow and lymphoid organs *(15)*.

Several oncogenes have been implicated in development of various types of leukemia, but their presumed role in leukemia-associated bone marrow and/or lymphoid angiogenesis remains conjectural. For example, in the experimental model of murine erythroleukemia, a disease induced by injection of the Friend virus complex into newborn mice, the process culminates in massive expansion of leukemic blasts in the spleen and lethality due to organ rupture *(257)*. This progressive leukemic splenomegaly leads to a tenfold enlargement of the spleen size, a change that could not conceivably occur without a significant rearrangement, expansion, and possibly angiogenesis within the vascular bed of this organ. It is implicit that sequential genetic alterations associated with Friend erythroleukemia (e.g., activation of oncoproteins such as Fli-1 and Spi-1, as well as loss of p53 tumor suppressor) are directly or indirectly involved in triggering such a massive vascular remodeling.

In human hematopoietic malignancies an impressive inventory of oncogenic changes has been compiled over the last two decades *(258–260)*. They include, for example: internal tandem duplications of FLT3 and mutations of the N-ras oncogenes in acute myeloid leukemia (AML) *(260)*, mutations of N-, or K-ras oncogenes in plasma cell leukemia, multiple myeloma, acute lymphoblastic leukemia (ALL), and chronic myelomonocytic leukemia (CML) *(260)*, expression of a hybrid *bcr-abl* oncogene in chronic myelogenous leukemia (CML) *(261)* and *PML/PLZF-RARα* oncogene in APL *(262,263)*, and probably many others. All these alterations, to one degree or another, are likely to play a causative role in progression of these respective malignancies. This notion is reinforced by the recently documented spectacular therapeutic efficacy in CML patients of the pharmacological inhibitor (Gleevec/STI571) targeted at the *bcr-abl* oncogene *(264)*. It remains an open question, whether the antileukemic effect of this signal transduction inhibitor, FTIs *(260)*, and other similar agents is strictly a result of inhibited proliferation, survival, increased differentiation, and other intrinsic properties of leukemic cells themselves, or, at least in part, involves suppression of oncogene-induced (bone marrow) angiogenesis (Table 4).

A hitherto rather unexpected contribution of the endothelial cell compartment to the oncogene-driven leukemogenesis can be inferred from recent studies on endothelial cell progenitors (EPCs) in CML patients *(265)*. Similarly to leukemic myeloid progenitors, these EPCs also carry the Philadelphia chromosome, a karyotypic signature of the *bcr-abl* oncogene *(265)*. The reasons for this unusual EPC involvement in CML could be related to the existence of a common *bcr-abl*-transformed presursor for both hematopoietic and endothelial lineages. Such transformed vascular cells may, in fact, carry features of genetic instability, malignancy, and drug resistance, thus far ascribed exclusively to cancer or leukemic cells themselves. In this context, targeting *bcr-abl* (with Gleevec) may result in both an indirect antiangiogenic effect, through inhibition of the angiogenic phenotype of CML cells, as well as more direct effect on *bcr-abl* postive EPCs.

10. ANTI-ANGIOGNIC EFFECTS OF ONCOGENE TARGETING SIGNAL TRANSDUCTION INHIBITING DRUGS

In 1995, we have postulated that pharmacological blockade of the mutant *ras* oncogene by using FTIs could contribute to the anticancer effects of these drugs *in vivo* by inhibiting VEGF expression and tumor angiogenesis *(89)*. Indeed, such an indirect anti-angiogenic effect could characterize many, if not all, signal transduction inhibitors and oncogene-targeting anticancer agents, inasmuch as oncogenes can be ascribed a general role in triggering tumor vascularization *(89,133)* (Tables 1 and 4). While this notion is awaiting rigorous clinical verification, preclinical observations seem to provide an increasing volume of affirmative evidence *(27)*.

Over the last two decades, the increasing understanding of the molecular causes and intricacies of malignant transformation stimulated parallel efforts to develop effective inhibitors of the oncogenic signaling pathways *(84,266,267)*. This massive undertaking yielded essentially two major classes of oncogene antagonists, both of which are currently either approved or being tested in clinical trials, namely: *(i)* inhibitors of protein prenylation (farnesylation and/or geranylgeranylation) directed against small membrane-associated proto-oncogenic GTPases (mainly Ras or Rho proteins) *(268);* and *(ii)* protein kinase inhibitors (PKIs) directed against a diverse group of enzymes, which act as generators or crucial transducers of intracellular oncogenic signals *(266,269)*. In both cases there is strong circumstantial preclinical evidence that angiogenesis inhibition may contribute to the therapeutic efficacy of these respective drugs *(6,27,89)*.

FTIs have originally been viewed as mainly cytostatic agents capable of merely reversing morphological transformation of cells harboring mutant *ras* (mainly the *H-ras* isoform) and inhibiting their mitogenesis *(270)*. More recently, however, this perception has been challenged by the results of animal studies, in which *H-ras*-expressing transgenic oncomice, which spontaneously develop mammary and parotid (salivary) gland carcinomas, have been put on a daily regimen of the FTI (L-744,832). This treatment, rather than inducing tumor stasis, resulted in remarkable regressions of even large established tumors *(82)*, an obvious indication of cytotoxic rather than cytostatic anticancer activity *in vivo*. While some direct proapoptotic effects were ascribed to FTIs *(143,236,271)*, the fact that cytotoxicity was mainly observed under *in vivo*, angiogenesis-dependent growth conditions suggested that blood vessel formation could also be affected by the FTI, e.g., due to down-regulation of VEGF and obliteration of other *ras*-dependent pro-angiogenic properties *(133)*.

Inhibitors of the oncogenic protein kinases may also act as both indirect and direct anti-agiogenics. In the first instance, blockade of the oncogenic action of the EGFR with specific monoclonal antibodies (e.g., IMC-C225/cetuximab, mAb806) *(104,272–276)* or small molecular weight inhibitors (e.g., ZD1839/Iressa) *(277)* was paralleled by a marked reduction in release from tumor cells of angiogenic growth factors, primarily VEGF, bFGF and IL-8, as well as by a commensurate inhibition of tumor growth and tumor vascularization. Indeed, similar anti-angiogenic activity could be part of the anticancer activity of other, possibly all other, kinase inhibitors currently in clinical development, including antagonists of HER-2/Erb-B2 (Herceptin/Trastuzumab), EGFR (Iressa, IMC-C225, Tarceva/OSI-744), NGFR (CEP-701), or bcr-abl (Gleevec/STI-571) *(269)* (Table 4). At least in the case of Herceptin, preclinical evidence in this regard is clearly affirmative *(104)* (also D. Slamon et al. unpublished observations). Again, as in the case of FTIs, this mode of action of PKIs can explain the disparity between their mild growth inhibitory effects against cancer cells in culture and the much more potent and cytotoxic effects of these oncogene targeting agents against tumors growing *in vivo*, i.e., in the context where access and generation of tumor blood vessels becomes an important *de facto* survival mechanism for cancer cells *(82,89,104)*. Naturally, the scope and the actual contribution of the angiogenesis inhibition to the overall antitumor activity of these respective compounds remains to be unequivocally established.

As mentioned already, like many other properties of cancer cells their angiogenic phenotype is likely to evolve with tumor progression as well *(15)* (Fig. 5). Under selective pressure such phenotype may become superfluous, redundant, and/or follow several alternative pathways *(197,199)*. This may lead to epigenetic forms of resistance/refractoriness to the anti-angiogenic effects of oncogene antagonists. An example of such an escape mechanism has been recently described in a study aimed at analysis of tumor relapses following treatment of SCID mice bearing A431 squamous cell carcinoma xenografts with a panel of neutralizing monoclonal antibodies (C225, mR3, hR3) directed against the EGFR oncogene *(272)*. In this case, rare recurrent tumors were removed, enzymatically dissociated, and drug resistant cancer cell variants were established in cell culture *(272)*. Interestingly, these variant cell lines were found to express significantly higher constitutive levels of VEGF than parental A431 cells *(272)*. Conversely, enforced overexpression of murine VEGF in the latter (A431) cell line led to expression of *in vivo* resistance/refractoriness to antiangiogenic and antitumor effects of EGFR antagonists *(272)*. Results such as these suggest that loss of sensitivity to signal transduction inhibitors may occur in cancer as a result, at least in part, of progression to a more angiogenic state and possibly due to acquisition of additional genetic changes.

In some instances, endothelial cells themselves may become a target for oncogene-directed signal transduction inhibitors. Thus, certain CAAX-FTIs (e.g., A-170634) have been shown to possess a direct anti-angiogenic effect *in vitro* and *in vivo*, in addition to blocking *ras*-dependent VEGF production in cancer cells *(145)*. Likewise, treatment of nude mice harboring orthotopic xenografts of human pancreatic carcinoma with a novel EGFR inhibitor (PKI-166) led to endothelial cell apoptosis, in part through down-regulation of angiogenic/survival growth factors (i.e., through an indirect mechanism), and in part through a presumed direct anti-endothelial activity of this agent *(278)*. Similar dual anti-angiogenic action seems to characterize some other inhibitors of intracellular signaling including antioxidants *(279)* or blockers of cyclooxygenase 2 activity *(280)*.

At least in the case of FTIs, the prospect of inhibiting angiogenesis-inducing pathways should be viewed with some caution. FTIs inhibit protein prenylation by acting on the cholesterol synthesis pathways downstream of HMG-CoA reductase *(281)*, an enzyme that is also inhibited by cholesterol lowering drugs known as statins *(268)*. Hence, certain similarities might exists between effects of these two groups of drugs. In fact, at least one statin (Lovastatin) has been used experimentally to inhibit *ras* farnesylation and proved effective in reducing VEGF synthesis by cancer cells *(282)*. However, statins also possess a direct pro-angiogenic activity *(281)* and are known to promote re-endothelialization of vascular grafts by mobilizing EPCs from the bone marrow *(283)*. It is not clear, whether such an effect could also be induced by FTIs and manifest itself in the context of cancer treatment, but if so, the release of EPCs could counteract some of the anti-angiogenic effects of FTIs.

Practical approaches to inhibit tumor angiogenesis in clinical settings will likely rely on using synergistic drug combinations rather than single agents.

11. SUMMARY

It is now recognized that the onset, maintenance, and progression of tumor angiogenesis is a central and indispensable element of tumor growth, invasion and metastasis *(10)*. Activated oncogenes are thought to play a key role in tumor-vascular interactions owing to one or more of the following influences: *(1)* direct induction of the pro-angiogenic phenotype in cancer cells; *(2)* indirect regulation of tumor angiogenesis through possible impact on: stromal cell recruitment, deregulation of hemostasis, and generation of circulating angiogenesis inhibitors; *(3)* possible influence upon positive selection of the angiogenic phenotype within the tumor cell population; and *(4)* regulation of the relative vascular/angiogenesis dependence of cancer cells.

Oncogene-directed signal transduction inhibitors represent a new generation of anti-cancer agents, which unlike traditional cytoreductive anticancer drugs, or direct angiogenesis inhibitors, are designed to act therapeutically in a causal rather than symptomatic or nonspecific manner. In this sense, these drugs are likely to exert their anticancer activity, at least in part, through disruption of the interrelationship between tumor cells and their adjacent angiogenic endothelium. Several possible complementary mechanisms of such action could be invoked, including: *(1)* attenuation of the oncogene-dependent pro-angiogenic phenotype of cancer cells, both constitutive and related to cancer cell hypersensitivity to epigenetic stimulation (e.g. hypoxia); *(2)* increase in vascular dependence of cancer cells and their possible sensitization to direct acting angiogenesis inhibitors; and *(3)* direct anti-angiogenic effects exerted on tumor-associated endothelium. Further studies are needed to understand the vascular targeting effects of these anticancer agents and define how they might be most effectively used in the clinic. One of the promising avenues in this regard is the inclusion of oncogene targeting agents in anticancer treatment regimens, e.g., those involving drugs developed as direct angiogenesis inhibitors.

ACKNOWLEDGMENTS

The authors are grateful for the continuing support and truly philosophical patience of their families without whom this work would not have been possible. J.R. would like to extend special thanks to his daughter Anna, who gave so much over the years and received so little. This work was supported by the Operating Grant and the Terry Fox Grant for New Investigators from the National Cancer Institute of Canada to J.R. and a grant from the Medical Research Council of Canada to R.S.K. We are also thankful to our colleagues including: Joanne Yu, Brenda Coomber, Alicia Viloria-Petit, Jennifer Tran, Petr and Giannoula Klement and many others who created an outstanding milieu for stimulating discussion, reflection, and experiments.

REFERENCES

1. Bishop JM. Cancer: the rise of the genetic paradigm. *Genes Dev* 1995; 9:1309–1315.
2. Hanahan D, Weinberg RA. The hallmarks of cancer. *Cell* 2000; 100:57–70.
3. Folkman J. What is the evidence that tumors are angiogenesis-dependent? *J Natl Canc Inst* 1990; 82:4–6.
4. Clark WH. Human cutaneous malignant melanoma as a model for cancer. *Cancer Metastasis Rev* 1991; 10:83–88.
5. Fearon ER, Vogelstein B. A genetic model for colorectal tumorigenesis. *Cell* 1990; 61:759–767.
6. Rak J, Yu JL, Klement G, Kerbel RS. Oncogenes and angiogenesis: signaling three-dimensional tumor growth [in process citation]. *J Investig Dermatol Symp Proc* 2000; 5:24–33.
7. Jain RK. Vascular and interstitial barriers to delivery of therapeutic agents in tumors. *Cancer Metastasis Rev* 1990; 9:253–266.
8. Holmgren L, O'Reilly MS, Folkman J. Dormancy of micrometastases: balanced proliferation and apoptosis in the presence of angiogenesis suppression. *Nat Med* 1995; 1:149–153.
9. Tannock IF. The relation between cell proliferation and the vascular system in a transplanted mouse mammary tumour. *Br J Cancer* 1968; 22:258–273.

10. Folkman J. Clinical applications of research on angiogenesis. *N Engl J Med* 1995; 333:1757–1763.
11. Mandriota SJ, Jussila L, Jeltsch M, Compagni A, Baetens D, Prevo R, et al. Vascular endothelial growth factor-C-mediated lymphangiogenesis promotes tumour metastasis. *EMBO J* 2001; 20:672–682.
12. Stacker SA, Caesar C, Baldwin ME, Thornton GE, Williams RA, Prevo R, et al. VEGF-D promotes the metastatic spread of tumor cells via the lymphatics. *Nat Med* 2001; 7:186–191.
13. Skobe M, Hawighorst T, Jackson DG, Prevo R, Janes L, Velasco P, et al. Induction of tumor lymphangiogenesis by VEGF-C promotes breast cancer metastasis. *Nat Med* 2001; 7:192–198.
14. Fidler IJ, Ellis LM. The implications of angiogenesis for the biology and therapy of cancer metastasis. *Cell* 1994; 79:185–188.
15. Rak J, Filmus J, Kerbel RS. Reciprocal paracrine interactions between tumor cells and endothelial cells. The "angiogenesis progression" hypothesis. *Eur J Cancer* 1996; 32A:2438–2450.
16. St Croix B, Rago C, Velculescu V, Traverso G, Romans KE, Montgomery E, et al. Genes expressed in human tumor endothelium. *Science* 2000; 289:1197–1202.
17. Rak JW, Hegmann EJ, Lu C, Kerbel RS. Progressive loss of sensitivity to endothelium-derived growth inhibitors expressed by human melanoma cells during disease progression. *J Cell Physiol* 1994; 159:245–255.
18. Li L, Nicolson GL, Fidler IJ. Direct in vitro lysis of metastatic tumor cells by cytoline- activated murine vascular endothelial cells. *Cancer Res* 1991; 51:245–254.
19. Nicosia RF, Tchao R, Leighton J. Angiogenesis-dependent tumor spread in reinforced fibrin clot culture. *Cancer Res* 1983; 43:2159–2166.
20. Skobe M, Rockwell P, Goldstein N, Vosseler S, Fusenig NE. Halting angiogenesis suppresses carcinoma cell invasion. *Nat Med* 1997; 3:1222–1227.
21. Brooks PC, Stromblad S, Klemke R, Visscher D, Sarkar FH, Cheresh DA. Antiintegrin αbβ3 blocks human breast cancer growth and angiogenesis in human skin. *J Clin Invest* 1995; 96:1815–1822.
22. Hamada J, Cavanaugh PG, Miki K, Nicolson GL. A paracrine migration-stimulating factor for metastatic tumor cells secreted by mouse hepatic sinusoidal endothelial cells: identification as complement component C3b. *Cancer Res* 1993; 53:4418–4423.
23. Rak J, St Croix B, Kerbel RS. Consequences of angiogenesis for tumor progression, metastasis and cancer therapy. *Anti-Cancer Drugs* 1995; 6:3–18.
24. Mangi MH, Newland AC. Angiogenesis and angiogenic mediators in haematological malignancies. *Br J Haematol* 2000; 111:43–51.
25. Perez-Atayde AR, Sallan SE, Tedrow U, Connors S, Allred E, Folkman J. Spectrum of tumor angiogenesis in the bone marrow of children with acute lymphoblastic leukemia. *Am J Pathol* 1997; 150:815–820.
26. Boehm T, Folkman J, Browder T, O'Reilly MS. Antiangiogenic therapy of experimental cancer does not induce acquired drug resistance. *Nature* 1997; 390:404–407.
27. Kerbel RS, Viloria-Petit A, Klement G, Rak J. 'Accidental' anti-angiogenic drugs. Anti-oncogene directed signal transduction inhibitors and conventional chemotherapeutic agents as examples. *Eur J Cancer* 2000; 36:1248–1257.
28. Kerbel RS. Tumor angiogenesis: past, present and the near future. *Carcinogenesis* 2000; 21:505–515.
29. McCarthy M. Targeted drugs take centre stage at US cancer meeting. *Lancet* 2001; 357:1593.
30. Risau W. Mechanisms of angiogenesis. *Nature* 1997; 386:671–674.
31. Carmeliet P. Mechanisms of angiogenesis and arteriogenesis. *Nat Med* 2000; 6:389–395.
32. Carmeliet P, Jain RK. Angiogenesis in cancer and other diseases. *Nature* 2000; 407:249–257.
33. Yancopoulos GD, Davis S, Gale NW, Rudge JS, Wiegand SJ, Holash J. Vascular-specific growth factors and blood vessel formation. *Nature* 2000; 407:242–248.
34. Sundberg C, Nagy JA, Brown LF, Feng D, Eckelhoefer IA, Manseau EJ, et al. Glomeruloid microvascular proliferation follows adenoviral vascular permeability factor/vascular endothelial growth factor-164 gene delivery. *Am J Pathol* 2001; 158:1145–1160.
35. Burri PH. Intussusceptive microvascular growth, a new mechanism of capillary network expansion. Angiogenesis, International Symposium, St. Gallen, March 1991; 13–15, 1991, Abstract:88.
36. Drake CJ, Little CD. VEGF and vascular fusion: implications for normal and pathological vessels. *J Histochem Cytochem* 1999; 47:1351–1356.
37. Asahara T, Murohara T, Sullivan A, Silver M, van der Zee R, Li T, et al. Isolation of putative progenitor endothelial cells for angiogenesis. *Science* 1997; 275:964–967.
38. Peichev M, Naiyer AJ, Pereira D, Zhu Z, Lane WJ, Williams M, et al. Expression of VEGFR-2 and AC133 by circulating human CD34(+) cells identifies a population of functional endothelial precursors. *Blood* 2000; 95:952–958.

39. Maniotis AJ, Folberg R, Hess A, Seftor EA, Gardner LM, Pe'er J, et al. Vascular channel formation by human melanoma cells in vivo and in vitro: vasculogenic mimicry. *Am J Pathol* 1999; 155:739–752.

40. McDonald DM, Munn L, Jain RK. Vasculogenic mimicry: how convincing, how novel, and how significant? *Am J Pathol* 2000; 156:383–388.

41. Folkman J. Tumor angiogenesis. *Adv Cancer Res* 1985; 43:175–203.

42. Holash J, Maisonpierre PC, Compton D, Boland P, Alexander CR, Zagzag D, et al. Vessel cooption, regression, and growth in tumors mediated by angiopoietins and VEGF. *Science* 1999; 284:1994–1998.

43. Benjamin LE, Golijanin D, Itin A, Pode D, Keshet E. Selective ablation of immature blood vessels in established human tumors follows vascular endothelial growth factor withdrawal. *J Clin Invest* 1999; 103:159–165.

44. Eberhard A, Kahlert S, Goede V, Hemmerlein B, Plate KH, Augustin HG. Heterogeneity of angiogenesis and blood vessel maturation in human tumors: implications for antiangiogenic tumor therapies. *Cancer Res* 2000; 60:1388–1393.

45. Denekamp J. Endothelial cell proliferation as a novel approach to targeting tumor therapy. *Br J Cancer* 1982; 45:136–139.

46. Plate KH, Breier G, Millauer B, Ullrich A, Risau W. Up-regulation of vascular endothelial growth factor and its cognate receptors in a rat glioma model of tumor angiogenesis. *Cancer Res* 1993; 53:5822–5827.

47. Kaipainen A, Vlaykova T, Hatva E, Bohling T, Jekunen A, Pyrhonen S, et al. Enhanced expression of the tie receptor tyrosine kinase mesenger RNA in the vascular endothelium of metastatic melanomas. *Cancer Res* 1994; 54:6571–6577.

48. Peters KG, Coogan A, Berry D, Marks J, Iglehart JD, Kontos CD. Expression of Tie2/Tek in breast tumor vasculature provides a new marker for evaluation of tumour angiogenesis. *Br J Cancer* 1998; 77:51–56.

49. Mustonen T, Alitalo K. Endothelial receptor tyrosine kinases involved in angiogenesis. *J Cell Biol* 1995; 129:895–898.

50. Rak JW, Hegmann EJ, Kerbel RS. The role of angiogenesis in tumor progression and metastasis. In: Heppner GH, ed. *Advances in Molecular and Cell Biology*. JAI Press, Greenwich, CT, 1993, pp. 205–251.

51. Contrino J, Hair G, Kreutzer DL, Rickles FR. In situ detection of tissue factor in vascular endothelial cells: correlation with the malignant phenotype of human breast disease [see comments]. *Nat Med* 1996; 2:209–215.

52. Veikkola T, Karkkainen M, Claesson-Welsh L, Alitalo K. Regulation of angiogenesis via vascular endothelial growth factor receptors. *Cancer Res* 2000; 60:203–212.

53. Ferrara N, Davis-Smyth T. The biology of vascular endothelial growth factor. *Endocr Rev* 1997; 18:4–25.

54. Ferrara N, Carver-Moore K, Chen H, Dowd M, Lu L, O'Shea KS, et al. Heterozygous embryonic lethality induced by targeted inactivation of the VEGF gene. *Nature* 1996; 380:439–442.

55. Carmeliet P, Ferreira V, Breier G, Pollefeyt S, Kieckens L, Gertsenstein M, et al. Abnormal blood vessel development and lethality in embryos lacking a single VEGF allele. *Nature* 1996; 380:435–439.

56. Carmeliet P, Collen D. Transgenic mouse models in angiogenesis and cardiovascular disease. *J Pathol* 2000; 190:387–405.

57. Carmeliet P, Ng YS, Nuyens D, Theilmeier G, Brusselmans K, Cornelissen I, et al. Impaired myocardial angiogenesis and ischemic cardiomyopathy in mice lacking the vascular endothelial growth factor isoforms VEGF164 and VEGF188. *Nat Med* 1999; 5:495–502.

58. Dvorak HF, Brown LF, Detmar M, Dvorak AM. Review: vascular permeability factor/vascular endothelial growth factor, microvascular hyperpermeability, and angiogenesis. *Am J Pathol* 1995; 146:1029–1039.

59. Hiratsuka S, Minowa O, Kuno J, Noda T, Shibuya M. Flt-1 lacking the tyrosine kinase domain is sufficient for normal development and angiogenesis in mice. *Proc Natl Acad Sci USA* 1998; 95:9349–9354.

60. Lannutti BJ, Gately ST, Quevedo ME, Soff GA, Paller AS. Human angiostatin inhibits murine hemangioendothelioma tumor growth in vivo. *Cancer Res* 1997; 57:5277–5280.

61. Carmeliet P, Moons L, Luttun A, Vincenti V, Compernolle V, De Mol M, et al. Synergism between vascular endothelial growth factor and placental growth factor contributes to angiogenesis and plasma extravasation in pathological conditions. *Nat Med* 2001; 7:575–583.

62. Friedlander M, Brooks PC, Shaffer RW, Kincaid CM, Varner JA, Cheresh DA. Definition of two angiogenic pathways by distinct α_v integrins. *Science* 1995; 270:1500.

63. Carmeliet P, Lampugnani MG, Moons L, Breviario F, Compernolle V, Bono F, et al. Targeted deficiency or cytosolic truncation of the VE-cadherin gene in mice impairs VEGF-mediated endothelial survival and angiogenesis. *Cell* 1999; 98:147–157.

64. Dumont DJ, Yamaguchi TP, Conlon RA, Rossant J, Breitman ML. tek, a novel tyrosine kinase gene located on mouse chromosome 4, is expressed in endothelial cells and their presumptive precursors. *Oncogene* 1992; 7:1471–1480.

65. Jones N, Iljin K, Dumont DJ, Alitalo K. Tie receptors: new modulators of angiogenic and lymphangiogenic responses. *Nat Rev Mol Cell Biol* 2001; 2:257–267.

66. Hanahan D. Signaling vascular morphogenesis and maintenance. *Science* 1997; 277:48–50.

67. Wang HU, Chen ZF, Anderson DJ. Molecular distinction and angiogenic interaction between embryonic arteries and veins revealed by ephrin-B2 and its receptor Eph-B4 [see comments]. *Cell* 1998; 93:741–753.

68. Folkman J. Tumor angiogenesis. In: Holland JF, Bast RC, Morton DL, Frei E, Kufe DW, Weichselbaum RR, eds. *Cancer Medicine, 4th ed.* Williams & Wilkins, Baltimore, 1997, pp. 181–204.

69. Hanahan D, Folkman J. Patterns and emerging mechanisms of the angiogenic switch during tumorigenesis. *Cell* 1996; 86:353–364.

70. Bouck N, Stellmach V, Hsu SC. How tumors become angiogenic. *Adv Cancer Res* 1996; 69:135–174.

71. Filleur S, Volpert OV, Degeorges A, Voland C, Reiher F, Clezardin P, et al. In vivo mechanisms by which tumors producing thrombospondin 1 bypass its inhibitory effects. *Genes Dev* 2001; 15:1373–1382.

72. Coussens LM, Raymond WW, Bergers G, Laig-Webster M, Behrendtsen O, Werb Z, et al. Inflammatory mast cells up-regulate angiogenesis during squamous epithelial carcinogenesis. *Genes Dev* 1999; 13:1382–1397.

73. Hlatky L, Tsionou C, Hahnfeld P, Coleman CN. Mammary fibroblasts may influence breast tumor angiogenesis via hypoxia-induced vascular endothelial growth factor up-regulation and protein expression. *Cancer Res.* 1994; 54:6083–6086.

74. Lyden D, Young AZ, Zagzag D, Yan W, Gerald W, O'Reilly R, et al. Id1 and Id3 are required for neurogenesis, angiogenesis and vascularization of tumour xenografts. *Nature* 1999; 401:670–677.

75. Rohan RM, Fernandez A, Udagawa T, Yuan J, D'Amato RJ. Genetic heterogeneity of angiogenesis in mice. *FASEB J* 2000; 14:871–876.

76. Kyriakides TR, Leach KJ, Hoffman AS, Ratner BD, Bornstein P. Mice that lack the angiogenesis inhibitor, thrombospondin 2, mount an altered foreign body reaction characterized by increased vascularity. *Proc Natl Acad Sci USA* 1999; 96:4449–4454.

77. Khosravi-Far R, Campbell S, Rossman KL, Der CJ. Increasing complexity of Ras signal transduction: involvement of Rho family proteins. *Adv Cancer Res* 1998; 172:57–107.

78. Minamoto, T, Sawaguchi K, Mai M, Yamashita N, Sugimura T, Esumi H. Infrequent K-*ras* activation in superficial-type (flat) colorectal adenomas and adenocarcinomas. *Cancer Res* 1994; 54:2841–2844.

79. Hasegawa H, Ueda M, Watanabe M, Teramoto T, Mukai M, Kitajima M. K-*ras* gene mutations in early colorectal cancer … flat elevated vs polyp-forming cancer … *Oncogene* 1995; 10:1413–1416.

80. Shirasawa S, Furuse M, Yokoyama N, Sasazuki T. Altered growth of human colon cancer cell lines disrupted at activated Ki-ras. *Science* 1993; 260:85–88.

81. Chin L, Tam A, Pomerantz J, Wong M, Holash J, Bardeesy N, et al. Essential role for oncogenic Ras in tumour maintenance. *Nature* 1999; 400:468–472.

82. Kohl NE, Omer CA, Conner MW, Anthony NJ, Davide JP, deSolms SJ, et al. Inhibition of farnesyltransferase induces regression of mammary and salivary carcinomas in *ras* transgenic mice. *Nat Med* 1995; 1:792–797.

83. Guha A, Feldkamp MM, Lau N, Boss G, Pawson A. Proliferation of human malignant astrocytomas is dependent on Ras activation. *Oncogene* 1997; 15:2755–2765.

84. Hunter T. Oncoprotein networks. *Cell* 1997; 88:333–346.

85. Chambers AF, Tuck AB. Ras-responsive genes and tumor metastasis. *Crit Rev Oncog* 1993; 4:95–114.

86. Bortner DM, Langer SJ, Ostrowski MC. Non-nuclear oncogenes and the regulation of gene expression in transformed cells. *Crit Rev Oncogen* 1993; 4:137–160.

87. Zuber J, Tchernitsa OI, Hinzmann B, Schmitz AC, Grips M, Hellriegel M, et al. A genome-wide survey of RAS transformation targets. *Nat Genet* 2000; 24:144–152.

88. Buick RN, Filmus J, and Quaroni A. Activated H-*ras* transforms rat intestinal epithelial cells with expression of α-TGF. *Exp Cell Res* 1987; 170:300–309.

89. Rak J, Mitsuhashi Y, Bayko L, Filmus J, Sasazuki T, and Kerbel RS. Mutant *ras* oncogenes upregulate VEGF/VPF expression: implications for induction and inhibition of tumor angiogenesis. *Cancer Res* 1995; 55:4575–4580.

90. Rak J, Mitsuhashi Y, Sheehan C, Tamir A, Viloria-Petit A, Filmus J, et al. Oncogenes and tumor angiogenesis: differential modes of vascular endothelial growth factor up-regulation in ras-transformed epithelial cells and fibroblasts. *Cancer Res* 2000; 60:490–498.

91. Rak J, Kerbel RS. Ras regulation of VEGF and angiogenesis. *Methods Enzymol,* 333:267–283.

92. Grugel S, Finkenzeller G, Weindel K, Barleon B, and Marme D. Both v-Ha-ras and v-raf stimulate expression of the vascular endothelial growth factor in NIH 3T3 cells. *J Biol Chem* 1995; 270:25915–25919.

93. Kerbel R, Viloria-Petit A, Okada F, Rak J. Establishing a link between oncogenes and tumor angiogenesis. *Mol Med* 1998; 4:286–295.

94. Bos JL. The ras gene family and human carcinogenesis. *Mutat Res* 1988; 195:255–271.

95. Brown LF, Detmar M, Claffey KP, Nagy JA, Feng D, Dvorak AM, et al. Vascular permeability factor/vascular endothelial growth factor: A multifunctional angiogenic cytokine. In; Goldberg ID, Goldberg REM, ed. *Regulation of Angiogenesis* Birkhauser Verlag, Basel/Switzerland, 1997; pp. 233–269.

96. Saleh M, Stacker SA, Wilks AF. Inhibition of growith of C6 glioma cells in vivo by expression of antisense vascular endothelial growth factor sequence. *Cancer Res* 1996; 56:393–401.

97. Ellis LM, Liu W, Wilson M. Down-regulation of vascular endothelial growth factor in human colon carcinoma cell lines by antisense transfection decreases endothelial cell proliferation. *Surgery* 1996; 120:871–878.

98. Masood R, Cai J, Zheng T, Smith DL, Naidu Y, Gill PS. Vascular endothelial growth factor/vascular permeability factor is an autocrine growth factor for AIDS-Kaposi sarcoma. *Proc Natl Acad Sci USA* 1997; 94:979–984.

99. Claffey KP, Brown LF, del Aguila LF, Tognazzi K, Yeo K-T, Manseau EJ, et al. Expression of vascular permeability factor/vascular endothelial growth factor melanoma cells increases tumor growth, angiogenesis, and experimental metastasis. *Cancer Res* 1996; 56:172–181.

100. Oku T, Tjuvajev JG, Miyagawa T, Sasajima T, Joshi A, Joshi R, et al. Tumor growth modulation by sense and antisense vascular endothelial growth factor gene expression: effects on angiogenesis, vascular permeability, blood volume, blood flow, fluorodeoxyglucose uptake, and proliferation of human melanoma intracerebral xenografts. *Cancer Res* 1998; 58:4185–4192.

101. Nguyen JT, Wu P, Clouse ME, Hlatky L, Terwilliger EF. Adeno-associated virus-mediated delivery of antiangiogenic factors as an antitumor strategy. *Cancer Res* 1998; 58:5673–5677.

102. Im SA, Gomez-Manzano C, Fueyo J, Liu TJ, Ke LD, Kim JS, et al. Antiangiogenesis treatment for gliomas: transfer of antisense-vascular endothelial growth factor inhibits tumor growth in vivo. *Cancer Res* 1999; 59:895–900.

103. Grunstein J, Masbad JJ, Hickey R, Giordano F, Johnson RS. Isoforms of vascular endothelial growth factor act in a coordinate fashion to recruit and expand tumor vasculature. *Mol Cell Biol* 2000; 20:7282–7291.

104. Viloria-Petit AM, Rak J, Hung M-C, Rockwell P, Goldstein N, Kerbel RS. Neutralizing antibodies against EGF and ErbB-2/*neu* receptor tyrosine kinases down-regulate VEGF production by tumor cells in vitro and in vivo: angiogenic implications for signal transduction therapy of solid tumors. *Am J Pathol* 1997; 151:1523–1530.

105. Kim KJ, Li B, Winer J, Armanini M, Gillett N, Phillips HS, et al. Inhibition of vascular endothelial growth factor-induced angiogenesis suppresses tumour growth in vivo. *Nature* 1993; 362:841–844.

106. Warren RS, Yuan H, Mati MR, Gillett NA, Ferrara N. Regulation by vascular endothelial growth factor of human colon cancer tumorigenesis in a mouse model of experimental liver metastasis. *J Clin Invest* 1995; 95:1789–1797.

107. Goldman CK, Kendall RL, Cabrera G, Soroceanu L, Heike Y, Gillespie GY, et al. Paracrine expression of a native soluble vascular endothelial growth factor receptor inhibits tumor growth, metastasis, and mortality rate. *Proc Natl Acad Sci USA* 1998; 95:8795–8800.

108. Lin P, Sankar S, Shan S, Dewhirst MW, Polverini PJ, Quinn TQ, et al. Inhibition of tumor growth by targeting tumor endothelium using a soluble vascular endothelial growth factor receptor. *Cell Growth Differ* 1998; 9:49–58.

109. Siemeister G, Schirner M, Weindel K, Reusch P, Menrad A, Marme D, et al. Two independent mechanisms essential for tumor angiogenesis: inhibition of human melanoma xenograft growth by interfering with either the vascular endothelial growth factor receptor pathway or the Tie-2 pathway. *Cancer Res* 1999; 59:3185–3191.

110. Millauer B, Longhi MP, Plate KH, Shawver LK, Risau W, Ullrich A, et al. Dominant-negative inhibition of Flk-1 suppresses the growth of many tumor types in vivo. *Cancer Res* 1996; 56:1615–1620.

111. Millauer B, Shawver LK, Plate KH, Risau W, Ullrich A. Glioblastoma growth inhibited in vivo by a dominant-negative Flk-1 mutant. *Nature* 1994; 367:576–579.

112. Witte L, Hicklin DJ, Zhu Z, Pytowski B, Kotanides H, Rockwell P, et al. Monoclonal antibodies targeting the VEGF receptor-2 (Flk1/KDR) as an anti-angiogenic therapeutic strategy. *Cancer Metastasis Rev* 1998; 17:155–161.

113. Shaheen RM, Davis DW, Liu W, Zebrowski BK, Wilson MR, Bucana CD, et al. Antiangiogenic therapy targeting the tyrosine kinase receptor for vascular endothelial growth factor receptor inhibits the growth of colon cancer liver metastasis and induces tumor and endothelial cell apoptosis. *Cancer Res* 1999; 59:5412–5416.

114. Fong TA, Shawver LK, Sun L, Tang C, App H, Powell TJ, et al. SU5416 is a potent and selective inhibitor of the vascular endothelial growth factor receptor (Flk-1/KDR) that inhibits tyrosine kinase catalysis, tumor vascularization, and growth of multiple tumor types. *Cancer Res* 1999; 59:99–106.

115. Okada F, Rak J, St Croix B, Lieubeau B, Kaya M, Roncari L, et al. Impact of oncogenes on tumor angiogenesis: mutant *K-ras* upregulation of VEGF/VPF is necessary but not sufficient for tumorigenicity of human colorectal carcinoma cells. *Proc Natl Acad Sci USA* 1998; 95:3609–3614.

116. Shi YP, Ferrara N. Oncogenic ras fails to restore an in vivo tumorigenic phenotype in embryonic stem cells lacking vascular endothelial growth factor (VEGF). *Biochem Biophys Res Commun* 1999; 254:480–483.

117. Grunstein J, Roberts WG, Mathieu-Costello O, Hanahan D, Johnson RS. Tumor-derived expression of vascular endothelial growth factor is a critical factor in tumor expansion and vascular function. *Cancer Res* 1999; 59:1592–1598.

118. Rosen K, Rak J, Leung T, Dean NM, Kerbel RS, Filmus J. Activated Ras prevents downregulation of Bcl-X(L) triggered by detachment from the extracellular matrix. A mechanism of Ras-induced resistance to anoikis in intestinal epithelial cells. *J Cell Biol* 2000; 149:447–456.

119. Robles AI, Rodriguez-Puebla ML, Glick AB, Trempus C, Hansen L, Sicinski P, et al. Reduced skin tumor development in cyclin D1-deficient mice highlights the oncogenic ras pathway in vivo. *Genes Dev* 1998; 12:2469–2474.

120. Kohl NE, Mosser SD, deSolms SJ, Giuliani EA, Pompliano DL, Graham SL, et al. Selective inhibition of *ras*-dependent transformation by a farnesyltransferase inhibitor. *Science* 1993; 260:1934–1942.

121. Tischer E, Mitchell R, Hartman T, Silva M, Gospodarowicz D, Fiddes JC. The human gene for vascular endothelial growth factor. *J Biol Chem* 1991; 266:11947–11954.

122. Shima DT, Kuroki M, Deutsch U, Ng YS, Adamis AP, D'Amore PA. The mouse gene for vascular endothelial growth factor. Genomic structure, definition of the transcriptional unit, and characterization of transcriptional and post-transcriptional regulatory sequences. *J Biol Chem* 1996; 271:3877–3883.

123. Levy AP, Levy NS, Goldberg MA. Post-transcriptional regulation of vascular endothelial growth factor by hypoxia. *J Biol Chem* 1996; 271:2746–2753.

124. Stein I, Neeman M, Shweiki D, Itin A, Keshet E. Stabilization of vascular endothelial growth factor mRNA by hypoxia and hypoglycemia and coregulation with other ischemia-induced genes. *Mol Cell Biol* 1995; 15:5363–5368.

125. Dibbens JA, Miller DL, Damert A, Risau W, Vadas MA, Goodall GJ. Hypoxic regulation of vascular endothelial growth factor mRNA stability requires the cooperation of multiple RNA elements. *Mol Biol Cell* 1999; 10:907–919.

126. Tober KL, Cannon RE, Spalding JW, Oberyszyn TM, Parrett ML, Rackoff AI, et al. Comparative expression of novel vascular endothelial growth factor/vascular permeability factor transcripts in skin, papillomas, and carcinomas of v-Ha-ras Tg.AC transgenic mice and FVB/N mice. *Biochem Biophys Res Commun* 1998; 247:644–653.

127. Kevil CG, De Benedetti A, Payne DK, Coe LL, Laroux FS, Alexander JS. Translational regulation of vascular permeability factor by eukaryotic initiation factor 4E: implications for tumor angiogenesis. *Int J Cancer* 1996; 65:785–790.

128. Stein I, Itin A, Einat P, Skaliter R, Grossman Z, Keshet E. Translation of vascular endothelial growth factor mRNA by internal ribosome entry: implications for translation under hypoxia. *Mol Cell Biol* 1998; 18:3112–3119.

129. DiSalvo J, Bayne ML, Conn G, Kwok PW, Trivedi PG, Soderman DD, et al. Purification and characterization of a naturally occurring vascular endothelial growth factor.placenta growth factor heterodimer. *J Biol Chem* 1995; 270:7717–7723.

130. Gangarosa LM, Sizemore N, Graves-Deal R, Oldham SM, Der CJ, Coffey RJ. A raf-independent epidermal growth factor receptor autocrine loop is necessary for Ras transformation of rat intestinal epithelial cells. *J Biol Chem* 1997; 272:18926–18931.

131. Hamilton M, Wolfman A. Oncogenic Ha-Ras-dependent mitogen-activated protein kinase activity requires signaling through the epidermal growth factor receptor. *J Biol Chem* 1998; 273:28155–28162.

132. Milanini J, Vinals F, Pouyssegur J, Pages G. p42/p44 MAP kinase module plays a key role in the transcriptional regulation of the vascular endothelial growth factor gene in fibroblasts. *J Biol Chem* 1998; 273:18165–18172.

133. Rak J, Filmus J, Finkenzeller G, Grugel S, Marme D, Kerbel RS. Oncogenes as inducers of tumor angiogenesis. *Cancer Metastasis Rev* 1995; 14:263–277.

134. Berra E, Pages G, Pouyssegur J. MAP kinases and hypoxia in the control of VEGF expression. *Cancer Metastasis Rev* 2000; 19:139–145.

135. Okajima E, Thorgeirsson UP. Different regulation of vascular endothelial growth factor expression by the ERK and p38 kinase pathways in v-ras, v-raf, and v-myc transformed cells. *Biochem Biophys Res Commun* 2000; 270:108–111.

136. Brondello JM, Brunet A, Pouyssegur J, McKenzie FR. The dual specificity mitogen-activated protein kinase phosphatase-1 and -2 are induced by the p42/p44MAPK cascade. *J Biol Chem* 1997; 272:1368–1376.

137. Pal S, Datta K, Khosravi-Far R, Mukhopadhyay D. Role of protein kinase czeta in ras-mediated transcriptional activation of vascular permeability factor/vascular endothelial growth factor expression. *J Biol Chem* 2001; 276:2395–2403.

138. Gille J, Swerlick RA, Caughman SW. Transforming growth factor-alpha-induced transcriptional activation of the vascular permeability factor (VPF/VEGF) gene requires AP-2-dependent DNA binding and transactivation. *EMBO J* 1997; 16:750–759.

139. Shields MJ, Der CJ. Mechanisms of Raf-independent Ras transformation Keystone Symposia X2, April 9–14, 1999 Abstract #3067, 203. 9-4-1999.

140. van Golen KL, Wu ZF, Qiao XT, Bao L, Merajver SD. RhoC GTPase overexpression modulates induction of angiogenic factors in breast cells. *Neoplasia* 2000; 2:418–425.

141. Lebowitz PF, Davide JP, Prendergast GC. Evidence that farnesyltransferase inhibitors suppress ras transformation by interfering with rho activity. *Mol Cell Biol* 1995; 15:6613–6622.

142. Lebowitz PF, Prendergast GC. Non-Ras targets of farnesyltransferase inhibitors: focus on Rho. *Oncogene* 1998; 17:1439–1445.

143. Feldkamp MM, Lau N, Guha A. Growth inhibition of astrocytoma cells by farnesyl transferase inhibitors is mediated by a combination of anti-proliferative, pro-apoptotic and anti-angiogenic effects. *Oncogene* 1999; 18:7514–7526.

144. Charvat S, Duchesne M, Parvaz P, Chignol MC, Schmitt D, Serres M. The up-regulation of vascular endothelial growth factor in mutated Ha-ras HaCaT cell lines is reduced by a farnesyl transferase inhibitor. *Anticancer Res* 1999; 19:557–561.

145. Gu WZ, Tahir SK, Wang YC, Zhang HC, Cherian SP, O'Connor S, et al. Effect of novel Caax peptidomimetic farnesyltransferase inhibitor on angiogenesis in vitro and in vivo. *Eur J Cancer* 1999; 35:1394–1401.

146. Bar-Sagi D, Hall A. Ras and Rho GTPases: a family reunion. *Cell* 2000; 103:227–238.

147. Garcia-Cardena G, Anderson KR, Mauri L, Gimbrone MA, Jr. Distinct mechanical stimuli differentially regulate the PI3K/Akt survival pathway in endothelial cells. *Ann NY Acad Sci* 2000; 902:294–297.

148. Riveline D, Zamir E, Balaban NQ, Schwarz US, Ishizaki T, Narumiya S, et al. Focal contacts as mechanosensors: externally applied local mechanical force induces growth of focal contacts by an mDial-dependent and ROCK-independent mechanism. *J Cell Biol* 2001; 153:1175–1186.

149. Alessi DR, Cuenda A, Cohen P, Dudley DT, Saltiel AR. PD 098059 is a specific inhibitor of the activation of mitogen- activated protein kinase kinase in vitro and in vivo. *J Biol Chem* 1995; 270:27489–27494.

150. Price LS, Collard JG. Regulation of the cytoskeleton by Rho-family GTPases: implications for tumour cell invasion. *Semin Cancer Biol* 2001; 11:167–173.

151. Irani K, Xia Y, Zweier JL, Sollott SJ, Der CJ, Fearon ER, et al. Mitogenic signaling mediated by oxidants in Ras-transformed fibroblasts. *Science* 1997; 275:1649–1652.
152. Kuroki M, Voest EE, Amano S, Beerepoot LV, Takashima S, Tolentino M, et al. Reactive oxygen intermediates increase vascular endothelial growth factor expression in vitro and in vivo. *J Clin Invest* 1996; 98:1667–1675.
153. White FC, Benehacene A, Scheele JS, Kamps M. VEGF mRNA is stabilized by ras and tyrosine kinase oncogenes, as well as by UV radiation—evidence for divergent stabilization pathways. *Growth Factors* 1997; 14:199–212.
154. Arbiser JL, Moses MA, Fernandez CA, Ghiso N, Cao Y, Klauber N, et al. Oncogenic H-ras stimulates tumor angiogenesis by two distinct pathways. *Proc Natl Acad Sci USA* 1997; 94:861–866.
155. Shweiki D, Itin A, Soffer D, Keshet E. Vascular endothelial growth factor induced by hypoxia may mediate hypoxia-initated angiogenesis. *Nature* 1992; 359:843–845.
156. Semenza GL. Hypoxia, clonal selection, and the role of HIF-1 in tumor progression. *Crit Rev Biochem Mol Biol* 2000; 35:71–103.
157. Mazure NM, Chen EY, Yeh P, Laderoute KR, Giaccia AJ. Oncogenic transformation and hypoxia synergistically act to modulate vascular endothelial growth factor expression. *Cancer Res* 1996; 56:3436–3440.
158. Mazure NM, Chen EY, Laderoute KR, Giaccia AJ. Induction of vascular endothelial growth factor by hypoxia is modulated by a phosphatidylinositol 3-kinase/Akt signaling pathway in Ha-ras-transformed cells through a hypoxia inducible factor-1 transcriptional element. *Blood* 1997; 90:3322–3331.
159. Zundel W, Schindler C, Haas-Kogan D, Koong A, Kaper F, Chen E, et al. Loss of PTEN facilitates HIF-1-mediated gene expression. *Genes Dev* 2000; 14:391–396.
160. Wen S, Stolarov J, Myers MP, Su JD, Wigler MH, Tonks NK, et al. PTEN controls tumor-induced angiogenesis. *Proc Natl Acad Sci USA* 2001; 98:4622–4627.
161. Zabrenetzky V, Harris CC, Steeg PS, Roberts DD. Expression of the extracellular matrix molecule thrombospondin inversely correlates with malignant progression in melanoma, lung and breast carcinoma cell lines. *Int J Cancer* 1994; 59:191–195.
162. Laderoute KR, Alarcon RM, Brody MD, Calaoagan JM, Chen EY, Knapp AM, et al. Opposing effects of hypoxia on expression of the angiogenic inhibitor thrombospondin 1 and the angiogenic inducer vascular endothelial growth factor [in process citation]. *Clin Cancer Res* 2000; 6:2941–2950.
163. Li J, Yen C, Liaw D, Podsypanina K, Bose S, Wang SI, et al. PTEN, a putative protein tyrosine phosphatase gene mutated in human brain, breast, and prostate cancer. *Science* 1997; 275:1943–1947.
164. Stambolic V, Suzuki A, de la Pompa JL, Brothers GM, Mirtsos C, Sasaki T, et al. Negative regulation of PKB/Akt-dependent cell survival by the tumor suppressor PTEN. *Cell* 1998; 95:29–39.
165. Jiang BH, Zheng JZ, Aoki M, Vogt PK. Phosphatidylinositol 3-kinase signaling mediates angiogenesis and expression of vascular endothelial growth factor in endothelial cells. *Proc Natl Acad Sci USA* 2000; 97:1749–1753.
166. Laughner E, Taghavi P, Chiles K, Mahon PC, Semenza GL. Her2 (neu) signaling increases the rate of hypoxia-inducible factor 1alpha (hif-1alpha) synthesis: novel mechanism for hif-1-mediated vascular endothelial growth factor expression. *Mol Cell Biol* 2001; 21:3995–4004.
167. Feldkamp MM, Lau N, Rak J, Kerbel RS, Guha A. Normoxic and hypoxic regulation of vascular endothelial growth factor (VEGF) by astrocytoma cells is mediated by Ras. *Int J Cancer* 1999; 81:118–124.
168. Richard DE, Berra E, Gothie E, Roux D, Pouyssegur J. p42/p44 mitogen-activated protein kinases phosphorylate hypoxia-inducible factor 1alpha (HIF-1alpha) and enhance the transcriptional activity of HIF-1. *J Biol Chem* 1999; 274:32631–32637.
169. Chen C, Pore N, Behrooz A, Ismail-Beigi F, Maity A. Regulation of glut1 mRNA by hypoxia-inducible factor-1. Interaction between H-ras and hypoxia. *J Biol Chem* 2001; 276:9519–9525.
170. Jiang BH, Agani F, Passaniti A, Semenza GL. V-SRC induces expression of hypoxia-inducible factor 1 (HIF-1) and transcription of genes encoding vascular endothelial growth factor and enolase 1: involvement of HIF-1 in tumor progression. *Cancer Res* 1997; 57:5328–5335.
171. Koong AC, Chen EY, Mivechi F, Denko NC, Stambrook P, Giaccia AJ. Hypoxic activation of nuclear factor-KB is mediated by a *ras* and *raf* signaling. *Cancer Res* 1994; 54:5273–5279.
172. Mukhopadhyay D, Tsiokas L, Zhou X-M, Foster D, Brugge JS, Sukhatme VP. Hypoxic induction of human vascular endothelial growth factor expression through c-Src activation. *Nature* 1995; 375:577–581.

173. Shima DT, Deutsch U, D'Amore PA. Hypoxic induction of vascular endothelial growth factor (VEGF) in human epithelial cells is mediated by increases in mRNA stability. *FEBS Lett* 1995; 370:203–208.

174. Kerbel R, Viloria-Petit A, Okada F, Rak J. The link between oncogenes, signal transduction therapy, and tumor angiogenesis. In: Voest EE, D'Amore P, eds. *Tumor Angiogenesis and Microcirculation.* Marcel Dekker, New York, 2001; pp. 285–307.

175. Graeber TG, Osmanian C, jacks T, Housman DE, Koch CJ, Lowe SW, et al. Hypoxia-mediated selection of cells with diminished apoptotic potential in solid tumours. *Nature* 1996; 379:88–91.

176. Dang CV, Semenza GL. Oncogenic alterations of metabolism. *Trends Biochem Sci* 1999; 24:68–72.

177. Los M, Voes EE. Genetic control of angiogenesis by tumor suppressor genes. In: Voes EE, D'Amore P, eds. *Tumor Angiogenesis and Microcirculation.* Marcel Dekker, New York, 2001; pp. 307–320.

178. Koura AN, Liu W, Kitadai Y, Singh RK, Radinsky R, Ellis LM. Regulation of vascular endothelial growth factor expression in human colon carcinoma cells by cell density. *Cancer Res* 1996; 56:3891–3894.

179. Mukhopadhyay D, Tsiokas L, Sukhatme VP. High cell density induces vascular endothelial growth factor expression via protein tyrosine phosphorylation. *Gene Expr* 1998; 7:53–60.

180. Sheta EA, Harding MA, Conaway MR, Theodorescu D. Focal adhesion kinase, Rap 1, and transcriptional induction of vascular endothelial growth factor. *J Natl Cancer Inst* 2000; 92:1065–1073.

181. Barker N, Morin PJ, Clevers H. The Yin-Yang of TCF/beta-catenin signaling. *Adv Cancer Res* 2000; 77:1–24.

182. Kolligs FT, Hu G, Dang CV, Fearon ER. Neoplastic transformation of RK3E by mutant beta-catenin requires deregulation of Tcf/Lef transcription but not activation of c-myc expression. *Mol Cell Biol* 1999; 19:5696–5706.

183. Novak A, Hsu SC, Leung-Hagesteijn C, Radeva G, Papkoff J, Montesano R, et al. Cell adhesion and the integrin-linked kinase regulate the LEF-1 and beta-catenin signaling pathways. *Proc Natl Acad Sci USA* 1998; 95:4374–4379.

184. Hahn WC, Counter CM, Lundberg AS, Beijersbergen RL, Brooks MW, Weinberg RA. Creation of human tumour cells with defined genetic elements [see comments]. *Nature* 1999; 400:464–468.

185. Serrano M, Lin AW, McCurrach ME, Beach D, Lowe SW. Oncogenic ras provokes premature cell senescence associated with accumulation of p53 and p16INK4a. *Cell* 1997; 88:593–602.

186. Holland EC, Hively WP, DePincho RA, Varmus HE. A constitutively active epidermal growth factor receptor cooperates with disruption of G1 cell-cycle arrest pathways to induce glioma-like lesions in mice. *Genes Dev* 1998; 12:3675–3685.

187. Ferbeyre G, de Stanchina E, Querido E, Baptiste N, Prives C, Lowe SW. PML is induced by oncogenic ras and promotes premature senescence. *Genes Dev* 2000; 14:2015–2027.

188. Harada H, Nakagawa K, Iwata S, Saito M, Kumon Y, Sakaki S, et al. Restoration of wild-type *p 16* down-regulates vascular endothelial growth factor expression and inhibits angiogenesis in human gliomas. *Cancer Res* 1999; 59:3783–3789.

189. Claudio PP, Stiegler P, Howard CM, Bellan C, Minimo C, Tosi GM, et al. RB2/p 130 gene-enhanced expression down-regulates vascular endothelial growth factor expression and inhibits angiogenesis in vivo. *Cancer Res* 2001; 61:462–468.

190. Schwarte-Waldhoff I, Volpert OV, Bouck NP, Sipos B, Hahn SA, Klein-Scory, S, et al. Smad4/DPC4-mediated tumor suppression through suppression of angiogenesis. *Proc Natl Acad Sci USA* 2000; 97:9624–9629.

191. Mukhopadhyay D, Tsiokas L, Sukhatme VP. Wild-type p53 and v-Src exert opposing influences on human vascular endothelial growth factor gene expression. *Cancer Res* 1995; 55:6161–6165.

192. Kieser A, Weich HA, Brandner G, Marme D, Kolch W. Mutant p53 potentiates protein kinase C induction of vascular endothelial growth factor expression. *Oncogene* 1994; 9:963–969.

193. Volpert OV, Dameron KM, Bouck N. Sequential development of an angiogenic phenotype by human fibroblasts progressing to tumorigenicity. *Oncogene* 1997; 14:1495–1502.

194. Bergers G, Javaherian K, Lo KM, Folkman J, Hanahan D. Effects of angiogenesis inhibitors on multistage carcinogenesis in mice. *Science* 1999; 284:808–812.

195. Ferrara N. The role of vascular endothelial growth factor in pathological angiogenesis. *Breast Cancer Res Treat* 1995; 36:127–137.

196. Fukumura D, Xavier R, Sugiura T, Chen Y, Park EC, Lu N, et al. Tumor induction of VEGF promoter activity in stromal cells. *Cell* 1998; 94:715–725.

197. Yoshiji H, Harris SR, Thorgeirsson UP. Vascular endothelial growth factor is essential for initial but not continued in vivo growth of human breast carcinoma cells. *Cancer Res* 1997; 57:3924–3928.

198. Rak J, Miguerol L, Lobe C, Nagy A, Gertsenstein M, Sheehan C, et al. Dependence of tumor angiogenesis on endogenous VEGF production as a function of tumor type. Keystone Symposia April 24-29, 2001, Angiogenesis and Chronic Diseases, Abstract #310, 61. 27-4-2001.

199. Relf M, LeJeune S, Scott PA, Fox S, Smith K, Leek R, et al. Expression of the angiogenic factors vascular endothelial cell growth factor, acidic and basic fibroblast growth factor, tumor growth factor beta-1, platelet-derived endothelial cell growth factor, placenta growth factor, and pleiotrophin in human primary breast cancer and its relation to angiogenesis. *Cancer Res* 1997; 57:963–969.

200. Dvorak HF, Dvorak AM, Manseau EJ, Wiberg L, Churchill WH. Fibrin gel investment associated with line 1 and line 10 solid tumor growth, angiogenesis, and fibroplasia in guinea pigs. Role of cellular immunity, myofibroblasts, microvascular damage, and infarction in line 1 tumor regression. *J Natl Cancer Inst* 1979; 62:1459–1472.

201. Dvorak FH. Abnormalities of hemostasis in malignant disease. In: Coleman RB, Hirsh J, Marder VJ, Salzman JB, eds. *Hemostasis and Thrombosis: Basic Principles and Clinical Practice, 3rd ed.* Lippincott, Philadelphia, 1994, pp. 1238–1254.

202. Rak J, Klement G. Impact of oncogenes and tumor suppressor genes on deregulation of hemostasis and angiogenesis in cancer. *Cancer Metastasis Rev* 2000; 19:93–96.

203. Mechtcheriakova D, Wlachos A, Holzmuller H, Binder BR, Hofer E. Vascular endothelial cell growth factor-induced tissue factor expression in endothelial cells is mediated by EGR-1. *Blood* 1999; 93:3811–3823.

204. Shoji M, Hancock WW, Abe K, Micko C, Casper KA, Baine RM, et al. Activation of coagulation and angiogenesis in cancer: immunohistochemical localization in situ of clotting proteins and vascular endothelial growth factor in human cancer. *Am J Pathol* 1998; 152:399–411.

205. Carmeliet P, Mackman N, Moons L, Luther T, Gressens P, Van VI, et al. Role of tissue factor in embryonic blood vessel development. *Nature* 1996; 383:73–75.

206. Zhang Y, Deng Y, Luther T, Muller M, Ziegler R, Waldherr R, et al. Tissue factor controls the balance of angiogenic and antiangiogenic properties of tumor cells in mice. *J Clin Invest* 1994; 94:1320–1327.

207. Coughlin SR. Thrombin signalling and protease-activated receptors. *Nature* 2000; 407:258–264.

208. Tallman MS. The thrombophilic state in acute promyelocytic leukemia. *Semin Thromb Hemost* 1999; 25:209–215.

209. Kini AR, Peterson LC, Tallman MS, Lingen MW. Angiogenesis in acute promyelocytic leukemia: induction by vascular endothelial growth factor and inhibition by all-trans retinoic acid. *Blood* 2001; 97:3919–3924.

210. Browder T, Folkman J, Pirie-Shephered S. The hemostatic system as a regulator of angiogenesis. *J Biol Chem* 2000; 275:1521–1524.

211. Dawson DW, Bouck NP. Thrombospondin as an inhibitor of angiogenesis. In: Teicher BA, ed. *Antiangiogenic Agents in Cancer Therapy.* Humana Press, Totowa, 1999, pp. 185–203.

212. Iruela-Arispe ML, Vazquez F, Ortega MA. Antiangiogenic domains shared by thrombospondins and metallospondins, a new family of angiogenic inhibitors. *Ann NY Acad Sci* 1999; 886:58–66.

213. Dawson DW, Volpert OV, Gillis P, Crawford SE, Xu H, Benedict W, et al. Pigment epithelium-derived factor: a potent inhibitor of angiogenesis. *Science* 1999; 285:245–248.

214. Van Meir EG, Polverini PJ, Chazin VR, Su Huang HJ, de Tribolet N, Cavenee WK. Release of an inhibitor of angiogenesis upon induction of wild type p53 expression in glioblastoma cells. *Nat Genet* 1994; 8:171–176.

215. Zhai Y, Ni J, Jiang GW, Lu J, Xing L, Lincoln C, et al. VEGI, a novel cytokine of the tumor necrosis factor family, is an angiogenesis inhibitor that suppresses the growth of colon carcinomas in vivo. *FASEB J* 1999; 13:181–189.

216. Nelson J, Allen WE, Scott WN, Bailie JR, Walker B, McFerran NV, et al. Murine epidermal growth factor (EGF) fragment (33-42) inhibits both EGF-and laminin-dependent endothelial cell motility and angiogenesis. *Cancer Res* 1995; 55:3772–3776.

217. Nishimori H, Shiratsuchi T, Urano T, Kimura Y, Kiyono K, Tatsumi K, et al. A novel brain-specific p53-target gene, BAI1, containing thrombospondin type 1 repeats inhibits experimental angiogenesis. *Oncogene* 1997; 15:2145–2150.

218. Zhang M, Volpert O, Shi YH, Bouck N. Maspin is an angiogenesis inhibitor. *Nat Med* 2000; 6:196–199.

219. O'Reilly MS, Boehm T, Shing Y, Fukai N, Vasios G, Lane WS, et al. Endostatin: an endogenous inhibitor of angiogenesis and tumor growth. *Cell* 1997; 88:277–285.

220. Brooks PC, Silletti S, von Schalscha TL, Friedlander M, Cheresh DA. Disruption of angiogenesis by PEX, a noncatalytic metalloproteinase fragment with integrin binding activity. *Cell* 1998; 92:391–400.

221. Colman RW, Jameson BA, Lin Y, Johnson D, Mousa SA. Domain 5 of high molecular weight kininogen (kininostatin) down-regulates endothelial cell proliferation and migration and inhibits angiogenesis. *Blood* 2000; 95:543–550.

222. Clapp C, Martial JA, Guzman RC, Rentier-Delrue F, Weiner RI. The 16-kilodalton N-terminal fragment of human prolactin is a potent inhibitor of angiogenesis. *Endocrinology* 1993; 133:1292–1299.

223. Homandberg GA, Williams JE, Grant D, Schumacher B, Eisenstein R. Heparin-binding fragments of fibronectin are potent inhibitors of endothelial cell growth. *Am J Pathol* 1985; 120:327–332.

224. Ramchandran R, Dhanabal M, Volk R, Waterman MJ, Segal M, Lu H, et al. Antiangiogenic activity of restin, NC10 domain of human collagen XV: comparison to endostatin. *Biochem Biophys Res Commun* 1999; 255:735–739.

225. Colorado PC, Torre A, Kamphaus G, Maeshima Y, Hopfer H, Takahashi K, et al. Anti-angiogenic cues from vascular basement membrane collagen. *Cancer Res* 2000; 60:2520–2526.

226. Kamphaus GD, Colorado PC, Panka DJ, Hopfer H, Ramchandran R, Torre A, et al. Canstatin, a novel matrix-derived inhibitor of angiogenesis and tumor growth. *J Biol Chem* 2000; 275:1209–1215.

227. Maeshima Y, Manfredi M, Reimer C, Holthaus KA, Hopfer H, Chandamuri B. et al. Identification of the anti-angiogenic site within vascular basement membrane-derived tumstatin. *J Biol Chem* 2001; 276:15240–15248.

228. Pike SE, Yao L, Jones KD, Cherney B, Appella E, Sakaguchi K, et al. Vasostatin, a calreticulin fragment, inhibits angiogenesis and suppresses tumor growth. *J Exp Med* 1998; 188:2349–2356.

229. O'Reilly MS, Holmgren L, Shing Y, Chen C, Rosenthal RA, Moses M, et al. Angiostatin: a novel angiogenesis inhibitor that mediates the suppression of metastases by a Lewis lung carcinoma. *Cell* 1994; 79:315–328.

230. O'Reilly MS, Pirie-Shepherd S, Lane WS, Folkman J. Antiangiogenic activity of the cleaved conformation of the serpin antithrombin [see comments]. *Science* 1999; 285:1926–1928.

231. Rak J. Possible role of tumour stem — end cell interaction in metastasis. *Med Hypoth* 1989; 29:17–19.

232. Nowell PC. The clonal evolution of tumor cell populations. *Science* 1976; 194:23–28.

233. Kerbel, RS. Growth dominance of the metastatic cancer cell: cellular and molecular aspects. *Adv Cancer Res* 1990; 55:87–132.

234. Jouanneau J, Moens G, Bourgeois Y, Poupon MF, Thiery JP. A minority of carcinoma cells producing acidic fibroblast growth factor induces a community effect for tumor progression. *Proc Natl Acad Sci USA* 1994; 91:286–290.

235. Miller FR, Heppner GH. Cellular interactions in metastasis. *Cancer Metastasis Rev* 1990; 9:21–34.

236. Rak J, Mitsuhashi Y, Erdos V, Huang S.-N., Filmus J, Kerbel RS. Massive programmed cell death in intestinal epithelial cells induced by three-dimensional growth conditions: suppression by expression of a mutant c-H-*ras* oncogene. *J Cell Biol* 1995; 131:1587–1598.

237. Rak J, Mitsuhashi Y, Sheehan C, Krestow JK, Florenes VA, Filmus J, et al. Collateral expression of proangiogenic and tumorigenic properties in intestinal epithelial cell variants selected for resistance to anoikis. *Neoplasia* 1999; 1:23–30.

238. Marshall CJ. Specificity of receptor tyrosine kinase signaling: transient versus sustained extracellular signal-regulated kinase activation. *Cell* 1995; 80:179–185.

239. Charoenrat P, Rhys-Evans P, Modjtahedi H, Eccles SA. Vascular endothelial growth factor family members are differentially regulated by c-erbB signaling in head and neck squamous carcinoma cells. *Clin Exp Metastasis* 2000; 18:155–161.

240. Rak J, Kerbel RS. Treating cancer by inhibiting angiogenesis: new hopes and potential pitfalls. *Cancer Metastasis Rev* 1996; 15:231–236.

241. Bedi A, Pasricha PJ, Akhtar AJ, Barber JP, Bedi GC, Giardiello FM, et al. Inhibition of apoptosis during development of colorectal cancer. *Cancer Res* 1995; 55:1811–1816.

242. Evan GI, Vousden KH. Proliferation, cell cycle and apoptosis in cancer. *Nature* 2001; 411:342–348.

243. Carmeliet P, Dor Y, Herbert JM, Fukumura D, Brusselmans K, Dewerchin M, et al. Role of HIF-1alpha in hypoxia-mediated apoptosis, cell proliferation and tumour angiogenesis [published erratum appears in Nature 1998 Oct 1;395(6701):525]. *Nature* 1998; 394:485–490.

244. Yu JL, Rak JW, Carmeliet P, Nagy A, Kerbel RS, Coomber BL. Heterogeneous vascular dependence of tumor cell populations. *Am J Pathol* 2001; 158:1325–1334.

245. Olive PL, Chaplin DJ, Durand RE. Pharmacokinetics, binding and distribution of Hoechst 33342 in spheroids and murine tumours. *Br J Cancer* 1985; 52:739–746.

246. Weidner N, Folkman J, Pozza F, Bevilacqua P, Allred EN, Moore DH, et al. Tumor angiogenesis: a new significant and independent prognostic indicator in early-stage breast carcinoma. *J Natl Cancer Inst* 1992; 84:1875–1887.

247. Abdalla SA, Behzad F, Bsharah S, Kumar S, Amini SK, O'Dwyer ST, et al. Prognostic relevance of microvessel density in colorectal tumours. *Oncol Rep* 1999; 6:839–842.
248. Teicher BA. Angiogenesis and cancer metastases: therapeutic approaches. *Crit Rev Onco Hematol* 1995; 20:9–39.
249. Browder T, Butterfield CE, Kraling BM, Shi B, Marshall B, O'Reilly MS, et al. Antiangiogenic scheduling of chemotherapy improves efficacy against experimental drug-resistant cancer. *Cancer Res* 2000; 60:1878–1886.
250. Klement G, Baruchel S, Rak J, Man S, Clark K, Hicklin DJ, et al. Continuous low-dose therapy with vinblastine and VEGF receptor-2 antibody induces sustained tumor regression without overt toxicity [in process citation]. *J Clin Invest* 2000; 105:R15–R24.
251. Padro T, Ruiz S, Bieker R, Burger H, Steins M, Kienast J, et al. Increased angiogenesis in the bone marrow of patients with acute myeloid leukemia. *Blood* 2000; 95:2637–2644.
252. Hussong JW, Rodgers GM, Shami PJ. Evidence of increased angiogenesis in patients with acute myeloid leukemia. *Blood* 2000; 95:309–313.
253. Katoh O, Tauchi H, Kawaishi K, Kimura A, Satow Y. Expression of the vascular endothelial growth factor (VEGF) receptor gene, KDR, in hematopoietic cells and inhibitory effect of VEGF on apoptotic cell death caused by ionizing radiation. *Cancer Res* 1995; 55:5687–5692.
254. Luo JC, Yamaguchi S, Shinkai A, Shitara K, Shibuya M. Significant expression of vascular endothelial growth factor/vascular permeability factor in mouse ascites tumors. *Cancer Res* 1998; 58:2652–2660.
255. Aguayo A, Kantarjian H, Manshouri T, Gidel C, Estey E, Thomas D, et al. Angiogenesis in acute and chronic leukemias and myelodysplastic syndromes. *Blood* 2000; 96:2240–2245.
256. Scappaticci FA, Smith R, Pathak A, Schloss D, Lum B, Cao Y, et al. Combination angiostatin and endostatin gene transfer induces synergistic antiangiogenic activity in vitro and antitumor efficacy in leukemia and solid tumors in mice. *Mol Ther* 2001; 3:186–196.
257. Ben-David Y. Bernstein A. Friend virus-induced erythroleukemia and the multistage nature of cancer. *Cell* 1991; 66:831–834.
258. Murray MJ, Cunningham JM, Parada LF, Dautry F, Lebowitz P, Weinberg, RA. The HL-60 transforming sequence: a ras oncogene coexisting with altered myc genes in hematopoietic tumors. *Cell* 1983; 33:749–757.
259. Adams J.M, Cory S. Oncogene co-operation in leukaemogenesis. *Cancer Surv* 1992; 15:119–141.
260. Reuter CW, Morgan MA, Bergmann L. Targeting the Ras signaling pathway: a rational, mechanism-based treatment for hematologic malignancies? *Blood* 2000; 96:1655–1669.
261. Druker BJ, Sawyers CL, Kantarjian H, Resta DJ, Reese SF, Ford JM, et al. Activity of a specific inhibitor of the BCR-ABL tyrosine kinase in the blast crisis of chronic myeloid leukemia and acute lymphoblastic leukemia with the Philadelphia chromosome. *N Engl J Med* 2001; 344:1038–1042.
262. Kakizuka A, Miller WH Jr., Umesono K, Warrell RP Jr., Frankel SR, Murty VV, et al. Chromosomal translocation t(15;17) in human acute promyelocytic leukemia fuses RAR alpha with a novel putative transcription factor, PML. *Cell* 1991; 66:663–674.
263. Pandolfi PP. Oncogenes and tumor suppressors in the molecular pathogenesis of acute promyelocytic leukemia. *Hum Mol Genet* 2001; 10:769–775.
264. Druker BJ, Talpaz M, Resta DJ, Peng, B, Buchdunger E, Ford, JM, et al. Efficacy and safety of a specific inhibitor of the BCR-ABL tyrosine kinase in chronic myeloid leukemia. *N Engl J Med* 2001; 344:1031–1037.
265. Gunsilius E, Duba HC, Petzer AL, Kahler CM, Grunewald K, Stockhammer G, et al. Evidence from a leukaemia model for maintenance of vascular endothelium by bone-marrow-derived endothelial cells. *Lancet* 2000; 355:1688–1691.
266. Blume-Jensen P, Hunter T. Oncogenic kinase signalling. *Nature* 2001; 411:355–365.
267. McCormick F. Signalling networks that cause cancer. *Trends Cell Biol* 1999; 9:M53–M56.
268. Sebti SM, Hamilton AD. Farnesyltransferase and geranylgeranyltransferase I inhibitors and cancer therapy: lessons from mechanism and bench-to-bedside translational studies. *Oncogene* 2000; 19:6584–6593.
269. Fletcher L. Approval heralds new generation of kinase inhibitors? *Nat Biotechnol* 2001; 19:599–600.
270. Gibbs JB, Oliff A, Kohl NE. Farnesyltransferase inhibitors: ras research yields a potential cancer therapeutic. *Cell* 1994; 77:175–178.
271. Lebowitz PF, Sakamuro D, Prendergast GC. Farnesyl transferase inhibitors induce apoptosis of Ras-transformed cells denied substratum attachment. *Cancer Res* 1997; 57:708–713.
272. Viloria-Petit A, Crombet T, Jothy S, Hicklin D, Bohlen P, Schlaeppi JM, et al. Acquired resistance to the antitumor effect of epidermal growth factor receptor-blocking antibodies in vivo: a role for altered tumor angiogenesis. *Cancer Res* 2001; 61:5090–5101.

273. Ciardiello F, Bianco R, Damiano V, Fontanini G, Caputo R, Pomatico G, et al. Antiangiogenic and antitumor activity of anti-epidermal growth factor receptor C225 monoclonal antibody in combination with vascular endothelial growth factor antisense oligonucleotide in human GEO colon cancer cells. *Clin Cancer Res* 2000; 6:3739–3747.

274. Ciardiello F, Damiano V, Bianco R, Bianco C, Fontanini G, De Laurentiis M, et al. Antitumor activity of combined blockade of epidermal growth factor receptor and protein kinase A. *J Natl Cancer Inst* 1996; 88:1770–1776.

275. Perrotte P, Matsumoto T, Inoue K, Kuniyasu H, Eve BY, Hicklin DJ, et al. Anti-epidermal growth factor receptor antibody C225 inhibits angiogenesis in human transitional cell carcinoma growing orthotopically in nude mice. *Clin Cancer Res* 1999; 5:257–265.

276. Mishima K, Johns TG, Luwor RB, Scott AM, Stockert E, Jungbluth AA, et al. Growth suppression of intracranial xenografted glioblastomas overexpressing mutant epidermal growth factor receptors by systemic administration of monoclonal antibody (mAb) 806, a novel monoclonal antibody directed to the receptor. *Cancer Res* 2001; 61:5349–5354.

277. Ciardiello F, Caputo R, Bianco R, Damiano V, Fontanini G, Cuccato S, et al. Inhibition of growth factor production and angiogenesis in human cancer cells by ZD1839 (Iressa), a selective epidermal growth factor receptor tyrosine kinase inhibitor. *Clin Cancer Res* 2001; 7:1459–1465.

278. Bruns CJ, Solorzano CC, Harbison MT, Ozawa S, Tsan R, Fan D, et al. Blockade of the epidermal growth factor receptor signaling by a novel tyrosine kinase inhibitor leads to apoptosis of endothelial cells and therapy of human pancreatic carcinoma. *Cancer Res* 2000; 60:2926–2935.

279. Cai T, Fassina G, Morini M, Aluigi MG, Masiello L, Fontanini G, et al. N-acetylcysteine inhibits endothelial cell invasion and angiogenesis. *Lab Invest* 1999; 79:1151–1159.

280. Gately S. The contributions of cyclooxygenase-2 to tumor angiogenesis. *Cancer Metastasis Rev* 2000; 19:19–27.

281. Lefer AM, Scalia R, Lefer DJ. Vascular effects of HMG CoA-reductase inhibitors (statins) unrelated to cholesterol lowering: new concepts for cardiovascular disease. *Cardiovasc Res* 2001; 49:281–287.

282. Feleszko W, Balkowiec EZ, Sieberth E, Marczak M, Dabrowska A, Giermasz A, et al. Lovastatin and tumor necrosis factor-alpha exhibit potentiated antitumor effects against Ha-ras-transformed murine tumor via inhibition of tumor-induced angiogenesis. *Int J Cancer* 1999; 81:560–567.

283. Isner JM. Recruitment of endothelial cell precursors in angiogenesis. Keystone Symposia Abstract Book Keystone Symposium X1, 4/24-29/2001(Angiogeesis and Chronic Disease), 31. 2001.

284. Slack JL, Bornstein P. Transformation by v-src causes transient induction followed by repression of mouse thrombospondin-1. *Cell Growth Differ* 1994; 5:1373–1380.

285. Bein K, Ware JA, Simons M. Myb-dependent regulation of thrombospondin 2 expression. Role of mRNA stability. *J Biol Chem* 1998; 273:21423–21429.

286. Meitar D, Crawford SE, Rademaker AW, Cohn SL. Tumor angiogenesis correlates with metastatic disease, N-myc amplification, and poor outcome in human neuroblastoma. *J Clin Oncol* 1996; 14:405–414.

287. Fotsis T, Breit S, Lutz W, Rossler J, Hatzi E, Schwab M, et al. Down-regulation of endothelial cell growth inhibitors by enhanced MYCN oncogene expression in human neuroblastoma cells. *Eur J Biochem* 1999; 263:757–764.

288. Hatzi E, Breit S, Zoephel A, Ashman K, Tontsch U, Ahorn H, et al. MYCN oncogene and angiogenesis: down-regulation of endothelial growth inhibitors in human neuroblastoma cells. Purification, structural, and functional characterization. *Adv Exp Med Biol* 2000; 476:239–248.

289. Breit S, Ashman K, Wilting J, Rossler J, Hatzi E, Fotsis T, et al. The N-myc oncogene in human neuroblastoma cells: down-regulation of an angiogenesis inhibitor identified as activin A. *Cancer Res* 2000; 60:4596–4601.

290. Schweigerer L., Schwab M, Fotsis T. Endothelial cell growth factors in human neuroblastoma cells transfected with the human MYCN oncogene. International Symposium on Angiogenesis. 1991.

291. Pelengaris S, Littlewood T, Khan M, Elia G, Evan G. Reversible activation of c-Myc in skin: induction of a complex neoplastic phenotype by a single oncogenic lesion. *Mol Cell* 1999; 3:565–577.

292. Yen L, You XL, Al Moustafa AE, Batist G, Hynes NE, Mader S, et al. Heregulin selectively upregulates vascular endothelial growth factor secretion in cancer cells and stimulates angiogenesis. *Oncogene* 2000; 19:3460–3469.

293. Fernandez A, Udagawa T, Schwesinger C, Beecken W, Achilles-Gerte E, McDonnell T, et al. Angiogenic potential of prostate carcinoma cells overexpressing bcl-2. *J Natl Cancer Inst* 2001; 93:208–213.

294. Sheibani N, Sorenson CM, Cornelius LA, Frazier WA. Thrombospondin-1, a natural inhibitor of angiogenesis, is present in vitreous and aqueous humor and is modulated by hyperglycemia. *Biochem Biophys Res Commun* 2000; 267:257–261.

295. Saez E, Rutberg SE, Mueller E, Oppenheim H, Smoluk J, Yuspa SH, et al. c-*fos* is required for malignant progression for skin tumors. *Cell* 1995; 82:721–732.

296. McGregor LM, McCune BK, Graff JR, McDowell PR, Romans KE, Yancopoulos GD, et al. Roles of trk family neurotrophin receptors in medullary thyroid carcinoma development and progression. *Proc Natl Acad Sci USA* 1999; 96:4540–4545.

297. Eggert A, Grotzer MA, Ikegaki N, Liu XG, Evans AE, Brodeur GM. Expression of neurotrophin receptor TrkA inhibits angiogenesis in neuroblastoma. *Med Pediatr Oncol* 2000; 35:569–572.

298. Le Buanec H, D'Anna R, Lachgar A, Zagury JF, Bernard J, Ittele D, et al. HPV-16 E7 but not E6 oncogenic protein triggers both cellular immunosuppression and angiogenic processes. *Biomed Pharmacother* 1999; 53:424–431.

299. Lopez-Ocejo O, Viloria-Petit A, Bequet-Romero M, Mukhopadhyay D, Rak J, Kerbel RS. Oncogenes and tumor angiogenesis: the HPV-16 E6 oncoprotein activates the vascular endothelial growth factor (VEGF) gene promoter in a p53 independent manner [in process citation]. *Oncogene* 2000; 19:4611–4620.

300. Zietz C, Rossle M, Haas C, Sendelhofert A, Hirschmann A, Sturzl M, et al. U. MDM-2 oncoprotein overexpression, p53 gene mutation, and VEGF up-regulation in angiosarcomas. *Am J Pathol* 1998; 153:1425–1433.

301. Auvinen M, Laine A, Paasinen-Sohns A, Kangas A, Kangas L, Saksela O, et al. Human ornithine decarboxylase-overproducing NIH3T3 cells induce rapidly growing, highly vascularized tumors in nude mice. *Cancer Res* 1997; 57:3016–3025.

302. Heaney AP, Horwitz GA, Wang Z, Singson R, Melmed S. Early involvement of estrogen-induced pituitary tumor transforming gene and fibroblast growth factor expression in prolactinoma pathogenesis. *Nat Med* 1999; 5:1317–1321.

303. Fu X, Roberts WG, Nobile V, Shapiro R, Kamps MP. mAngiogenin-3, a target gene of oncoprotein E2a-Pbx1, encodes a new angiogenic member of the angiogenin family. *Growth Factors* 1999; 17:125–137.

304. Bais C, Santomasso B, Coso O, Arvanitakis L, Raaka EG, Gutkind JS, et al. G-protein-coupled receptor of Kaposi's sarcoma-associated herpesvirus is a viral oncogene and angiogenesis activator [see comments] [published erratum appears in Nature 1998 Mar 12;392(6672):210]. *Nature* 1998; 391:86–89.

305. Sodhi A, Montaner S, Patel V, Zohar M, Bais C, Mesri EA, et al. The Kaposi's sarcoma-associated herpes virus G protein-coupled receptor up-regulates vascular endothelial growth factor expression and secretion through mitogen-activated protein kinase and p38 pathways acting on hypoxia-inducible factor 1alpha. *Cancer Res* 2000; 60:4873–4880.

306. Iberg N, Rogelj S, Fanning P, Klagsbrun M. Purification of 18-and 22-kDa forms of basic fibroblast growth factor from rat cells transformed by the ras oncogene. *J Biol Chem* 1989; 264:19951–19955.

307. Chotani MA, Touhalisky K, Chiu IM. The small GTPases Ras, Rac, and Cdc42 transcriptionally regulate expression of human fibroblast growth factor 1. *J Biol Chem* 2000; 275:30432–30438.

308. Marshall CJ, Vousden K, Ozanne B. The involvement of activated ras genes in determining the transformed phenotype. *Proc R Soc Lond B Biol Sci* 1985; 226:99–106.

309. Glick AB, Sporn MB, Yuspa SH. Altered regulation of TGF-beta 1 and TGF-alpha in primary keratinocytes and papillomas expressing v-Ha-ras. *Mol Carcinog* 1991; 4:210–219.

310. Castelli C, Sensi M, Lupetti R, Mortarini R, Panceri P, Anichini A, et al. Expression of interleukin 1 alpha, interleukin 6, and tumor necrosis factor alpha genes in human melanoma clones is associated with that of mutated N-RAS oncogene. *Cancer Res* 1994; 54:4785–4790.

311. Demetri GD, Ernst TJ, Pratt II ES, Zenzle BW, Rheinwald JG, Griffin J. D. Expression of *ras* oncogenes in cultured human cells alters the transcriptional posttranscriptional regulation of cytokine genes. *J Clin Invest* 1990; 86:1261–1269.

312. Dickson RB, Kasid A, Huff KK, Bates SE, Knabbe C, Bronzert D, et al. Activation of growth factor secretion in tumorigenic states of breast cancer induced by 17β-estradiol or v-Ha-*ras* oncogene. *Proc Natl Acad Sci USA* 1987; 84:837–841.

313. Bowen-Pope DF, Vogel A, Ross R. Production of platelet-derived growth factor-like molecules and reduced expression of platelet-derived growth factor receptors accompany transformation by a wide spectrum of agents. *Proc Natl Acad Sci USA* 1984; 81:2396–2400.

314. Craig AM, Nemir M, Mukherjee BB, Chambers AF, Denhardt DT. Identification of the major phosphoprotein secreted by many rodent cell lines as 2ar/osteopontin: enhanced expression in H-ras-transformed 3T3 cells. *Biochem Biophys Res Commun* 1988; 157:166–173.

315. Cohen RL, Niclas J, Lee WM, Wun TC, Crowley CW, Levinson AD, et al. Effects of cellular transformation on expression of plasminogen activator inhibitors 1 and 2. Evidence for independent regulation. *J Biol Chem* 1989; 264:8375–8383.

316. Arbiser JL, Petros J, Klafter R, Govindajaran B, McLaughlin ER, Brown LF, Cohen C, Moses M, Kilroy S, Arnold RS, Lambeth JD. Reactive oxygen generated by NOX-1 triggers the angiogenic switch. *Proc Natl Acad Sci USA* 2002; 2:715–720.

317. LeCouter J, Kowalski J, Foster J, Hass P, Zhang Z, Dillard-Telm L, Frantz G, Rangell L, De Guzman L, Keller GA, Peale F, Gurney A, Hillan KJ, Ferrara N. Identification of an angiogenic mitogen selective for endocrine gland endothelium. *Nature* 2001; 6850:877–884.

318. Izumi Y, Xu L, di tomaso E, Fukumura D, Jain RV. Tumor biology: herceptin acts as anti-angigenic cocktail. *Nature* 2002; 6878:279–280.

319. Yu JL, Rak JW, Coomber BL, Hicklin DJ, Kerbel RS. Effect of p53 status on tumor espons to autoangiogenic therapy. *Science* 2002; 295, 559, 1526–1528.

320. Rak J, Yu JL, Kerbel RS, Coomber BL. What do oncogenic mutations have to do with angiogenesis/vascular dependence of tumors? *Cancer Res* 2002, 62;7:1931–1934.

11 Oncogenes as Therapeutic Targets to Prevent Metastasis

Ann F. Chambers, PhD
and Hemanth J. Varghese, BSc

CONTENTS

1. INTRODUCTION

Oncogenes, including activated ras, have been shown to induce metastatic ability in appropriate cell types. This response is most likely due to downstream changes in expression of genes that contribute to the metastatic phenotype. Some of these Ras-responsive, metastasis-associated genes, including osteopontin, cathepsins, calcyclin, and vascular endothelial growth factor, have been identified. Because of their association with metastatic ability, oncogenes would appear to be promising targets for antimetastatic therapeutic strategies. Studies on mechanisms of metastasis using in vivo video microscopy, coupled with quantitative assessment of which steps in the metastatic process contribute to metastatic inefficiency, have suggested that regulation of cancer cell growth in a secondary site is crucial to determining whether or not clinically relevant metastases form. Studies on the stages of metastasis affected by Ras suggest that the ability of cancer cells to grow in a secondary site can be significantly affected by activated Ras-signaling. Because oncogene expression can markedly influence the growth phase of the metastatic process, inhibition of onco-

From: *Oncogene-Directed Therapies*
Edited by: J. W. Rak © Humana Press Inc., Totowa, NJ

gene action offers a clinically and biologically appropriate therapeutic strategy to combat metastasis.

Tumor metastasis is the spread of cancer from a primary site and the establishment of secondary tumors in distant locations *(1–4)*. Metastasis is responsible for most deaths due to cancer, and tumors that have not metastasized are generally easier to treat. Thus, it is imperative that the mechanisms of metastasis be better understood and that therapeutic targets to prevent deaths due to metastasis be identified. In this context, oncogene-based therapy offers much promise. Oncogenes were linked in early studies to metastatic ability, and recent studies on the biological mechanisms of metastasis suggest that therapies that target oncogene signal pathways may be useful in preventing and treating metastases.

2. Ras ONCOGENES, TUMOR PROGRESSION, AND INDUCTION OF THE METASTATIC PHENOTYPE

In the late 1970s and early 1980s, genomic DNA transfection into normal murine NIH 3T3 fibroblasts led to the discovery that the H-*ras* oncogene was able to morphologically transform these cell in vitro *(5–8)*. This identification of a transforming oncogene in cellular DNA firmly linked human and animal cancer with the growing field of study on retroviral oncogenes *(9)*. In addition to showing altered morphology in vitro, *ras*-transformed NIH 3T3 cells were shown to be able to form tumors in nude mice *(10–12)*. Moreover, in 1985, it was reported that *ras*-transformed NIH 3T3 cells also were metastatic *(13–15)*. This effect was shown to be related to expression levels of the activated Ras oncoprotein, suggesting a direct causative effect *(16)*. Later studies confirmed that NIH 3T3, as well as some other cell lines, could acquire metastatic ability by transfection with a single gene, members of the *ras* family of oncogenes *(17,18)*. This was not always the case, however, and some cell lines were found to be resistant to Ras-mediated induction of metastatic ability *(14,19–21)*. Furthermore, oncogenes other than *ras* were also shown to induce metastatic ability in some cell types *(22,23)*. Together, these studies raised important questions about regulation of the metastatic phenotype.

Tumor progression has been known to be a multistep process, clinically, pathologically, and at the molecular level as well. The general paradigm developed by Vogelstein and colleagues for progression in colon cancer *(24,25)* appears to hold true for other cancers as well. The progression from a normal colonic cell through to a metastatic colon cancer required a series of genetic alterations, which include loss of tumor suppressor gene function (e.g., APC and p53 genes), as well as gain of activating mutations in oncogenes (e.g., K-*ras*). The specific oncogenes and tumor suppressor genes involved in tumor progression will vary for individual types of cancer, but the overall concept appears to apply to many cancer types. Interestingly, in this scheme, the genetic changes responsible for the final stage of progression to metastatic ability remain unknown. As genetic changes that are unique to metastasis have not been identified, it may be that "the" metastatic phenotype is, in fact, simply the accumulation of sufficient genetic and epigenetic changes to produce the phenotypic changes necessary to give rise to sufficiently efficient metastatic cells.

How can this scheme of tumor progression be reconciled with the induction of a fully metastatic phenotype in NIH 3T3 cells by a single gene such as an activated *ras* oncogene? This was particularly puzzling, in that ras mutation in colon cancer progression can occur as a relatively early event, with over 60% of intermediate adenomas having mutated ras *(24)*. Furthermore, members of the *ras* oncogene family are mutated in a very high proportion of human cancers of many types *(26)*. It is thus apparent that activation of a single oncogene, *ras* or other, is usually not sufficient to render the cell metastatic. However, in a cell carrying appropriate alterations in other genes (both oncogenes and tumor suppressor genes), Ras activation may, in some cases, be sufficient to convert the cell to a metastatic phenotype. Evidence suggests that NIH 3T3 cells are in that category, and were a good model in which to test the role of a specific oncogene change in malignancy.

Even in appropriate cells such as NIH 3T3 cells, which are receptive to a single oncogene change, how does a single gene, such as an activated ras oncogene, alone make the cells capable of metastasis? Here the answer seems to lie in the nature of oncogene-encoded proteins and the molecular pathways that they control.

3. Ras SIGNALING PATHWAYS CAN LEAD TO CHANGES IN GENE EXPRESSION ASSOCIATED WITH METASTATIC ABILITY

Oncogenes are genes that, almost by definition, code for proteins that regulate growth control and responsiveness to environmental signals *(27,28)*. When these control mechanisms are constitutively activated in the absence of external growth signals, the unregulated growth of cancer can occur. The molecular details of these signaling pathways are increasingly becoming understood, and it is clear that these pathways provide a complex mechanism by which a cell can sense its environment and respond appropriately. A hallmark of cancer is obviously the lack of appropriate response to growth control signals, leading to unregulated and progressive growth. Members of the *ras* oncogene family provide an example of how activated oncogenes can lead to phenotypic changes that promote metastatic behavior, via changes in downstream gene expression.

Ras genes code for a family of membrane-bound small GTP binding proteins. These proteins act as cellular transducers relaying ligand-mediated signals from cell surface receptors into the cytoplasm, where they participate in signaling cascades regulating expression of sets of genes *(29–32)*. These downstream genes are involved in many cellular properties, including growth, differentiation, and apoptosis, depending on the cell type and on cross-talk between other signaling pathways that also are activated. Ras proteins are activated by association with guanine nucleotide exchange factors (GEFs), which convert the inactive GDP-bound form of Ras to its active GTP-bound form, and inactivated by GTPase-activating proteins (GAPs), which terminate Ras signaling through the reverse process. Activated *ras* oncogenes have been shown to contain point mutations that result in a loss of GTPase sensitivity, which leads to constitutive stimulation of downstream effectors and deregulation of signal transduction pathways. Ras proteins associate with many downstream effector proteins (i.e., Raf, PI3K), activating different signaling cascades, and regulating expression of genes affecting various cellular responses, including metastatic potential. The general mechanism by which activated Ras can induce metastasis in some cell types appears to be via induction of changes in expression various genes important to the metastatic phenotype *(33,34)*, as diagramed in Fig. 1. The net effect of these changes in expression of metastasis-associated genes is to induce the cell behavioral phenotypic changes that lead to metastatic ability.

A number of Ras-induced genes, whose protein products play a functional role in metastasis have been identified *(33,34)*. These include the secreted integrin-binding

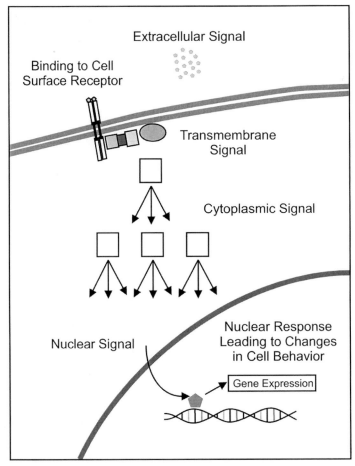

Fig. 1. Regulation of gene expression by signal transduction pathways. Oncogene activation of signal transduction pathways can lead to changes in expression of genes that contribute functionally to the metastatic phenotype, as well as to other changes in cell behavior (e.g., apoptosis, differentiation, growth, etc.), depending on the cell type and other signaling pathways activated in the cell.

protein osteopontin (OPN) *(35–37)*, the cysteine proteinases Cathepsins L and B *(38,39)*, and calcyclin *(40)*, among others, and each of these has been shown to contribute functionally to the metastatic phenotype. In addition, vascular endothelial growth factor (VEGF) has been shown to be induced by *ras* oncogene activation *(41,42)*. VEGF can promote angiogenesis, which can contribute to metastasis both via promoting the escape of cancer cells from a primary tumor, as well as through maintenance and growth of metastases. In some cases, the mechanism by which activated Ras can lead to induction of these genes has been determined (e.g., the Ras-responsive sequence in the OPN promoter, identified by Guo et al. *[43]*). Inhibition of expression of individual Ras-induced genes has also been shown to be able to reduce metastatic ability of the cells, as shown by studies of antisense OPN expression *(44–47)*. This finding suggests that inhibition of Ras signaling, or of individual downstream Ras-induced genes, may be sufficient to interfere with the metastatic process. While the mechanisms by which each of the many Ras-induced metastasis-associated genes contributes functionally to metastasis varies, overall, the set of genes induced by Ras signaling can lead to phenotypic changes that result in metastatic behavior of cells. Interestingly, Webb et al. *(48)* used Ras effector domain mutants and found that metastasis was induced only by an activated MEK/ERK pathway, suggesting that the details of which specific Ras pathways are activated is important for induction of the metastatic phenotype. A feature of an activated *ras* or other oncogene, in appropriate cells, is to render them capable of growth that is unresponsive to growth regulatory environmental signals. As will be discussed below, this aspect of metastasis is crucial in the establishment and growth of tumors in secondary sites.

4. METASTATIC PROCESS AND THE IMPORTANCE OF GROWTH REGULATION IN SECONDARY SITES

Metastasis is the process of formation of tumors at sites distant from the location of the primary tumor. The process consists of a series of sequential steps (see refs. *1–4,49,50* for reviews), beginning with the escape of cancer cells from a primary tumor, their entry into the blood or lymphatic circulation (intravasation), their transport via the circulation to distant organs, their arrest in the microcirculation of these organs, escape from the circulation (extravasation), and growth in the new site. Only metastases that complete all of these steps and grow sufficiently large to cause physiological effects of metastatic growth to the patient are clinically relevant.

The metastatic process is known to be inherently inefficient, with many cells that may be shed from a primary tumor (or injected into the circulation of an experimental animal) resulting in few overt macrometastases *(4,49–51)*. We have developed research strategies to quantify metastatic inefficiency and to determine which steps in the process contribute to the overall loss of cells through the sequential steps in the process. These approaches have included use of in vivo videomicroscopy, to observe and quantify the success of cells at each step in the process, and a "cell accounting" procedure, to permit calculation of the efficiency at each step.

Our studies, on cells that have been injected into the circulation, suggest that events in the secondary organ are then crucial in determining numbers of metastases that form *(2,3,49,50)*. Regulation of survival and growth of cancer cells in the secondary organ contributes significantly to the overall metastatic efficiency. Our findings have suggested that early steps in hematogenous metastasis are quite efficient, with most cells able to complete this phase of the process once they have entered into the circulation. (In contrast, the intravasation process also has been shown, in other models, to be inefficient *[52]*). Efficient steps of hematogenous metastasis include survival in the circulation, arrest in the first capillary bed encountered by size restriction, and extravasation into host tissue. For the several cell types and organs we have studied experimentally, more than 80% of cells delivered to the circulation successfully complete these steps. Inefficiency of subsequent steps is then responsible for overall metastatic inefficiency. These inefficient steps include the initiation of growth in secondary sites by a small subset of cells and the persistence of growth of a subset of the cells that had initiated growth. Therefore, regulation of growth in a secondary site is crucial for determining whether or not clinically relevant macroscopic metastases develop. Thus, this phase of the metastatic process offers a biologically relevant therapeutic target.

The growth phase of the metastatic process also offers the most promising therapeutic target from a clinical standpoint (see refs. *2* and *50* for discussion). When cancer is diagnosed, either it has metastasized or not. If not, it can often be successfully treated by local therapy (e.g., surgery). If metastasis has already occurred and clinically detectable metastases are present, treatment for systemic disease can be initiated (e.g., chemotherapy). Uncertainty arises when it is not known if metastasis has been initiated, and then prognostic factors in the primary tumor are used to assess the probability of undetectable metastases being present and to determine the probability that systemic treatment may be of benefit. In some cases, for example in breast cancer, evidence of metastasis may not occur for years after apparently successful treatment of the primary cancer. Treatment of metastatic disease, either of known metastases or to prevent appearance of metastases in the future, offers a broad therapeutic time window via inhibition of growth in the secondary site. Any therapy that prevents metastases from growing to a point where they cause physiological harm to the patient is of potential clinical utility. It is in this context that oncogene-based therapies offer an attractive therapeutic approach.

5. Ras-TRANSFORMATION OF NIH 3T3 CELLS RESULTS IN MAINTENANCE OF GROWTH OF MICROMETASTASES

Based on this knowledge of the steps in metastasis, coupled with knowledge about Ras-mediated signal transduction, we have begun to ask which steps in the metastatic process are affected by activated Ras signaling, using a pair of cell lines (control NIH 3T3 cells and a *ras*-transformed metastatic NIH 3T3 cell line called PAP2 *[16]*). Our findings to date are summarized in Fig. 2. These cell lines differ in their tumorigenic and metastatic properties, with only the PAP2 cells being able to form tumors from subcutaneous injection in nude mice and to metastasize to the lungs in either spontaneous or experimental metastasis assays in mice or chick embryos *(16,53)*. We thus are comparing the abilities of the two cell lines to complete the sequential steps in the metastatic process. Initially, we asked whether these cells differed in their ability to survive in the circulation and to extravasate, using a chick embryo chorioallantoic membrane metastasis assay and in vivo videomicroscopy analyses *(54)*. Unexpectedly, in that study we found that both cell lines were equally able to extravasate, with approx 90% of observed cells from each cell line having fully completed extravasation by 24 h after intravenous injection. After extravasation, cells of both cell lines also showed the same initial behavior, preferentially migrating towards arterioles, rather than venules or lymphatic vessels, and interacting with the outer surfaces of arterioles. This study suggested that the ras-transformed and control NIH 3T3 cells, therefore, must differ in their metastatic ability because of differences in subsequent steps in the metastatic process, namely some aspect of growth in the secondary site *(53)*.

In more recent studies, using in vivo videomicroscopy and cell accounting analyses, we are extending these studies to murine liver metastases and to aspects of the growth phases of the metastatic process *(55)*. Our findings indicate that both cell lines can complete early stages of hematogenous metastasis to the liver with equal efficiency (see Fig. 2). The difference between the cell lines in end point in metastatic ability, or

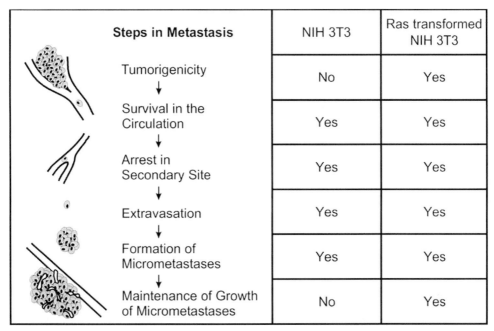

Steps in Metastasis	NIH 3T3	Ras transformed NIH 3T3
Tumorigenicity	No	Yes
Survival in the Circulation	Yes	Yes
Arrest in Secondary Site	Yes	Yes
Extravasation	Yes	Yes
Formation of Micrometastases	Yes	Yes
Maintenance of Growth of Micrometastases	No	Yes

Fig. 2. Ability of ras-transformed and control NIH 3T3 fibroblasts to complete sequential steps in metastasis. Using in vivo videomicroscopy and quantitative measurements of metastatic efficiency, we determined the fate of NIH 3T3 fibroblasts and ras transformed fibroblasts, at each stage of the metastatic process. Data summarized from Koop et al. *(54)* and Varghese et al. *(55)*.

the ability to form macroscopic metastases, arises from Ras-induced maintenance of the growth of micrometastases. This finding is consistent with the concept, discussed above, that anti-oncogene therapy directed at the growth phase of metastases may offer a promising target for treatment.

6. ONCOGENES AS THERAPEUTIC TARGETS TO PREVENT METASTASIS

Oncogene expression has the potential to affect most steps in the metastatic process via induction of downstream genes that affect processes such as growth, apoptosis, motility, adhesion, and proteolytic activity (see Table 1). As illustrated by studies on the effects of activated Ras in NIH 3T3 cells, discussed above, oncogene expression may contribute more to some steps in the metastatic process than to others. Clinically, however, the step most amenable to therapeutic intervention is the final broad phase of growth of metastatic lesions in a secondary site. This phase is sensitive to activated oncogene expression, for the maintenance and progressive growth of metastases. Oncogene-based therapies, either targeting the signal pathways activated by an oncogene or targeting one or more oncogene-induced downstream effector proteins, offer a promising and clinically relevant therapeutic approach to prevent the growth of metastases and the physiological consequences of this growth to the patient.

Table 1
Possible Contributions of Oncogenes to Steps in the Metastatic Process

Steps in metastasis	Affected by oncogene expression?	Promising therapeutic target?
Intravasation	Yes–e.g., effects on cell motility, proteinases, etc.	No–limited opportunity clinically
Survival in circulation	Unlikely, since highly efficient, but perhaps via proteinase induction	Unlikely–limited opportunity clinically
Arrest in secondary site	Unlikely, since highly efficient, but perhaps via adhesive changes	Unlikely–limited opportunity clinically
Extravasation	Perhaps, via induction of proteinases or motility, but already quite efficient	Unlikely–limited opportunity clinically
Initiation of growth by a subset of cells	Yes–e.g. via effects on proliferation/apoptosis balance	Yes–promising target, biologically and clinically
Maintenance of growth of micrometastases	Yes–e.g. via effects on proliferation/apoptosis balance, angiogenic factors	Yes–promising target, biologically and clinically

Oncogenes likely can contribute to all steps in the metastatic process, through various mechanisms that include induction of proteinases, adhesion molecules, motile behavior, induction of angiogenic factors, effects on proliferation and protection from apoptosis. Clinically, however, the later steps in the process offer more accessible targets for treatment. Thus, inhibition of oncogene-mediated growth ability of cancer cells in a secondary site offers a clinically useful therapeutic target with a broad time window for treatment.

ACKNOWLEDGMENTS

We thank members of our research team and especially Drs. Alan Groom and Ian MacDonald for helpful discussions. Supported by grants (to A.F.C.) No. 42511 from the Canadian Institutes for Health Research and No. 012078 from the Canadian Breast Cancer Research Initiative and a Pre-doctoral Studentship (to H.J.V.) from the Canadian Institutes for Health Research.

REFERENCES

1. Fidler IJ. The biology of human cancer metastasis. *Acta Oncol* 1991; 30:668–675.
2. Chambers AF. The metastatic process: basic research and clinical implications. *Oncol Res* 1999; 11:161–168.
3. Chambers AF, MacDonald IC, Schmidt EE, Morris VL, Groom AC. Clinical targets for anti-metastasis therapy. *Adv Cancer Res* 2000; 79:91–121.
4. Yoshida BA, Sokoloff MM, Welch DR, Rinker-Schaeffer CW. Metastasis-suppressor genes: a review and perspective on an emerging field. *J Natl Cancer Inst* 2000; 92:1717–1730.
5. Shih C, Shilo BZ, Goldfarb MP, Dannenberg A, Weinberg RA. Passage of phenotypes of chemically transformed cells via transfection of DNA and chromatin. *Proc Natl Acad Sci USA* 1979; 76:5714–5718.
6. Tabin CJ, Bradley SM, Bargmann CI, Weinberg RA, Papageorge AG, Scolnick EM, et al. Mechanism of activation of a human oncogene. *Nature* 1982; 300:143–149.
7. Parada LF, Tabin CJ, Shih C, Weinberg RA. Human EJ bladder carcinoma oncogene is homologue of Harvey sarcoma virus ras gene. *Nature* 1982; 297:474–478.

8. Shih C, Weinberg RA. Isolation of a transforming sequence from a human bladder carcinoma cell line. *Cell* 1982; 29:161–169.
9. Bishop JM. The molecular genetics of cancer. *Science* 1987; 235:305–311.
10. Blair DG, Cooper CS, Oskarsson MK, Eader LA, Vande Woude GF. New method for detecting cellular transforming genes. *Science* 1982; 218:1122–1125.
11. Chang EH, Furth ME, Scolnick EM, Lowy DR. Tumorigenic transformation of mammalian cells induced by a normal human gene homologous to the oncogene of Harvey murine sarcoma virus. *Nature* 1982; 297:479–483.
12. Fasano O, Birnbaum D, Edlund L, Fogh J, Wigler M. New human transforming genes detected by a tumorigenicity assay. *Mol Cell Biol* 1984; 4:1695–1705.
13. Bondy GP, Wilson S, Chambers AF. Experimental metastatic ability of H-ras-transformed NIH3T3 cells. *Cancer Res* 1985; 45:6005–6009.
14. Muschel RJ, Williams JE, Lowy DR, Liotta LA. Harvey ras induction of metastatic potential depends upon oncogene activation and the type of recipient cell. *Am J Pathol* 1985; 121:1–8.
15. Thorgeirsson UP, Turpeenniemi-Hujanen T, Williams JE, Westin EH, Heilman CA, Talmadge JE, et al. NIH/3T3 cells transfected with human tumor DNA containing activated ras oncogenes express the metastatic phenotype in nude mice. *Mol Cell Biol* 1985; 5:259–262.
16. Hill SA, Wilson S, Chambers AF. Clonal heterogeneity, experimental metastatic ability, and p21 expression in H-ras-transformed NIH 3T3 cells. *J Natl Cancer Inst* 1988; 80:484–490.
17. Chambers AF, Tuck AB. Oncogene transformation and the metastatic phenotype. *Anticancer Res* 1988; 8:861–871.
18. Wright JA, Egan SE, Greenberg AH. Genetic regulation of metastatic progression. *Anticancer Res* 1990; 10:1247–1255.
19. Tuck AB, Wilson SM, Chambers AF. Resistance of murine LTA cells to oncogene-mediated progression from tumorigenic to metastatic phenotype. *Anticancer Res* 1990; 10:1507–1514.
20. Tuck AB, Wilson SM, Chambers AF. ras transfection and expression does not induce progression from tumorigenicity to metastatic ability in mouse LTA cells. *Clin Exp Metastasis* 1990; 8:417–431.
21. Tuck AB, Wilson SM, Khokha R, Chambers AF. Different patterns of gene expression in ras-resistant and ras-sensitive cells. *J Natl Cancer Inst* 1991; 83:485–491.
22. Chambers AF, Wilson S. Cells transformed with a ts viral src mutant are temperature sensitive for in vivo growth. *Mol Cell Biol* 1985; 5:728–733.
23. Egan SE, McClarty GA, Jarolim L, Wright JA, Spiro I, Hager G, et al. Expression of H-ras correlates with metastatic potential: evidence for direct regulation of the metastatic phenotype in 10T1/2 and NIH 3T3 cells. *Mol Cell Biol* 1987; 7:830–837.
24. Fearon ER, Vogelstein B. A genetic model for colorectal tumorigenesis. *Cell* 1990; 61:759–767.
25. Kinzler KW, Vogelstein B. Lessons from hereditary colorectal cancer. *Cell* 1996; 87:159–170.
26. Bos JL. Ras oncogenes in human cancer: a review. *Cancer Res* 1989; 49:4682–4689.
27. Bishop JM. Molecular themes in oncogenesis. *Cell* 1991; 64:235–248.
28. Hanahan D, Weinberg RA. The hallmarks of cancer. *Cell* 2000; 100:57–70.
29. Campbell SL, Khosravi-Far R, Rossman KL, Clark GJ, Der CJ. Increasing complexity of Ras signaling. *Oncogene* 1998; 17:1395–1413.
30. Shields JM, Pruitt K, McFall A, Shaub A, Der CJ. Understanding Ras: 'it ain't over 'til it's over'. *Trends Cell Biol* 2000; 10:147–154.
31. Frame S, Balmain A. Integration of positive and negative growth signals during ras pathway activation in vivo. *Curr Opin Genet Dev* 2000; 10:106–113.
32. Wasylyk B, Hagman J, Gutierrez-Hartmann A. Ets transcription factors: nuclear effectors of the Ras-MAP-kinase signaling pathway. *Trends Biochem Sci* 1998; 23:213–216.
33. Chambers AF, Tuck AB. Ras-responsive genes and tumor metastasis. *Crit Rev Oncog* 1993; 4:95–114.
34. Chambers AF. Mechanisms of oncogene-mediated alterations in metastatic ability. *Biochem Cell Biol* 1992; 70:817–821.
35. Craig AM, Nemir M, Mukherjee BB, Chambers AF, Denhardt DT. Identification of the major phosphoprotein secreted by many rodent cell lines as 2ar/osteopontin: enhanced expression in H-ras-transformed 3T3 cells. *Biochem Biophys Res Commun* 1988; 157:166–173.
36. Craig AM, Bowden GT, Chambers AF, Spearman MA, Greenberg AH, Wright JA, et al. Secreted phosphoprotein mRNA is induced during multi-stage carcinogenesis in mouse skin and correlates with the metastatic potential of murine fibroblasts. *Int J Cancer* 1990; 46:133–137.
37. Chambers AF, Behrend EI, Wilson SM, Denhardt DT. Induction of expression of osteopontin (OPN; secreted phosphoprotein) in metastatic, ras-transformed NIH 3T3 cells. *Anticancer Res* 1992; 12:43–47.

38. Denhardt DT, Greenberg AH, Egan SE, Hamilton RT, Wright JA. Cysteine proteinase cathepsin L expression correlates closely with the metastatic potential of H-ras-transformed murine fibroblasts. *Oncogene* 1987; 2:55–59.

39. Chambers AF, Colella R, Denhardt DT, Wilson SM. Increased expression of cathepsins L and B and decreased activity of their inhibitors in metastatic, ras-transformed NIH 3T3 cells. *Mol Carcinog* 1992; 5:238–245.

40. Guo XJ, Chambers AF, Parfett CL, Waterhouse P, Murphy LC, Reid RE, et al. Identification of a serum-inducible messenger RNA (5B10) as the mouse homologue of calcyclin: tissue distribution and expression in metastatic, ras-transformed NIH 3T3 cells. *Cell Growth Differ* 1990; 1:333–338.

41. Rak J, Mitsuhashi Y, Bayko L, Filmus J, Shirasawa S, Sasazuki T, et al. Mutant ras oncogenes upregulate VEGF/VPF expression: implications for induction and inhibition of tumor angiogenesis. *Cancer Res* 1995; 55:4575–4580.

42. Grugel S, Finkenzeller G, Weindel K, Barleon B, Marme D. Both v-Ha-Ras and v-Raf stimulate expression of the vascular endothelial growth factor in NIH 3T3 cells. *J Biol Chem* 1995; 270:25915–25919.

43. Guo X, Zhang YP, Mitchell DA, Denhardt DT, Chambers AF. Identification of a ras-activated enhancer in the mouse osteopontin promoter and its interaction with a putative ETS-related transcription factor whose activity correlates with the metastatic potential of the cell. *Mol Cell Biol* 1995; 15:476–487.

44. Behrend EI, Craig AM, Wilson SM, Denhardt DT, Chambers AF. Reduced malignancy of ras-transformed NIH 3T3 cells expressing antisense osteopontin RNA. *Cancer Res* 1994; 54:832–837.

45. Gardner HA, Berse B, Senger DR. Specific reduction in osteopontin synthesis by antisense RNA inhibits the tumorigenicity of transformed Rat1 fibroblasts. *Oncogene* 1994; 9:2321–2326.

46. Su L, Mukherjee AB, Mukherjee BB. Expression of antisense osteopontin RNA inhibits tumor promoter-induced neoplastic transformation of mouse JB6 epidermal cells. *Oncogene* 1995; 10:2163–2169.

47. Feng B, Rollo EE, Denhardt DT. Osteopontin (OPN) may facilitate metastasis by protecting cells from macrophage NO-mediated cytotoxicity: evidence from cell lines down-regulated for OPN expression by a targeted ribozyme. *Clin Exp Metastasis* 1995; 13:453–462.

48. Webb CP, Van Aelst L, Wigler MH, Vande Woude GF. Signaling pathways in Ras-mediated tumorigenicity and metastasis. *Proc Natl Acad Sci USA* 1998; 95:8773–8778.

49. Chambers AF, MacDonald IC, Schmidt EE, Morris VL, Groom AC. Preclinical assessment of anti-cancer therapeutic strategies using in vivo videomicroscopy. *Cancer Metastasis Rev* 1998–99; 17:263–269.

50. Chambers AF, Naumov GN, Vantyghem SA, Tuck AB. Molecular biology of breast cancer metastasis: Clinical implications of experimental studies on metastatic inefficiency. *Breast Cancer Res* 2000; 2:400–407.

51. Weiss L. Metastatic inefficiency. *Adv Cancer Res* 1990; 54:159–211.

52. Wyckoff JB, Jones JG, Condeelis JS, Segall JE. A critical step in metastasis: in vivo analysis of intravasation at the primary tumor. *Cancer Res* 2000; 60:2504–2511.

53. Chambers AF, Denhardt GH, Wilson SM. ras-transformed NIH 3T3 cell lines, selected for metastatic ability in chick embryos, have increased proportions of p21-expressing cells and are metastatic in nude mice. *Invasion Metastasis* 1990; 10:225–240.

54. Koop S, Schmidt EE, MacDonald IC, Morris VL, Khokha R, Grattan M, et al. Independence of metastatic ability and extravasation: metastatic ras-transformed and control fibroblasts extravasate equally well. *Proc Natl Acad Sci USA* 1996; 93:11080–11084.

55. Varghese HJ, Davidson MTM, MacDonald IC, Wilson SM, Nadkarni KV, Groom AC, Chambers AF. Activated ras regulates the proliferation/apoptosis balance and early survival of developing micrometastases. *Cancer Res* 2002; 62:887–891.

12   The Impact of Oncogenes on Tumor Maintenance

Senji Shirasawa, MD, PhD,
and Takehiko Sasazuki, MD, PhD

CONTENTS

1. INTRODUCTION

It is now widely accepted that cancer results from an accumulation of genetic alterations, including subtle sequence changes, alterations in chromosome number, chromosomal translocation, and gene amplifications *(1)*. These alterations result in a gain of function of oncogenes and a loss of function of tumor suppressor genes, leading to uncontrolled growth, differentiation, and apoptosis. The number of mutations required for a tumor to develop in human populations is age-dependent, and seven or eight acquired mutations in a cell are required in commonly occurring solid tumors before an overt malignancy becomes evident *(2)*. The ectopic expression of the telomerase catalytic subunit, in combination with two oncogenes, the simian virus 40 large T and an oncogenic allele of Ha-*ras,* lead to direct tumorigenic conversion of normal human cells *(3)*. Therefore, there is a succession of genetic alterations, each of which conferring one or another type of growth advantages, lead to the transformation of normal

From: *Oncogene-Directed Therapies*
Edited by: J. W. Rak © Humana Press Inc., Totowa, NJ

cells into malignant tissue *(4)*. Cancer cell genotypes are a manifestation of six essential alterations in cell physiology that collectively dictate malignant growth through various mechanistic strategies: self-sufficiency in growth signals, insensitivity to growth-inhibitory signals, evasion of apoptosis, limitless replicative potential, sustained angiogenesis, and tissue invasion and metastasis *(4)*. This classification is needed for a better understanding of molecular mechanisms involved in tumorigenesis and for designing appopriate therapy.

Ras has been implicated in controlling cell proliferation, differentiation, and apoptosis. The activated *ras* oncogenes can transform mammalian cells in culture and have been implicated in the formation of a high proportion of human tumors *(5,6)*. Activated Ki-*ras* oncogenes were found in the majority of exocrine pancreas carcinomas *(7)* and in a high frequency of colorectal tumors and lung adenocarcinoma, whereas the N-*ras* gene was frequently mutated in myeloid leukemia, indicating a possible correlation between tumor type and *ras* gene mutation *(6)*. Furthermore, Ki-*ras,* but not H- or N-*ras,* was found to be essential for normal development in mice *(8,9),* and Ki-Ras4B possesses distinct COOH-terminal modification *(10)*. Taken together, these results suggest that Ki-Ras has specific functions in signal transductions and that these are not shared by other family members. Although ectopic expression of H-, Ki-, or N-*ras* gene in rat fibroblasts resulted in a similar expression pattern in cells transformed by other mutated *ras* isoforms, isoform-specific downstream targets did exist *(11)*. While these experiments were done using fibroblasts, we have identified differential expressed genes, using a suppression polymerase chain reaction (PCR)-cDNA subtraction library between human colon cancer HCT116 cells and its derived activated Ki-*ras* disrupted HKe3 cells. Some of the genes up-regulated by activated Ki-*ras* in fibroblasts were down-regulated in HCT116 cells, which suggested that activated Ki-Ras-mediated signaling depended on the cells examined, levels of Ras-expression, and the conditions. To address the function and biological meaning of activated Ki-*ras* in human colon cancer cells, we should probably analyze colon cancer cells harboring Ki-*ras* mutation, but not other types of cells. Based on this concept, we earlier disrupted activated Ki-*ras* in human colon cancer cell lines, HCT116 and DLD-1 cells, through gene targeting in order to analyze the function of activated Ki-*ras* by comparing parental cells and cells disrupted at activated Ki-*ras* *(12)*. Here, we review the impact of Ki-*ras* oncogene on tumor maintenance, utilizing this system.

2. REDUCED TUMORIGENICITY OF HUMAN COLON CANCER CELLS DISRUPTED AT ACTIVATED Ki-*ras*

Human colon cancer cells, HCT116 and DLD-1 cells, were used to elucidate the biological meaning of activated Ki-*ras* in human colorectal tumorigenesis. Genetic alterations of these cells are summarized in Table 1. Both lines of cells have a Ki-*ras* mutation at codon 13, mismatch repair enzyme MLH1 and GTBP mutation *(13,14),* and transforming growth factor (TGF)-β receptor II mutation *(15)*. HCT116 cells have a deleted in colon cancer (DCC) mutation and β-catenin mutation *(16),* whereas DLD-1 cells have p53 and adenomatous polyposis coli (APC) mutations *(17)*. These findings coincide with the multistep carcinogenesis that occurs in colorectal tumors. The accumulation of genetic alterations is vitally important for tumorigenesis, however, cancer cells that once gain the malignant potential can lose or reduce their malignant characteristics when one of the mutations in tumor cells functionally disappears. To address this question, we established clones of HCT116- and DLD-1-derived cells disrupted at

Table 1
Genetic Alterations of Human Colon Cancer Cells HCT116 and DLD-1

HCT116		DLD-1	
Ki-*ras*	+(Gly13Asp)	Ki-*ras*	+(Gly13Asp)
p53	WT	p53	+(Ser241Pro)
DCC	+	DCC	WT
APC	WT	APC	+
β-catenin	+(Ser45-deletion)	β-catenin	WT
MLH1	+	GTBP	+
TGFβ-RII	+(A10tract)	TGFβ-RII	+(Leu452Pro)

+, mutation-positive; WT, mutation-netagive.

Table 2
Properties of Parental Cells and Ki-*ras* Disrupted Clones

Cell line	Ki-ras disruption[a]	Tumorigenicity in nude mice[b]	Soft agar cloning efficiency (%)	Expression of c-myc[c]
DLD-1	Parental	5/5	20.0	3.6
DKs-5	NHR	5/5	21.8	3.9
DK0-1	HR-N	5/5	24.0	3.6
DK0-3	HR-M	0/7	0.0	0.3
DK0-4	HR-M	0/7	0.0	0.4
DKs-8	HR-M	0/7	0.0	0.8
HCT 116	Parental	5/5	18.6	10.6
HK2-10	NHR	3/3	19.3	9.2
HK2-8	HR-M	0/4	2.1	1.1
HKe-3	HR-M	0/7	0.9	0.3
HKh-2	HR-M	0/7	0.0	1.1

[a] NHR, nonhomologous recombination; HR-N, homologous recombination at the normal Ki-*ras* allele; HR-M, homologous recombination at the mutant Ki-*ras* allele.

[b] The fraction of mice showing evident tumors after 2 mo.

[c] Expression was determined by the relative radioactivity of c-*myc* and β-*tubulin* mRNA bands on Northern blots. The ratio of these mRNAs in normal colon epithelium was 0.4:0.6.

activated Ki-*ras (12),* and we found that these activated Ki-*ras*-disrupted cells lost or had a reduced tumorigenicity in nude mice and anchorage-independent growth assayed by soft-agar colony formation, with reduction of c-*myc* mRNA expression to the level seen in the normal colonic epithelium (Table 2). This finding not only demonstrated that somatic cell knock-out strategy is a useful tool to analyze the function of the cancer-related genes, but also that the function of activated Ki-*ras* oncogene in colon cancer is not redundant, but rather is essential for maintenance of the tumorigenic phenotype. Thus efforts were made to target *ras* in human cancer.

3. GROWTH FACTORS REGULATED BY ACTIVATED Ki-Ras

Normal cells require growth signals from the extracellular environment to maintain an active proliferative state. Most of these signals are transmitted by transmembrane

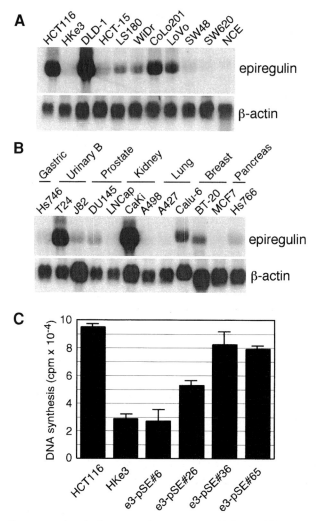

Fig. 1. (A) Epiregulin expression in human colon cancer cell lines. **(B)** Epiregulin expression in human cancer cell lines. **(C)** Epiregulin activities in conditioned media of the HKe3 cells expressing exogenous epiregulin on 32D cells expressing EGFR. ³H-thymidine incorporated into the DNA was measured using scintillation counter. In the case of 32D cells, the extent of DNA synthesis was less than 1000 cpm in all cases of conditioned media samples.

receptors through binding distinctive types of signaling molecules. Tumor cells show a reduced dependence on exogenous growth stimulation, as they generate many of their own growth signals, alterations of extracellular growth signals, transcellular transducers, or alterations in intracellular signaling pathways. Cell surface receptors transducing growth signals into the cell are targets of deregulation of tumorigenesis. Epiregulin, a member of epidermal growth factor (EGF) family *(18)* is expressed in many kinds of human cancer cell lines (Fig. 1A,B), whereas expression is rare in human adult tissues except for peripheral blood lymphocytes *(19)*. Although epiregulin can be a potent pan ErbB ligand *(20)*, the biological significance in tumorigenesis still remains unknown. We found that the expression of epiregulin is up-regulated by activated Ki-Ras in HCT116 cells *(21)*. TGF-α, EGF, or heparin binding EGF-like growth factor was rarely expressed in HCT116 cells. We then determined whether or not secreted epiregulin could stimulate growth of 32D cells expressing the EGF receptor (EGFR) (DER cells), as the growth of 32D cells is dependent on interleukin (IL)-3. Depending on expression level of exogenous epiregulin (e3-pSE#6 expressed little; e3-pSE#26 expressed a middle level; and e3-pSE#36 and e3-pSE#65 expressed highest epiregulin, respectively). The conditioned medium of HKe3 transfectants expressing epiregulin stimulated EGFR in DER cells, resulting in DNA synthesis without IL-3 (Fig. 1C), whereas 32D cells had little DNA synthesis when conditioned medium was used. Furthermore, HKe3 cells expressing epiregulin led to tumors in nude mice, although their growth rate in vivo were much slower than that seen with HCT116 cells. These results, taken together, suggested that activated Ki-Ras is one factor contributing to overexpression of epiregulin in human colon cancer cells, and that epiregulin plays a critical role in human tumorigenesis in vivo.

4. DEREGULATED CONTROLS OF PRB, c-Myc, AND JNK SIGNALING PATHWAY BY ACTIVATED Ki-*Ras*

The c-*myc* gene is amplified in various human cancers, including lung and breast carcinoma *(22,23)*, and expression is up-regulated in almost one-third of breast and colon carcinomas *(24,25)*. APC negatively regulates β-catenin, and β-catenin is a coactivator for the transcriptional factor TCF, which activates c-*myc* expression, suggesting that deregulated c-*myc* expression is central to signal transduction through APC *(26)*. c-Myc induces both neoplastic formation and apoptosis. c-Myc will be a key switch for induction of telomerase activity contributing to the immortality of tumor cells, as well as expression of the catalytic subunit of telomerase *(27)*. In collaboration with activated Ras, c-Myc is able to transform primary fibroblasats, in which c-Myc appears to inactivate cellular responses that are normally required for Ras-mediated growth inhibition, resulting in switching the gene for Ras into a growth-promoting gene *(28)*. Reciprocally, Ras can inhibit Myc-mediated apoptosis *(29)*. Numerous studies have demonstrated the growth-regulated accumulation of c-*myc* mRNA resulting from increases both in c-*myc* transcription and c-*myc* mRNA stability. Furthermore, posttranslational control of c-Myc levels contributes to the deregulated accumulation of c-Myc activity *(30)*.

In most of human colon cancers, over expression of c-*myc* mRNA is observed without amplification of the c-*myc* gene. Although APC will be one of the main factors contributing to this deregulated expression of c-*myc,* activated Ki-Ras will be also one of the key factors involved in c-*myc* expression *(12)*. As shown in Table 2, levels of c-*myc* mRNA were dramatically reduced in HR-M clones, and Fig. 2 shows that the levels of c-Myc proteins are greatly reduced in HKe3 cells more than in HCT116, and HKe3 cells re-expressing activated Ki-*ras* regains over expression of c-Myc, despite of existence of β-catenin mutation. These results suggested that activated Ki-Ras will be critically involved in c-*myc* expression, degradation, or c-Myc stabilization, resulting in the uncontrolled cell growth in these cells.

The retinoblastoma protein (pRB) family is thought to inactivate E2F by physically blocking the action of the transcription activation domain of E2F. Formation of E2F-pRB complexes are inhibited by phosphorylation of several different clusters of sites of pRB, with cyclin D-dependent kinase acting first and cyclin E- or cyclin A-dependent kinases acting later *(31)*. Many antiproliferative signals are transmitted to the pRB family, including pRB, p107, and p130. pRB/p107/p130-triple knock-out mouse

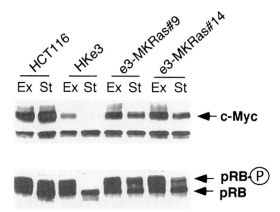

Fig. 2. Western blot analysis of c-Myc expression and the state of phosphorylation of pRB. e3-MKRas#9 and #14 are the HKe3-derived cells expressing activated Ki-Ras. Ex, exponential growth; St, serum starved condition; P, hyper-phosphorylated.

embryonic fibroblasts has a shorter cell cycle and were resistant to G1 arrest following DNA damage and were insensitive to G1 arrest signals *(32,33),* thus confirming that the essential role of the pRB family in the control of G1/S transition. Hypophosphorylated pRB blocks proliferation by sequestering and altering the function of E2F transcription factors that control the expression of genes essential for progression from G1 to S phase. Deregulated pRB pathway renders cells that are insensitive to antigrowth signals. One of the factors by which pRB is maintained in the hypophosphorylated state is TGF-β-mediated signals. The phosphorylation of pRB, governed by TGF-β-mediated signals, is disrupted in variety of ways in many kinds of human tumors, for example, down-regulation of TGF-β receptors or dysfunctional receptors *(34,35).* Indeed, both HCT116 and DLD-1 have mutations of the TGF-β receptor II, probably caused by abnormality of mismatch repair enzymes (Table 1) and leading to deregulation of TGF-β-mediated antigrowth signals. However, activated Ki-Ras is also critically involved in the state of phosphorylation of pRB. When fetal calf serum was scanty in the culture medium in HCT116, HKe3, and HKe3 cells expressing activated Ki-Ras, HKe3 cells showed only the hypophosphorylated from of pRB, whereas HCT116 cells and HKe3 cells expressing activated Ki-Ras showed both forms as observed under exponential growth conditions with calf serum (Fig. 2). These results suggest that activated Ki-Ras-mediated signals culminates in a *deregulated state of* phosphorylation of pRB, thus leading to uncontrolled growth of human cancers.

The Ras-mediated signaling pathway is complex and depends on the cells used and the environmental factors *(36).* Oncogenic Ha-Ras causes a marked increase in transcriptional activity of c-Jun through phosphorylation of c-Jun at Ser-63 and Ser-73, which is phosphorylated by c-Jun NH$_2$-terminal kinases (JNKs) *(37–39).* To determine how activated Ki-Ras is involved in the JNK signaling pathway in HCT116 cells, c-*jun* expression, phosphorylation of c-Jun, activity of JNKs, and activity of SEK1 were analyzed under conditions stimulated by 12-*O*-tetradecanoylphorbol 13-acetate (TPA) *(40).* With nonstimulating conditions, exponential growth and serum-starved conditions, neither HCT116 nor HKe3 cells expressed c-*jun* or show activation of the SEK1-

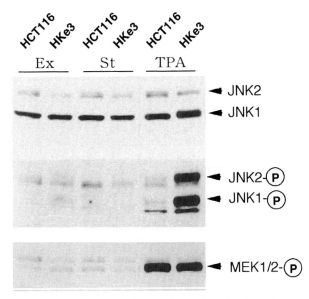

Fig. 3. Inhibition of TPA-induced JNK activation in HCT116 cells. Ex, exponential growth; St, serum starved; TPA, 1 h after TPA stimulation; and P, phosphorylated forms.

JNK pathway. However, when stimulated by TPA, only HKe3 cells showed strong c-*jun* induction, phosphorylation of c-Jun, through the SEK1-JNK pathway (Fig. 3). This phenomenon was also observed in all HCT116-derived activated Ki-*ras*-disrupted cells. These results, taken together, suggest that activated Ki-Ras suppresses TPA-induced activation of SEK1-JNK. However, the inhibitor for PI3K did not inhibit TPA-induced SEK1-JNK activation in HKe3 cells *(40)*, which means that activation of PI3K may not be involved in this pathway, and the imbalance between ERK and JNK activity caused by activated Ki-Ras may play critical roles in human tumorigenesis.

5. Ki-Ras AND APOPTOSIS

The potential of tumor cells to expand is determined not only by the rate of cell proliferation, but also by the rate of apoptosis. Activated Ras have either positive or negative effects on the regulation of apoptosis, depending on cell types, cellular circumstances, and environmental factors *(41)*. These opposing effects on apoptosis by activated Ras relate to Ras-mediated multiple effector pathways. For example, activated Ras has clearly been shown to protect cells from apoptosis either through activation of Akt or through NF-κB activation *(42,43)*. Caspase-9 (Casp9) and caspase-3 (Casp3) are intracellular proteases functioning as initiators and effectors of apoptosis, respectively. Most of the apoptotic stimuli release of cytochrome c (cyto c) from mitochondria into the cytosol, where it binds to the Apaf-1 *(44)*. This complex between cyto c and Apaf-1 induces the binding to pro-Casp9, and then induces proteolytic processing and the activation of pro-Casp9. Active Casp9 cleaves pro-Casp3, then active Casp3 initiates a cascade of caspase activation that culminates in apoptosis. Prostate epithelial cells (267) expressing exogenous activated Ki-Ras showed resistance to apoptotic stimuli causing cyto c release, and cytosolic extracts derived from these cells were resistant to cyto c-induced caspase activa-

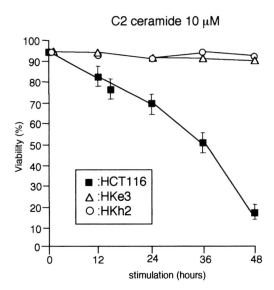

Fig. 4. Viability of HCT116 cells, HKe3 cells, and HKh2 cells following treatment of C2 ceramide.

tion. The reduced caspase activity correlated with the inhibition of proteolytic processing of pro-Casp3 *(45–47)*. Furthermore, a farnesyl transferase inhibitor reversed the resistance of cytosolic extracts to cyto c in 267 prostate cells expressing activated Ki-Ras, and DLD-1 cells displayed a similar resistance to cyto c, whereas DK0-3 cells and DKs-8 cells showed a reversion of resistance to cyto c *(48)*. Pro-Casp9 proteolytic processing in response to cyto c was impaired in cytosolic extracts derived from 267 cells expressing activated Ki-Ras. The mechanism of resistance to cyto c-induced pro-Casp9 by activated Ki-Ras is due to the activation of Akt through PI3K pathway and activated Akt phosphorylates pro-Casp9, resulting in inhibition of its proteolytic activity *(48)*. Thus, activated Ki-Ras is involved in protection from cyto c-induced apoptosis.

Ceramide acts as a second messenger to mediate effects on cell differentiation, growth inhibition, and apoptosis *(49)*. Activation of JNK is essential for stress- and ceramide-induced apoptosis in certain cells. TPA-induced JNK activation is inhibited in HCT116 cells. Ceramide-induced apoptosis, JNK and ERK activity, as initiated by ceramide, was analyzed using HCT116, HKe3, and HKh2 *(50)*. In HKe3 and HKh2 cells, the activity of JNK increased significantly within 60 min following C2 ceramide stimulation, and some apoptosis followed (Fig. 4). On the other hand, C2 ceramide caused a marked apoptosis in HCT116 cells, but activation of JNK was not observed. C2 ceramide did not activate ERK in any of the cells. These results suggest that activated Ki-Ras contributes to the sensitivity of ceramide-induced apoptosis, without JNK or ERK activation, and other signaling pathways involved in ceramide-induced apoptosis may be present. These results also show that the effect of activated Ki-Ras on apoptosis depends on the conditions analyzed.

6. LIMITLESS REPLICATIVE POTENTIAL

Most types of tumor cells in culture appear to be immortalized, and this limitless replicative potential is essential for development of a malignant growth state. Telom-

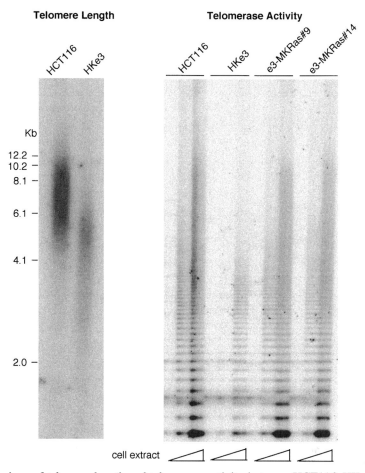

Fig. 5. Comparison of telomere length and telomerase activity between HCT116, HKe3, and HKe3 expressing activated Ki-Ras.

eres are the ends of chromosomes and are composed of several thousand repeats of hexanucleotide. The 50–100 bp of telomeric DNA from the ends of every chromosome are lost during even one replication. With this progressive erosion of telomeres through successive cycles of replication, eventually they lose their potential to protect the ends of chromosomal DNA and cell death follows. Telomere maintenance is evident in all types of malignant cells *(51)*, and most of these mechanisms maintaining telomeres are through activation of telomerase enzymes, which adds hexanucleotide repeats onto the ends of telomeric DNA *(52)*.

To determine if activated Ki-Ras-mediated signaling affects telomere length and/or telomerase activity in these cells, telomere length and telomerase activity in vitro was analyzed (Fig. 5). HCT116 cells have much longer telomeres than do HKe3, and telomerase activity of HCT116 was much higher than that of HKe3. Furthermore, HKe3 cells re-expressing activated Ki-Ras showed a higher telomerase activity than did HKe3 cells. HCT116 cell also expresses much c-Myc, whereas HKe3 cells express little c-Myc. These results, taken together, suggest that activated Ki-Ras may affect telomerase activity through the regulation of c-Myc expression.

7. SUSTAINED ANGIOGENESIS

Oxygen and nutrients supplied by the vasculature are crucial for cell function and survival. Positive and negative signals for angiogenesis are regulated by soluble factors, such as vascular endothelial growth factor (VEGF) and fibroblast growth factors (FGFs) and their receptors on the surface of endothelial cells. Tumors appear to activate the angiogenic switch, from vascular quiescence to sustained angiogenesis, by changing the balance of angiogenesis inducers and inhibitors *(53)*. One angiogenesis inhibitor is thrombospondin-1, which binds to CD36, a transmembrane receptor on endothelial cells coupled to intracellular tyrosine kinases *(54)*. The inhibitor thrombospondin-1 is positively regulated by p53 in some cell types *(55)*. Many human cancers have the p53 mutations, therefore, the loss of p53 function may also be involved in tumorigenesis through sustained angiogenesis. We and others also found that thrombospondin-1 is down-regulated by activated Ki-Ras *(11)*. HKe3 cells showed expression of thrombospondin-1, whereas HCT116 cells and HKe3 cells expressing activated Ki-Ras showed little expression, which suggests that activated Ki-Ras is involved in tumorigenesis through down-regulation of the angiogenesis inhibitor thrombospondin-1.

In terms of positive signals for angiogenesis, Rak et al. reported that VEGF mRNA expression in DLD-1 and HCT116 were higher than that in DKs-8 and HKh2, respectively *(56)*, suggesting that activated Ki-Ras-mediated signals induce VEGF mRNA expression. Further studies by Okada et al., who used the HCT116- and DLD-1-derived transfectants expressing antisense VEGF and KHh-2, and DKs-8-derived transfectants expressing sense VEGF, respectively, showed that reduced expression of VEGF by antisense markedly inhibited the tumorigenesis in nude mice for HCT116 cells and DLD-1 cells, and induction of expression of VEGF in HKh2 cells and DKs-8 cells led to tumors in nude mice, albeit their growth rate in vivo being much slower than that seen in HCT116 cells and DLD-1 cells *(57)*. Thus, activated Ki-Ras-dependent VEGF expression is necessary, but not sufficient, for progressive tumor growth in vivo, and the relative contribution of activated Ki-*ras* to the process of tumor angiogenesis is given increasing attention.

8. TISSUE INVASION AND METASTASIS

The character of tissue invasion and metastasis demands thorough investigations. Invasion and metastasis are complex processes involving changes in physical coupling of cells to their microenvironment and activation of extracellular proteases. Tissue invasion processes include cell–cell adhesion molecules, some of which also link cells to extracellular matrix substrates. E-cadherin, ubiquitously expressing on epithelial cells, serves as a widely acting suppressor of invasion and metastasis *(58)*. The bridges of E-cadherin between adjacent cells result in the transmission of antigrowth and other signals through cytoplasmic contacts with β-catenin to intracellular signaling. Tissue invasion and metastasis processes involve activation of extracellular proteases by up-regulation of protease genes and down-regulation of protease inhibitor ones. The urokinase-type plasminogen activator (u-PA) is a serine protease that converts inert zymogen plasminogen to active plasmin. Urokinase binds to a glycosylated cell surface receptor,u-PA receptor (u-PAR), which is thought to play a critical role in invasion and metastasis. Colon cancer patients with a high u-PAR expression had a poorer prognosis, and colon cancer cell lines expressing a large number of u-PAR at the cell surface

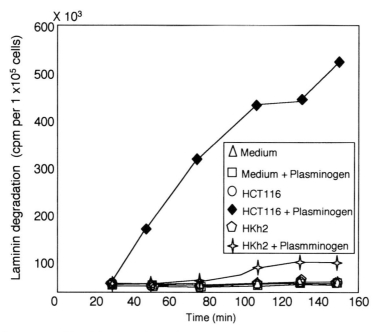

Fig. 6. A slower rate of laminin degradation in HKh2 cells than HCT116 cells. Cells were plated onto radioactive laminin-coated dishes, then supplemented with or without plasminogen. Culture supernatant were counted for radioactivity at the indicated times.

were more invasive in vitro compared with other colon cancer cells with a lesser degree of expression of u-PAR. HCT116 cell-derived activated Ki-*ras*-disrupted cells expressed 50–85% less u-PAR protein compared with the parental HCT116 cells *(59)*. One of the functions of the u-PAR is to facilitate plasminogen-dependent proteolysis. HCT116 cells rapidly degrade laminin, which is one of the major elements of basement membranes, whereas HKh2 cells showed only 80% less laminin degradation in vitro (Fig. 6). These findings suggested that activated Ki-Ras is involved in u-PAR-directed proteolysis and tissue invasion and metastasis through up-regulation of α-PAR ensues.

9. OTHER FACTORS CONTRIBUTING TO TUMORIGENESIS

p53 gene mutation is thought to be one of the most frequent genetic alterations in human cancers. In response to DNA damage, p53 elicits either cell cycle arrest to allow for DNA repair or apoptosis if the damage is excessive, the result being that the genome is protected from accumulating excess mutations. Cells lacking functional p53 are more genetically unstable. Genes involved in sensing and repairing DNA damage are lost in human cancers *(60)*. This genome instability provides cells with selective advantages for growth by acquiring accumulation of genetic alterations. INK4a exhibits loss of function in a variety of human cancers at a high incidence. INK4a encodes two distinct growth inhibitors, the cyclin-dependent kinase (CDK) inhibitor p16 and the tumor suppressor p19arf. The former product is linked to the pRB-pathway, through the inhibition of CDK4-directed phosphorylation of pRB. The latter is linked to the p53-pathway, through interacting Mdm2 (a transcriptional target of p53), the result being neutralization of Mdm2's inhibition of p53 *(61)*. Although Mdm2 is a

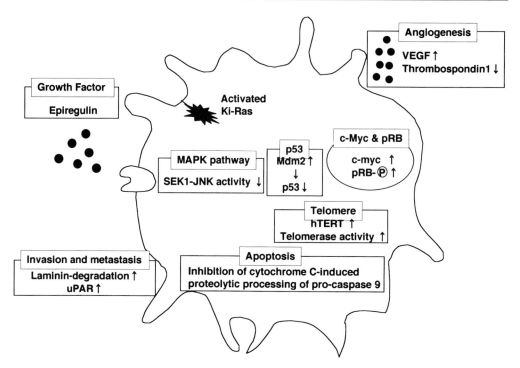

Fig. 7. Gene products regulated by activated Ki-Ras in human colon cancer cells.

transcriptional target of p53, resulting in a negative feedback loop through which p53 itself initiates its own destruction *(62)*, p53-independent pathways triggered by growth factors also regulate Mdm2 expression.

Ries et al. *(63)* determined if Ras-mediated radioresistance is dependent on p53, using HCT116, HCT116-p53–/– *(64)*, HKe3, DLD-1, and DK0-4 cells. HKe3 expressed less Mdm2 and more p53 than HCT116, and p53 accumulated at higher levels in HKe3 cells after γ-irradiation because of lower levels of Mdm2, and the radiosensitivity of these cells increased dramatically. Furthermore, the inhibition of MEK in the parental HCT116 cells through addition of U0126 resulted in a radiosensitive phenotype similar to that seen with HKe3 cells. Treatment of p53-deficient HCT116 cells with U0126 revealed no significant difference, and there was no difference of radioresistance between DLD-1 and DK0-4 cells harboring the mutant p53, which thus indicates that Ras-mediated radioresistance depends on p53.

10. CONCLUDING REMARKS

In human colorectal cancers, mutations of the Ki-*ras* gene are frequent. To address the function of activated Ki-Ras in human colon cancers, we established the human colon cancer cell HCT116- and DLD-1-derived activated Ki-*ras*-disrupted cells through homologous recombination. The tumorigenicity in vitro and in vivo in these cells was reduced dramatically. These cells have been extensively analyzed by the collaborators and functions of activated Ki-Ras in tumor maintenance were elucidated. Activated Ki-Ras in human colon cancer cells analyzed revealed: (i) self-sufficiency in growth signals through epiregulin; (ii) insensitivity to growth-inhibitory signals through deregulation of c-Myc and pRB; (iii) evasion of apoptosis through phosphorylation of Caspase-9; (iv) limitless replicative potential through expression of hTERT, (v) sustained angiogenesis through VEGF expression and the reduced expression of thrombospondin-1; and (vi) tissue invasion and metastasis through uPAR expression (Fig. 7). Therefore, these findings demonstrate that activated Ki-Ras manifests six essential alterations in cell physiology *(4)* and malignant growth occurs.

ACKNOWLEDGMENTS

We thank M. Ohara for language assistance. We are indebted to our collaborators utilizing our system to analyze the functions of activated Ki-Ras in human tumorigenesis. We acknowledge not citing many original papers directly, but rather through the reviews. Our studies are supported by a Grant-in-Aid for Scientific Research on Priority Areas (C) from the Ministry of Education, Science, Technology, Sports,and Culture of Japan.

REFERENCES

1. Lengauer C, Kinzler KW, Vogelstein B. Genetic instabilities in human cancers. *Nature* 1998; 396:643–649.
2. Renan MJ. How many mutations are required for tumorigenesis? Implications from human cancer data. *Mol Carcinogenesis* 1993; 7:139–146.
3. Hahn WC, Counter CM, Lundberg AS, Beijersbergen RL, Brooks MW, Weinberg RA. Creation of human tumour cells with defined genetic elements. *Nature 1999; 400:464–468.*
4. Hanahan D, Weinberg RA. The hallmarks of cancer. *Cell* 2000; 100:57–70.
5. Barbacid M. ras genes. *Annu Rev Biochem* 1987; 56:779–827.
6. Bos JL. ras oncogenes in human cancer: a review. *Cancer Res* 1989; 49:4682–4689.
7. Almoguera C, Shibata D, Forrester K, Martin J, Arnheim N, Perucho M. Most human carcinomas of the exocrine pancreas contain mutant c-Ki-ras genes. *Cell* 1988; 53:549–554.
8. Koera K, Nakamura K, Nakao K, et al. K-ras is essential for the development of the mouse embryo. *Oncogene* 1997; 15:1151–1159.
9. Johnson L, Greenbaum D, Cichowski K, et al. K-ras is an essential gene in the mouse with partial functional overlap with N-ras. *Genes Dev* 1997; 11:2468–2481.
10. James GL, Goldstein JL, Brown MS. Polylysine and CVIM sequences of K-RasB dictate specificity of prenylation and confer resistance to benzodiazepine peptidomimetic in vitro. *J Biol Chem* 1995; 270:6221–6226.
11. Zuber J, Tchernitsa OI, Hinzmann B, et al. A genome-wide survey of RAS transformation targets. *Nat Genet* 2000; 24:144–152.
12. Shirasawa S, Furuse M, Yokoyama N, Sasazuki T. Altered growth of human colon cancer cell lines disrupted at activated Ki-ras. *Science* 1993; 260:85–88.
13. Papadopoulos N, Nicolaides NC, Wei YF, et al. Mutation of a mutL homolog in hereditary colon cancer. *Science* 1994; 263:1625–1629.
14. Papadopoulos N, Nicolaides NC, Liu B, et al. Mutations of GTBP in genetically unstable cells. *Science* 1995; 268:1915–1917.
15. Ilyas M, Efstathiou JA, Straub J, Kim HC, Bodmer WF. Transforming growth factor β stimulation of colorectal cancer cell lines: type II receptor bypass and changes in acdhesion molecule expression. *Proc Natl Acad Sci USA* 1999; 96:3087–3091.
16. Morin PJ, Sparks AB, Korinek V, Barker N, Clevers H, Vogelstein B, et al. Activation of β-catenin-Tcf signaling in colon cancer by mutations in β-catenin or APC. *Science* 1997; 275:1787–1790.
17. Korinek V, Barker N, Morin PJ, et al. Constitutive transcriptional activation by a β-catenin-Tcf complex in APC$^{-/-}$ colon carcinoma. *Science* 1997; 275:1784–1787.
18. Massague J, Pandiella A. Membrane-anchored growth factors. *Annu Rev Biochem* 1993; 62:515–541.
19. Toyoda H, Komurasaki T, Uchida D, Morimoto S. Distribution of mRNA for human epiregulin, a differentially expressed member of the epidermal growth factor. *Biochem J* 1997; 326:69–75.
20. Shelly M, Pinkas-Kramarski R, Guarino BC, et al. Epiregulin is a potent pan-ErbB ligand that preferentially activates heterodimeric receptor complexes. *J Biol Chem* 1998; 273:10496–10505.

21. Baba I, Shirasawa S, Iwamoto R, et al. Involvement of deregulated epiregulin expression in tumorigenesis in vivo through activated Ki-ras signaling pathway in human colon cancer cells. *Cancer Res* 2000; 60:6886–6889.

22. Little CD, Nau MM, Carney DN, Gazdar AF, Minna JD. Amplification and expression of the c-myc oncogene in human lung cancer cell lines. *Nature* 1983; 306:194–196.

23. Mariani-Costantini R, Escot C, Theillet C, et al. In situ c-myc expression and genomic status of the c-myc locus in infiltrating ductal carcinomas of the breast. *Cancer Res* 1988; 48:199–205.

24. Erisman MD, Rothberg PG, Diehl RE, Morse CC, Spandorfer JM, Astrin SM. Deregulation of c-myc gene expression in human colon carcinoma is not accompanied by amplification or rearrangement of the gene. *Mol Cell Biol* 1985; 5:1969–1976.

25. Escot C, Theilletet C, Lidereau R, et al. Genetic alteration of the c-myc protooncogene (MYC) in human primary breast carcinomas. *Proc Natl Acad Sci USA* 1986; 83:4834–4838.

26. He T-C, Sparks AB, Rago C, et al. Identification of c-MYC as a target of the APC pathway. *Science* 1998; 281:1509–1512.

27. Wang J, Xie LY, Allan S, Breach D, Hannon GJ. Myc activates telomerase. *Genes Dev* 1998; 12:1769–1774.

28. Serrano M, Lin AW, McCurrach ME, Beach D, Lowe SW. Oncogenic ras provokes premature cell senescence associated with accumulation of p53 and p16INK4a. *Cell* 1997; 88:593–602.

29. Evan G, Littlewood T. A matter of life and cell death. *Science* 1998; 281:1317–1322.

30. Sears R, Nuckolls F, Haura E, Taya Y, Tamai K, Nevins JR. Multiple Ras-dependent phosphorylation pathways regulate Myc protein stability. *Genes Dev* 2000; 14:2501–2514.

31. Dyson N. The regulation of E2F by pRB-family proteins. *Genes Dev* 1998; 12:2245–2262.

32. Sage J, Mulligan GJ, Attardi LD, et al. Targeted disruption of the three Rb-related genes leads to loss of G_1 control and immortalization. *Genes Dev* 2000; 14:3037–3050.

33. Dannenberg J-H, van Rossum A, Schuijff L, te Riele H. Ablation of the retinoblastoma gene family deregulates G_1 control causing immotralization and increased cell turnover under growth-restricting conditions. *Genes Dev* 2000; 14:3051–3064.

34. Fynan TM, Reiss M. Resistance to inhibition of cell growth by transforming growth factor-β and its role in oncogenesis. *Crit Rev Oncog* 1993; 4:493–540.

35. Markowitz S, Wang J, Meyeroff L, et al. Inactivation of the type II TGF-β receptor in colon cancer cells with microsatellite instability. *Science* 1995; 268:1336–1338.

36. Campbell SL, Khosravi-Far R, Rossman KL, Clark GJ, Der CJ. Increasing complexity of Ras signaling. *Oncogene* 1998; 17:1395–1413.

37. Binetruy B, Smeal T, Karin M. Ha-Ras augments c-Jun activity and stimulates phosphorylation of its activation domain. *Nature* 1991; 351:122–127.

38. Smeal T, Binétruy B, Mercola DA, Birrer M, Karin M. Oncogenic and transcriptional cooperation with Ha-Ras requires phosphorylation of c-Jun on serines 63 and 73. *Nature* 1991; 354:494–496.

39. Hibi M, Lin A, Smeal T, Minden A, Karin M. Identification of an oncoprotein- and UV-responsive protein kinase that binds and potentiates the c-Jun activation domain. *Genes Dev* 1993; 7:2135–2148.

40. Okumura K, Shirasawa S, Nishioka M, Sasazuki T. Activated Ki-Ras suppresses 12-*O*-tetradecanoylphorbol-13-acetate-induced activation of the c-Jun NH_2-terminal kinase pathway in human colon cancer cells. *Cancer Res* 1999; 59:2445–2450.

41. Downward J. Ras signalling and apoptosis. *Curr Opin Genet Dev* 1998; 8:49–54.

42. Khwaja A, Rodriguez-Viciana P, Wennström S, Warne PH, Downward J. Matrix adhesion and Ras transformation both activate a phosphoinositide 3-OH kinase and protein kinase B/Akt cellular survival pathway. *EMBO J* 1997; 16:2783–2793.

43. Mayo MW, Wang C-Y, Cogswell PC, et al. Requirement of NK-κB activation to suppress p53-independent apoptosis induced by oncogenic Ras. *Science* 1997; 278:1812–1815.

44. Green DR, Reed JC. Mitochondria and apoptosis. *Science* 1998; 281:1309–1312.

45. Yang J, Liu X, Bhalla K, et al. Prevention of apoptosis by Bcl-2: release of cytochrome c from mitochondria blocked. *Science* 1997; 275:1129–1132.

46. Kluck RM, Bossy-Wetzel E, Green DR, Newmeyer DD. The release of cytochrome c from mitochondria: a primary site for Bcl-2 regulation of apoptosis. *Science* 1997; 275:1132–1136.

47. Bossy-Wetzel E, Newmeyer DD, Green DR. Mitochondrial cytochrome c release in apoptosis occurs upstream of DEVD-specific caspase activation and independently of mitochondrial transmembrane depolarization. *EMBO J* 1998; 17:37–49.

48. Cardone MH, Roy N, Stennicke HR, et al. Regulation of cell death protease caspase-9 by phosphorylation. *Science* 1998; 282:1318–1321.

49. Hannun YA, Obeid LM. Ceramide: an intracellular signal for apoptosis. *Trends Biochem Sci* 1995; 20:73–77.

50. Ohmori M, Shirasawa S, Furuse M, Okumura K, Sasazuki T. Activated Ki-ras enhances sensitivity of ceramide-induced apoptosis without c-Jun NH_2-terminal kinase/stress-activated protein kinase or extracellular signal-regulated kinase activation in human colon cancer cells. *Cancer Res* 1997; 57:4714–4717.

51. Shay JW, Bacchetti S. A survey of telomerase activity in human cancer. *Eur J Cancer* 1997; 33:787–791.

52. Bryan TM, Cech TR. Telomerase and the maintenance of chromosome ends. *Curr Opin Cell Biol* 1999; 11:318–324.

53. Hanahan D, Folkman J. Patterns and emerging mechanisms of the angiogenic switch during tumorigenesis. *Cell* 1996; 86:353–364.

54. Bull HA, Brickell PM, Dowd PM. Src-related protein tyrosine kinases are physically associated with the surface antigen CD36 in human dermal microvascular endothelial cells. *FEBS Lett* 1994; 351:41–44.

55. Demeron KM, Volpert OV, Tainsky MA, Bouck N. Control of angiogenesis in fibroblasts by p53 regulation of thrombospondin-1. *Science* 1994; 265:1582–1584.

56. Rak J, Mitsuhashi Y, Bayko L, et al. Mutant ras oncogenes upregulate VEGF/VPF expression: implications for induction and inhibition of tumor angiogenesis. *Cancer Res* 1995; 55:4575–4580.

57. Okada F, Rak JW, Croix BS, et al. Impact of oncogenes in tumor angiogenesis: mutant K-ras up-regulation of vascular endothelial growth factor/vascular permeability factor is necessary, but not sufficient for tumorigenicity of human colorectal carcinoma cells. *Proc Natl Acad Sci USA* 1998; 95:3609–3614.

58. Christofori G, Semb H. The role of the cell-adhesion molecule E-cadherin as a tumour-suppressor gene. *Trends Biochem Sci* 1999; 24:73–76.

59. Allgayer H, Wang H, Shirasawa S, Sasazuki T, Boyd D. Targeted disruption in an invasive colon cancer cell line down-regulates urokinase receptor expression and plasminogen-dependent proteolysis. *Br J Cancer* 1999; 80:1884–1891.

60. Levine AJ. p53, the cellular gatekeeper for growth and division. *Cell* 1997; 88:323–331.

61. Pomerantz J, Schreiber-Agus N, Liégeois NJ, et al. The Ink4a tumore suppressor gene product, p19[Art], interacts with MDM2 and neutralizes MDM2's inhibition of p53. *Cell* 1998; 92:713–723.

62. Picksley SM, Lane DP. The p53-mdm2 autoregulatory feedback loop: a paradigm for the regulation of growth control by p53. *Bioessays* 1993; 15:689–690.

63. Ries S, Biederer C, Woods D, et al. Opposing effects of ras on p53: transcriptional activation of mdm2 and induction of p19[ARF]. *Cell* 2000; 103:321–330.

64. Bunz F, Dutriaux A, Lengauer C, et al. Requirement for p53 and p21 to sustain G2 arrest after DNA damage. *Science* 1998; 282:1497–1501.

13 Primary and Secondary Events in Oncogene-Driven Tumor Development

Lessons from Transgenic Model Systems

Michaela Herzig, PhD,
and Gerhard Christofori, PhD

CONTENTS

1. INTRODUCTION

Molecular analysis of multistage carcinogenesis in patients is mainly hampered by the inavailability of biopsies from early tumor stages. In contrast, mouse models of tumor development offer the means to reproducibly isolate different stages of tumor progression, which then are amenable to pathological, genetic, and biochemical analyses. Moreover, tumor cell lines derived from the different tumor stages are useful tools in experimentally addressing many cancer-related questions. Finally, genetic modulation of gene function by overexpression in transgenic mice (gain of function) or by genetic ablation in knock-out mice (loss of function) provide the opportunity to determine whether observed genetic changes are cause or consequence of tumor development. Hence, murine models of carcinogenesis have been instrumental in identifying cancer-related genes and in unraveling their causal role in carcinogenesis.

However, simple overexpression of an oncogene in a particular tissue of a transgenic mouse or ablation of the function of a tumor suppressor gene in knock-out mice, although it may result in tumor formation, does not necessarily recapitulate the genetics and biology of human cancer, and in the majority of mouse models generated up to date, the comparison of mouse and human tumorigenesis reveals certain inconsistencies.

From: *Oncogene-Directed Therapies*
Edited by: J. W. Rak © Humana Press Inc., Totowa, NJ

(1) Transgenic approach   **(2) Knock-out approach**

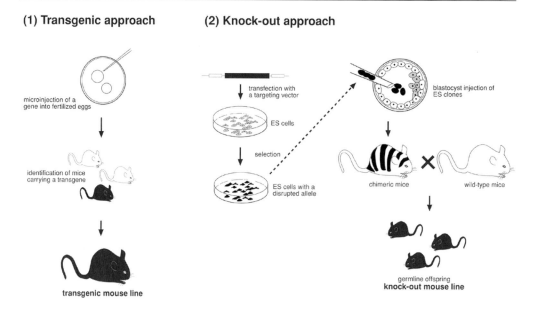

Fig. 1. Schematic outline of the generation of (1) transgenic mouse lines by DNA injection and (2) knock-out mice by gene targeting. Germline transmission is indicated by one offspring in the transgenic approach and by three offspring in the knock-out approach (*see* text for details).

Some of the still unresolved issues and limitations of mouse models are owing to species-specific pecularities of cancer-associated genes, the tissue specificity of cancer predispositions, and the low frequency of metastasis in mice.

To improve and optimize the use of mouse models for cancer research, three major challenges have to be tackled:

1. Modulating biological activities in a way that the outcome resembles human cancer (rebuilding cancer). Of course, this goal is hampered by a number of obstacles, including differences in gene function between human and mouse or by redundancies within gene families.
2. Molecular dissection of tumor progression. Rebuilding human cancer in mouse models may not be possible unless all players are known, including mild genetic modifiers. This is a rate-limiting step and bears a major challenge for the future, because genetic modifiers may not be the same between mouse and human.
3. Development of murine models as tools for testing specific therapeutic approaches. Mouse models that precisely recapitulate human carcinogenesis can be used to experimentally evaluate both broad range and highly specific therapeutic approaches.

1.1. Manipulating the Mouse Genome

Generation of a transgenic mouse that carries in its germ line exogenously added genetic information (transgene) is performed by physically microinjecting the DNA construct into the male pronucleus of the fertilized one-cell mouse embryo (Fig. 1). The microinjected constructs usually consist of a tissue- or cell type-specific promoter, a cDNA encoding the gene product of interest, and mRNA processing sequences, such as a polyadenylation site and introns, to ensure accurate and efficient gene expression (Fig. 2). To accurately recapitulate temporal and spatial expression patterns of genes, in

Transgenic Approaches

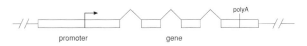

Classical Transgene

YAC or BAC

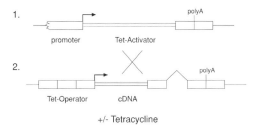

Inducible Expression

Tet-system:

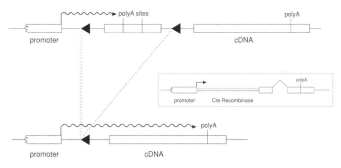

Cre Recombinase:

Fig. 2. Schematic representation of different transgene constructs that are commonly used to generate transgenic mouse lines expressing a gene of interest. Constitutive expression in a tissue of choice is achieved by the use of a short promoter region that is sufficient to convey cell type-specific expression (classical transgene). Temporal and spatial expression of an endogeneous gene is accurately recapitulated by expressing a gene of interest under the control of the entire regulatory region cloned, for example, in YACs or BACs. Inducible expression of a trangene can be achieved by using the tetracycline-inducible system or Cre-recombinase mediated activation of transgene expression (for details *see* text).

recent years short promoter constructs have been replaced by genomic regions containing the entire regulatory region of a gene, for example by using yeast artificial chromosomes (YACs) or bacterial artificial chromosomes (BACs) for generating the transgene construct of interest (Fig. 2).

In many cases, transgene expression may interfere with embryonic development and, hence, is sought to be under temporal or spatial control. For this purpose, a number of inducible systems have been adapted for the use in the generation of transgenic mice. One aproach utilizes the bacteria-derived tetracycline-inducible system (Fig. 2) *(1)*. Two mouse lines are usually generated; one line expresses the gene of interest under the control of a promoter region (Tet-operator) that binds and responds to the tetracycline-dependent transcriptional regulator (Tet-activator). The second mouse line expresses the Tet-activator protein that specifically binds the Tet-operator sequence. The Tet-activator protein has been engineered to transactivate either in the absence of tetracycline (Tet-Off system) or in the presence of tetracycline (Tet-On system). Appropriate choice of the promoter expressing the Tet-activator will decide in which tissue or in which cell type expression of the gene of interest will be modulated. The two mouse lines are then intercrossed to generate bitransgenic mice that carry both transgenes. Tetracycline is provided in the drinking water or by other means, resulting in repression of gene expression in case of the Tet-Off system and activation of gene expression in the Tet-On system *(2)*.

While transgenic mouse lines have been instrumental in the gain of function approach, in particular to learn about the oncogenic potential of genes, inactivation of gene function by stable genetic ablation (knock-out mice) was crucial to learn about the tumor suppressing capabilities of genes. Knock-out mouse lines are generated with the help of embryonic stem (ES) cells, which are totipotent cells that can be cultured in vitro and that are able to contribute to the development of mice, including the germ cells (Fig. 1). In order to inactivate a gene of interest, targeting vectors are constructed in a way that transfection of the vector in ES cells results in homologous recombination and the removal of important regions, mainly coding exons, of the gene (Fig. 3). Positive and negative selection strategies are used to isolate ES cell clones that carry one inactivated allele of the gene. These cells are injected into wild-type blastocyst stage embryos, which are subsequently implanted into a foster mother. Resulting chimeric mice are born in which the manipulated ES cells may have contributed to a majority of the mouse tissue including the germ cells, thus establishing a stable knock-out mouse line heterozygous for the inactivated allele. Intercrosses between these mice will produce mice in which both alleles are inactivated (homozygous knock-out). Dependent on the function of the gene, complete loss of function may result in a variety of developmental or physiological phenotypes, ranging from early embryonic lethal to barely detectable. Early embryonic lethality of knock-out mice is an unwanted complication in cancer research. For example, analysis of the molecular function in carcinogenesis of some important tumor suppressor genes, including the retinoblastoma protein (pRb) or adenomatous polyposis coli (APC), is precluded by early death of the deficient mice. Hence, an inducible or conditional way of ablating gene function has been developed (conditional knock-out) (Fig. 3). Homologous recombination in ES cells is used to introduce phage P1 (loxP) recombination recognition sites in a way that they flank the exon(s) to be deleted. Mice are then generated that carry these "floxed" alleles in their germline. These mice are then crossed to transgenic mice that express phage P1 recombinase Cre, the recombinase that specifically recognizes loxP sites and excises the flanked exon(s) by homologous recombination (Fig. 3). Choosing cell type-specific or inducible promoters to drive expression of Cre offers the opportunity to inactivate gene function at desired time points and/or within tissues of choice. Floxed alleles and Cre recombinase in ES cells in culture are also routinely used to replace a whole coding area of a gene by a cDNA encoding another gene, so as to utilize the regulatory region of one gene to drive expression of another gene (knock-in) (Fig. 3). Targeting of large

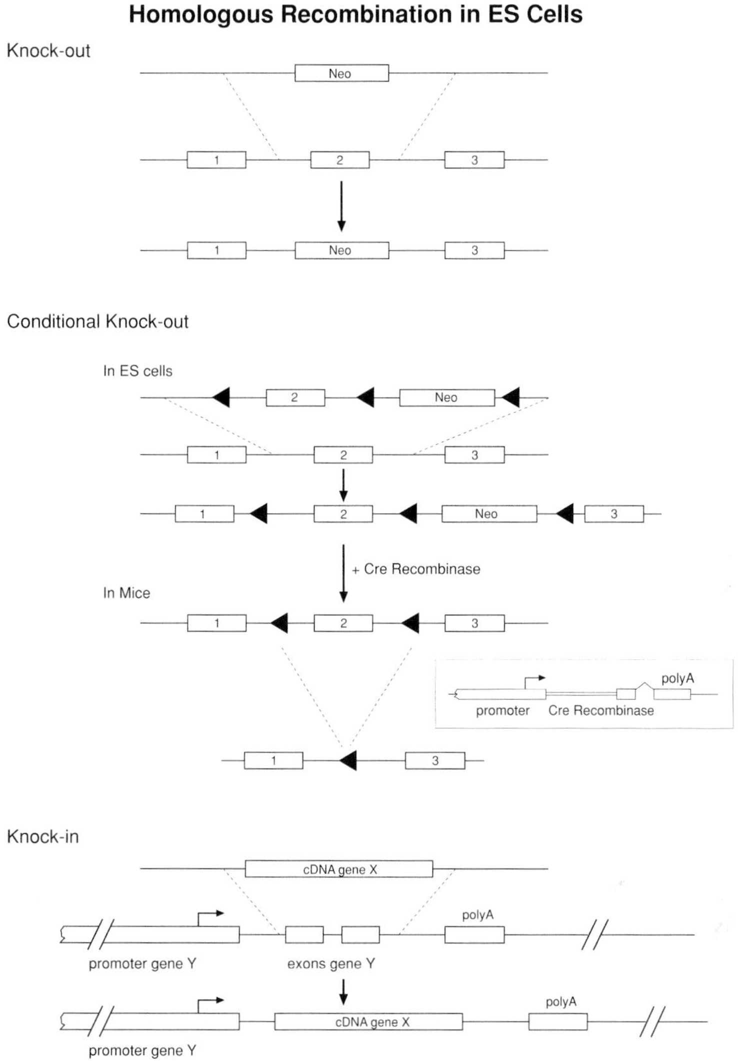

Homologous Recombination in ES Cells

Fig. 3. Examples of experimental strategies to generate mutant mice by homologous recombination in ES cells. Mice are subsequently generated by injecting the modified ES cells into blastocysts (Fig. 1) (for details *see* text).

chromosomal areas with loxP sites and subsequent recombination with Cre recombinase is also used to rebuild chromosomal aberrations, such as deletions, duplications, translocations, and gene conversions in mice. Among many other variations to this scheme, a combination of knock-out/knock-in and transgenic strategies allows inducible expression of a gene of interest by inserting several floxed polyadenylation sites between the promoter region and the coding region of the transgene coding region (Fig. 2). In the presence of the polyadenylation sites, mRNAs encoding the transgene are not produced. Upon expression of Cre recombinase the polyadenylation sites are removed by homologous recombination, and the transgene is expressed. This approach offers dual specificity: both the promoter driving the blocked transgene and the pro-

Table 1
Genes that Act as Tumor Suppressors in Human and Mouse

Gene	Gene function	Mouse tumors (knock-out mouse)	Human tumors (loss of function)	References
pRb	Cell cycle regulator	Pituitary adenocarcinoma, pheochromocytoma, thyroid medullary carcinoma.	Retinoblastoma, osteosarcoma.	26,27,245,246
p53	Control of growth arrest and apoptosis	Lymphoma, sarcoma, and others.	Sarcoma, breast/brain tumors.	49,50,247,248
NF1	Ras-GAP	Pheochromocytoma, myeloid leukemia, neurofibroma in chimeras.	Neurofibroma, sarcoma, glioma.	222,225
NF2	Cytoskeletal regulator (Merlin)	Sarcoma, metastases in $p53^{-/-}$.	Schwannoma, meningioma.	226,249
APC[Min] (aa850) APC[Δ716] APC[Δ580]	Component of Wnt signaling	Multiple intestinal polyps. Intestinal adenocarcinoma. Multiple intestinal polyps.	Colorectal cancer, brain.	145,250 252 148
Ink4a locus (p16;p19/ARF)	p16:CDK inhibitor, p19:stabilizer of p53	Lymphoma, sarcoma, 5carcinoma, glioma.	Melanoma, pancreatic cancer, ALL, glioma.	33
p19/ARF	p19 stabilizer of p53	Lymphoma, sarcoma, carcinoma, glioma.	ALL.	34
Patched	Sonic hedgehog receptor	Medulloblastoma.	Basal cell carcinoma, medulloblastoma.	162
DPC4/Smad4	Transducer of TGF-β signaling	JPS.	Pancreatic/colon cancer, hamartoma, JPS.	253
PTEN	Dual specificity phosphatase	Lymphoma, thyroid, endometrium, prostate.	Glioblastoma, prostate, breast cancer.	130,131,132
MSH2	MMR	Lymphoma, colon/skin carcinoma.	Colorectal cancer, HNPCC.	254,255
MLH1	MMR	Lymphoma, intestinal adenoma/carcinoma.	Colorectal cancer, HNPCC.	77,256
PMS2	MMR	Lymphoma, sarcoma.	Non-polyposis colorectal cancer.	81
MSH6	MMR	Lymphoma, intestinal adenoma/carcinoma.	Colorectal cancer, HNPCC.	75,76
ATM	DNA repair	Lymphoma.	Lymphoma, leukemia.	92

Table 2
Genes that Act as Tumor Suppressors in Mouse

Gene	Gene function	Mouse tumors (knock-out mouse)	Human tumors (loss of function)	References
Smad3	Transducer of TGF-β signaling	Colorectal cancer.	none	140
E2F1	Transcription factor	Lymphoma, lung, reproductive tract.	none	42
p27/KIP1	CDK inhibitor	Multiple tissue hyperplasia, pituitary tumors, retinal dysplasia.	none	35,36,257
p18/Ink4c	CDK inhibitor	Pituitary tumor.	none	38
ATR	DNA repair	Tumor prone.	none	93
Tcf-1	Transcription factor, transducer of β-catenin signaling	Mammary gland and intestinal tumors, cooperates with APC in intestinal tumor formation.	none	154

Table 3
Genes that Act as Tumor Suppressors in Human

Gene	Gene function	Mouse tumors (knock-out mouse)	Human tumors (loss of function)	References
WT1	Transcriptional regulator	none	Nephroblastoma.	258
VHL	Regulator of proteolysis	none	Hemangioma, renal, pheochromocytoma.	259,260
BRCA1	DNA repair	none	Breast/ovarian tumors.	261,262,263
BRCA2	DNA repair	none	Breast/ovarian tumors.	264,265,266
PMS1	MMR	none	Colorectal cancer.	81
DPC4/ Smad4	Transducer of TGF-β signaling	none	Pancreatic/colon cancer, hamartoma.	267
DCC	Receptor of netrin-1	none	Colorectal cancer	268

moter controlling Cre recombinase expression can be chosen according to the experimental needs.

In the near future, these sophisticated technologies will be used at even more advanced levels to generate mouse models of carcinogenesis that mimic cancer in man as closely as possible. Faced with the huge number of mouse lines that develop tumors and that have been generated over the years by purpose or by coincidence, in this book chapter, we will restrict ourselves to mouse models that gave major insights into the molecular mechanisms of tumor progression. In particular, we will present experiments that used mouse genetics to proof molecular principles of mouse tumor development that are most likely also valid in human cancerogenesis. Some of the transgenic and knock-out mouse lines that, at least in part, are used as models for human carcinogenesis are summarized in Tables 1–5.

Table 4
Examples of Cooperativity Between Tumor Suppressor Genes in Mouse

Gene	Tumor phenotype of composite knock-out mouse	References
APC, p53	Pancreatic neoplasia, without increasing intestinal tumor formation.	146
Patched, p53	Medulloblastoma.	163
NF1, p53	Astrocytoma, glioblastoma.	225
DPC4, p53	Pancreatic cancer.	203
pRb, p53	Pinealoblastoma, islet cell tumors, bronchial epithelial hyperplasia, retinal dysplasia, and others.	28
DPC4, APC	Cooperates with Apc$^{\Delta716}$ in colorectal carcinoma.	253
Tcf-1, APC	Cooperates with APC^{Min} in intestinal tumor formation.	154
PMS2, APC	Cooperates with APC^{Min} in intestinal tumor formation.	82
MHL1, APC	Cooperates with APC(1638n) in intestinal tumor formation.	77,251
MSH2, APC	Cooperates with APC^{Min} in intestinal tumor formation.	80
MMP-7, APC	Decrease in intestinal polyp formation of APC.^{Min}	110
MTase, APC	Decrease in intestinal polyp formation.	106
pRb, E2F-1	Decreased frequency of pituitary and thyroid tumors.	43
pRb, p107	Retinoblastoma.	29
p18/Ink4c, p27	Pituitary tumors.	38
PTEN, p27	Prostate cancer.	133

Table 5
Transgenic Tumor Models

Tumor type	Promoter	Oncogene	References
Skin tumors			
Squamous cell carcinoma			
TG.AC mouse	ζ-globin	v-Ha-Ras	10
	K5	E2F-1	46
	K14	HPV16-E6/7	175
Melanoma (ocular)			
	Tyr	v-Ha-Ras	169
	Tyr	Ret	170
	Tyr	T antigen	168,269
Melanoma (invasive)			
INK4a$^{-/-}$ background	Tyr	v-Ha-Ras	13
Metastatic	Tyr	HGF/SF	8
Basal cell carcinoma			
	K14	Sonic hedgehog	156,270
	K5	mutant smoothened	157
	K5	Gli-2	158
BCC, trichoepitheliomas pilomatricoma	K5	Gli-1	159
	K5	truncated β-catenin	152
Breast cancer			
	MMTV	Py-MT	271
Bitransgenic	MMTV MMTV	c-Myc v-Ha-Ras	178
	MMTV	TGF-α	272

Table 5
(*Continued*)

Tumor type	Promoter	Oncogene	References
	MMTV	c-Neu	*179*
	MMTV	Activated c-Neu	*178*
	Neu	c-Neu	*180*
	Neu	Activated c-Neu	*180*
	MMTV	Cyclin D1	*41*
	WAP	T antigen	*273*
Lymphoid malignancies			
	MRP8	PML-RARα/PML-RARαm4	*274,275, 276*
	Cathepsin G	PML-RARα	*277*
	Knock-in cathepsin G locus	PML-RARα	*278*
	Cathepsin G	PLZF-RARα	*232*
	Eμ	c-Myc	*279*
	Eμ	N-Myc	*280,281*
	Eμ	v-Abl	*282*
	Eμ	Bcr-v-Abl	*283*
	Eμ	Ha-Ras	*234*
	Eμ	Bcl-2	*289*
Retinoblastoma			
	Mouse IRBP	T-Antigen	*284*
	Human IRBP	T-Antigen	*31*
	IRBP, p53$^{-/-}$	HPV-E7	*32*
	LH	T-Antigen	*285*
Lung cancer			
	SPC	T-Antigen	*218*
	K19	T-Antigen	*220*
Bitransgenic	SPC	c-myc	*221*
	SPC	EGF	
Rhabdomyosarcoma			
	β-globin	T-Antigen	*287*
Prostate cancer			
	MTT	HGF/SF	*288*
TRAMP mouse	probasin	T-Antigen	*191*
	C3(1)	T-Antigen	*197*
	Fetal-globin	T-Antigen	*201*
	Cryptidin	T-Antigen	*200*
Pancreatic carcinoma			
	Elastase I	K-Ras	*202*
	Elastase I	TGF-α	*203*
Hepatocellular carcinoma			
	Antithrombin-III	T-antigen	*204*
	Albumin	T antigen	*205*
	MT	Growth hormone	*208*
Bitransgenic	MT	TGF-α	*21*
	albumin	c-Myc	
	HBx	HBx	*217*

2. GROWTH CONTROL

Cancer cells bear an indefinite proliferative capacity being able to elude the commitment to terminal differentiation and quiescence that normally regulate tissue homeostasis in the organism. To achieve this property, tumor cells become independent from external growth stimuli either by replacing external growth signals with autocrine growth factors and/or with constitutive activation of signal transduction cascades or by deregulating cell cycle control.

2.1. Autocrine Growth Stimulation

Many cancer cells, such as glioblastoma and sarcoma cells, produce their own growth factors, platelet-derived growth factor (PDGF) and transforming growth factor (TGF)-α, respectively, that are normally produced by stromal cells *(3)*. Similarly, melanoma cells produce high levels of fibroblast growth factor (FGF)-2 and are dependent on this growth factor for proliferation *(4)*. Alternatively, tumor cells become self-sufficient in regulating mitogenic pathways by either overexpression or mutation of signal transduction molecules. Examples are the up-regulated expression of growth factor receptors, such as epidermal growth factor receptor (EGFR) or HER-2neu *(5)*. Moreover, tyrosine-kinase receptors, such as EGFR, are frequently found mutated or truncated in a way that they are constitutively active independently from ligand binding *(6)*. Finally, 25% of human tumors present activating mutations in Ras, resulting in persistent signal transduction via the mitogen-activated protein kinase (MAPK) pathway, the phosphoinositol 3 kinase (PI3K) pathway, and possibly other downstream effector pathways.

Several mouse models have confirmed a role of growth factor/receptor tyrosine kinase signaling in carcinogenesis. For example, during skin tumorigenesis, overexpression of the EGF family member TGF-α in basal keratinocytes induces skin papillomas at sites of wounding or mechanical stress *(7)*. Similarly, ectopic expression of HGF/SF in melanocytes induces the development of spontaneous/cutaneous melanoma of about 20% of the mice with ultimate progression to metastasis after a year *(8)*. Transgenic modulation of signal transduction molecules that act downstream of receptor tyrosine kinases also results in tumor development. For example, transgenic mice expressing Ha-Ras in suprabasal keratinocytes develop benign papillomas *(9)*, whereas the more potent viral oncogene v-Ha-Ras initiates skin tumors that eventually convert to squamous carcinoma *(10,11)*. EGFR activation leads to association of the adapter proteins Grb2 and Sos, the latter a Ras-specific guanine nucleotide exchange factor that catalyzes activation of Ras by facilitating the GTP-GDP exchange. Expression of a consitutive-active Sos in basal keratinocytes of transgenic mice induces spontaneous papillomas with 100% penetrance *(12)*. Notably, tumor development is impaired when Sos tumors arise in a EGFR hypomorphic background, suggesting that a survival signal independent from the Ras signal is activated upon EGFR stimulation.

In tumor-prone *Ink4a*-deficient mice, expression of an activated Ha-Ras is sufficient to induce melanoma formation *(13,14)*. Notably, the maintenance of the transformed state is dependent on Ras activity, since tumor growth is reversed when expression of the oncogene is abolished. Similarly to Ras, induction of c-Myc expression in skin or T lymphocytes leads to neoplasia in a reversible fashion *(15,16)*. These experiments indicate that the sole activation of an oncogene can instruct cells to proliferate and prevent them from differentiation, growth arrest, or apoptosis. Nonetheless, tumor cells seem to retain the capability of returning to normal regulatory responses, when the oncogene is inactivated. In contrast to these results, simian virus 40 (SV40) T antigen-mediated transformation of pancreatic β cells could not be reversed after a certain time point *(17)*. These experiments solicit questions about the number and nature of additional genetic or epigenetic changes that render tumor cells irreversibly malignant.

One approach to identify cooperative effects between oncogenes is the genetic complementation of transgenic mouse lines that overexpress two different genes of interest in the same target cell, resulting in increased incidence of tumor formation, accelerated tumor progression, or higher degree of malignancy. For example, co-expression of Ha-Ras and c-Myc, or Wnt-1 plus FGF3, in mammary epithelial cells of bitransgenic animals results in an earlier appearance and a higher frequency of solid tumors, as compared to expression of either of the transgenes alone *(18,19)*. A similar cooperative effect has been demonstrated in liver oncogenesis, where combinations of SV40 T antigen and c-Myc, T antigen and Ha-Ras, or c-Myc plus Ha-Ras resulted in acceleration of tumorigenesis and formation of tumors with more malignant phenotypes *(20,21)*. In a different set of transgenic mice, cooperative effects between TGF-α and either c-Myc or SV40 T antigen has been revealed in liver and pancreas tumorigenesis *(22)*. A variation on this theme has been demonstrated with transgenic mice that overexpress v-Ha-Ras in the epidermal layer of the skin. Expression of v-Ha-Ras obviated the need for classical carcinogens as initiators of tumorigenesis, since application of tumor promotors such as phorbol 12-myristate-13-acetate (PMA) to the skin of the mice resulted in the formation of skin papillomas *(10)*. This approach has been also used to show that TGF-α can bypass the need for a Ras mutation in the chemical carcinogenesis of skin papillomas *(23)*. In a similar cooperative fashion, exposure to UV light results in enhanced melanoma formation in transgenic mice that express SV40 large T antigen oncoprotein in melanocytes *(24)*.

2.2. Cell Cycle Control

Cellular quiescence and tissue homeostasis is maintained by multiple antiproliferative signals in normal tissue. Most antiproliferative signals are transduced via the pRb and its family members p107 and p130. Upon phosphorylation, these proteins release the otherwise tightly bound transcription factor E2F thereby activating expression of genes essential for G1 to S phase transition. Hence, any disruption of the pRb pathway renders cells insensitive to antigrowth signals that normally block progression from G1 to S phase *(25)*.

In human cancer, inactivating mutations of pRb have been documented in sporadic and familial retinoblastoma, cancers of the lung, breast, prostate, and bladder, and papillomavirus-associated cervical tumors. In addition, a large percentage of human cancers carry a mutation in one of the components of the pRb pathway, all of which lead to phosphorylation of pRb and disruption of cell cycle control. These alterations include amplifications of the genes encoding *cyclin D1* and cyclin-dependent kinase 4 *(CDK4)* and loss of the CDK-inhibitor p16/Ink4a. However, no alterations in the transcription factor *E2F* gene have been found to date.

Inactivation of both copies of Rb in the mouse germ line results in early embryonic lethality due to neuronal cell death and defective erythropoiesis. Heterozygous animals are predisposed to the development of tumors of the pituitary gland and the thyroid, but not to retinoblastoma. Similar to human retinoblastoma, most of these tumors show loss of the second allele of *pRb (26–28)*. Hence, the wide range of tumors arising in humans and especially familial retinoblastoma are not detected in the murine model.

Since mice with targeted deletion of *pRb* fail to show a retinal phenotype as suggested from human studies, it was interesting to investigate pRb family members p107 and p130 in respect to their tumor suppressive function. Mice carrying a targeted deletion of the *Rb* family members p107 and p130 develop normally and do not exhibit any cancer predisposition in either heterozygous or homozygous state. Loss of p107 in the $Rb^{+/-}$ background, however, leads to bilateral multifocal retinal hyperplasia with high penetrance and suggests tumor suppressive function of p107 and moreover overlapping function of pRb and p107 in the murine retina *(29,30)*. Interestingly, no other combination of mutations in the pRb family members, including $Rb^{+/-}$ $p130^{-/-}$, $p130^{+/-}$ $p107^{-/-}$, or $p107^{+/-}$ $p130^{-/-}$, has resulted in retinal abnormalities or any other tumor phenotype suggesting that loss of both p107 and p130 is insufficient to promote tumor progression in the mouse.

Expression of viral oncogenes in the murine retina demonstrates that disruption of the pRb pathway as well as inactivation of p53 is crucial in the development of retinoblastoma. As expected, mice expressing T antigen specifically in the retina, thereby inactivating pRb as well as p53, develop retinoblastoma *(31)*. In contrast, transgenic mice expressing only the human papilloma virus (HPV) E7 gene product do not exhibit retinal hyperplasia, because inactivation of pRb by E7 protein in the presence of functional p53 leads of massive apoptosis. However, mice expressing HPV E7 in the retina and simultaneously lack p53 develop retinoblastoma *(32)*. Similar results were obtained in $Rb^{+/-}$ animals: while p53 wild-type animals do not show retinal abnormalities, p53-deficient mice succumb to retinal dysplasia, pinealoblastoma, islet cell tumors, and bronchial hyperplasia. Consistent with the cooperative effect between the loss of pRb and the loss pf p53 functions, analysis of mice heterozygous for both Rb and p53 revealed a broader spectrum of tumors than the single deletions underlining also the importance of the two major pathways affected during cancerogenesis *(25)*.

The tumor suppressor pRb is one of the major targets of CDKs and their inhibitors (CDK inhibitors). As expected, targeted deletion of the *Ink4a* locus, encoding the CDK inhibitor p16 and p19/ARF, results in a cancer prone condition *(33,34)*. Notably, loss of Ink4a function cooperates with v-Ha-Ras in the induction of melanoma with loss of the second *Ink4a* allele in heterozygous *Ink4a* tumors *(13)*. Targeted inactivation of the CDK inhibitor p27 leads to increased body size, hyperplasia of ovaries, testes, and throid, retinal dysplasia, and pituitary tumors *(35,36)*. A significant increase in the onset of pituitary and thyroid tumors has been observed in $Rb^{+/-}$ $p27^{-/-}$ animals, with loss of the remaining wild-type *pRb* allele *(37)*, suggesting cooperatitvity between pRb and p27. A similar cooperative effect has been observed between two CDK inhibitors, p27 and p18, in context of suppression of pituitary tumorigenesis *(38)*. Loss of p18, like loss of p27, leads to pituitary hyperplasia and adenoma with high penetrance, whereas mice deficient in both p18 and p27 exhibited a significant acceleration of tumor development. In contrast, targeted inactivation of the CDK inhibitor, p21, a major transcriptional target of p53, does not result in tumor formation *(39,40)*.

Cyclin D1 has been identified as a candidate oncogene and is suspected to contribute to a variety of neoplasms including breast cancer. To evaluate the potential of cyclin D1 to promote tumorigenesis in vivo, cyclin D1 was overexpressed in mammary epithelium of transgenic mice using the mouse mammary tumor virus (MMTV) long terminal repeat (LTR) regulatory region. MMTV-cyclin D1 transgenic mice display abnormal proliferation of the mammary epithelium and develop multifocal mammary adenocarcinomas *(41)*.

Mice lacking the transcription factor E2F1 are viable and susceptible to a variety of tumors, which indicates, surprisingly, a tumor suppressive function of E2F1 *(42)*. Within one year, homozygous animals develop testicular atrophy and exocrine gland hyperplasia and tumors of the reproductive tract, lung and lymphomas at low incidence. The tumor spectrum of pRb$^{+/-}$ animals differs from the one observed in E2F1$^{-/-}$ mice. Tumors of the pituitary and thyroid arising in pRb heterozygous animals are not observed in mice lacking E2F1. Furthermore, pRb$^{+/-}$ animals develop only low levels of bronchial lung hyperplasia, while E2F1$^{-/-}$ mice develop lung adenoma. pRb$^{+/-}$E2F1$^{-/-}$ double mutant mice show reduced frequency of both thyroid and pituitary tumors in comparison to pRb$^{+/-}$ animals. In addition, the lifespan of pRb$^{+/-}$ is significantly extended, suggesting that upon loss of pRb function, E2F1 acts as an oncogene *(43)*.

Expression of human E2F1 under control of the keratin-5 (K5) promoter induced hyperproliferation, hyperplasia and p53-dependent apoptosis in the epidermis of transgenic mice. Moreover, up-regulated E2F1 promotes spontaneous skin tumor development upon loss of p53 and also cooperates with v-Ha-Ras in the formation of benign skin papillomas *(44,45)*. On the other hand, the K5-E2F1 transgenic mice are resistant to chemically induced skin carcinogenesis, probably due to apoptosis early at the initiation stage of tumor development *(46)*. Hence, E2F1 exhibits both oncogenic and tumor suppressive properties dependent upon the experimental context.

In contrast to the results obtained by overexpression of E2F1, up-regulation of E2F4 in the epidermis of mice does not induce spontaneous skin tumors *(47)*. Also in contrast to E2F1, E2F4 cooperates with chemical skin carcinogenesis, but not with loss of p53.

2.3. Checkpoint Control

Once cells have entered the cell cycle, for example by activating growth factor-induced signal transduction cascades, additional controls are installed to assure accurate DNA replication, mitosis, and cell division. Checkpoints are thought to exist at several phases of the cell cycle, including the transition from G0 to G1, from G1 to S, from anaphase to telophase and at cell division. Loss of any of these checkpoints can result in disturbed DNA replication, DNA repair, and chromosome segregation and thus in genomic instability and an increased mutational rate. Loss of such controls are regularly observed in cancer cells.

The most frequent genetic alteration in human cancer is loss of function of the tumor suppressor gene product p53; more than 50% of all human cancer types harbor mutations in the p53 gene *(48)*. The tumor suppressor gene *p53* encodes a sequence specific transcription factor which in response to DNA damage or other stress-related signals promotes growth arrest and, in cases of irreversible DNA damage, induces apoptosis. Consistent with its biochemical function, with its frequent inactivation in human cancers and with Li-Fraumeni syndrome, where *p53* is mutated in the germ line, p53 knock-out mice rapidly develop malignant tumors, predominantly lymphomas and rare cases of sarcomas *(49,50)*. In the majority of tumors in mice heterozygous for the deletion of p53, the second allele is found to be lost. Moreover, in all cases where p53 knock-out mice have been intercrossed with tumor-bearing transgenic mouse lines, tumorigenesis was dramatically accelerated. Together the data from transgenic mouse experiments emphasize the pivotal role of *p53* as a tumor suppressor gene.

A recently identified regulator of p53, Mdm2, is itself oncogenic and targets p53 for ubiquitin-mediated degradation. *Mdm2* gene amplifications and overexpression have been reported in human sarcomas and various other malignancies, however, they have been exclusively observed in tumors with functional p53 *(51,52)*. Further evidence that p53 and Mdm2 may act in the same pathway comes from experiments where the embryonic lethality of Mdm2 knock-out mice can be completely rescued by ablation of p53 function *(53,54)*. Moreover, Mdm2/p53 double knock-out mice exhibit spontaneous tumor development that is indistinguishable from the tumor spectrum and tumor rate observed in p53 knock-out mice *(55)*.

Overexpression of Mdm2 in the mammary epithelium of transgenic mice was found to inhibit proper mammary gland development by stimulation of multiple rounds of S phase without completion of mitosis *(56,57)*. A small number of mice developed mammary tumors late in life, indicating that Mdm2 may play a role in induction of epithelial tumors. Overexpression of Mdm2 under control of its native promoter in transgenic mice causes the development of lymphomas and sarcomas *(58)*. The high incidence of Mdm-2 induced sarcoma that are not observed in p53 null mice argue for a p53-independent mechanism of Mdm2 during tumorigenesis. Thus, overcoming p53-induced suppression of tumor cell growth seems one but not the only function of Mdm2.

Crosstalk between the pRb and p53 pathway occurs on several levels. p21, for example, is a transcriptional target of p53 and induces cell cycle arrest by interfering with phosphorylation of pRb. Direct physical interaction is elicited through Mdm2 that associates with both tumor suppressors p53 and pRb, thereby targeting the first for degradation and inhibiting the repressor function of the second, consequently resulting in cell cycle progression. Finally, p19/ARF links the pRb cell cycle control pathway and the p53 DNA damage pathway. The *Ink4a* locus encodes two unrelated proteins, the cell cycle inhibitor p16/Ink4a and p19/ARF, a stabilizer of p53. Upon loss of p16, cyclin-dependent kinase 4 and 6 are no more repressed, they hyperphosphorylate pRb resulting in the release of E2F transcription factors and unscheduled entry into S phase. On the other hand, p19ARF efficiently induces a G1/G2 arrest by sequestration of Mdm2, thereby preventing Mdm2-mediated p53 degradation. In mice, knock-out of the whole *Ink4a* locus or of only p19/ARF generates a strong cancer prone condition *(33,34)*. Hence, appropriate function of these two pathways is fundamental for tumor suppression, consistent with the fact that basically all tumor cells eliminate the function of either of these pathways. Moreover, many tumor viruses encode for proteins that efficiently disrupt the function of both pRb and p53. Because of their high transforming potential, these viral oncoproteins, such as SV40 large T antigen, human papilloma virus 16 (HPV) E6 and E7 gene products, or adenovirus E1A and E1B gene products, have been and still are extensively used as transforming agents in mouse models of carcinogenesis.

2.4. Immortalization

At first sight, deregulation of proliferation and evasion from programmed cell death (apoptosis) seems sufficient to enable a cancer cell to grow to a cell population comprising a tumor mass. However, growth inhibition and apoptosis are not the only mechanisms that counteract tumor progression. Cells have also developed a device, based on their telomere length, to count the number of cell doublings. Normal cells enter crisis after a limited number of divisions (60–70 for human cells) resulting in cell cycle arrest and/or apoptosis. Telomerase, the enzyme that is responsible to maintain proper telomere length, is not active in normal human somatic cells, however, its activity is found to be up-regulated in approximately 80% of cancer cells *(59)*, prolonging their life span and allowing them to circumvent crisis and senescence *(60)*.

The functional role of telomerase in tumorigenesis has been assessed in experiments in which tumor-prone Ink4a-deficient mice have been crossed with telomerase-deficient mice (mTR–/–). In the absence of telomerase activity, tumor incidence is greatly reduced *(61)*, indicating that the gain of telomerase activity indeed favors tumor progression. On the other hand, two observations contradict this conclusion and complicate the evaluation of telomerase as a target for therapeutic intervention. First, telomerase-deficient mice, when bred up to the sixth generation, exhibit a significant tumor predisposition *(62)*. Secondly, embryonic fibroblasts deficient for both p53 and telomerase have a higher transformation rate than p53-deficient cells *(63)*. In both cases, the lack of telomerase activity correlates with a high rate of chromosomal damage and overall genomic instability. Telomere erosion is now known to be recognized by DNA damage-sensing systems resulting in the induction of p53 *(64)*. Notably, p53 deficient mice, who predominantly develop soft tissue sarcomas and lymphomas, develop tumors in the self-renewing compartments of the skin, breast, and intestine, when crossed to telomerase-deficient mice *(65)*. Therefore, it can be speculated, that in the absence of p53, cells do not arrest upon DNA damage and continue to accumulate chromosomal abnormalities, thus promoting tumor progression. Hence, pharmacological inhibitors of telomerase activity may have two distinct effects: they are likely to regress advanced tumors, however, on the other hand they may enhance progression of early tumors by accelerating the accumulation of intolerable genomic disarray.

2.5. Apoptosis/Survival

Programmed cell death (apoptosis) is a fundamental property of all multicellular organisms, and it is not surprising that virtually all cell types of the human body carry a latent form of the apoptotic program, which can be triggered upon a variety of physiological signals. Extrinsic signals, such as Fas ligand binding the Fas receptor or tumor necrosis factor-α (TNF-α) binding to its receptors, lead via a number of receptor/adaptor molecules to the activation of cascade of cysteine proteases, caspases, first by activation of an upstream caspase, which in return, activates downstream effector caspases and the execution of cell death *(66)*. In contrast, intrinsic stimuli of apoptosis activate the release of cytochrome C from the mitochondria which via activation of another upstream caspase results in the activation of downstream caspases. The latter process is induced, for example, by the p53 target gene Bax which favors release of cytochrome C from the mitochondria. In contrast, prominent anti-apoptotic members of the same family of genes, such as Bcl-2 and Bcl-x, prevent cytochrome C-induced execution of apoptosis and thus maintain survival even in the presence of apoptotic stimuli *(67)*.

As described in the previous paragraphs, oncogene-induced proliferation via up-regulation of p19/ARF results in the activation of p53, cell cycle arrest and, in cases of irreversible DNA damage, in apoptosis. In addition, there are a number of p53-independent pathways that are activated in tumor cells and that lead to apoptosis, for example the up-regulation of Fas receptor and Fas ligand on tumor cells. Hence, in order to give rise to massive tumors, tumor cells need to overcome these pro-apoptotic pathways and to escape cell death. Resistance to apoptosis can be acquired by different means. Of course, the most frequent event seen in human and mouse tumors involves mutational inactivation of p53. Fas ligand-induced apoptosis is frequently overcome by the tumor cells' expression of a nonsignaling decoy receptor that antagonizes the Fas signal by sequestration of the ligand *(66)*.

Some mouse models nicely exemplify the functional role of anti-apoptotic oncogenes in tumor progression. Most notably is the acceleration of c-Myc-induced lymphomagenesis by the apoptosis suppressor Bcl-2 *(22)*. In a similar manner, c-Myc transgene-induced massive apoptosis of pancreatic β cells is rescued by expression of Bcl-2 leading to β cell tumor formation *(68)*. On the other hand, sensitivity to apoptosis can be overcome by the up-regulated expression of survival factors, such as insulin-like growth factors (IGFs), EGFs, PDGFs, or interleukin-3. Using a transgenic mouse model of β cell carcinogenesis (Rip1Tag2), it has been demonstrated that IGF-II acts as a survival factor during tumorigenesis in vivo *(69)*. In this transgenic mouse model, expression of IGF-II is up-regulated concomitant with the onset of tumor cell hyperproliferation. Upon crossing Rip1Tag2 transgenic mice with IGF-II knock-out mice, tumor outgrowth is dramatically reduced, and this can be accounted for by an increase in tumor cell apoptosis. These experiments have clearly demonstrated the survival function of classical growth factor signal transduction pathways. However, the molecular details of how these signals repress the execution of tumor cell apoptosis remain to be elucidated.

3. GENOMIC INSTABILITY

Most of the molecular changes described above reflect genetic alterations of specific genes. Genomic integrity, however, is ensured by a complex machinery of DNA monitoring and repair enzymes making mutations of specific genes or chromosomal aberrations an unlikely event. Yet, human cancers do arise with substantial frequency, raising the question of what causes the high genomic instability found in cancer cells. Increased rates of mutations and chromosomal aberrations may be explained by the deficiencies in components of the genomic caretaker system. The most prominent example is loss of function of the tumor supressor p53 that occurs in more than 50% of all human malignancies. Proteins with similar caretaker functions are currently identified with ever increasing numbers and some of them are indeed impaired in cancer cells. Loss of function of these bona fide tumor suppressor genes promotes genomic instability subsequently leading to the generation of tumor cells with selective advantages.

3.1. Mutator Phenotype: HNPCC

In patients with hereditary non-polyposis colorectal cancer (HNPCC), most tumors show microsatellite instability (MIN). Microsatellites are highly repetitive DNA sequences that are prone to accumulate errors (mismatches) during DNA replication. In HNPCC patients, the failure to repair these mismatches is due to inactivating mutations in genes involved in postreplicative mismatch repair (MMR) *(70)*. *MMR* genes are highly conserved throughout evolution. They are all derived from the prototype bacterial *mutS* and *mutL* genes. Eukaryotic homologues are named *MSH* for mutS homologue and *MLH* for mutL homologue *(71)*. Probably six human *MSH* genes exist (1–6), where MSH2/MSH6 function in the repair of single base mismatches and MSH2/MSH/3 in the repair of two to four base insertion/deletions. Of the mutL homologues, *MLH* genes are implicated in mitotic repair, whereas MSH4 and 5 and PMS2 are involved in postmeiotic repair and MSH1 is involved in mitochondrial genome repair. Defects in the mismatch repair system can shift the spontaneous mutation rate from 10^{-6} to 10^{-3}–10^{-2}, resulting in a mutator phenotype characterized by an increased frequency of mutations in tumor suppressor genes and oncogenes. Indeed, microsatellites have been found within the coding regions of genes that are known to play important roles in cellular transformation, including APC, TGF-β receptor II, IGF-2 receptor, Tcf-4, Bax, and MMR genes themselves *(72,73)*. A failure to repair replication errors within these microsatellites invariably leads to a loss of the tumor suppressing functions of these genes.

Loss of MLH1 and MSH2 function has been implicated in HNPCC. Knock-out mice of MSH2 are fertile and develop normally. However, they exhibit a reduced life span, development of T cell lymphomas, and with older age, also skin and gastrointestinal (GI) tract tumors of benign and malignant characteristics *(74)*. MSH6 knock-out mice are fertile, and similar to MSH2 knock-out mice, they are prone to the development of B and T cell lymphomas and GI tract tumors at older age, however, they live longer than MSH2 knock-out mice *(75)*. While MSH6$^{-/-}$ mice are deficient in single MMR, insertion/deletions are still repaired, hence the longer life span. While MSH6 knock-out mice can serve as an attenuated model of HNPCC, inactivation of MSH3 was not seen in HNPCC and knock-out mice do not develop tumors *(76)*. In contrast, MLH1 knock-out mice are infertile and they are predisposed to the development of T cell lymphomas and GI tract tumors *(77)*. Although rare, MLH1 mutations are also found in patients who died very early of leukemias, lymphomas, or neurofibromatosis type 1 *(78,79)*. As expected, when MMR-deficient mice are crossed to other mouse models of tumorigenesis, tumor development is dramatically accelerated. For example, MLH1-deficiency in a truncated APC(1638n) background results in a higher incidence of GI tract tumors and in accelerated progression to malignant stages *(77)*. Intercrosses between MSH2 knock-out mice and APC-deficient (Min) mice also accelerate tumorigenesis *(80)*. Interestingly, the wild-type allele of APC is lost in both cases, most likely due to the fact that there is actually a microsatellite region within the coding region of APC that makes APC itself a target of the MIN phenotype. PMS2 knock-out mice exhibit male infertility, lymphomas, and some rare type tumors, however no GI tract tumors *(81)*. When crossed with APC^{Min} mice, an increased number of GI tumors, but no further progression to tumor malignancy, is apparent *(82)*. PMS1 knock-out mice do not develop tumors at all *(81)*.

3.2. Chromosomal Instability

In contrast to the MIN caused by MMR defects, chromosomal instability (CIN) is characterized by chromosomal rearrangements, including large deletions, fusions, and translocation *(83)*. CIN is easily recognized in tumor cells by their aneuploid DNA content. On a molecular level, a first report indicates a correlation between aneuploidy and mutations in molecules responsible for chromosome separation during mitosis *(84)*, however, a causal role of these mutations in tumor initiation is still unclear.

3.2.1. DOUBLESTRAND BREAK REPAIR

Evidence for an involvement of chromosomal instability in cancer comes from studies on DNA repair in response to double-strand DNA breaks. Familial syndromes, such as ataxia telangiectasia (AT), Nijmwegen breakage syndrome (NBS) and Li-Fraumeni (loss of p53 function) or individuals with mutations in the breast cancer susceptibility genes *BRCA1* and 2, have indicated that defects in chromosomal homeostasis predispose to cancer.

AT is a complex autosomal recessive disorder characterized by cerebellar ataxia and dilation of blood vessels within the eyes and parts of the facial regions. Patients suffer from recurrent infections due to immunodeficiencies and are predisposed to develop cancer, predominantly lymphomas and leukemias *(85)*. The gene mutated in *At* patients *(ATM)* and a closely related gene *(ATR)* have been subsequently cloned and characterized *(86)*. ATM and ATR are protein kinases that are involved in DNA damage responses. One of the substrates of ATM kinase activity is the product of the gene deleted in Nijmwegen breakage syndrome (*NBS1* or nibrin), an autosomal recessive genetic disorder characterized by an excessively high risk for the development of lymphatic tumors and an extreme sensitivity towards ionizing radiation *(87)*.

Based on the identification of these genes and their functional characterization, major insights into DNA repair mechanisms have been gained: double-strand breaks in the DNA double helix, caused for example by γ-irradiation, usually induce activation of p53 via the kinases ATM, ATR, DNA-dependent protein kinase (DNA-PK), or alternatively of the p53 family member p73 via ATM and c-Abl, resulting in growth arrest or apoptosis *(86,88)*.

DNA-PK is a molecule responsible for double-strand break repair and for specific V(D)J recombination. DNA-PK knock-out mice exhibit high susceptibility to tumor development *(89,90)*. Moreover, mice deficient for both DNA-PK and poly(ADP-ribose)polymerase (PARP), another DNA-damage sensing molecule, develop thymic lymphomas *(91)*.

ATM knock-out mice are resistant to γ-irradiation and, similar to patients, exhibit a predisposition to the development of thymic lymphomas *(92)*. Disruption of the function of ATR results in early embryonic lethality, however, in the heterozygous state a predisposition to tumor development is observed *(93)*. Inactivation of *NBS1* in mice results in embryonic lethality indicating that NBS1 mediates essential functions during proliferation in the absence of externally induced damage *(94)*.

Inheritance of mutations in the *BRCA* genes predisposes individuals to a high lifetime risk of breast and ovarian cancer *(95)*. Surprisingly, unlike other tumor supressor genes, mutations in the *BRCA* genes are not found in sporadic forms of breast cancer. BRCA1 and BRCA2 are multifunctional proteins involved in homologous recombination and transcription coupled double-strand break repair, thereby maintaining genomic integrity. Both are interacting with transcriptional regulators and repair proteins such as Rad51, which is required for recombination and recombinational repair of double-strand DNA breaks.

Homozygous deletion of BRCA1, BRCA2, and Rad51 in mice leads to early embryonic lethality and, unexpectedly, heterozygous animals develop normally and do not seem to be susceptible to the development of mammary tumors *(86,88)*. In contrast, mice that carry a truncated version of BRCA2 develop lymphoma that aquire mutations in p53, Bub1, and Mad3L, thereby losing the mitotic spindle checkpoint and ability to repair DNA *(96)*. Moreover, embryonic fibroblasts derived from BRCA1 knock-out mice are unable to arrest at the G2-M checkpoint, resulting in abnormal chromosome segregation, aneuploidy, and amplification of centrosomes, suggesting that mutant BRCA might induce genetic instability by disruption of regulation of centrosome duplication.

3.2.2. CHROMOSOME SEGREGATION

Proper separation of chromosomes during mitosis is monitored by a checkpoint that leads to cell cycle arrest if chromosomes are not correctly aligned and attached to the mitotic spindle. Loss of this checkpoint has been shown to result in chromosome mis-segregation and may contribute to genomic instability observed in many types of cancer *(97)*. The checkpoint that controls the metaphase to anaphase transition involves a number of proteins that have all been identified in yeast cell cycle regulation. In mammalian cells, most of these components are highly conserved: Mad1-3, Bub1, BubR1, and Bub3 have been shown to play a role in mitotic checkpoint control. Mammalian Bub1 and BubR1 are kinases that are active during mitosis and upon spindle checkpoint arrest. Bub1 has been shown to phosphorylate Mad1 in vitro. Mad2 has been found at decreased levels in a breast cancer cell line *(98)* and in colon cancer cell lines *(99)*. A dominant-negative version of Bub1 causes loss of checkpoint and chromosomal instability, indicating a correlation between the loss of checkpoint control genes and CIN *(84)*. However, these proteins are not found to be completely absent in human cancers. Disruption of Bub1 in *Drosophila* and Mad2 in *Caenorhabitis elegans* and in mice results in embryonic lethality with increased chromosomal aberrations and apoptosis, indicating that checkpoint control genes are important during normal mitosis even without mutational challenge *(100–102)*. Most notably, haploinsufficiency of the Mad2 locus by targeted inactivation is associated with aneuploidy in human cancer cells and in mouse embryonic fibroblasts *(103)*. Consequently, in Mad2$^{+/-}$ mice elevated chrommsome missegregation coincides with tumor development *(102)*.

3.3. Epigenetics

Besides mutation or deletion, tumor suppressor genes can also be disabled by silencing their promoters. Recent studies have demonstrated that in many different tumor cell types, CpG islands in the promoter region of many tumor suppressor genes are hypermethylated, thereby preventing their expression *(104)*. The frequency of this CpG island methylator phenotype (CIMP) accounts for most of the tumor cases in which mutations or chromosomal aberrations affecting tumor suppressor genes could not be detected. Tumor suppressor genes that are inactivated by CIMP include the von Hippel Lindau gene *(VHL)*, the cell cycle inhibitor *p16/Ink4a,* and the cell adhesion molecule *E-cadherin (105)*. Curiously, the MMR gene *MLH1* has also been found inactivated by hypermethylation, suggesting that CIMP may lead to the MIN mutator phenotype *(105)*. Hypermethylation does not appear to be a random process, since some promoters seem to be predisposed. However, the molecular mechanisms by which promoter hypermethylation is achieved and how its specificity is acquired are not known. There is only indirect evidence that alterations in DNA methylase (Mtase) activity could account for CIMP. Mtase activity is frequently found to be increased in various human malignancies, including colon cancer, hematopoietic cancers, and lung cancer *(104)*. Inhibition of Mtase activity in mice, which by the mutation of the *APC* tumor suppressor gene are predisposed to colon cancer (Min mice), have markedly reduced tumor incidence *(106)*. Other epigenetic events, for example the role chromatin regulation could play in carcinogenesis, have just started to be investigated in mouse models of tumorigenesis. On the other hand, similar to human cancers, e.g., Wilms' tumor, imprinting of specific genes is also lost during tumor progression in mouse models of tumorigenesis *(107)*, providing a experimental tool to elucidate the molecular mechanisms involved in this epigenetic event.

4. TUMOR PROGRESSION

Cancer is a disease of dynamic genetic and epigenetic changes resulting in gain and loss of function of genes that are able to modulate tumor growth. The transformation of a normal cell to a malignant tumor cell is, therefore, dependent upon a number of molecular changes. As a consequence, tumor development occurs in multiple pathological stages, including hyperplasia with high an incidence of proliferation, the formation of new blood vessels (tumor angiogenesis), extensive tissue remodeling, invasion of tumor cells into surrounding tissue and, finally, dissemination of tumor cells to form metastases. Thus, each of the molecular changes appears to be a rate-limiting, stochastic event towards malignancy, and the genes that are involved in them are of course the target of intensive investigations.

4.1. Tissue Remodeling

Altered regulation of cell–cell and cell–matrix interactions are found whenever tumor cells invade their environment. Extra-cellular matrix (ECM)-degrading proteinases regulate cellular behavior by remodeling stromal and cell surface proteins and are widely expressed during all stages of tumor development, especially the members of the matrix metalloproteinase family (MMPs) and the plasminogen activator system. Proteases are often produced as inactive zymogens deposited in the ECM closely associated with the cell surface or even in association with cell surface proteins.

To address the question whether MMPs have an implication in tumor initiation, transgenic mice have been generated expressing MMP3/stromelysin-1 specifically in the mammary gland *(108)*. Surprisingly, the mere expression of MMP3 is sufficient to initiate and promote the development of malignant mammary lesions that show epithelial to mesenchymal transition and distant metastases. Induction of neoplasia was due to proteolytic activity of MMP3 as overexpression of the MMP inhibitor TIMP-1 repressed tumor formation.

Transgenic mice expressing MMP7/matrilysin specifically in the breast epithelium develop premalignant hyperplastic nodules in older females *(109)*. Moreover, expression of MMP7 in these mice enhances the onset of primary mammary tumors of MMTV-Neu mice, however, does not significantly increase the incidence of late stage tumors and metastasis, again linking the function of a MMP to the early stages of tumor progression. A similar effect on early stage of tumorigenesis has been observed when MMP7 knock-out mice were crossed to APC[Min] mice, resulting in a significant decrease in polyp number and size without a change in invasive behavior *(110)*.

An influence of MMPs on both early and late stage tumorigenesis has been reported in a model of skin carcinogenesis. Transgenic mice expressing the early region of HPV16, specifically in basal keratinocytes, develop invasive squamous cell carcinoma of the epidermis *(111)*. Extensive remodeling of the ECM occurs early in neoplastic progression, and gelatinase B/MMP9 is already detected as active protein in hyperplastic tissue. Concomitant with this observation, HPV16 mice that lack MMP9 show a markedly delay in the development of hyperplastic and dysplastic lesions and a reduced incidence of malignancy *(112)*. Notably, MMP9 is predominantly expressed by cells of the stromal compartment, rather than by the tumor cells themselves. Bone-marrow reconstitution experiments restore the characteristic HPV16 phenotype in MMP9 knock-out mice and, moreover, demonstrate that inflammatory cells expressing MMP9 can be co-conspirators in skin carcinogenesis *(112)*.

The importance of gelatinase A/MMP2 and gelatinase B/MMP9 in tumor formation has been further elucidated in the Rip1Tag2 model of pancreatic β cell carcinogenesis *(113)*. Crossing Rip1Tag2 transgenic mice with MMP9 knock-out mice results in an impaired onset of angiogenesis and, as a consequence, in reduced tumor incidence and tumor growth *(114)*. A possible mechanism involves the MMP9-mediated activation of the angiogenic factor vascular endothelial growth factor (VEGF), which is constitutively expressed even by normal β cells, but sequestered in a latent form in the ECM. In contrast, crossing Rip1Tag2 transgenic mice with MMP2 knock-out mice has resulted in impaired tumor progression without affecting angiogenesis, suggesting that MMP2 with similar substrate specificities may have distinct functions *(114)*.

4.2. Angiogenesis

The formation of new blood vessels (angiogenesis) is critical for the growth and persistence of primary solid tumors and their metastases. Furthermore, angiogenesis is also required for metastatic dissemination, since an increase in vascular density facilitates access of tumor cells to the circulation. Induction of angiogenesis precedes the formation of malignant tumors, and increased vascularization seems to correlate with the invasive properties of tumors and thus with the malignant tumor phenotype. In the last few years, the discovery and characterization of tumor-derived angiogenesis modulators greatly contributed to our understanding of how tumors regulate angiogenesis *(115,116)*. Some of the best characterized angiogenic factors that are secreted by tumor cells include VEGF, FGFs, and angiopoietins. By binding their cognate receptors on endothelial cells, these angiogenic factors induce migration, proliferation, and tube formation of endothelial cells. Inhibition of neovascularization by anti-angiogenic compounds, such as endostatin, angiostatin, thrombospondin, platelet factor-4, TNP 470, and others, as well as the inhibition of the function of angiogenic factors, for example by neutralizing antibodies against VEGF by soluble growth factor receptors or by specific pharmaceutical inhibitors have demonstrated that angiogenesis is absolutely required for tumor outgrowth and that angiogenic factors are responsible for the onset of tumor angiogenesis *(115)*.

Mouse models have been instrumental in investigating the molecular mechanisms of tumor angiogenesis and in testing angiostatic compounds. For example, the onset of tumor angiogenesis, the angiogenic switch, has been first characterized in the Rip1Tag2 transgenic mouse model of pancreatic β cell carcinogenesis *(117)*. In these experiments, tissue biopsies from the different stages of tumor development are co-cultured with endothelial cells in a 3-dimensional collagen matrix. While endothelial cells do not respond to the presence of an early, nonangiogenic tumor stage, in the presence of a tumor stage with active angiogenesis, endothelial cells respond by migration and proliferation. These experiments have also indicated that soluble angiogenic factors are secreted by tumor cells. The Rip1Tag2 tumor model has also been instrumental to demonstrate that MMP9 is functionally involved in the onset of tumor angiogenesis by releasing latent VEGF from ECM *(114)* (see above) and that FGFs are functionally involved in tumor angiogenesis by inhibiting the angiogenic switch with soluble FGF receptors *(118)*.

In the past years, many inhibitors of angiogenesis have been identified and characterized, either protein factors or small chemical entities *(115)*. Of course, transgenic mouse models are frequently used to evaluate the efficacy of these compounds in the inhibition of tumor angiogenesis and thus tumor growth. For example, among many other assay systems, Rip1Tag2 transgenic mice have also been used to demonstrate the anti-angiogenic activities of endostatin, angiostatin, interferon α, or TNP 470 *(119,120)*.

4.3. Metastasis

Outgrowth of a solid tumor mass in late stage tumorigenesis often generates pioneer cells that move out of the primary tumor mass and invade surrounding tissue. Eventually, tumor cells intravasate into blood vessels, disseminate through the bloodstream, and extravasate at distant sites to settle and form metastases. Although only a small number of tumor cells succeed to survive this journey, 90% of all human cancer deaths are caused by metastases. Moreover, human tumors often exhibit an organ-specific pattern of metastasis. This preference of tumor cells to specifically home to a distant organ may reflect expression of specific tumor cell surface proteins that may interact with proteins on the endothelial cell surface of a particular organ. Consistent with this notion, redirection of tumor cell metastasis has been achieved in mouse models by forced expression of $\alpha_4\beta_1$ intregin or L-selectin on the surface of tumor cells *(121,122)*.

4.3.1. Loss of Cell Adhesion and Invasion

Development of malignant tumors, in particular the transition from benign lesions to invasive, metastatic cancer, is characterized by a tumor cell's ability to overcome cell–cell adhesion and to invade surrounding tissue, and changes in the expression of many cell adhesion molecules have been implicated in tumor progression. The majority of human cancers (approx 80–90%) originate from epithelial cells. Normally, epithelial cells are tightly interconnected through several junctional structures, including tight junctions, adherens-type junctions, and desmosomes. The establishment and maintenance of these junctional complexes depends on Ca^{2+}-dependent homophilic interactions mediated by the cell-adhesion molecule E-cadherin in the zonula adherens *(123)*. Critical for the activity of E-cadherin is its interaction with the catenins (α, β, and γ catenin [plakoglobin]), which link E-cadherin to the actin cytoskeleton, and any disruption of the intracellular E-cadherin-catenin complex concomitantly causes loss of cell adhesion.

Recently, it has been shown that expression of E-cadherin is lost during the transition from well-differentiated adenoma to invasive carcinoma in the Rip1Tag2 transgenic mouse model of pancreatic β cell carcinogenesis *(113)*. To assess whether loss of E-cadherin-mediated cell adhesion is a cause or a consequence of tumor progression in vivo, Rip1Tag2 mice have been crossed with transgenic mice that either express wild-type E-cadherin or a dominant-negative form of E-cadherin specifically in pancreatic β cells *(124)*. Maintenance of E-cadherin expression during β-cell tumorigenesis results in arrest of tumor development at the adenoma stage, whereas expression of a dominant-negative E-cadherin induces early in vasion and metastasis. These results demonstrate that loss of E-cadherin-mediated cell–cell adhesion is one rate-limiting step in the progression from adenoma to carcinoma in vivo.

Other cell–cell adhesion molecules that seem to play a role in tumor cell invasion and metastasis include the immunoglobulin superfamily of cell adhesion molecules (CAM). In many human cancers, including Wilm's tumor, colon carcinoma, melanoma, Ewing sarcoma, neuroblastoma, small-cell lung cancer, and multiple myeloma, re-expression of the embryonal isoforms NCAM 140, and NCAM 180 concomitant with the loss of NCAM 120 is observed. Moreover, in human pancreatic and colorectal cancer reduced levels of NCAM expression appeared to correlate with increased tumor malignancy *(125)*. NCAM's functional contribution to tumor development is still only partially understood. A first answer to this question has come also from experiments with Rip1Tag2 trangenic mice *(125)*. Similar to the development of many human cancers, expression of NCAM in Rip1Tag2 transgenic mice changes from the 120 kDa isoform in normal tissue to the 140/180 kDa isoforms in tumor tissue. To assess the role of NCAM during tumor progression, Rip1Tag2 mice have been crossed with NCAM knock-out mice. In NCAM-deficient Rip1Tag2 mice a dramatic increase in tumor metastasis was observed, predominantly metastases to local lymph nodes. In contrast, other tumor stages, in particular the transition from adenoma to carcinoma, were not affected by the loss of NCAM function, suggesting that the loss of NCAM function is one rate-limiting step in the actual metastatic dissemination of β tumor cells.

4.3.2. LYMPHANGIOGENESIS

Very recent experiments revealed that lymphangiogenesis, the formation of new lymphatic vessels, plays an important role in tumor metastasis. With the discovery of specific markers that are exclusively expressed on lymphatic endothelial cells, it has been possible to correlate increased lymphatic vessel density with progressive malignancy and metastasis *(126,127)*. Moreover, members of the VEGF family of factors, VEGF-C and -D have been identified to bind to VEGF receptor-3, a tyrosine kinase receptor that, in the adult, is exclusively expressed on lymphatic endothelial cells. Subsequently, it has been demonstrated that VEGF-C and -D are able to induce lymphangiogenesis, for example by expression of these factors in transgenic mice. Finally, the causal role of lymphangiogenesis in tumor metastasis has been demonstrated by expressing VEGF-C or VEGF-D either in xenografted tumor cell lines or in transgenic mouse models of tumorigenesis, such as Rip1Tag2 transgenic mice *(126,127)*. Expression of the lymphangiogenic factors during tumor outgrowth leads to active lymphangiogenesis, increased lymphatic vessel density in the tumor tissue and to metastatic dissemination of tumor cells.

5. TUMOR MODELS

5.1. Molecular Pathways

5.1.1. PTEN

Loss of heterozygosity at chromosome 10q23 is frequently found in a number of different human tumors, including glioblastoma, melanoma, small-cell lung carcinoma, meningioma, and cancers of the kidney, breast, endometrium, and prostate. The recently identified candidate tumor supressor gene in this region is termed *PTEN* for "phosphate and tensin homologue deleted on chromosome ten" *(128)*. Both alleles of *PTEN* are inactivated in advanced stages of glioblastomas and prostate carcinoma, but also in early stages of endometrial tumors. Moreover, germ line mutations in PTEN cause several autosomal dominant inherited cancer syndromes, such as Cowden disease, and predispose individuals to multiple benign tumors and malignancies of the breast and thyroid. PTEN is a dual specificity phosphatase, it can dephosphorylate both phosphoproteins and phospholipids, in particular the product of PI3K, phosphoinositol-3 phosphates. PTEN has been shown to exert an important function in cell cycle arrest and programmed cell death. Overexpression of PTEN in glioma and breast cancer cells induces apoptosis via inhibition of protein kinase B/Akt. Deregulation of the Akt/PI3K survival pathway upon loss of PTEN may explain its tumor suppressive role and association with late-stage more aggressive and metastatic tumors *(129)*.

Loss of function mutation in mice by targeting the catalytic domain of PTEN causes early embryonic lethality *(130–132)*. Heterozygous animals develop a variety of different tumors, including lymphoma, dysplastic intestinal polyps, endometrial atypical complex hyperplasia, prostatic neoplasia, and thyroid follicular carcinoma. In all cases, carcinomas arising in PTEN heterozygous animals were well differentiated and did not show signs of invasion or metastasis, indicating that additional genetic alterations may be necessary for malignant conversion. Consistent with the tumor suppressive function of PTEN, loss of heterozygosity was frequently observed in mouse lymphomas. In contrast, using a different strategy to inactivate PTEN, a different tumor spectrum, including tumors of the skin and testes, and a remaining wild-type allele of PTEN in hyperplastic colon mucosa and intestinal polyps of PTEN heterozygotes mice has been observed *(133)*. Biallelic inactivation of PTEN and down-regulation of the CDK inhibitor p27 are frequent events in human metastatic prostate cancer, and a similar cooperativity between these two tumor suppressors has also been observed in prostate tumors of PTEN $^{+/-}$ p27$^{-/-}$ mice, thus recapitulating the etiology of human cancer *(133)*.

Loss of PTEN cooperates also with other oncogenic events. For example, MMTV-Wnt-1 transgenic mice develop ductal carcinoma in the mammary gland, however, upon mutation of one allele of PTEN, tumors appear significantly earlier than in mice carrying either alteration alone *(134)*. The majority of these tumors exhibit loss of the wild type allele of PTEN indicating a growth advantage for tumors upon complete inactivation of PTEN.

5.1.2. TGF-ʙ Signaling

TGF-β is a potent inhibitor of epithelial cell growth and modulator of cellular phenotype. TGF-β transduces its signal via Smad proteins, a family of intracellular proteins that become phosphorylated upon TGF-β receptor activation and subsequently translocate into the nucleus, where in combination with cofactors they act as transcriptional regulators *(135)*.

Mutations within the TGF-β pathway have been found in various human tumors, including pancreatic and colorectal cancer. The role of TGF-β1 in skin carcinogenesis has been addressed in transgenic mice expressing TGF-β1 specifically in keratinocytes *(136)*. Induction of skin tumors by the tumor initiator/promoter protocol DMBA/TPA has revealed that keratinocyte-derived TGF-β1 acts as inhibitor of keratinocyte growth, thus reducing outgrowth of benign tumors. In contrast, TGF-β1 seemed to promote tumorigenesis in late stages as judged by the appearance of early carcinoma and an increase in absolute numbers of malignant spindle cell carcinoma. These studies indicate distinct roles for TGF-β1 in early and late stage tumorigenesis: it acts as tumor suppressor of benign tumor outgrowth, but as a tumor promoter in the progression to invasive carcinoma.

However, mice heterozygous for deletions of TGF-βs, TGF-β type II receptor, Smad2, or Smad4 do not develop colorectal cancer (137,138). In a homozygous state, these mice are embryonic or postnatal lethal, thus precluding tumor formation. For one of the TGFs, TGF-β1, a tumor suppressive function has been documented upon treatment of TGF-β1 heterozygous animals with carcinogens; tumors in TGF-β1 mutant mice occurred at higher multiplicity and were more malignant than in wild-type animals (139). In contrast, another component of the TGF-β signaling, Smad3, has been found to play a critical role in the formation of colorectal adenocarcinomas, since 100% of mice with homozygous deletion of Smad3 develop highly invasive, metastasizing colorectal cancer, with great similarity to the human disease (140). APC function is not lost in these tumors, rather it appears that inactivation of the TGF-β signaling pathway in these mice blocks the differentiation of epithelial cells and keeps them in their proliferative state. Consistent with this notion, overexpression of Smad3 inhibits proliferation of epithelial cells (138).

5.1.3. WNT SIGNALING: FAMILIAL ADENOMATOUS POLYPOSIS

The proto-oncogene *Wnt-1* has been identified by its oncogenic properties activated through insertion of MMTV (Int-1) (141,142). Since then, the number of *Wnt* family members is ever increasing. Most of the members of the family activate Wnt signaling by binding to their receptor Frizzled, which results via the adaptor protein Dishevelled and casein kinase II in the inhibition of glycogen synthetase kinase 3β (GSK-3β). One of the substrates of GSK-3β is β-catenin. β-catenin is usually sequestered in the E-cadherin adherens junction or in tight-junction complexes. Nonsequestered free β-catenin is rapidly phosphorylated by GSK-3β in a complex that comprises, in addition to GSK-3β and β-catenin, the scaffolding proteins axin or conductin and the tumor suppressor protein APC. Phosphorylated β-catenin is subsequently degraded by the ubiquitin-proteasome pathway. If APC is nonfunctional or GSK-3β activity is blocked by the activated Wnt signaling pathway, β-catenin accumulates at high levels in the cytoplasm. Subsequently, it translocates to the nucleus, where it binds to a member of the Tcf/Lef-1 family of transcription factors and possibly activates the expression of Tcf/Lef-1-target genes, such as *c-Myc* and *cyclin D1* (141,142). Hence, up-regulated Wnt signaling plays an important role in the induction of cellular proliferation.

The tumor supressor gene *APC* has been initially identified by genetic analysis of familial adenomatous polyposis (FAP) characterized by thousands of benign colorectal polyps, some of which will progress to a malignant state if not removed. APC has also been found to be mutated in a large fraction of sporadic colon cancers, mainly truncating mutations (143,144). The convergence of the Wnt signaling pathway and APC function has been a very exciting issue in the past few years, and the functional roles of APC and β-catenin have been investigated in great detail, mainly in the etiology of colon carcinoma and melanoma.

A mouse model of FAP has been generated by random mutation, resulting in a mouse line called the Min mice for multiple intestinal neoplasia (APC[Min]). These mice carry a nonsense mutation at the region corresponding to codon 850 of the human APC gene. Heterozygous APC^{Min} mice mimic FAP remarkably well, but develop polyps of the small intestine rather than in the colon *(145)*. Unlike human colorectal cancer, intestinal polyps in the APC^{Min} mice rarely progress to malignancy. Still, these mice have been frequently used for genetic complementation experiments to study the function of genes of interest during tumorigenesis. For example, crossing APC^{Min} mice with DNA methylase knock-out mice has resulted in a reduction of tumor load *(106)*, and combinaton of p53 knock-out mice with APC^{Min} mice resulted in pancreatic neoplasia *(146)*.

Similar to the phenotype of the APC^{Min} mouse, truncation of APC at amino acid 716 causes early embryonic lethality in the homozygous state and formation of multiple intestinal polyps in heterozygous animals *(147)*. Conditional APC knock-out mice have refined this model, for example, recombinant adenovirus expressing Cre recombinase is used to specifically generate alleles of APC, which are truncated at aa 580 in colonic crypt cells and, consequently, induce the development of numerous polyps that eventually progressed to malignancy *(148)*. While loss of the wild-type allele of *APC* is observed in the polyps of these mice, unlike human colorectal cancer, mutations of *K-Ras* or loss of p53 have not been found *(149,150)*.

Mice carrying a truncation of APC at aa 1638 are viable and tumor-free and, importantly, regulation of β-catenin appears unaffected *(151)*. APC$^{\Delta1638}$ proteins lack the carboxy-terminal binding sites for tubulin, DLG, EB1, and possibly p34^{cdc2}, but retain the β-catenin and conductin/axin binding motifs. These data provide strong evidence for the importance of β-catenin in tumor formation. Mutations in β-catenin are also described in desmoid tumors, gastric cancers, thyroid cancers, hepatoblastoma, and tumors of the hair follicle *(141)*. These mutations affect mainly the N-terminal phosphorylation sites of β-catenin, resulting in stabilization of the protein and constitutive activation of downstream signals. Such constitutive-active β-catenin mutants have been expressed in a number of tissue types, however, thus far, only the expression in the skin of transgenic mice has resulted in tumor formation, namely epitheloid cysts and differentiated hair tumors morphological similar to human trichofolliculomas and pilomatricomas *(152)*. In contrast, overexpression of the transcription factor Lef-1 in the epidermis does not induce tumor formation, but leads to misorientation of hair follicles *(153)*. However, not all Tcf/Lef-1 transcription factors seem to cooperate with β-catenin in its oncogenic action. For example, mice deficient for the transcription factor Tcf-1 develop spontaneous mammary and colon carcinoma and, when crossed to APC^{Min} mice, these animals display 10× more intestinal polyps as compared to Tcf-1$^{+/+}$ littermates, raising the possibility that Tcf-1 is a repressor of the Wnt signaling pathway *(154)*.

5.1.4. Hedgehog Pathway: Basal Cell Carcinoma

Deregulation of the developmental signaling pathway involving mammalian homologues of the *Drosophila* segment polarity genes Hedgehog (*Hh*) and Patched (*Ptc*) contributes to tumor formation in various tissues *(155)*. The importance of the Hh pathway in the development of basal cell carcinoma (BCC) is supported by the identification of the Ptc receptor as defective gene in an autosomal dominant disease, called basal cell nevus syndrome (BCNS). BCNS or Gorlic's syndrome are characterized by developmental defects, skeletal abnormalities, and predisposition to certain tumors, including BCC, medulloblastoma, and meningiomas. The Hh signal transduction pathway constitutes an important developmental pathway as first delineated for *Drosophila* Hh and later for the mammalian homologues Sonic Hh, Indian Hh, and Desert hedgehog Hh (Shh, Ihh, and Dhh, respectively). Inactivation of the Ptc receptor or constitutive activation of the Hh pathway results in transcriptional activation of the proto-oncogene *Gli* and, subsequently, in the activation of the TGF-β and Wnt signaling pathways thereby influencing embryonic patterning and cell polarity. While rare cases of human BCC, medulloblastoma, and breast cancer samples exhibit Shh mutations, the majority of cancers analyzed contains inactivating mutations of Ptc or oncogenic activating mutations of Smoothened (Smo), which are the two antagonistic receptors regulating Shh signaling *(155)*.

Transgenic expression of Shh in skin leads to epidermal proliferation, loss of differentiation and epidermal lesions that detach from the basal membrane due to lack of certain cell adhesion molecules, altogether characteristics of human BCC *(156)*. Moreover, expression of a mutant variant of Smo provokes a similar skin phenotpe in late embryonic skin *(157)*. All components of the Hh pathway seem to contribute to the formation of BCC. For example, transgenic expression of Gli2 in cutaneous keratinocytes results in a practical model of spontaneous BCC in adult mice *(158)*. Similarly, expression of human *Gli1* induces formation of several types of spontaneous skin tumors, including BCC, cylindroma, and trichoblastoma *(159)*. The *Gli1* cDNA used in this study has been originally identified as an amplified oncogene in human glioma *(160)*. However, in contrast to human epithelial malignancies, where mutations in the *p53* and *Ha-Ras* genes are frequently found, neither of them has been affected during Gli-induced tumorigenesis.

Targeted deletion of the Ptc receptor leads to skin tumors in heterozygous animals only upon irradiation *(161)*, although inactivation of Ptc1 is a major event in sporadic and familial basal cell carcinoma in patients. However, animals heterzygous for Ptc resemble some features of BCNS, in that they exhibit larger body size, skeletal abnormalities, and cerebellar tumors *(162)*. Somatic mutations in the Ptc gene are frequently found in medulloblastoma and germline mutations in the Ptc gene in BCNS predispose individuals to a number of different tumors, including medulloblastoma. Consistent with these observations, heterozygous Ptc knock-out mice exhibit several characteristics of the human disease and about 15% of animals develop cerebellar tumors. Moreover, high levels of *Gli1* observed in the mouse medulloblastoma indicate activation of the Hh pathway or reduced Ptc activity in the tumor cells. Interestingly, tumors retain one wild-type Ptc allele and also express the protein, thus arguing that haploinsufficiency of Ptc$^{+/-}$ is sufficient to promote tumor formation. Interestingly, lack of p53 in the Ptc$^{+/-}$ animals dramatically accelerates tumor development and increases the incidence of tumors form 15% in p53 wild-type mice to more than 95% in mice lacking p53 *(163)*. Finally, a small subset of Ptc$^{+/-}$ mice develop neoplasms resembling human rhabdomyosarcomas with an up-regulation of IGF-II expression *(164)*.

5.2. Some More Tumor Type-Specific Models

5.2.1. MELANOMA

Melanoma involves multiple genetic and epigenetic events; it affects a younger population and it is notorious for its propensity to metastasize early in the course of the disease. The discovery of genes that are almost exclusively expressed in melanocytes, such as tyrosinase and tyrosinase-related protein-1 and -2 (TRP-1 and -2), and the subsequent cloning and characterization of their promoter regions allowed specific expression of oncogenes in melanocytes. However, early expression of these melanocyte-specific genes in the presumptive retinal pigmental epithelium (RPE) has resulted in the formation of RPE tumors *(165)*. The resulting death of the animals prevents analysis of melanoma development which is only possible by transplantation to syngeneic hosts *(166,167)*. Such ocular melanoma and melanocytic lesions have been obtained by expression of SV40 T antigen, viral Ha-Ras, or the Ret oncogene *(13,168–170)*. In contrast, expression of hepatocyte growth factor/scatterfactor (HGF/SF) has resulted in an autocrine activation of the c-Met receptor in melanocytes leading to full blown melanoma development, including metastasis to the liver *(8)*.

The search for genetic loci linked to melanoma predisposition has yielded some prominent candidates, such as loss of the tumor supressors Ink4a (Mts-1) and PTEN as well as amplification of the EGF receptor. As described above, the *Ink4a* locus encodes the two unrelated proteins, the cell cycle inhibitor p16 and the p53 stabilizer p19/ARF. In mice, deletion of the entire *Ink4a* locus or the exclusive inactivation of p19/ARF generates a strong cancer prone condition *(33,34)*. When crossed to transgenic mice that express v-Ha-Ras under the control of tyrosinase promoter, these mice develop amelanotic, invasive, and highly vascular tumors *(13)*. Notably, when v-Ha-Ras is expressed under the control of the tetracycline-inducible system, restraining of transgene expression results in the complete regression of melanoma, indicating that oncogenic Ras is not only required for tumor initiation but also for tumor maintenance *(14)*.

5.2.2. Squamous Cell Carcinoma

For many decades, chemical carcinogenesis in mouse skin has been used as a model for squamous cell cancer, and from these studies the definition of tumor initiation, promotion, and malignant conversion has arisen. To mimic skin cancer, transgenic mice have been generated predominantly by using keratin promoters to drive expression of v-Ha-Ras, which is frequently mutated in epidermal hyperplasias and papillomas *(171)*. However, the rate and frequency of tumorigenesis is limited in these mice, and additional events seem to be required for full blown tumorigenesis. One of these transgenic mouse lines, the TG.AC mice, expressing activated viral Ha-Ras under control of the ζ-globin promoter in an FVB/N background *(10)* is routinely used in chemical skin carcinogenesis experiments or in genetic complementation experiments. For example, when crossed to transgenic mice that specifically express the angiogenic factor VEGF in keratinocytes, TG.AC tumorigenesis is accelerated *(172)*. Moreover, in a Fos knockout background, malignant progression upon tumor promoter treatment is prevented, indicating that Fos is required for tumor progression *(173)*. v-Ha-Ras expression in TG.AC mice also cooperates with p53 deficiency or overexpression of Mdm2 *(174)*.

Among many other transgenic mouse lines that develop skin cancer, expression of E2F1 under the control of the keratin-5 promoter (K5-E2F1) nicely demonstrates the oncogenic and tumor suppressor function of E2F: these mice are predisposed to spontaneous tumors in a variety of epithelia, however, they are resistant to chemical carcinogenesis at the initiation stage due to an induction of apoptosis *(46)*.

Finally, multistage development of squamous cell carcinoma (SCC) is faithfully recapitulated in a transgenic mouse line that carries the HPV 16 E6 and E7 genes under the control of the keratin-14 promoter. Expression of the viral oncogenes in basal keratinocytes of the skin results in epidermal hyperplasia after 1 mo. dysplasia after 3–6 mo, and, in an FVB/N background, invasive carcinoma by 8–12 mo *(175)*. Reminiscent of human cervical cancers, estrogen profoundly induces cervical and vaginal SCC *(176)*.

5.2.3. BREAST CANCER

Already in the early days of mouse breeding spontaneous formation of breast tumors has been observed in C3H/HeJ females after several cycles of pregancy and regression. Subsequently, it has been found that this strain carries a latent infection of MMTV and that the expression of genes which are located nearby the integration sites are activated by the strong enhancer contained in the long terminal repeat (LTR) of the virus *(177)*. Molecular characterization of these genes has lead to the discovery of a number of proto-oncogenes, the so-called Int-genes, comprising a number of now well-studied oncogenes (see *Section 5.3.*). Subsequently, the hormone-dependent tissue-specific activity of the MMTV promoter in mammary epithelial cell and in prostate epithelial cells has been used for the generation of transgenic mouse models of mammary carcinogenesis.

In 20–30% of human breast cancers, the proto-oncogene *Neu/ErbB-2,* a member of the EGFR gene family, has been found to be amplified and, hence, the wild-type and an activated form of this tyrosine kinase receptor have been used to generate mouse model of mammary carcinogenesis. In transgenic mouse lines that express activated Neu under the control of the MMTV LTR (MMTV-Neu), female mice reproducibly develop poorly differentiated adenocarcinomas of the epithelia of the mammary gland, whereas MMTV-c-Myc or MMTV-v-Ha-Ras mice only stochastically develop tumors *(178,179)*.

The role of the *Neu* oncogene has been recently confirmed by transgenic expression of the wild-type or the activated from of Neu under the control of the endogeneous Neu-promoter. In both cases, malignant foci form during multiple rounds of pregnancy *(180)*. Similarly, conditional expression of activated Neu under its own promoter leads to focal malignancies after a long latency period *(181)*. However, expression of activated Neu under normal transcriptional control does not seem to be sufficient for tumor formation; amplification of the transgene and, with it, elevated levels of the Neu protein is observed in these tumors.

In many transgenic approaches undertaken to mimic mammary carcinogenesis, the MMTV promoter, the whey acidic protein or the β-lactoglobulin promoter have been used to drive transgenic expression of a number of potential oncogenes, including SV40 T antigen, v-Ha-Ras, c-Myc, Bcl-2, cyclin E, and many others, all leading by themselves or in combination with each other to the development of mammary adeno-carcinomas *(177,182)*. Consistent with the insertion/activation mechanism of MMTV-induced carcinogenesis, MMTV-driven transgenic expression of Int-genes results into oncogenesis by themselves, for example Int-3 (Notch) *(183)*, or in cooperation with other oncogenes, for example Int-1 (Wnt-1) with other integration events of MMTV *(184)*, or Int-1 with TGF-α or PTEN-deficiency *(185)*.

The 5′ flanking region of the C3 (1) component of the rat prostate steroid binding protein (PSBP) has also been used to target expression of SV40 T antigen to the epithelium of the mammary gland *(186)* and the prostate (see *Section 5.2.4.*). However, unlike most of the other models, these mice develop tumors already in virgin females with a clear hormone independence during the formation of invasive carcinomas.

Some of these mouse models have been further employed to investigate subsequent genetic aberrations that may be causally involved in breast carcinogenesis. Cooperative effects have been found with mutations in p53, with genomic instability or loss of heterozygosity *(187,188)*. Notably, although p53-deficient mice predominantly develop soft tissue sarcomas and lymphomas, when crossed to telomerase-deficient mice, they develop epithelial cancers with high incidence by a process involving genomic instability *(65)*. The role of genomic instability in mouse breast carcinogenesis has also been demonstrated by ablating BRCA1 specifically in the mammary gland, resulting in tumor formation with very long latency and at low frequency. However, when combined with p53-deficiency, tumors form with high incidence *(189)*. Finally, transgenic mice expressing a dominant-negative form of p53 (p53 172R-H) under the control of the WAP promoter exhibit a significantly reduced resistance to chemically induced carcinogenesis of the mammary epithelium *(182)*.

5.2.4. Prostate Carcinoma

In human patients, two pathological situations are distinguished in the prostate: prostate intraepithelial neoplasia (PIN) vs benign prostatic hyperplasia (BPH), with PIN being most likely the precursor for cancer. Malignant prostate cancers are further differentiated into androgen-dependent earlier lesions, which are amenable to androgen-ablation therapy, and androgen-independent progressive disease. Many genes have been implicated in the etiology of PIN, including *MXII, PTEN, pRb, BRCA1, Bcl-2, DCC,* and *DPC4,* however, thus far no master regulator, such as APC in colorectal cancer, has been found for PIN.

Since the mouse prostate is anatomically not quite comparable to the human prostate, xenograft transplantation experiments have been popular to study prostate carcinogenesis. More recently, with the discovery of prostate-specific promoters, several transgenic mouse lines have been generated which develop prostate cancer. The probasin ligand carrier family of proteins is specifically expressed in epithelial cell nuclei and the ducts of the dorsolateral and ventral prostate *(190)*. Their expression is dependent on androgens and, to a lesser degree, on glucocorticoids. A short fragment of the probasin promoter combined with chicken lysozyme MAR sequences has been used to target expression of SV40 T antigen to the prostate epithelium. These mice, subsequently called the TRAMP (transgenic adenocarcinoma mouse prostate) model, develop prostate cancer in a multistep tumorigenesis pathway *(191,192)*. Focal adenocarcinomas form between 10 and 20 weeks of age with 100% incidence, and advanced stages recapitulate metastasis to lymph nodes and lung and to bone in an FVB/N genetic background. This model is now frequently used to study the molecular events involved in multistage tumorigenesis, for example the IGF axis *(193)*, and for therapeutic tests, such as for androgen-ablation experiments or immunotherapy *(194–196)*. In contrast to the expression of SV40 T antigen, probasin promoter-driven expression of Ha-Ras has only resulted in epithelial and stromal hyperplasia, but not in neoplasia *(192)*.

Other promoters have also been used to target prostate epithelial cells in transgenic mice. For example, the C3(1) androgen-regulated promoter that usually drives expression of the ventral prostate secretory protein PSBP has been used to express SV40 T-antigen; while females develop mammary adenocarcinomas, males develop prostate cancer *(197)*. Stepwise tumor progression from low grade to high grade PIN is nicely recapitulated in these mice; similar to human PIN, tumors also show mutations of the Ras gene *(198)*. In contrast, expression of Bcl-2 under the control of the C3(1) promoter has resulted in hypertrophy, but not in neoplasia *(199)*.

Neuroendocrine cells, the rarest cell type in the prostate have been targeted by the expression of T antigen using the mouse cryptidin promoter. These mice rapidly developed progressive metastasizing cancer which is even androgen-independent, hence providing a useful model for prostate cancer with neuroendocrine origin *(200)*. Finally, fetal globin-T antigen transgenic mice develop prostate tumors at high frequency and short latency with neuroendocrine and epithelial features and, thus, are a model for late stage metastazing cancer that is not androgen-dependent *(201)*.

5.2.5. PANCREATIC CARCINOMA

Human pancreatic adenocarcinomas frequently exhibit activating mutations of K-Ras and loss of function for p53, Ink4a, and Smad4. However, transgenic expression of K-Ras in acinar cells of exocrine pancreas result in tumors with acinar characteristics that do not resemble human ductal pancreatic adenocarcinoma *(202)*.

Recently, a mouse model of ductal pancreatic cancer has been generated by overexpression of TGF-α under control of the rat elastase promoter *(203)*. Persistent activation of the EGF receptor by TGF-α results in elevated levels of Ras activity as well as other signaling pathways througout adulthood, eventually leading to premalignant lesions of tubular structure. Furthermore, induction of p53 and its direct target p21 in tubular complexes of TGF-α transgenic mice indicates that p53 acts as tumor suppressor in pancreatic tumor progression. When crossed to p53 knock-out mice, the incidence of pancreatic tumors increases significantly in p53$^{+/-}$ mice and reaches 100% penetrance in p53$^{-/-}$ mice, suggesting that the loss of p53 is indeed a rate-limiting step in pancreatic carcinogenesis. A critical role of p53 in pancreatic tumorigenesis has also been confirmed by the surprising observation that APC^{Min} mice, null for p53, are predisposed to pancreatic acinar cell adenocarcinoma *(146)*. Loss of heterozygosity analyses have revealed additional genetic alterations, such as loss of the *Ink4a* and *Smad4* locus in about 30% of cases. Hence, these TGF-α transgenic mice develop pancreatic tumors similar to the human disease with regard to cellular differentiation, growth characteristics, and genetic alterations.

5.2.6. HEPATOCELLULAR CARCINOMA

A number of genes are specifically expressed in hepatocytes, and their promoter regions have been used to target expression of various oncogenes to the liver of transgene mice. For example, expression of SV40 T antigen under the control of the albumin or the antithrombin III promoter leads to the development of multifocal hepatocellular carcinoma (HCC) at remarkable synchrony *(204,205)*. In contrast, varying results have been obtained with the use of the α-1-antitrypsin promoter to express SV40 T antigen. Some lines develop liver tumors exclusively, while other lines exhibit gastric neoplasias, pancreatic carcinoma or kidney hyperplasia *(206)*. Similarly, depending on the transgenic line, expression of v-Ha-Ras under control of the L-type pyruvate kinase promoter results not only in HCC, but also in polycystic kidney disease and epididymis hyperplasia *(207)*. Surprisingly, HCC sporadically develops in mice that express growth hormone under the control of the metallothionein promoter *(208)*. Some of these mouse models have been used to assess the involvement of cooperating factors in liver carcinogenesis. For example, T antigen transgenic mice have been used to demonstrate that tissue inhibitor of metalloproteinase-1 (TIMP-1) interferes with tumor cell proliferation and with tumor vascularization *(209)*.

Cooperation between oncogenes in the induction of hepatocellular carcinogenesis has also been nicely exemplified in transgenic mice that express c-Myc under the control of the albumin promoter and TGF-α under control of the metallothionein promoter. Co-expression of the two transgenes dramatically accelerated the development of HCC as compared to the neoplastic lesions caused by the transgenes alone *(21)*. Moreover, multistage tumorigenesis with a number of subsequent genetic and epigenetic changes is observed in the doubletransgenic mice, thus resembling human HCC *(210)*. Notably, co-expression of HGF inhibits c-Myc-induced carcinogenesis *(211)*. These mice have been also instrumental in the molecular dissection of multistage tumorigenesis. For example, they have been employed to demonstrate that the disruption of the pRB/E2F pathway and inhibition of apoptosis are major oncogenic events during hepatocellular carcinogenesis *(212)*.

Mutational analysis of two different HCC mouse models suggests that deregulated β-catenin might serve as a second hit in tumor progression cooperating with a distinct tumor pathway. For example, c-Myc-induced liver tumors display a significant fraction of β-catenin mutations *(213)*. In contrast, T-antigen induced hepatocellular tumors do not gain activating mutations of β-catenin *(214)*. Since T-antigen itself disrupts the cell cycle efficiently by sequestration of pRb, a T-antigen induced tumor may not require additional mutations in β-catenin.

Chronic infection with hepatitus B virus (HBV) can cause liver cancer in humans, and experimental approaches that employed the liver-specific expression of HBV genes in transgenic mice have helped to shed some light into the etiology of HBV-dependent liver carcinogenesis. Transgenic mice that express the major envelope protein of HBV, HBV surface antigen, represent an experimental model for chronic infection with HBV, manifested by prolonged hepatocelluar injury, necrosis, hyperplasia, and elavated incidence of liver cancer after some latency *(215)*. Intercrossing these mice with TGF-α transgenic mice has resulted in accelerated liver carcinogenesis in males but not in females *(216)*. Expression of the HBV regulatory protein HBx under its own regulatory element has resulted in the stepwise development of HCC, thereby nicely resembling HBV-induced liver carcinogenesis, again with faster kinetic in males than in females *(217)*.

5.2.7. LUNG CANCER

Mutations in oncogenes and loss of tumor suppressor genes are also found in the different types of lung cancer in patients; most frequently are mutations in K-Ras and p53, overexpression of cyclin D1, Bcl-2, or ErbB2/Neu, and loss of Ink4a or pRb. With the cloning of genes that are specifically expressed in lung epithelia, such as the human surfactant protein C (SPC) in alveolar type II pneumocytes and the Clara cell reactive 10 kDa protein (CC10) gene in Clara cells, it is possible to target expression of cocogenes to pulmonary epithelium and to generate transgenic mouse models of lung carcinogenesis. Examples are expression of SV40 T antigen *(218)* or c-Raf-1 kinase *(219)* under control of the SPC promoter. Moreover, expression of T antigen under the control of the keratin-19 promoter develop bronchiolar papillary tumors with progression to lung adenocarcinomas *(220)*. Cooperative effects between different oncogenes in lung carcinogenesis have also been demonstrated, for example in SPC-c-Myc and SPC-EGF bitransgenic mice *(221)*. However, specific transgenic mouse models that attempt to mimic the molecular changes observed during human lung carcinogenesis, in particular mutations in K-Ras and overexpression of cyclin D1 in a p53-, Ink4a-, or pRb-deficient background, have yet to be generated.

5.2.8. Neurofibromatosis Type 1

Neurofibromatosis type 1 (NF1) is an autosomal dominant disorder characterized by tumors of the neural crest, including benign neurofibromas and malignant neurosarcomas. Loss of NF1 activates Ras signaling and cooperates with inactivating mutations of p53 during tumorigenesis. The NF1 gene neurofibromin encodes a guanosine triphosphate activating protein (GAP) that negatively regulates signaling by the GTPase Ras. Mice carrying a targeted disruption in one allele of the *NF1* gene are tumor prone and develop tumors associated with NF1: pheochromocytomas and myeolid leukemias, thereby confirming the tumor suppressive function of NF1 *(222)*. In both tumor types, loss of the wild-type allele is found with high frequency. Additional genetic alterations, however, are difficult to detect due to the heterogeneity of the cell types within the tumor samples.

Although NF1$^{+/-}$ mice are cancer prone, they do not develop neurofibromas and, therefore, do not recapitulate the etiology of neural crest tumors. Loss of the remaining wild-type allele as a rate limiting step in the formation of neurofibromas in mice was proven in chimeric animals composed in part of NF1$^{-/-}$ cells *(223)*. In addition, mutations of p53 predispose NF1 heterozygous animals to wider spectrum of tumors, including soft tissue sarcomas and neural crest-derived malignanacies *(223,224)*. Interestingly, NF1 and p53 genes are linked in humans and mice and all tumor cell lines established from these mice exhibited loss of heterozygosity at both the NF1 and the p53 locus. Finally, combined loss of both tumor suppressors, NF1 and p53 induces a multistage tumor progression pathway, ranging from low-form astrocytoma to glioblastoma multiforme, thereby accurately recapitulating human glioma formation *(225)*.

5.2.9. Neurofibromatosis Type 2

NF2 is a rare dominantly inherited disorder associated with tumors of the nervous systems, including schwannomas, meningiomas, and ependymomas. NF2 is a classic tumor suppressor gene; NF2 patients carry one defective NF2 allele in their germline and lose the second allele during tumor progression. Moreover, somatic inactivation of both NF2 alleles is found in the majority of sporadic schwannomas and meningiomas. The NF2 locus encodes for a protein of the ERM family of cytoskeleton-membrane linker proteins, called merlin. Reorganization of the actin-cytoskeleton is dependent on functional ERM proteins, and connected with adhesion and migration of cells, merlin activity is often altered during tumor progression.

Targeted mutation of the NF2 locus leads to the development of a wide spectrum of metastatic tumors in heterozygous animals, with loss of the second allele is tumor cells *(226)*. In contrast to human NF2 patients that develop benign tumors of the nervous system, heterozygous NF2 mice develop osteosarcomas, fibrosarcomas, and HCC after a long latency period. The metastasizing potential of these tumors is striking, since most other mouse models fail to establish secondary tumors at distant sites, and since human schwannomas and meningiomas of NF2 patients are relatively benign. Considering the cellular function of the cytoskeletal linker protein merlin, however, a loss of function mutation might promote tumor cell migration and the subsequent formation of metastasis.

Transgenic mice expressing a mutated from of merlin under a Schwann cell-specific promoter have been generated *(227)*. The mutation used in these transgenic mice is found in NF2 patients and may function as a dominant-negative version of merlin, thus interfering with the function of the endogenous protein. Indeed, many of these mice develop Schwann cell hyperplasia and schwannomas and prove a causal role for merlin in tumorigenesis of the nervous system. Finally, specific ablation of merlin function by conditional knock-out technique in Schwann cells results in characteristics of human NF2, including schwannomas, Schwann cell hyperplasia, cataract, and osseous metaplasia. Hence, the tumor suppressor function of NF2 in context of murine schwannomas has been established, and failure of the heterozygous NF2 mice to form schwannomas can be explained by an insufficient loss of the second allele.

5.2.10. ACUTE PROMYELOCYTIC LEUKEMIA

Acute promyelocytic leukemia (APL) is a subtype of acute nonlymphocytic leukemia (ANLL), characterized by uncontrolled expansion of cells at the promyelocytic stage of neutrophilic differentiation. A receprocal translocation of chromosomes 15 and 17, t(15;17)(q22;q21), has been identified to tightly correlate with APL *(286)*. The gene encoding retinoic acid receptor *(RARα)* has been found within the breakpoint region of chromosome 17 and to be fused to a gene within the breakpoint of chromosome 15, named *PML.* The translocation creates two fusion proteins, RARα-PML and PML-RARα. RARs are members of the superfamily of nuclear hormone receptors, which act in heterodimers with retinoid-X-receptors (RXR). In the absence of retinoic acid (RA), by binding to co-repressors, RARs act as transcriptional repressors. RA causes the dissociation of the co-repressors and the recruitment of co-activators, resulting into activation of gene expression. PML is a member of the RING finger family of protein, localized to nuclear bodies, but with unknown function. In more rare cases of APL, RARα has been found to be fused by reciprocal translocations to other partners, including the zinc finger protein *(PLZF)* gene, the nucleophosmin *(NPM)* gene, and the nuclear mitotic apparatus *(NuMA)* gene located on chromosomes 11, 5, or 11 *(228,229).* Most notably, RA induces remission of the disease by stimulating the differentiation of tumor cells *(230),* and APL has become a paradigm for therapeutic approaches utilizing differentiation agents (differentiation therapy). Such defined genetic aberrations have been a opportunity to mimic the disease in transgenic mouse models *(228,229).*

Using either the human cathepsin-G promoter or the human MRP8 promoter and human PML-RARα cDNA as a transgene, mice developed leukemia with high frequency, demonstrating the causal role of the fusion protein in the etiology of APL. However, there are still significant differences in the pathology of the disease between the different transgenic mouse lines and human disease. Moreover, full-blown leukemia does not develop at birth and is preceded by a preleukemic period of variable length, suggesting that other events are required for leukemogenesis.

Detailed mutational analysis of the fusion proteins by transgene expression also revealed major insights into the mode of action of the deregulated activity of RARα. These experiments also revealed that the PML moiety of the fusion protein plays an important role. PML is a component of nuclear bodies that are composed of multiple proteins and associate with the nuclear matrix. While the function of PML in the nuclear bodies remains to be elucidated, it may affect the regulation of cell proliferation and survival by suppressing cell growth. Notably, targeted inactivation of PML in mice results in the formation of a variety of tumors *(231).*

Recently, transgenic mice expressing all four fusion proteins have been generated to compare the contribution of the different fusion partners. By comparison, there are slight differences in the timing of leukemia development and in the actual phenotype. For example, the PLZF-RARα fusion gene is not sufficient to provide the block of neutrophil development at the promelocytic stage, a hallmark of APL. The reverse fusion partner, RARα-PLZF, may be required as well, and the X-RARα fusion proteins, despite their identity in the RARα protion, do not seem to be identical in their function.

Transgenic expression of the reciprocal fusion partners by themselves, for example the transactivation domain of RARα fused to the C terminus of PML, alone does not cause leukemia. However, when crossed to PML-RARα transgenic mice, an increase in penetrance and earlier onset of leukemia development is observed. RARα-PLZF by itself is also not sufficient to, induce leuemogenesis but can impair myelopoiesis *(232)*.

Of course, the translocation in human cancers also results in a heterozygous situation for the nonaffected alleles of PML and RARα, and the contribution of the fusion protein itself and/or the potential haploinsufficient effect of the translocation have to be distinguished. Simple overexpression of the fusion proteins, hence, can not completely recapitulate APL of human patients. Research is underway, mainly pioneered by the laboratory of Pier-Paolo Pandolfi (Memorial Sloan Kettering Cancer Center), to accurately recapitulate APL by combining mice that express various fusion proteins, knockout mice to modulate gene dosage of the remaining alleles, knock-in mice to mimic expression patterns, and the Cre/LoxP inducible recombination system to generate APL-specific chromosomal aberrations. These complex approaches will certainly help to understand the detailed molecular mechanisms involved in APL and will offer a better chance in developing efficacious treatment for this neoplastic disease.

5.2.11. LYMPHOMA

Lymphoid neoplasias often involve translocation of cellular protooncogene, such as *c-Myc, Bcl-2,* and *cyclin D1,* to an immunoglobulin locus resulting in deregualted expression of the oncogene. A number of transgenic mice have been generated that utililize enhancers from the immunoglobulin heavy chain locus to drive expression of these or other oncogenes. The availablity of promoters that specifically target expression to lymphocytes together with the accessibility of the cells for phenotypic and molecular analyses have made these transgenic mice a valuable tool not only for studying lymphomagenesis, but also for investigating cooperative effects between genes of various oncogenic potential.

Mice bearing *c-Myc, Bcl-2, cyclin D1, c-Abl, Ras,* and *Bmi* oncogenes have been generated. The main promoter used is the Eμ heavy chain enhancer which drives expression of the transgene throughout the B-lymphoid lineage including very early stages, sometimes also the T-cell lineage and myeloid cells *(233)*. Expression of c-Myc under control of the Eμ enhancer results in aggressive pre-B- or B-cell lymphoma and lymphoblastic leukemia that randomly arise as clonal tumors. Moreover, the lack of transplantability of these tumors and additional mutations in the genes for *N-Ras* or *K-Ras* suggests that c-Myc itself is not sufficient for full-blown lymphomagenesis *(233,234)*.

Chronic myeloid leukemia and some cases of acute lymphoblastic leukemia show translocations between chromosomes 9 and 22, where the 5′ portion of *c-Abl* is fused to the *Bcr* gene. Similarly, a *gag-abl* fusion carried by the Abelson murine leukemia virus generates pre-B and T lymphomas and potentiates the development of plasmacyotmas in pristane treated Balb/C mice. Transgenic expression of v-Abl under control of the Eμ enhancer provokes the formation of higly tumorigenic pre-B cell lymphomas and plasmacytomas. Eighty percent of the plasmacytomas evidence translocations of *c-Myc,* and consistent with an involvement of c-Myc in lymphomagenesis, bitransgenic c-Myc/Abl mice develop plasmacytomas very rapidly *(234).* N-Ras is mutated in certain forms of leukemia, particularly in acute myeloid leukemia. Eμ-N-Ras transgenic mice by themselves develop thymic T cell lymphomas and histiocytic sarcomas, however, when crossed to Eμ-Myc transgenic mice, they develop B cell lymphomas *(234).*

In follicular B-cell lymphoma and in some chronic lymphocytic leukemias, the *Bcl-2* gene is translocated to the immunoglobulin locus, t(14;18). Consistent with its role in anti-apoptosis, Bcl-2 transgenic mice exhibit elevated B cell numbers, and the progressive increase in plasma cells results in autommiune disease *(234).* These cells are arrested in the G_0 phase of the cell cycle and, hence, do not proliferate, but are resistant to apoptosis. In direct comparison to c-Myc, the Bcl-2 transgene is much less oncogenic; only few pre-B-cell lymphomas and plasmacytomas form that contain a rearranged *c-Myc* allele, indicating a cooperative effect between the two oncogenes. Myc induces proliferation with a high incidence of apoptosis, whereas Bcl-2 prevents the execution of apoptosis resulting in a high incidence of malignant disease *(234).* Other proteins that regulate apoptosis have been modulated in transgenic mouse models to study their role in tumorigenesis, such as the use of caspase-8 or -9 knock-out mice, Fas receptor-or Fas ligand-deficient mice, or transgenic expression of anti-apoptotic proteins, such as the cowpox virus *crmA* gene. While Bcl-2 affects lymphomagenesis by inhibiting the apoptosis pathway that is induced by DNA damage or physiological events (intrinsic pathway), changes in death receptor signaling also affect tumorigenesis. For example, *Lpr* mice lacking Fas receptor develop plasmacytoma with age and, when crossed to Eμ-Myc mice, exhibit an accelerated onset of lymphoma development *(234).*

In mantle cell lymphomas cyclin D1 is frequently found to be translocated to the immunoglobulin heavy chain locus, but Eμ-cyclin D1 transgenic mice do not develop spontaneous tumors. However, in Eμ-c-Myc transgenic mice upregulated expression of cyclin D1 is observed in tumor cells and a cooperative effect between c-Myc and cycline D1 is found in bitransgenic mice *(234).*

5.3. *Insertional Mutagenesis*

One route to the identification of genes that cooperate with oncogenes and/or that are able to modulate tumor phenotypes is their identification by retroviral insertional mutagenesis. Certain retroviruses appear to integrate at preferential not spot in the genome. Some of these integration events result in the upregulation of genes that lie nearby. If such up-regulation can contribute to the transformed phenotype, that cell will be selected and clonally expanded. For example, MMTV reproduceably integrates in the vicinity of the genes encoding for *Int-1/Wnt-1, Int-2/FGF-3, Int-3/Notch, Int-4/Wnt-3,* and *hst/FGF-4,* thereby up-regulating expression of these genes and enhancing mammary carcinogenesis *(185).* Cooperative effects between Int-1 and Int-2, or between Int-1 and hst/FGF-4, have also been demonstrated by infecting transgenic mice that express an *Int-1* transgene in mammary epithelial cells with MMTV. Integration of the MMTV proviral DNA resulted in up-regulation of Int-2 or hst/FGF-4 expression and, consequently, in acceleration of tumor development.

A similar mechanism has been revealed for Moloney murine leukemia virus (MuLV), which upon integration can up-regulate expression of c-Myc, Pim-1, or other genes in lymphocytes. This phenomenon has been used to identify a whole series of genes involved in lymphomagenesis *(235)*. For example, transgenic animals that specifically express c-Myc in lymphocytes have been infected with MuLV. In the resulting lymphomas, Pim-1 and Pim-2, which are Ser/Thr kinases, have been found at elevated levels. Transgenic expression of Pim-1 has revealed again the cooperative partners and in addition the zinc finger protein Bmi-1 *(235)*. Overexpression of Bmi-1, as a member of the polycomb group of homeobox genes, causes homeotic transformations and promotes the immortalization of fibroblasts by down-regulating the p16/ARF locus, which is normally induced by p53. Bim-1 may thus provide an escape route from senescence. In the reverse case, infection of *Pim-1* transgenic animals with MuLV results in high levels of c-Myc or N-Myc expression and, consequently, in increased lymphoma development. These cooperative effects have also been shown by the construction of bitransgenic animals, for example with *c-Myc* and *Pim-1 (235)* or *c-Myc* and *Bmi-1 (236)*. Insertional mutagenesis with Eμ-N-Ras transgenic mice has revealed *c-Myc* and *N-Myc* in T cell lymphomas *(237)*, and experiments with Eμ v-Abl transgenic have recovered *c-Myc, N-Myc,* and *Pim-1* genes *(238)*.

5.4. Modifier Genes

In addition to environmental and epigenetic factors, phenotypic variation of tumors is also due to the expression of genes that modify the cancerous phenotype, termed modifier genes. Identification of relevant cancer modifier loci in humans is an extremely difficult task and requires linkage studies of large and fully phenotyped pedigrees of individuals who carry specific mutations. However, evidence for the existence of modifier loci has also been obtained in rodent models that have been characterized for their genetic susceptibility to spontaneous or induced tumor formation. Crosses between susceptible and resistant strains have lead to the conclusion that susceptibility can be a dominant trait.

For example, in the A/J strain of mice, a polymorphism in the second intron of *K-Ras* is responsible for the development of lung tumors with old age *(239)*. Another prominent example is the APC[Min] mouse carrying a mutation in the tumor suppressor gene *APC* (see *Section 5.1.3.*). When heterozygous for the mutation, these mice develop spontaneous intestinal tumors with high penetrance. Multiplicity and size of the tumors, however, decreases upon inheritance of the *Mom1* (modifier of Min) locus. Linkage analysis suggested that the *Mom1* gene may be *Pla2g2a* and encodes a secretory phospholipase A2 that is involved in the synthesis of prostaglandins. Interestingly, inhibition of prostaglandin synthesis reduces the rate of incidence and the size of colorectal tumors in mice and humans. In exploring the phoshpholipase hypothesis, APC[Min] mice, which overexpress the *Pla2g2a* gene, show a significant decrease in tumor load and tumor size *(240)*.

In addition to single modifier genes, loci have been reported that genetically interact with each other, thereby affecting tumor development. For example, in a mouse model of lung carcinoma the tumor initiation is counteracted by the presence of several *Par* resistance loci, impairing the initiation of lung tumors *(241)*. Not only tumor initiation but also tumor growth can be affected by modifier loci, as shown for the *Hcr* resistance locus which prevents growth of liver tumors arising as consequence of the *Hcs* (hepatocacinogen sensitivity) locus *(242)*. Interspecific crosses, for example between *mus spretus* and *mus musculus* have revealed a number of loci that interact with each other in the modulation of skin tumorigenesis *(243)*. Therefore, animal models represent a useful tool to identify cancer modifier genes, however, these genes may be specific to experimental models and may not necessarily play an important role in human tumor development.

5.5. Rebuilding Cancer: the TVA System

Most mouse models, thus far, have employed only few genetic changes in an attempt to mimic human cancer. As it is well-established that human cancer development requires many genetic and epigenetic events, it seems necessary to find technical ways to accurately recapitulate the etiology of cancers in man. One of the strategies to allow many genetic manipulations in one mouse is based on a combination of classical transgene/knock-out technology with viral gene delivery and has been pioneered mainly by the laboratory of Harold Varmus (Sloan Kettering Cancer Institute) *(244)*.

The cell surface receptor for the subgroup-A avian leukosis virus, TVA, is expressed under the control of a cell-type (tumor-type)-specific promoter in transgenic mice. Expression of this receptor on the surface of cells is then sufficient to mediate retroviral infection by subgroup-A avian sarcoma leukosis virus (ASLV), other mouse cells will not be infected. Modified retroviral vectors have been constructed by removing the *v-Src* gene from Rous Sarcoma Virus (RSV) and replacing it with a multicloning site. These recombinant retroviruses infect TVA expressing mammalian cells with high efficiency, the viral genome integrates into the host genome, and no infectious particles will be made to spread to other cells. TVA receptors are not blocked by the virus, so multiple rounds of infection can be performed. These viruses are now used to deliver genes of interest to be expressed. Such technology is currently used to mimic the multiple known genetic changes occuring during carcinogenesis in patients.

For example, to generate a mouse model of glioblastoma, TVA is expressed under the control of the glial fibrillary acidic protein (GFAP) promoter or the nestin promoter in astrocytes and glial precursor cells. Retroviral transduction of the *bFGF* gene has revealed that bFGF, as suspected in human gliomas, induced proliferation and migration of of glial cells. Combinations with gain of function and loss of function mice, for example retroviral overexpression of Cdk4 and a constitutive active from of EGFR in a p53- or Ink4a-deficient background, theoretically reconstitutes at least part of the genetic changes in human glioblastoma. Initial results show that activated EGFR does not induce tumors, however, in an Ink4a knock-out background glioma-like lesions develop. Moreover, in p53-deficient mice constitutive EGFR does not provoke neoplastic lesions, unless Cdk4 is overexpressed as well *(244)*.

Using a number of cell type-specific promoters to express TVA, similar experiments have been initiated to rebuild breast cancer, lung cancer, melanoma, and others. One major disadvantage of this approach is the fact that retroviral infection/integration requires cell proliferation and, hence, attempts are underway to adapt this approach to lentiviruses that can infect nonproliferating cells by engineering the ASLV envelope protein into lentivirus vectors. These experimental approaches will be an important tool to systematically study multicooperative effects between genes and are expected to give major insights into the genetic interaction between genes during multistage tumorigenesis. In particular, in times of major efforts to identify cancer susceptibility/modifier genes, this technology will be instrumental for functional studies.

ACKNOWLEDGMENTS

We apologize to those colleagues whose work we could not cite due to space restrictions. We are grateful to Erwin Wagner for Fig. 1 and Hannes Tkadletz for artwork. The work in the laboratory of the authors is supported by Boehringer Ingelheim, by the Austrian Industrial Research Promotion Fund (FFF), and by the Austrian Science Foundation (FWF).

REFERENCES

1. Kistner A, Gossen M, Zimmermann F, et al. Doxycycline-mediated quantitative and tissue-specific control of gene expression in transgenic mice. *Proc Natl Acad Sci USA* 1996; 93:10933–10938.
2. Saez E, No D, West A, Evans RM. Inducible gene expression in mammalian cells and transgenic mice. *Curr Opin Biotechnol* 1997; 8:608–616.
3. Fedi P, Tronick SR, Aaronson SA. Growth factors. In: Holland JF, Bast RC, Morton DL, Frei E, Kufe DW, Weichselbaum RR, eds. Cancer Medicine. Williams and Wilkins, Baltimore, 1997, pp. 41–64.
4. Becker D, Meier CB, Herlyn M. Proliferation of human malignant melanomas is inhibited by antisense oligodeoxynucleotides targeted against basic fibroblast growth factor. *EMBO J* 1989; 8:3685–3691.
5. Yarden Y, Ullrich A. Molecular analysis of signal transduction by growth factors. *Biochemistry* 1988; 27:3113–3119.
6. Alimandi M, Wang LM, Bottaro D, et al. Epidermal growth factor and betacellulin mediate signal transduction through co-expressed ErbB2 and ErbB3 receptors. *EMBO J* 1997; 16:5608–5617.
7. Vassar R, Fuchs E. Transgenic mice provide new insights into the role of TGF-alpha during epidermal development and differentiation. *Genes Dev* 1991; 5:714–727.
8. Otsuka T, Takayama H, Sharp R, et al. c-Met autocrine activation induces development of malignant melanoma and acquisition of the metastatic phenotype. *Cancer Res* 1998; 58:5157–5167.
9. Bailleul B, Surani MA, White S, et al. Skin hyperkeratosis and papilloma formation in transgenic mice expressing a ras oncogene from a suprabasal keratin promoter. *Cell* 1990; 62:697–708.
10. Leder A, Kuo A, Cardiff RD, Sinn E, Leder P. v-Ha-ras transgene abrogates the initiation step in mouse skin tumorigenesis: effects of phorbol esters and retinoic acid. *Proc Natl Acad Sci USA* 1990; 87:9178–9182.
11. Brown K, Strathdee D, Bryson S, Lambie W, Balmain A. The malignant capacity of skin tumours induced by expression of a mutant H-ras transgene depends on the cell type targeted. *Curr Biol* 1998; 8:516–524.
12. Sibilia M, Fleischmann A, Behrens A, et al. The EGF receptor provides an essential survival signal for SOS-dependent skin tumor development. *Cell* 2000; 102:211–220.
13. Chin L, Pomerantz J, Polsky D, et al. Cooperative effects of INK4a and ras in melanoma susceptibility in vivo. *Genes Dev* 1997; 11:2822–2834.
14. Chin L, Tam A, Pomerantz J, et al. Essential role for oncogenic Ras in tumour maintenance. *Nature* 1999; 400:468–472.
15. Felsher DW, Bishop JM. Reversible tumorigenesis by MYC in hematopoietic lineages. *Mol Cell* 1999; 4:199–207.
16. Pelengaris S, Littlewood T, Khan M, Elia G, Evan G. Reversible activation of c-Myc in skin: induction of a complex neoplastic phenotype by a single oncogenic lesion. *Mol Cell* 1999; 3:565–577.
17. Ewald D, Li M, Efrat S, et al. Time-sensitive reversal of hyperplasia in transgenic mice expressing SV40 T antigen. *Science* 1996; 273:1384–1386.
18. Sinn E, Muller W, Pattengale P, Tepler I, Wallace R, Leder P. Coexpression of MMTV/v-Ha-ras and MMTV/c-myc genes in transgenic mice: synergistic action of oncogenes in vivo. *Cell* 1987; 49:465–475.
19. Kwan H, Pecenka V, Tsukamoto A, et al. Transgenes expressing the Wnt-1 and int-2 proto-oncogenes cooperate during mammary carcinogenesis in doubly transgenic mice. *Mol Cell Biol* 1992; 12:147–154.
20. Sandgren EP, Quaife CJ, Pinkert CA, Palmiter RD, Brinster RL. Oncogene-induced liver neoplasia in transgenic mice. *Oncogene* 1989; 4:715–724.

21. Murakami H, Sanderson ND, Nagy P, Marino PA, Merlino G, Thorgeirsson SS. Transgenic mouse model for synergistic effects of nuclear oncogenes and growth factors in tumorigenesis: interaction of c-myc and transforming growth factor alpha in hepatic oncogenesis. *Cancer Res* 1993; 53:1719–1723.

22. Adams JM, Cory S. Transgenic models of tumor development. *Science* 1991; 254:1161–1167.

23. Vassar R, Hutton ME, Fuchs E. Transgenic overexpression of transforming growth factor alpha bypasses the need for c-Ha-ras mutations in mouse skin tumorigenesis. *Mol Cell Biol* 1992; 12:4643–4653.

24. Larue L, Dougherty N, Mintz B. Genetic predisposition of transgenic mouse melanocytes to melanoma results in malignant melanoma after exposure to a low ultraviolet B intensity nontumorigenic for normal melanocytes. *Proc Natl Acad Sci USA* 1992; 89:9534–9538.

25. Vooijs M, Berns A. Developmental defects and tumor predisposition in Rb mutant mice. *Oncogene* 1999; 18:5293–5303.

26. Jacks T, Fazeli A, Schmitt EM, Bronson RT, Goodell MA, Weinberg RA. Effects of an Rb mutation in the mouse. *Nature* 1992; 359:295–300.

27. Hu N, Gutsmann A, Herbert DC, Bradley A, Lee WH, Lee EY. Heterozygous Rb-1 delta 20/+mice are predisposed to tumors of the pituitary gland with a nearly complete penetrance. *Oncogene* 1994; 9:1021–1027.

28. Williams BO, Remington L, Albert DM, Mukai S, Bronson RT, Jacks T. Cooperative tumorigenic effects of germline mutations in Rb and p53. *Nat Genet* 1994; 7:480–484.

29. Robanus-Maandag E, Dekker M, van der Valk M, et al. p107 is a suppressor of retinoblastoma development in pRb-deficient mice. *Genes Dev* 1998; 12:1599–1609.

30. Lee MH, Williams BO, Mulligan G, et al. Targeted disruption of p107: functional overlap between p107 and Rb. *Genes Dev* 1996; 10:1621–1632.

31. al-Ubaidi MR, Font RL, Quiambao AB, et al. Bilateral retinal and brain tumors in transgenic mice expressing simian virus 40 large T antigen under control of the human interphotoreceptor retinoid-binding protein promoter. *J Cell Biol* 1992; 119:1681–1687.

32. Howes KA, Ransom N, Papermaster DS, Lasudry JG, Albert DM, Windle JJ. Apoptosis or retinoblastoma: alternative fates of photoreceptors expressing the HPV-16 E7 gene in the presence or absence of p53. *Genes Dev* 1994; 8:1300–1310.

33. Serrano M, Lee H, Chin L, Cordon-Cardo C, Beach D, DePinho RA. Role of the INK4a locus in tumor suppression and cell mortality. *Cell* 1996; 85:27–37.

34. Kamijo T, Zindy F, Roussel MF, et al. Tumor suppression at the mouse INK4a locus mediated by the alternative reading frame product p19ARF. *Cell* 1997; 91:649–659.

35. Nakayama K, Ishida N, Shirane M, et al. Mice lacking p27(Kip1) display increased body size, multiple organ hyperplasia, retinal dysplasia, and pituitary tumors. *Cell* 1996; 85:707–720.

36. Fero ML, Rivkin M, Tasch M, et al. A syndrome of multiorgan hyperplasia with features of gigantism, tumorigenesis, and female sterility in p27(Kip1)-deficient mice. *Cell* 1996; 85:733–744.

37. Park MS, Rosai J, Nguyen HT, Capodieci P, Cordon-Cardo C, Koff A. p27 and Rb are on overlapping pathways suppressing tumorigenesis in mice. *Proc Natl Acad Sci USA* 1999; 96:6382–6387.

38. Franklin DS, Godfrey VL, Lee H, et al. CDK inhibitors p18(INK4c) and p27(Kip1) mediate two separate pathways to collaboratively suppress pituitary tumorigenesis. *Genes Dev* 1998; 12:2899–2911.

39. Deng C, Zhang P, Harper JW, Elledge SJ, Leder P. Mice lacking p21CIP1/WAF1 undergo normal development, but are defective in G1 checkpoint control. *Cell* 1995; 82:675–684.

40. Brugarolas J, Chandrasekaran C, Gordon JI, Beach D, Jacks T, Hannon GJ. Radiation-induced cell cycle arrest compromised by p21 deficiency. *Nature* 1995; 377:552–557.

41. Wang TC, Cardiff RD, Zukerberg L, Lees E, Arnold A, Schmidt EV. Mammary hyperplasia and carcinoma in MMTV-cyclin D1 transgenic mice. *Nature* 1994; 369:669–671.

42. Yamasaki L, Jacks T, Bronson R, Goillot E, Harlow E, Dyson NJ. Tumor induction and tissue atrophy in mice lacking E2F-1. *Cell* 1996; 85:537–548.

43. Yamasaki L, Bronson R, Williams BO, Dyson NJ, Harlow E, Jacks T. Loss of E2F-1 reduces tumorigenesis and extends the lifespan of Rb1(+/–) mice. *Nat Genet* 1998; 18:360–364.

44. Pierce AM, Gimenez-Conti IB, Schneider-Broussard R, Martinez LA, Conti CJ, Johnson DG. Increased E2F1 activity induces skin tumors in mice heterozygous and nullizygous for p53. *Proc Natl Acad Sci USA* 1998; 95:8858–8863.

45. Pierce AM, Fisher SM, Conti CJ, Johnson DG. Deregulated expression of E2F1 induces hyperplasia and cooperates with ras in skin tumor development. *Oncogene* 1998; 16:1267–1276.

46. Pierce AM, Schneider-Broussard R, Gimenez-Conti IB, Russell JL, Conti CJ, Johnson DG. E2F1 has both oncogenic and tumor-suppressive properties in a transgenic model. *Mol Cell Biol* 1999; 19:6408–6414.

47. Wang D, Russell JL, Johnson DG. E2F4 and E2F1 have similar proliferative properties but different apoptotic and oncogenic properties in vivo. *Mol Cell Biol* 2000; 20:3417–3424.

48. Ko LJ, Prives C. p53: puzzle and paradigm. *Genes Dev* 1996; 10:1054–1072.

49. Donehower LA, Harvey M, Slagle BL, et al. Mice deficient for p53 are developmentally normal but susceptible to spontaneous tumours. *Nature* 1992; 356:215–221.

50. Jacks T, Remington L, Williams BO, et al. Tumor spectrum analysis in p53-mutant mice. *Curr Biol* 1994; 4:1–7.

51. Bueso-Ramos CE, Manshouri T, Haidar MA, Huh YO, Keating MJ, Albitar M. Multiple patterns of MDM-2 deregulation in human leukemias: implications in leukemogenesis and prognosis. *Leuk Lymphoma* 1995; 17:13–18.

52. Momand J, Jung D, Wilczynski S, Niland J. The MDM2 gene amplification database. *Nucleic Acids Res* 1998; 26:3453–3459.

53. Jones SN, Roe AE, Donehower LA, Bradley A. Rescue of embryonic lethality in Mdm2-deficient mice by absence of p53. *Nature* 1995; 378:206–208.

54. Montes de Oca Luna R, Wanger DS, Lozano G. Rescue of early embryonic lethality in mdm2-deficient mice by deletion of p53. *Nature* 1995; 378:203–206.

55. Jones SN, Sands AT, Hancock AR, et al. The tumorigenic potential and cell growth characteristics of p53- deficient cells are equivalent in the presence or absence of Mdm2. *Proc Natl Acad Sci USA* 1996; 93:14106–14111.

56. Lundgren K, Montes de Oca Luna R, McNeill YB, et al. Targeted expression of MDM2 uncouples S phase from mitosis and inhibits mammary gland development independent of p53. *Genes Dev* 1997; 11:714–725.

57. Reinke V, Bortner DM, Amelse LL, et al. Overproduction of MDM2 in vivo disrupt S phase independent of E2F1. *Cell Growth Differ* 1999; 10:147–154.

58. Jones SN, Hancock AR, Vogel H, Donehower LA, Bradley A. Overexpression of Mdm2 in mice reveals a p53-independent role for Mdm2 in tumorigenesis. *Proc Natl Acad Sci USA* 1998; 95:15608–15612.

59. Holt SE, Shay JW. Role of telomerase in cellular proliferation and cancer. *J Cell Physiol* 1999; 180:10–18.

60. Bodnar AG, Ouellette M, Frolkis M, et al. Extension of life-span by introduction of telomerase into normal human cells. *Science* 1998; 279:349–352.

61. Greenberg RA, Chin L, Femino A, et al. Short dysfunctional telomeres impair tumorigenesis in the INK4a(delta2/3) cancer-prone mouse. *Cell* 1999; 97:515–525.

62. Rudolph KL, Chang S, Lee HW, et al. Longevity, stress response, and cancer in aging telomerase-deficient mice. *Cell* 1999; 96:701–712.

63. Chin L, Artandi SE, Shen Q, et al. p53 deficiency rescues the adverse effects of telomere loss and cooperates with telomere dysfunction to accelerate carcinogenesis. *Cell* 1999; 97:527–538.

64. Karlseder J, Broccoli D, Dai Y, Hardy S, de Lange T. p53- and ATM-dependent apoptosis induced by telomeres lacking TRF2. *Science* 1999; 283:1321–1325.

65. Artandi SE, Chang S, Lee SL, et al. Telomere dysfunction promotes non-reciprocal translocations and epithelial cancers in mice. *Nature* 2000; 406:641–645.

66. Ashkenazi A, Dixit VM. Apoptosis control by death and decoy receptors. *Curr Opin Cell Biol* 1999; 11:255–260.

67. Kroemer G, Reed JC. Mitochondrial control of cell death. *Nat Med* 2000; 6:513–519.

68. Pelengaris S, Rudolph B, Littlewood T. Action of Myc in vivo—proliferation and apoptosis. *Curr Opin Genet Dev* 2000; 10:100–105.

69. Christofori G, Naik P, Hanahan D. A second signal supplied by insulin-like growth factor II in oncogene-induced tumorigenesis. *Nature* 1994; 369:414–418.

70. Peltomaki P. DNA mismatch repair gene mutations in human cancer. *Environ Health Perspect* 1997; 105(Suppl 4):775–780.

71. Kolodner R. Biochemistry and genetics of eukaryotic mismatch repair. *Genes Dev* 1996; 10:1433–1442.

72. Duval A, Iacopetta B, Ranzani GN, Lothe RA, Thomas G, Hamelin R. Variable mutation frequencies in coding repeats of TCF-4 and other target genes in colon, gastric and endometrial carcinoma showing microsatellite instability. *Oncogene* 1999; 18:6806–6809.

73. Schwartz S Jr, Yamamoto H, Navarro M, Maestro M, Reventos J, Perucho M. Frameshift mutations at mononucleotide repeats in caspase-5 and other target genes in endometrial and gastrointestinal cancer of the microsatellite mutator phenotype. *Cancer Res* 1999; 59:2995–3002.

74. Reitmair AH, Redston M, Cai JC, et al. Spontaneous intestinal carcinomas and skin neoplasms in Msh2-deficient mice. *Cancer Res* 1996; 56:3842–3849.

75. Edelmann W, Yang K, Umar A, et al. Mutation in the mismatch repair gene Msh6 causes cancer susceptibility. *Cell* 1997; 91:467–477.

76. de Wind N, Dekker M, Claij N, et al. HNPCC-like cancer predisposition in mice through simultaneous loss of Msh3 and Msh6 mismatch-repair protein functions. *Nat Genet* 1999; 23:359–362.

77. Edelmann W, Yang K, Kuraguchi M, et al. Tumorigenesis in Mlh1 and Mlh1/Apc1638N mutant mice. *Cancer Res* 1999; 59:1301–1307.

78. Ricciardone MD, Ozcelik T, Cevher B, et al. Human MLH1 deficiency predisposes to hematological malignancy and neurofibromatosis type 1. *Cancer Res* 1999; 59:290–293.

79. Wang Q, Lasset C, Desseigne F, et al. Neurofibromatosis and early onset of cancers in hMLH1-deficient children. *Cancer Res* 1999; 59:294–297.

80. Reitmair AH, Cai JC, Bjerknes M, et al. MSH2 dificiency contributes to accelerated APC-mediated intestinal tumorigenesis. *Cancer Res* 1996; 56:2922–2926.

81. Prolla TA, Baker SM, Harris AC, et al. Tumour susceptibility and spontaneous mutation in mice deficient in Mlh1, Pms1 and Pms2 DNA mismatch repair. *Nat Genet* 1998; 18:276–279.

82. Baker SM, Harris AC, Tsao JL, et al. Enhanced intestinal adenomatous polyp formation in Pms2–/–;Min mice. *Cancer Res* 1998; 58:1087–1089.

83. Lengauer C, Kinzler KW, Vogelstein B. Genetic instabilities in human cancers. *Nature* 1998; 396:643–649.

84. Cahill DP, Lengauer C, Yu J, et al. Mutations of mitotic checkpoint genes in human cancers. *Nature* 1998; 392:300–330.

85. Lavin MF, Shiloh Y. The genetic defect in ataxia-telangiectasia. *Annu Rev Immunol* 1997; 15:177–202.

86. Khanna KK, Jackson SP. DNA double-strand breaks: signaling, repair and the cancer connection. *Nat Genet* 2001; 27:247–254.

87. Featherstone C, Jackson SP. DNA repair: the Nijmegen breakage syndrome protein. *Curr Biol* 1998; 8:R622–R625.

88. Dasika GK, Lin SC, Zhao S, Sung P, Tomkinson A, Lee EY. DNA damage-induced cell cycle checkpoints and DNA strand break repair in development and tumorigenesis. *Oncogene* 1999; 18:7883–7899.

89. Gu Y, Seidl KJ, Rathbun GA, et al. Growth retardation and leaky SCID phenotype of Ku70-deficient mice. *Immunity* 1997; 7:653–656.

90. Li GC, Ouyang H, Li X, et al. Ku70: a candidate tumor suppresor gene for murine T cell lymphoma. *Mol Cell* 1998; 2:1–8.

91. Morrison C, Smith GC, Stingl L, Jackson SP, Wagner EF, Wang ZQ. Genetic interaction between PARP and DNA-PK in V(D)J recombination and tumorigenesis. *Nat Genet* 1997; 17:479–482.

92. Canman CE, Lim DS. The role of ATM in DNA damage responses and cancer. *Oncogene* 1998; 17:3301–3308.

93. Brown EJ, Baltimore D. ATR disruption leads to chromosomal fragmentation and early embryonic lethality. *Genes Dev* 2000; 14:397–402.

94. Zhu J, Petersen S, Tessarollo L, Nussenzweig A. Targeted disruption of the Nijmegen breakage syndrome gene NBS1 leads to early embryonic lethality in mice. *Curr Biol* 2001; 11:105–109.

95. Scully R, Puget N, Vlasakova K. DNA polymerase stalling, sister chromatid recombination and the BRCA genes. *Oncogene* 2000; 19:6176–6183.

96. Lee H, Trainer AH, Friedman LS, et al. Mitotic checkpoint inactivation fosters transformation in cells lacking the breast cancer susceptibility gene, Brca2. *Mol Cell* 1999; 4:1–10.

97. Wassmann K, Benezra R. Mitotic checkpoints: from yeast to cancer. *Curr Opin Genet Dev* 2001; 11:83–90.

98. Li Y, Benezra R. Identification of a human mitotic checkpoint gene: hsMAD2. *Science* 1996; 274:246–248.

99. Cahill DP, da Costa LT, Carson-Walter EB, Kinzler KW, Vogelstein B, Lengauer C. Characterization of MAD2B and other mitotic spindle checkpoint genes. *Genomics* 1999; 58:181–187.

100. Basu J, Bousbaa H, Logarinho E, et al. Mutations in the essential spindle checkpoint gene bub1 cause chromosome missegregation and fail to block apoptosis in *Drosophila*. *J Cell Biol* 1999; 146:13–28.

101. Kitagawa R, Rose AM. Components of the spindle-assembly checkpoint are essential in *Caenorhabditis elegans. Nat Cell Biol* 1999; 1:514–521.

102. Dobles M, Liberal V, Scott ML, Benezra R, Sorger PK. Chromosome missegregation and apoptosis in mice lacking the mitotic checkpoint protein Mad2. *Cell* 2000; 101:635–645.

103. Michel LS, Liberal V, Chatterjee A, et al. MAD2 haplo-insufficiency causes premature anaphase and chromosome instability in mammalian cells. *Nature* 2001; 409:355–359.

104. Toyota M, Issa JP. CpG island methylator phenotypes in aging and cancer. *Semin Cancer Biol* 1999; 9:349–357.

105. Herman JG. p16(INK4): involvement early and often in gastrointestinal malignancies. *Gastroenterology* 1999; 116:483–485.

106. Laird PW, Jackson-Grusby L, Fazeli A, et al. Suppression of intestinal neoplasia by DNA hypomethylation. *Cell* 1995; 81:197–205.

107. Feinberg AP. DNA methylation, genomic imprinting and cancer. *Curr Top Microbiol Immunol* 2000; 249:87–99.

108. Sternlicht MD, Lochter A, Sympson CJ, et al. The stromal proteinase MMP3/stromelysin-1 promotes mammary carcinogenesis. *Cell* 1999; 98:137–146.

109. Rudolph-Owen LA, Chan R, Muller WJ, Matrisian LM. The matrix metalloproteinase matrilysin influences early-stage mammary tumorigenesis. *Cancer Res* 1998; 58:5500–5506.

110. Wilson CL, Heppner KJ, Labosky PA, Hogan BL, Matrisian LM. Intestinal tumorigenesis is suppressed in mice lacking the metalloproteinase matrilysin. *Proc Natl Acad Sci USA* 1997; 94:1402–1407.

111. Coussens LM, Hanahan D, Arbeit JM. Genetic predisposition and parameters of malignant progression in K14- HPV16 transgenic mice. *Am J Pathol* 1996; 149:1899–1917.

112. Coussens LM, Tinkle CL, Hanahan D, Werb Z. MMP-9 supplied by bone marrow-derived cells contributes to skin carcinogenesis. *Cell* 2000; 103:481–490.

113. Hanahan D. Heritable formation of pancreatic beta-cell tumours in transgenic mice expressing recombinant insulin/simian virus 40 oncogenes. *Nature* 1985; 315:115–122.

114. Bergers G, Brekken R, McMahon G, et al. Matrix metalloproteinase-9 triggers the angiogenic switch during carcinogenesis. *Nat Cell Biol* 2000; 2:737–744.

115. Ferrara N, Alitalo K. Clinical applications of angiogenic growth factors and their inhibitors. *Nat Med* 1999; 5:1359–1364.

116. Carmeliet P, Jain RK. Angiogenesis in cancer and other diseases. *Nature* 2000; 407:249–257.

117. Folkman J, Watson K, Ingber D, Hanahan D. Induction of angiogenesis during the transition from hyperplasia to neoplasia. *Nature* 1989; 339:58–61.

118. Compagni A, Wilgenbus P, Impagnatiello MA, Cotten M, Christofori G. Fibroblast growth factors are required for efficient tumor angiogenesis. *Cancer Res* 2000; 60:7163–7169.

119. Bergers G, Hanahan D, Coussens LM. Angiogenesis and apoptosis are cellular parameters of neoplastic progression in transgenic mouse models of tumorigenesis. *Int J Dev Biol* 1998; 42:995–1002.

120. Parangi S, O'Reilly M, Christofori G, et al. Antiangiogenic therapy of transgenic mice impairs de novo tumor growth. *Proc Natl Acad Sci USA* 1996; 93:2002–2007.

121. Matsuura N, Puzon-McLaughlin W, Irie A, Morikawa Y, Kakudo K, Takada Y. Induction of experimental bone metastasis in mice by transfection of integrin alpha 4 beta 1 into tumor cells. *Am J Pathol* 1996; 148:55–61.

122. Qian F, Hanahan D, Weissman IL. L-selectin can facilitate metastasis to lymph nodes in a transgenic mouse model of carcinogenesis. *Proc Natl Acad Sci USA* 2001; 98:3976–3981.

123. Aberle H, Schwartz H, Kemler R. Cadherin-catenin complex: protein interactions and their implications for cadherin function. *J Cell Biochem* 1996; 61:514–523.

124. Perl AK, Wilgenbus P, Dahl U, Semb H, Christofori G. A causal role for E-cadherin in the transition from adenoma to carcinoma. *Nature* 1998; 392:190–193.

125. Perl AK, Dahl U, Wilgenbus P, Cremer H, Semb H, Christofori G. Reduced expression of neural cell adhesion molecule induces metastic dissemination of pancreatic beta tumor cells. *Nat Med* 1999; 5:286–291.

126. Pepper MS. Lymphangiogenesis and tumor metastasis: myth or reality? *Clin Cancer Res* 2001; 7:462–468.

127. Plate K. From angiogenesis to lymphangiogenesis. *Nat Med* 2001; 7:151–152.

128. Simpson L, Parsons R. Pten: life as a tumor suppressor. *Exp Cell Res* 2001; 264:29–41.

129. Vazquez F, Sellers WR. The PTEN tumor suppressor protein: an antagonist of phosphoinositide 3-kinase signaling. *Biochim Biophys Acta* 2000; 1470:M21–M35.

130. Podsypanina K, Ellenson LH, Nemes A, et al. Mutation of Pten/Mmac 1 in mice causes neoplasia in multiple organ systems. *Proc Natl Acad Sci USA* 1999; 96:1563–1568.

131. Di Cristofano A, Pesce B, Cordon-Cardo C, Pandolfi PP. Pten is essential for embryonic development and tumour suppression. *Nat Genet* 1998; 19:348–355.

132. Suzuki A, de la Pompa JL, Stambolic V, et al. High cancer susceptibility and embryonic lethality associated with mutation of the PTEN tumor suppressor gene in mice. *Curr Biol* 1998; 8:1169–1178.

133. Di Cristofano A, De Acetis M, Koff A, Cordon-Cardo C, Pandolfi PP. Pten and p27KIP1 cooperate in prostate cancer tumor suppression in the mouse. *Nat Genet* 2001; 27:222–224.

134. Li Y, Podsypanina K, Liu X, et al. Deficiency of Pten accelerates mammary oncogenesis in MMTV-Wnt-1 transgenic mice. *BMC Mol Biol* 2001; 2:2.

135. Attisano L, Wrana JL. Smads as transcriptional co-modulators. *Curr Opin Cell Biol* 2000; 12:235–243.

136. Cui W, Fowlis DJ, Bryson S, et al. TGFbetal inhibits the formation of benign skin tumors, but enhances progression to invasive spindle carcinomas in transgenic mice. *Cell* 1996; 86:531–542.

137. Hata A, Shi Y, Massague J. TGF-beta signaling and cancer: structural and functional consequences of mutations in Smads. *Mol Med Today* 1998; 4:257–262.

138. Datto M, Wang XF. The Smads: transcriptional regulation and mouse models. *Cytokine Growth Factor Rev* 2000; 11:37–48.

139. Tang B, Bottinger EP, Jakowlew SB, et al. Transforming growth factor-betal is a new form of tumor suppressor with true haploid insufficiency. *Nat Med* 1998; 4:802–807.

140. Zhu Y, Richardson JA, Parada LF, Graff JM. Smad3 mutant mice develop metastatic colorectal cancer. *Cell* 1998; 94:703–714.

141. Barker N, Clevers H. Catenins, Wnt signaling and cancer. *Bioessays* 2000; 22:961–965.

142. Polakis P. Wnt signaling and cancer. *Genes Dev* 2000; 14:1837–1851.

143. van Es JH, Giles RH, Clevers HC. The many faces of the tumor suppressor gene APC. *Exp Cell Res* 2001; 264:126–134.

144. Bienz M, Clevers H. Linking colorectal cancer to Wnt signaling. *Cell* 2000; 103:311–320.

145. Su LK, Kinzler KW, Vogelstein B, et al. Multiple intestinal neoplasia caused by a mutation in the murine homolog of the APC gene. *Science* 1992; 256:668–670.

146. Clarke AR, Cummings MC, Harrison DJ. Interaction between murine germline mutations in p53 and APC predisposes to pancreatic neoplasia but not to increased intestinal malignancy. *Oncogene* 1995; 11:1913–1920.

147. Oshima M, Oshima H, Kobayashi M, Tsutsumi M, Taketo MM. Evidence against dominant negative mechanisms of intestinal polyp formation by Apc gene mutations. *Cancer Res* 1995; 55:2719–2722.

148. Shibata H, Toyama K, Shioya H, et al. Rapid colorectal adenoma formation initiated by conditional targeting of the Apc gene. *Science* 1997; 278:120–123.

149. Luongo C, Moser AR, Gledhill S, Dove WF. Loss of Apc+ in intestinal adenomas from Min mice. *Cancer Res* 1994; 54:5947–5952.

150. Smits R, Kartheuser A, Jagmohan-Changur S, et al. Loss of Apc and the entire chromosome 18 but absence of mutations at the Ras and Tp53 genes in intestinal tumors from Apc1638N, a mouse model for Apc-driven carcinogenesis. *Carcinogenesis* 1997; 18:321–327.

151. Smits R, Kielman MF, Breukel C, et al. Apc1638T: a mouse model delineating critical domains of the adenomatous polyposis coli protein involved in tumorigenesis and development. *Genes Dev* 1999; 13:1309–1321.

152. Gat U, DasGupta R, Degenstein L, Fuchs E. De Novo hair follicle morphogenesis and hair tumors in mice expressing a truncated beta-catenin in skin. *Cell* 1998; 95:605–614.

153. Zhou P, Byrne C, Jacobs J, Fuchs E. Lymphoid enhancer factor 1 directs hair follicle patterning and epithelial cell fate. *Genes Dev* 1995; 9:700–713.

154. Roose J, Huls G, van Beest M, et al. Synergy between tumor suppressor APC and the beta-catenin-Tcf4 target Tcf1. *Science* 1999; 285:1923–1926.

155. Ruiz I, Altaba A. Gli proteins and Hedgehog signaling: development and cancer. *Trends Genet* 1999; 15:418–425.

156. Oro AE, Higgins KM, Hu Z, Bonifas JM, Epstein EH, Scott MP. Basal cell carcinomas in mice over-expressing sonic hedgehog. *Science* 1997; 276:817–821.

157. Xie J, Murone M, Luoh SM, et al. Activating Smoothened mutations in sporadic basal-cell carcinoma. *Nature* 1998; 391:90–92.

158. Grachtchouk M, Mo R, Yu S, et al. Basal cell carcinomas in mice overexpressing Gli2 in skin. *Nat Genet* 2000; 24:216–217.

159. Nilsson M, Unden AB, Krause D, et al. Induction of basal cell carcinomas and trichoepitheliomas in mice overexpressing GLI-1. *Proc Natl Acad Sci USA* 2000; 97:3438–3443.

160. Kinzler KW, Ruppert JM, Bigner SH, Vogelstein B. The GLI gene is a member of the Kruppel family of zinc finger proteins. *Nature* 1988; 332:371–374.

161. Aszterbaum M, Epstein J, Oro A, et al. Ultraviolet and ionizing radiation enhance the growth of BCCs and trichoblastomas in patched heterozygous knockout mice. *Nat Med* 1999; 5:1285–1291.

162. Wetmore C, Eberhart DE, Curran T. The normal patched allele is expressed in medulloblastomas from mice with heterozygous germ-line mutation of patched. *Cancer Res* 2000; 60:2239–2246.

163. Wetmore C, Eberhart DE, Curran T. Loss of p53 but not ARF accelerates medulloblastoma in mice heterozygous for patched. *Cancer Res* 2001; 61:513–516.

164. Hahn H, Wojnowski L, Zimmer AM, Hall J, Miller G, Zimmer A. Rhabdomyosarcomas and radiation hypersensitivity in a mouse model of Gorlin syndrome. *Nat Med* 1998; 4:619–622.

165. Mintz B, Klein-Szanto AJ. Malignancy of eye melanomas orginating in the retinal pigment epithelium of transgenic mice after genetic ablation of choroidal melanocytes. *Proc Natl Acad Sci USA* 1992; 89:11421–11425.

166. Mintz B, Silvers WK. Transgenic mouse model of malignant skin melanoma. *Proc Natl Acad Sci USA* 1993; 90:8817–8821.

167. Mintz B, Silvers WK, Klein-Szanto AJ. Histopathogenesis of malignant skin melanoma induced in genetically susceptible transgenic mice. *Proc Natl Acad Sci USA* 1993; 90:8822–8826.

168. Penna D, Schmidt A, Beermann F. Tumors of the retinal pigment epithelium metastasize to inguinal lymph nodes and spleen in tyrosinase-related protein 1/SV40 T antigen transgenic mice. *Oncogene* 1998; 17:2601–2607.

169. Powell MB, Hyman P, Bell OD, et al. Hyperpigmentation and melanocytic hyperplasia in transgenic mice expressing the human T24 Ha-ras gene regulated by a mouse tyrosinase promoter. *Mol Carcinog* 1995; 12:82–90.

170. Iwamoto T, Takahashi M, Ito M, et al. Aberrant melanogenesis and melanocytic tumour development in transgenic mice that carry a metallothionein/ret fusion gene. *EMBO J* 1991; 10:3167–3175.

171. Greenhalgh DA, Rothnagel JA, Quintanilla MI, et al. Induction of epidermal hyperplasia, hyperkeratosis, and papillomas in transgenic mice by a targeted v-Ha-ras oncogene. *Mol Carcinog* 1993; 7:99–110.

172. Larcher F, Murillas R, Bolontrade M, Conti CJ, Jorcano JL. VEGF/VPF overexpression in skin of transgenic mice induces angiogenesis, vascular hyperpermeability and accelerated tumor development. *Oncogene* 1998; 17:303–311.

173. Saez E, Rutberg SE, Mueller E, et al. c-fos is required for malignant progression of skin tumors. *Cell* 1995; 82:721–732.

174. Ganguli G, Abecassis J, Wasylyk B. MDM2 induces hyperplasia and premalignant lesions when expressed in the basal layer of the epidermis. *EMBO J* 2000; 19:5135–5147.

175. Arbeit JM, Munger K, Howley PM, Hanahan D. Progressive squamous epithelial neoplasia in K14-human papillomavirus type 16 transgenic mice. *J Virol* 1994; 68:4358–4368.

176. Arbeit JM, Howley PM, Hanahan D. Chronic estrogen-induced cervical and vaginal squamous carcinogenesis in human papillomavirus type 16 transgenic mice. *Proc Natl Acad Sci USA* 1996; 93:2930–2935.

177. Callahan R. MMTV-induced mutations in mouse mammary tumors: their potential relevance to human breast cancer. *Breast Cancer Res Treat* 1996; 39:33–44.

178. Muller WJ, Sinn E, Pattengale PK, Wallace R, Leder P. Single-step induction of mammary adenocarcinoma in transgenic mice bearing the activated c-neu oncogene. *Cell* 1988; 54:105–115.

179. Bouchard L, Lamarre L, Tremblay PJ, Jolicoeur P. Stochastic appearance of mammary tumors in transgenic mice carrying the MMTV/c-neu oncogene. *Cell* 1989; 57:931–936.

180. Weinstein EJ, Kitsberg DI, Leder P. A mouse model for breast cancer induced by amplification and overexpression of the neu promoter and transgene. *Mol Med* 2000; 6:4–16.

181. Andrechek ER, Hardy WR, Siegel PM, Rudnicki MA, Cardiff RD, Muller WJ. Amplification of the neu/erbB-2 oncogene in a mouse model of mammary tumorigenesis. *Proc Natl Acad Sci USA* 2000; 97:3444–3449.

182. Li B, Murphy KL, Laucirica R, Kittrell F, Medina D, Rosen JM. A transgenic mouse model for mammary carcinogenesis. *Oncogene* 1998; 16:997–1007.

183. Gallahan D, Jhappan C, Robinson G, et al. Expression of a truncated Int3 gene in developing secretory mammary epithelium specifically retards lobular differentiation resulting in tumorigenesis. *Cancer Res* 1996; 56:1775–1785.

184. Shackleford GM, MacArthur CA, Kwan HC, Varmus HE. Mouse mammary tumor virus infection accelerates mammary carcinogenesis in Wnt-1 transgenic mice by insertional activation of int-2/Fgf-3 and hst/Fgf-4. *Proc Natl Acad Sci USA* 1993; 90:740–744.

185. Li Y, Hively WP, Varmus HE. Use of MMTV-Wnt-1 transgenic mice for studying the genetic basis of breast cancer. *Oncogene* 2000; 19:1002–1009.

186. Green JE, Shibata MA, Yoshidome K, et al. The C3(1)/SV40 T-antigen transgenic mouse model of mammary cancer: ductal epithelial cell targeting with multistage progression to carcinoma. *Oncogene* 2000; 19:1020–1027.

187. Radany EH, Hong K, Kesharvarzi S, Lander ES, Bishop JM. Mouse mammary tumor virus/v-Ha-ras transgene-induced mammary tumors exhibit strain-specific allelic loss on mouse chromosome 4. *Proc Natl Acad Sci USA* 1997; 94:8664–8669.

188. Murphy KL, Rosen JM. Mutant p53 and genomic instability in a transgenic mouse model of breast cancer. *Oncogene* 2000; 19:1045–1051.

189. Deng CX, Scott F. Role of the tumor suppressor gene Brcal in genetic stability and mammary gland tumor formation. *Oncogene* 2000; 19:1059–1064.

190. Greenberg NM, DeMayo FJ, Sheppard PC, et al. The rat probasin gene promoter directs hormonally and developmentally regulated expression of a heterologous gene specifically to the prostate in transgenic mice. *Mol Endocrinol* 1994; 8:230–239.

191. Greenberg NM, DeMayo F, Finegold MJ, et al. Prostate cancer in a transgenic mouse. *Proc Natl Acad Sci USA* 1995; 92:3439–3443.

192. Gingrich JR, Barrios RJ, Morton RA, et al. Metastatic prostate cancer in a transgenic mouse. *Cancer Res* 1996; 56:4096–4102.

193. Kaplan PJ, Mohan S, Cohen P, Foster BA, Greenberg NM. The insulin-like growth factor axis and prostate cancer: lessons from the transgenic adenocarcinoma of mouse prostate (TRAMP) model. *Cancer Res* 1999; 59:2203–2209.

194. Gingrich JR, Barrios RJ, Kattan MW, Nahm HS, Finegold MJ, Greenberg NM. Androgen-independent prostate cancer progression in the TRAMP model. *Cancer Res* 1997; 57:4687–4691.

195. Foster BA, Gingrich JR, Kwon ED, Madias C, Greenberg NM. Characterization of prostatic epithelial cell lines derived from transgenic adenocarcinoma of the mouse prostate (TRAMP) model. *Cancer Res* 1997; 57:3325–3330.

196. Kwon ED, Hurwitz AA, Foster BA, et al. Manipulation of T cell costimulatory and inhibitory signals for immunotherapy of prostate cancer. *Proc Natl Acad Sci USA* 1997; 94:8099–8103.

197. Maroulakou IG, Anver M, Garrett L, Green JE. Prostate and mammary adenocarcinoma in transgenic mice carrying a rat C3(1) simian virus 40 large tumor antigen fusion gene. *Proc Natl Acad Sci USA* 1994; 91:11236–11240.

198. Shibata MA, Ward JM, Devor DE, Liu ML, Green JE. Progression of prostatic intraepithelial neoplasia to invasive carcinoma in C3(1)/SV40 large T antigen transgenic mice: histopathological and molecular biological alterations. *Cancer Res* 1996; 56:4894–4903.

199. Zhang X, Chen MW, Ng A, et al. Abnormal prostate development in C3(1)-bcl-2 transgenic mice. *Prostate* 1997; 32:16–26.

200. Garabedian EM, Humphrey PA, Gordon JI. A transgenic mouse model of metastatic prostate cancer originating from neuroendocrine cells. *Proc Natl Acad Sci USA* 1998; 95:15382–15387.

201. Perez-Stable C, Altman NH, Brown J, Harbison M, Cray C, Roos BA. Prostate, adrenocortical, and brown adipose tumors in fetal globin/T antigen transgenic mice. *Lab Invest* 1996; 74:363–373.

202. Quaife CJ, Pinkert CA, Ornitz DM, Palmiter RD, Brinster RL. Pancreatic neoplasia induced by ras expression in acinar cells of transgenic mice. *Cell* 1987; 48:1023–1034.

203. Wagner M, Greten FR, Weber CK, et al. A murine tumor progression model for pancreatic cancer recapitulating the genetic alterations of the human disease. *Genes Dev* 2001; 15:286–293.

204. Bennoun M, Rissel M, Engelhardt N, Guillouzo A, Briand P, Weber-Benarous A. Oval cell proliferation in early stages of hepatocarcinogenesis in simian virus 40 large T transgenic mice. *Am J Pathol* 1993; 143:1326–1336.

205. Kitagawa T, Hino O, Lee GH, et al. Multistep hepatocarcinogenesis in transgenic mice harboring SV40 T-antigen gene. *Princess Takamatsu Symp* 1991; 22:349–360.

206. Sepulveda AR, Finegold MJ, Smith B, et al. Development of a transgenic mouse system for the analysis of stages in liver carcinogenesis using tissue-specific expression of SV40 large T-antigen controlled by regulatory elements of the human alpha-1-antitrypsin gene. *Cancer Res* 1989; 49:6108–6117.

207. Gilbert E, Morel A, Tulliez M, et al. In vivo effects of activated H-ras oncogene expressed in the liver and in urogenital tissues. *Int J Cancer* 1997; 73:749–756.

208. Orian JM, Tamakoshi K, Mackay IR, Brandon MR. New murine model for hepatocellular carcinoma: transgenic mice expressing metallothionein-ovine growth hormone fusion gene. *J Natl Cancer Inst* 1990; 82:393–398.

209. Martin DC, Sanchez-Sweatman OH, Ho AT, Inderdeo DS, Tsao MS, Khokha R. Transgenic TIMP-1 inhibits simian virus 40 T antigen-induced hepatocarcinogenesis by impairment of hepatocellular proliferation and tumor angiogenesis. *Lab Invest* 1999; 79:225–234.

210. Santoni-Rugiu E, Jensen MR, Factor VM, Thorgeirsson SS. Acceleration of c-myc-induced hepatocarcinogenesis by co-expression of transforming growth factor (TGF)-alpha in transgenic mice is associated with TGF-beta1 signaling disruption. *Am J Pathol* 1999; 154:1693–1700.

211. Santoni-Rugiu E, Nagy P, Jensen MR, Factor VM, Thorgeirsson SS. Evolution of neoplastic development in the liver of transgenic mice co-expressing c-myc and transforming growth factor-alpha. *Am J Pathol* 1996; 149:407–428.

212. Santoni-Rugiu E, Jensen MR, Thorgeirsson SS. Disruption of the pRb/E2F pathway and inhibition of apoptosis are major oncogenic events in liver constitutively expressing c-myc and transforming growth factor alpha. *Cancer Res* 1998; 58:123–134.

213. de La Coste A, Romagnolo B, Billuart P, et al. Somatic mutations of the beta-catenin gene are frequent in mouse and human hepatocellular carcinomas. *Proc Natl Acad Sci USA* 1998; 95:8847–8851.

214. Umeda T, Yamamoto T, Kajino K, Hino O. beta-catenin mutations are absent in hepatocellular carcinomas of SV40 T-antigen transgenic mice. *Int J Oncol* 2000; 16:1133–1136.

215. Chisari FV, Klopchin K, Moriyama T, et al. Molecular pathogenesis of hepatocellular carcinoma in hepatitis B virus transgenic mice. *Cell* 1989; 59:1145–1156.

216. Jakubczak JL, Chisari FV, Merlino G. Synergy between transforming growth factor alpha and hepatitis B virus surface antigen in hepatocellular proliferation and carcinogenesis. *Cancer Res* 1997; 57:3606–3611.

217. Kim CM, Koike K, Saito I, Miyamura T, Jay G. HBx gene of hepatitis B virus induces liver cancer in transgenic mice. *Nature* 1991; 351:317–320.

218. Wikenheiser KA, Clark JC, Linnoila RI, Stahlman MT, Whitsett JA. Simian virus 40 large T antigen directed by transcriptional elements of the human surfactant protein C gene produces pulmonary adenocarcinomas in transgenic mice. *Cancer Res* 1992; 52:5342–5352.

219. Kerkhoff E, Fedorov LM, Siefken R, Walter AO, Papadopoulos T, Rapp UR. Lung-targeted expression of the c-Raf-1 kinase in transgenic mice exposes a novel oncogenic character of the wild-type protein. *Cell Growth Differ* 2000; 11:185–190.

220. Lebel M, Webster M, Muller WJ, Royal A, Gauthier J, Mes-Masson AM. Transgenic mice bearing the polyomavirus large T antigen directed by 2.1 kb of the keratin 19 promoter develop bronchiolar papillary tumors with progression to lung adenocarcinomas. *Cell Growth Differ* 1995; 6:1591–1600.

221. Ehrhardt A, Bartels T, Geick A, Klocke R, Paul D, Halter R. Development of pulmonary bronchioloalveolar adenocarcinomas in transgenic mice overexpressing murine c-myc and epidermal growth factor in alveolar type II pneumocytes. *Br J Cancer* 2001; 84:813–818.

222. Jacks T, Shih TS, Schmitt EM, Bronson RT, Bernards A, Weinberg RA. Tumour predisposition in mice heterozygous for a targeted mutation in Nf1. *Nat Genet* 1994; 7:353–361.

223. Cichowski K, Shih TS, Schmitt E, et al. Mouse models of tumor development in neurofibromatosis type 1. *Science* 1999; 286:2172–2176.

224. Vogel KS, Klesse LJ, Velasco-Miguel S, Meyers K, Rushing EJ, Parada LF. Mouse tumor model for neurofibromatosis type 1. *Science* 1999; 286:2176–2179.

225. Reilly KM, Loisel DA, Bronson RT, McLaughlin ME, Jacks T. Nf1;Trp53 mutant mice develop glioblastoma with evidence of strain-specific effects. *Nat Genet* 2000; 26:109–113.

226. McClatchey AI, Saotome I, Mercer K, et al. Mice heterozygous for a mutation at the Nf2 tumor suppressor locus develop a range of highly metastatic tumors. *Genes Dev* 1998; 12:1121–1133.

227. Giovannini M, Robanus-Maandag E, Niwa-Kawakita M, et al. Schwann cell hyperplasia and tumors in transgenic mice expressing a naturally occurring mutant NF2 protein. *Genes Dev* 1999; 13:978–986.

228. He LZ, Merghoub T, Pandolfi PP. In vivo analysis of the molecular pathogenesis of acute promyelocytic leukemia in the mouse and its therapeutic implications. *Oncogene* 1999; 18:5278–5292.

229. Kogan SC, Bishop JM. Acute promyelocytic leukemia: from treatment to genetics and back. *Oncogene* 1999; 18:5261–5267.

230. Huang ME, Ye YC, Chen SR, et al. Use of all-trans retinoic acid in the treatment of acute promyelocytic leukemia. *Blood* 1988; 72:567–572.

231. Wang ZG, Ruggero D, Ronchetti S, et al. PML is essential for multiple apoptotic pathways. *Nat Genet* 1998; 20:266–272.

232. He LZ, Guidez F, Tribioli C, et al. Distinct interactions of PML-RARalpha and PLZF-RARalpha with co-repressors determine differential responses to RA in APL. *Nat Genet* 1998; 18:126–135.
233. Strasser A, Harris AW, Bath ML, Cory S. Novel primitive lymphoid tumours induced in transgenic mice by cooperation between myc and bcl-2. *Nature* 1990; 348:331–333.
234. Adams JM, Harris AW, Strasser A, Ogilvy S, Cory S. Transgenic models of lymphoid neoplasia and development of a pan- hematopoietic vector. *Oncogene* 1999; 18:5268–5277.
235. Berns A. Tumorigenesis in transgenic mice: identification and characterization of synergizing oncogenes. *J Cell Biochem* 1991; 47:130–135.
236. Haupt Y, Bath ML, Harris AW, Adams JM. bmi-1 transgene induces lymphomas and collaborates with myc in tumorigenesis.*Oncogene* 1993; 8:3161–3164.
237. Haupt Y, Harris AW, Adams JM. Retroviral infection accelerates T lymphomagenesis in E mu-N-ras transgenic mice by activating c-myc or N-myc. *Oncogene* 1992; 7:981–986.
238. Haupt Y, Harris AW, Adams JM. Moloney virus induction of T-cell lymphomas in a plasmacytomagenic strain of E mu-v-abl transgenic mice. *Int J Cancer* 1993; 55:623–629.
239. You M, Wang Y, Lineen AM, Gunning WT, Stoner GD, Anderson MW. Mutagenesis of the K-ras protooncogene in mouse lung tumors induced by N-ethyl-N-nitrosourea or N-nitrosodiethylamine. *Carcinogenesis* 1992; 13:1583–1586.
240. Cormier RT, Hong KH, Halberg RB, et al. Secretory phospholipase Pla2g2a confers resistance to intestinal tumorigenesis. *Nat Genet* 1997; 17:88–91.
241. Pataer A, Nishimura M, Kamoto T, Ichioka K, Sato M, Hiai H. Genetic resistance to urethan-induced pulmonary adenomas in SMXA recombinant inbred mouse strains. *Cancer Res* 1997; 57:2904–2908.
242. Lee GH, Drinkwater NR. The Hcr (hepatocarcinogen resistance) loci of DBA/2J mice partially suppress phenotypic expression of the Hcs (hepatocarcinogen sensitivity) loci of C3H/HeJ mice. *Carcinogenesis* 1995; 16:1993–1996.
243. Nagase H, Mao JH, de Koning JP, Minami T, Balmain A. Epistatic interactions between skin tumor modifier loci in interspecific (spretus/musculus) backcross mice. *Cancer Res* 2001; 61:1305–1308.
244. Fisher GH, Orsulic S, Holland E, et al. Development of a flexible and specific gene delivery system for production of murine tumor models. *Oncogene* 1999; 18:5253–5260.
245. Lee EY, Chang CY, Hu N, et al. Mice deficient for Rb are nonviable and show defects in neurogenesis and haematopoiesis. *Nature* 1992; 359:288–294.
246. Clarke AR, Maandag ER, van Roon M, et al. Requirement for a functional Rb-1 gene in murine development. *Nature* 1992; 359:328–330.
247. Harvey M, McArthur MJ, Montgomery CA Jr, Butel JS, Bradley A, Donehower LA. Spontaneous and carcinogen-induced tumorigenesis in p53-deficient mice. *Nat Genet* 1993; 5:225–229.
248. Purdie CA, Harrison DJ, Peter A, et al. Tumour incidence, spectrum and ploidy in mice with a large deletion in the p53 gene. *Oncogene* 1994; 9:603–609.
249. Giovannini M, Robanus-Maandag E, van der Valk M, et al. Conditional biallelic Nf2 mutation in the mouse promotes manifestations of human neurofibromatosis type 2. *Genes Dev* 2000; 14:1617–1630.
250. Moser AR, Pitot HC, Dove WF. A dominant mutation that predisposes to multiple intestinal neoplasia in the mouse. *Science* 1990; 247:322–324.
251. Fodde R, Edelmann W, Yang K, et al. A targeted chain-termination mutation in the mouse Apc gene results in multiple intestinal tumors. *Proc Natl Acad Sci USA* 1994; 91:8969–8973.
252. Oshima H, Oshima M, Kobayashi M, Tsutsumi M, Taketo MM. Morphological and molecular processes of polyp formation in Apc(delta716) knockout mice. *Cancer Res* 1997; 57:1644–1649.
253. Takaku K, Miyoshi H, Matsunaga A, Oshima M, Sasaki N, Taketo MM. Gastric and duodenal polyps in Smad4 (Dpc4) knockout mice. *Cancer Res* 1999; 59:6113–6117.
254. Reitmair AH, Schmits R, Ewel A, et al. MSH2 deficient mice are viable and susceptible to lymphoid tumours. *Nat Genet* 1995; 11:64–70.
255. de Wind N, Dekker M, Berns A, Radman M, te Riele H. Inactivation of the mouse Msh2 gene results in mismatch repair deficiency, methylation tolerance, hyperrecombination, and predisposition to cancer. *Cell* 1995; 82:321–330.
256. Baker SM, Plug AW, Prolla TA, et al. Involvement of mouse Mlh1 in DNA mismatch repair and meiotic crossing over. *Nat Genet* 1996; 13:336–342.
257. Kiyokawa H, Kineman RD, Manova-Todorova KO, et al. Enhanced growth of mice lacking the cyclin-dependent kinase inhibitor function of p27 (Kip1). *Cell* 1996; 85:721–732.
258. Kreidberg JA, Sariola H, Loring JM, et al. WT-1 is required for early kidney development. *Cell* 1993; 74:679–691.

259. Duan DR, Pause A, Burgess WH, et al. Inhibition of transcription elongation by the VHL tumor suppressor protein. *Science* 1995; 269:1402–1406.

260. Kibel A, Iliopoulos O, DeCaprio JA, Kaelin WG Jr. Binding of the von Hippel-Lindau tumor suppressor protein to Elongin B and C. *Science* 1995; 269:1444–1446.

261. Gowen LC, Johnson BL, Latour AM, Sulik KK, Koller BH. Brca1 deficiency results in early embryonic lethality characterized by neuroepithelial abnormalities. *Nat Genet* 1996; 12:191–194.

262. Hakem R, de la Pompa JL, Sirard C, et al. The tumor suppressor gene Brca1 is required for embryonic cellular proliferation in the mouse. *Cell* 1996; 85:1009–1023.

263. Liu CY, Flesken-Nikitin A, Li S, Zeng Y, Lee WH. Inactivation of the mouse Brca1 gene leads to failure in the morphogenesis of the egg cylinder in early postimplantation development. *Genes Dev* 1996; 10:1835–1843.

264. Suzuki A, de la Pompa JL, Hakem R, et al. Brca2 is required for embryonic cellular proliferation in the mouse. *Genes Dev* 1997; 11:1242–1252.

265. Connor F, Bertwistle D, Mee PJ, et al. Tumorigenesis and a DNA repair defect in mice with a truncating Brca2 mutation. *Nat Genet* 1997; 17:423–430.

266. Sharan SK, Morimatsu M, Albrecht U, et al. Embryonic lethality and radiation hypersensitivity mediated by Rad51 in mice lacking Brca2. *Nature* 1997; 386:804–810.

267. Sirard C, de la Pompa JL, Elia A, et al. The tumor suppressor gene Smad4/Dpc4 is required for gastrulation and later for anterior development of the mouse embryo. *Genes Dev* 1998; 12:107–119.

268. Fazeli A, Dickinson SL, Hermiston ML, et al. Phenotype of mice lacking functional deleted in colorectal cancer (Dcc) gene. *Nature* 1997; 386:796–804.

269. Bradl M, Klein-Szanto A, Porter S, Mintz B. Malignant melanoma in transgenic mice. *Proc Natl Acad Sci USA* 1991; 88:164–168.

270. Fan H, Oro AE, Scott MP, Khavari PA. Induction of basal cell carcinoma features in transgenic human skin expressing Sonic Hedgehog. *Nat Med* 1997; 3:788–792.

271. Lifsted T, Le Voyer T, Williams M, et al. Identification of inbred mouse strains harboring genetic modifiers of mammary tumor age of onset and metastatic progression. *Int J Cancer* 1998; 77:640–644.

272. Halter SA, Dempsey P, Matsui Y, et al. Distinctive patterns of hyperplasia in transgenic mice with mouse mammary tumor virus transforming growth factor-alpha. Characterization of mammary gland and skin proliferations. *Am J Pathol* 1992; 140:1131–1146.

273. Li M, Lewis B, Capuco AV, Laucirica R, Furth PA. WAP-TAg transgenic mice and the study of dysregulated cell survival, proliferation, and mutation during breast carcinogenesis. *Oncogene* 2000; 19:1010–1019.

274. Brown D, Kogan S, Lagasse E, et al. A PMLRARalpha transgene initiates murine acute promyelocytic leukemia. *Proc Natl Acad Sci USA* 1997; 94:2551–2556.

275. He LZ, Tribioli C, Rivi R, et al. Acute leukemia with promyelocytic features in PML/RARalpha transgenic mice. *Proc Natl Acad Sci USA* 1997; 94:5302–5307.

276. Kogan SC, Hong SH, Shultz DB, Privalsky ML, Bishop JM. Leukemia initiated by PMLRARalpha: the PML domain plays a critical role while retinoic acid-mediated transactivation is dispensable. *Blood* 2000; 95:1541–1550.

277. Grisolano JL, Wesselschmidt RL, Pelicci PG, Ley TJ. Altered myeloid development and acute leukemia in transgenic mice expressing PML-RAR alpha under control of cathepsin G regulatory sequences. *Blood* 1997; 89:376–387.

278. Westervelt P, Ley TJ. Seed versus soil: the importance of the target cell for transgenic models of human leukemias. *Blood* 1999; 93:2143–2148.

279. Adams JM, Harris AW, Pinkert CA, et al. The c-myc oncogene driven by immunoglobulin enhancers induces lymphoid malignancy in transgenic mice. *Nature* 1985; 318:533–538.

280. Dildrop R, Ma A, Zimmerman K, et al. IgH enhancer-mediated deregulation of N-myc gene expression in transgenic mice: generation of lymphoid neoplasias that lack c-myc expression. *EMBO J* 1989; 8:1121–1128.

281. Rosenbaum H, Webb E, Adams JM, Cory S, Harris AW. N-myc transgene promotes B lymphoid proliferation, elicits lymphomas and reveals cross-regulation with c-myc. *EMBO J* 1989; 8:749–755.

282. Rosenbaum H, Harris AW, Bath ML, et al. An E mu-v-abl transgene elicits plasmacytomas in concert with an activated myc gene. *EMBO J* 1990; 9:897–905.

283. Hariharan IK, Harris AW, Crawford M, et al. A bcr-v-abl oncogene induces lymphomas in transgenic mice. *Mol Cell Biol* 1989; 9:2798–2805.

284. Howes KA, Lasudry JG, Albert DM, Windle JJ. Photoreceptor cell tumors in transgenic mice. *Invest Opthalmol Vis Sci* 1994; 35:342–351.

285. Windle JJ, Albert DM, O'Brien JM, et al. Retinoblastoma in transgenic mice. *Nature* 1990; 343:665–669.

286. Rowley JD, Golomb HM, Dougherty C. 15/17 translocation, a consistent chromosomal change in acute promyelocytic leukemia. *Lancet* 1977; 1:549–550.

287. Teitz T, Chang JC, Kitamura M, Yen TS, Kan YW. Rhabdomyosarcoma arising in transgenic mice harboring the beta-globin locus control region fused with simian virus 40 large T antigen gene. *Proc Natl Acad Sci USA* 1993; 90:2910–2914.

288. Takayama H, LaRochelle WJ, Sharp R, et al. Diverse tumorigenesis associated with aberrant development in mice overexpressing hepatocyte growth factor/scatter factor. *Proc Natl Acad Sci USA* 1997; 94:701–706.

289. Strasser A, Harris AW, Cory S. E mu-bcl-2 transgene facilitates spontaneous transformation of early pre-B and immunoglobulin-secreting cells but not T cells. *Oncogene* 1993; 8:1–9.

III ONCOGENES AS TARGETS FOR ANTICANCER THERAPY IN VIVO

14 Targeting Oncogenes in Hematopoietic Malignancies

Michael E. O'Dwyer, MD
and Brian J. Druker, MD

CONTENTS

1. INTRODUCTION

The development of the first successful treatments for leukemia owed much more to empiric observation than rational drug design in an era when the biology of leukemia was poorly understood. While cytotoxic chemotherapeutic drugs have played, and continue to play, an essential role in cancer management, their relative lack of specificity and the frequency of resistance have been a limit to this approach. This has prompted a search for targeted therapies, with the goal of maximizing responses while minimizing toxicity. This first requires the identification of good targets, and it is only relatively recently that we have had the necessary tools to undertake this process. To be considered a good target, an oncogene product should be clearly responsible for the molecular pathogenesis of the disease. It should be a protein that is mutated or aberrantly expressed with that event being critical to the malignant process. Advances in the fields of cytogenetics, molecular genetics, and biochemistry over the past half century have greatly advanced our understanding of leukemia pathogenesis and helped identify candidate targets. We now know that oncogenic activation can result from several different mechanisms, including chromosomal translocations, activating mutations, loss of function mutations, and deletions. This chapter will show how the application of this knowledge has aided in the development of molecularly based treatment approaches, in particular the *Bcr-Abl* tyrosine kinase inhibitor STI571.

From: *Oncogene-Directed Therapies*
Edited by: J. W. Rak © Humana Press Inc., Totowa, NJ

2. IDENTIFYING THE TARGETS

2.1. Chromosomal Translocations

The identification of the Philadelphia (Ph) chromosome as the first consistent chromosomal abnormality in a human malignancy and the subsequent discovery that many types of leukemia and lymphoma were associated with recurrent chromosomal translocations suggested that these chromosomal abnormalities could play a role in the pathogenesis of these diseases *(1)*. Numerous recurrent chromosomal translocations have since been identified, and the molecular consequences of some of these are now well characterized *(2)*. Chromosomal translocations result in cellular transformation by one of two principal mechanisms. In the first, juxtaposition to a transcriptionally active region of the genome leads to increased expression of the target gene. This is more commonly seen in lymphoid malignancies where target genes are translocated to the immunoglobulin or T cell receptor loci in the case of B and T cell malignancies, respectively. In the case of follicular lymphoma, the t(14;18) leads to increased expression of the anti-apoptotic protein Bcl-2 as a result of the juxtaposition of the *bcl-2* gene on chromosome 18 with the immunoglobulin heavy chain locus on chromosome 14 *(3,4)*. A similar mechanism operates in both Burkitt's lymphoma as a consequence of t(8;14) and mantle cell lymphoma as a consequence of t(11;14), with overexpression of the *c-myc* and *cyclin D1* genes, respectively *(5–7)*. The second mechanism, which is more common in leukemia, results in the generation of chimeric oncogenes, which alter the phenotype of the affected cell.

The production of chimeric oncogenes involving transcription factors can disrupt the normal function of these factors leading to altered cellular differentiation. In acute promyelocytic leukemia (APL) associated with the (15;17) translocation, the normal response of the retinoic acid receptor-α (RAR-α) to its ligand, retinoic acid (RA), is disrupted in the fusion protein, promyelocytic leukemia (PML)-RAR-α. RAR-α normally functions as a ligand inducible transcription factor. In the absence of RA, it recruits the nuclear co-repressor complex (N-CoR), which in turn recruits *Sin3* and histone deacetylase, thus repressing transcription. Once RA binds to its receptor, the repressor complex is released, co-activators with histone acetyltransferase activity are recruited to the transcription complex, and transcription of RA response elements ensues. PML-RAR-α, unlike normal RAR-α does not release the co-repressor complex in response to physiologic levels of RA resulting in a blockade in myeloid differentiation. However, pharmacologic doses of RA (1 μM) are capable of relieving this repression, restoring normal cellular differentiation *(8–11)*. RA therapy may also lead to degradation of PML-RAR-α by a proteolytic pathway, contributing to its ability to restore normal differentiation *(12)*.

The therapeutic efficacy of RA was first demonstrated in China with all-*trans* retinoic acid (ATRA) producing differentiation and remission in patients with APL with less toxicity than conventional chemotherapy *(13)*. This was a major advance and the first example of a small molecule successfully targeting the underlying molecular lesion in a form of leukemia. However, this was an empiric discovery, as at that time, the molecular basis of APL had not yet been elucidated. Further experience with ATRA in APL showed that the vast majority of patients relapsed if treated with ATRA alone. Subsequent clinical trials have now refined the treatment of this disease, and by utilizing a combination of chemotherapy and ATRA, high rates of durable remission are seen. In one recently reported study, a complete remission (CR) rate of 92% and relapse-free survival rate of 86% were seen *(14)*. For APL patients who fail therapy with ATRA, arsenic trioxide can induce CR in approximately 80% of patients *(15)*. Therefore, with current therapy, the vast majority of APL patients should survive their disease. Disruption of the transcription factor, known as core binding factor (CBF), is a common theme in several different types of leukemia. CBF is a heterodimeric protein consisting of AML1 (also known as CBFa2), the DNA-binding component, and CBFβ, which binds to AML1 and stabilizes its binding to DNA *(16)*. Approximately 12% of cases of acute myeloid leukemia (AML) have a translocation between chromosomes 8 and 21, t(8;21) *(17)*. This translocation generates a dominant negative AML1/ETO fusion protein, which interferes with the normal transactivating function of AML1 *(18)*. The AML1 protein regulates the expression of genes crucial for normal hematopoietic development, differentiation, and function, including the genes for myeloperoxidase, neutrophil elastase, interleukin 3, and granulocyte macrophage colony-stimulating factor (GM-CSF). The ETO fusion partner binds to the N-CoR, which then recruits Sin3 and histone deacetylase. This complex inhibits the expression of normal AML1-responsive genes, disrupting hematopoiesis *(19)*. A related form of AML, associated with inv *(16)*, is also characterized by abnormal AML1/CBFβ-dependent transcriptional regulation. In this case, the fusion protein CBFβ-MYH11 also functions as a dominant repressor, again recruiting a co-repressor with histone deacetylase activity *(20)*. CBFβ-MYH11 transcripts have been detected in up to 10% of patients with newly diagnosed AML *(21)*. Finally, the most frequent chromosomal translocation seen in childhood acute lymphoblastic leukemia (ALL), t(12;21), accounting for approximately 25% of cases of ALL, results in the generation of a TEL-AML1 chimeric protein. It appears that TEL-AML1 contributes to leukemogenesis through the recruitment of a nuclear co-repressor complex with histone deacetylase activity *(22)*. Therefore, a shared theme between t(8;21), inv(16), t(12;21), and APL is that of transcriptional repression related to excessive histone deacetylase activity.

Another common consequence of translocation events is activation of a tyrosine kinase. In those translocations involving genes encoding tyrosine kinases, the partner gene usually encodes a dimerization motif, which leads to constitutive activation of the tyrosine kinase. Chronic myelogenous leukemia (CML) is the classic example of this. The Ph chromosome, a shortened chromosome 22, was the first consistent chromosomal abnormality identified in a human malignancy (1). With the development of improved chromosomal banding techniques in the early 1970s, it became apparent that the Ph chromosome was the result of a reciprocal translocation between the long arms of chromosomes 9 and 22, t(9;22)(q34;q11) *(23)*. The molecular consequences of this translocation were subsequently shown to be the juxtaposition of the *c-Abl* oncogene from chromosome 9 with sequences from chromosome 22, the breakpoint cluster region (*Bcr*), giving rise to a fusion *bcr-abl* gene *(24)*. The size of the protein generated by the fusion gene varies depending on where the breakpoint occurs in the Bcr region. A210-kDa fusion protein (p210) is seen in approximately 95% of patients with CML and up to 20% of adult patients with ALL. A 185-kDa fusion protein (p185) is seen in 10% of adults with ALL and is the predominant Bcr-Abl fusion protein in Ph positive pediatric ALL patients, which accounts for approximately 5% of such cases. The product of this fusion gene is a constitutively active tyrosine kinase with markedly enhanced enzymatic activity compared to the Abl kinase. This enhanced tyrosine kinase activity is critical for its transforming potential *(25)*. Other examples of translocations involving genes encoding tyrosine kinases include t(5;12), producing a TEL-platelet-derived growth factor receptor (PDGFR) fusion tyrosine kinase associated with some cases of chronic myelomonocytic leukemia (CMML) and t(2;5), producing a nucleophosmin–anaplastic lymphoma kinase (NPM-ALK) fusion tyrosine kinase associated with T cell anaplastic large cell lymphoma (ALCL) *(26,27)*.

2.2. Activating Mutations

Activating mutations in cytokine receptors, specifically receptor tyrosine kinases, are being increasingly recognized as a means of cellular transformation in hematopoietic malignancies. Activating mutations of two members of the class III receptor tyrosine kinases, c-kit and Flt3, have been documented in leukemic cells from patients with AML. An internal tandem duplication (ITD) of the juxtamembrane coding region of the Flt3 gene on chromosome 13 has been reported in up to 30% of adult AML patients and up to 16.5% of pediatric AML patients *(28–31)*. More recently, another 7% of AML and 3% of myelodysplasia patients were found to have a point mutation in the activation loop of the Flt3 kinase domain *(32)*. Consequently, mutant Flt3 receptors dimerize in the absence of ligand with constitutive tyrosine kinase activation, resulting in growth factor independence. Clinically, the presence of Flt3-ITD is associated with poor prognosis, and affected patients have lower rates of CR following induction chemotherapy and higher relapse rates. Activating mutations in c-kit are less common and appear to occur predominantly in patients with CBF-related AML *(33,34)*. These could be important "second-hits" in the development of these subtypes of leukemia (see *below*).

3. VALIDATING THE TARGETS
3.1. Models of Leukemogenesis

To be considered a good target for directed therapy, an oncogene must be shown to be clearly responsible for malignant transformation. Retroviral expression of the oncogene in cell lines conferring growth factor independence is supportive, but the strongest evidence comes from animal models where knock-in (translocations or activating mutations) or knock-out (deletions or loss of function mutations) strategies can recapitulate the human disease. In the case of CML, experiments in transgenic mice and murine recipients of Bcr-Abl-transduced hematopoietic stem cells demonstrate that expression of Bcr-Abl alone can induce leukemia *(35,36)*. Similarly, retroviral insertion of the *NPM-ALK* gene into murine hematopoietic cells followed by transplantation into lethally irradiated recipients causes lymphoid malignancy in mice *(37)*. Lastly, transfection of the murine interleukin (IL) 3-dependent cell line, 32D, with a mutant *Flt3* gene results in growth factor independence and transplantation into syngeneic mice leads to the development of leukemia within 5 wk *(38)*. Whether hematopoietic progenitors expressing a similar Flt3 mutant would rapidly develop leukemia, needs to be determined. The situation may be more complex for some other oncogenes. Transgenic mice expressing PML-RAR-α develop APL, although with relatively long latency, but co-expression of the reciprocal translocation partner, RAR-α-PML, leads to a murine disease resembling APL with much shorter latency *(39)*. Experiments in mice expressing chimeric CBF proteins also indicate that these abnormalities alone may be insufficient to induce leukemia.

When AML1 was replaced by AML1-ETO in mice using a knock-in strategy, a block in hematopoiesis was seen, but mouse embryos died in mid-gestation due to development of severe central nervous system hemorrhage (40). To overcome this embryonal lethality, subsequent experiments employed a model in which the AML1-ETO expression was inducible, under the control of a tetracycline-responsive element. Despite high expression of AML1-ETO in the bone marrow cells of these mice, no leukemia was seen during 24 mo of observation, though a partial block of myeloid differentiation was seen (41). Although mice expressing AML1-ETO do not develop leukemia, they are at much higher risk of developing leukemia when compared to control mice, following exposure to alkylating agents (42). Similarly, mice expressing CBFβ-MYH11 did not develop leukemia, but, following exposure to low dose alkylating agents, had a high rate of leukemic transformation, whereas no cases of leukemia were seen in similarly treated control mice (43). This suggests that secondary mutations cooperate with AML1-ETO to induce leukemia and that AML1-ETO induced leukemia may be a multistep process. In the case of Burkitt's lymphoma, transgenic mice overexpressing c-myc develop lymphomas (44). However, it is likely that other abnormalities cooperate with c-myc to induce lymphoma. Up to 80% of cases of Burkitt's lymphoma exhibit mutations in the p53 tumor suppressor gene, and when wild-type p53 is expressed in a Burkitt's lymphoma cell expressing a mutated form of p53, rapid cell death by apoptosis ensues (45). In fact, enforced expression of c-myc causes apoptosis in the absence of secondary abnormalities that circumvent apoptosis, such as bcl-2 overexpression or p53 mutations (46,47).

4. HITTING THE TARGET

For maximal utility as a single agent, the identification of crucial, early events in malignant progression is the first step in the successful development of a targeted therapy. An equally important issue is the selection of patients for clinical trials based on the presence of the appropriate target. Finally, to avoid toxicity, the ideal target should be dispensable for normal cellular function.

4.1. Histone Deacetylase Inhibitors and Differentiating Agents

Histone deacetylase inhibitors may relieve the transcriptional repression associated with certain types of leukemia, thus enhancing differentiation. By loosening the contacts between DNA and histones, histone acetylation opens up chromatin making it more accessible to transcription factors, leading to increased gene expression (48). Corepressor complexes with histone deacetylase activity, on the other hand, will inhibit gene expression. Several years ago, Warrell et al. (49) reported the successful use of the histone deacetylase inhibitor, sodium phenylbutyrate, in a patient with t(15,17) APL resistant to ATRA. The addition of phenylbutyrate to ATRA resulted in a molecular remission coinciding with an increase in histone acetylation in blood and marrow mononuclear cells (49). Phenylbutyrate and another histone deacetylase inhibitor, trichostatin A, have been shown to induce differentiation in AML cells expressing AML1-ETO along with increased histone acetylation. Additive effects on differentiation were seen with the combination of phenylbutyrate and G- or GM-CSF (50). This was postulated to be due to the release of AML1-ETO inhibition of wild-type AML1 function, allowing activation of myeloid cell-specific promoters, including those for cytokine receptors. The addition of dexamethasone to phenylbutyrate increased induction of apoptosis *(50)*. Based on these results, a clinical trial is currently in progress evaluating the efficacy of the combination of phenylbutyrate, dexamethasone, and GM-CSF in patients with relapsed or refractory t(8;21) AML. AML cells (ranging from French-American-British class M0 to M7) not expressing AML1-ETO or PML-RAR-α have also been shown to undergo differentiation when exposed to trichostatin A alone or in combination with other differentiating agents such as ATRA *(51)*. ATRA appears to augment the cytostatic and differentiating activity of phenylbutyrate permitting administration of lower doses of the histone deacetylase inhibitors *(52)*. This is important, as the levels of phenylbutyrate necessary for single agent in vitro activity (1 to 2 μM) may be difficult to achieve in vivo due to toxicity. Finally, a recent report showed that histone deacetylase inhibitor treatment of AML cells had immunomodulatory effects, with up-regulation of the co-stimulatory molecule CD86 and the adhesion molecule ICAM-1 *(53)*. AML cells induced to up-regulate co-stimulatory/adhesion molecules were shown to provoke a more vigorous allogeneic mixed leukocyte reaction. Potentially, histone deacetylase inhibitors could have a dual therapeutic benefit of inducing differentiation and increasing the immunogenicity of leukemia cells.

4.2. Signal Transduction Inhibitors

The final approach to be discussed is that of signal transduction inhibition. This approach utilizes small molecular weight inhibitors of enzymes, such as tyrosine kinases, which are critical to the oncogenic process. Since deregulated tyrosine kinase activity is involved in the pathogenesis and disease progression of CML, CMML associated with t(15;12), ALCL associated with t(2;5) and AML associated with ITD's of Flt3, these diseases are obvious choices for the development of specific signal transduction inhibitors. The following discussion will focus on the development of STI571 for the treatment of CML, as this serves as a paradigm for the development of similar therapies.

4.2.1. CML

CML accounts for 20% of all cases of leukemia with an annual incidence of 1 to 1.5 cases per 100,000. The median age of onset is approx 60 yr, but all age groups are affected *(54)*. Three clinical phases are recognized: a chronic phase lasting 4–6 yr, an accelerated phase lasting 6–18 mo, and a blast phase lasting 3–6 mo. The chronic phase is characterized by a massive proliferation of maturing myeloid cells, white cells, and frequently platelets. As the disease progresses, the malignant clones loses the capacity to differentiate until eventually the disease terminates in an acute leukemia, termed blast crisis. The accelerated phase is an intermediate phase characterized by increasing myeloid immaturity, systemic symptoms, and refractoriness to therapy. The only therapy known to cure CML is allogeneic stem cell transplantation, but since most patients are too old or lack suitable donors, this option is available to less than a third of patients. The 5–10 yr survival following allogeneic stem cell transplantation is 65%, with significant procedural related morbidity and mortality. Oral chemotherapy agents, such as hydroxyurea or busulfan, can control blood counts in most chronic phase patients, but do not delay the onset of blast crisis *(55)*. The use of interferon-α is associated with a definite survival advantage when compared to chemotherapy with patients living on average 2 yr longer *(56)*. The best survival advantage is seen in those patients who achieve a major cytogenetic response (a reduction in the percentage of marrow metaphases containing the Ph chromosome to less than 35%), although this occurs in less than one third of patients. Moreover, as many as 20% of patients discontinue interferon-α therapy due to intolerable toxicity. The addition of subcutaneous ara-C has been shown to increase response rates but at the cost of increased toxicity *(57)*. These shortcomings provided the impetus for the development of a more effective less toxic therapy for CML.

4.2.2. Bcr-Abl: the Ideal Target

Bcr-Abl impacts on numerous downstream signaling pathways in the CML cell affecting cell growth, adhesion, and survival *(58)*. However, since all of these events are dependent on the tyrosine kinase activity of the fusion protein, it is clear that inhibition of the enzymatic activity of Bcr-Abl should be an effective treatment of CML, since Bcr-Abl is present in the majority of patients with CML and is the causative abnormality of the disease, with its kinase activity being essential for transformation. Moreover, since Abl knock-out mice are viable, it is likely that Abl kinase activity would be dispensable for normal cellular function suggesting that targeting of Abl kinases would have a relatively selective effect on Bcr-Abl expressing cells *(59)*.

4.2.3. Developing an Inhibitor of the Bcr-Abl Tyrosine Kinase

Tyrosine kinases, such as Bcr-Abl, catalyze the transfer of phosphate from adenosine triphosphate (ATP) to selected tyrosine residues on substrate proteins. With their tyrosine residues in the phosphorylated form, substrate proteins assume conformational changes leading to association with other downstream effectors, propagating signal transduction. Tyrosine kinases thus play a vital role in cell growth, differentiation, and survival. Since all protein kinases use ATP as a phosphate donor, and as there is a high degree of conservation among kinase domains, particularly in the ATP binding sites, it was thought that inhibitors of ATP binding would lack sufficient target specificity to be clinically useful. This was the case with the first tyrosine kinase inhibitors identified, such as herbimycin-A, which were all natural plant derivatives. However, in 1988, Yaish et al. published a series of compounds, known as tyrphostins, that demonstrated that specific tyrosine kinase inhibitors could be developed *(60)*. Around the same time, scientists at Ciba Geigy (now Novartis) were performing high-throughput screens of chemical libraries searching for compounds with kinase inhibitory activity. They eventually identified a lead compound with kinase inhibitory activity of the 2-phenylaminopyrimidine class. Though of low potency and poor specificity, this served as a base compound from which a series of related compounds were synthesized. By analyzing the relationship between structure and activity, this series of compounds were optimized to inhibit a variety of targets *(61)*. One series of compounds, optimized against the PDGFR, proved to be equally active against the Abl tyrosine kinase. STI571 (formerly CGP57148, now Gleevec, imatinib mesylate) emerged as the lead compound for clinical development based on its superior in vitro selectivity against CML cells and its drug-like properties, including pharmacokinetics and formulation properties *(61)*.

4.2.3.1. Preclinical Studies. Experiments in our laboratory showed that STI571 was a potent and selective inhibitor of the Abl tyrosine kinases, including Bcr-Abl *(62)*. The concentration (IC50) of STI571 that resulted in a 50% reduction in substrate phosphorylation and cellular tyrosine phosphorylation induced by Bcr-Abl was 0.025 and 0.25 μM, respectively. The only other tyrosine kinase we found to be inhibited by STI571, besides Abl and the PDGFR, was c-kit. STI571 specifically inhibited the proliferation of myeloid cell lines containing Bcr-Abl. Colony-forming assays from CML patients showed a marked decrease (92–98%) in the number of Bcr-Abl colonies with no inhibition of normal colony formation when grown in the presence of 1μM STI571. Similar results were reported elsewhere *(63)*. Long-term marrow culture experiments showed that prolonged exposure to STI571 exerted a sustained inhibitory effect on CML progenitors with little toxicity to normal progenitors, again demonstrating its selective nature *(64)*. Subsequent experiments showed that p185 and p210 expressing cells were sensitive to the STI571 *(65,66)*. Dose-dependent inhibition of tumor growth was seen in Bcr-Abl-innoculated mice treated with STI571, but a once daily dosing schedule failed to eradicate the tumors *(62)*. Gambacorti and colleagues subsequently showed a 3×/day dosing schedule with oral administration of STI571 effectively eradicated Bcr-Abl containing tumors in nude mice *(67)*. Since the half-life of STI571 in mice is approx 4 h, it seemed likely that continuous exposure to STI571 would be required for optimal antileukemic effects.

4.2.3.2. Clinical Trials of STI571 in CML. Based on the efficacy of STI571 in a variety of preclinical models and an acceptable animal toxicology profile, a phase I clinical trial with STI571 started in June 1998 *(68)*. This was a dose escalation study, designed to establish the maximum tolerated dose (MTD), with clinical efficacy as a secondary endpoint. Patients were enrolled in 14 successive dose cohorts ranging from 25–1000 mg of STI571. Patients were eligible if they were in the chronic phase of CML and had failed therapy with interferon-α. STI571 was administered as a once daily oral therapy, and no other cytoreductive agents were allowed. Once doses of 300 mg or greater were reached, 53 out of 54 patients had a complete hematologic response. Responses were typically seen within the first 3 wk of therapy and have been maintained in 96% of patients with a median duration of follow up of 310 d. At this dose level (>300 mg), major cytogenetic responses were seen in 31% of patients, with 13% achieving a complete cytogenetic response. Side-effects have been minimal, with no dose-limiting toxicities encountered. Grade 2 and 3 myelosuppression were observed at a dose > 300 mg in 21 and 8% of patients, respectively. Myelosuppression is likely consistent with a therapeutic effect as the Ph-positive clone contributes the majority of hematopoiesis in these patients. Pharmacokinetic studies showed that the half-life of STI571 is 13–16 h, which is sufficiently long to permit once daily dosing. Although the follow-up on this group of patients is relatively short (median 1 yr), these data indicate that an Abl-specific tyrosine kinase inhibitor has significant activity in CML, even in interferon refractory patients.

Given the effectiveness of STI571 in chronic phase patients who had failed interferon, the Phase I studies were expanded to include CML patients in myeloid and lymphoid blast crisis and patients with relapsed or refractory Ph chromosome positive ALL *(69)*. Patients have been treated with daily doses of 300–1000 mg of STI571. Twenty-one out of thirty-eight patients (55%) in myeloid blast crisis responded to therapy, which was defined by a decrease in percentage of marrow blasts to less than 15%. Eight out of 38 patients (21%) had marrow blasts cleared to <5%. Seven out of thirty-eight of the myeloid blast crisis patients (18%) have remained in remission on STI571 with follow-up ranging from 101–349 d. Fourteen out of twenty patients with lymphoid phenotype disease (70%), CML in lymphoid blast crisis, or Ph-positive ALL responded with 11 out of 20 patients (55%) clearing their marrows to <5% blasts.

Unfortunately, all but one of the lymphoid phenotype patients have relapsed between d 42 and 123. Thus, STI571 has remarkable single-agent activity in CML blast crisis and Ph positive ALL, but responses tend not to be durable. However, these studies demonstrate that in the majority of cases, the leukemic clone in Bcr-Abl positive acute leukemias, including CML blast crisis, remains at least partially dependent on Bcr-Abl kinase activity for survival.

To confirm the positive results seen in the phase I studies, phase II studies with STI571 were initiated towards the end of 1999, encompassing all phases of CML. These studies were designed to evaluate the safety and efficacy of STI571 in larger cohorts of patients. Chronic phase (having failed interferon), accelerated, and blast crisis patients were enrolled in these studies at 27 institutions in 6 countries. Evaluation of response and pharmacokinetic data from the Phase I study indicated that doses of 400–600 mg should be optimal for phase II testing *(70)*. Between December 1999 and May 2000, 532 chronic phase patients who were refractory to or intolerant of interferon-α were treated with STI571 at a dose of 400 mg daily *(71)*. After a median exposure of 8.5 mo, 47 and 28% of patients achieved major and complete cytogenetic responses, respectively. Only 3% of patients discontinued treatment due to disease progression, with only 2% of all patients stopping therapy due to adverse events. Of 233 accelerated phase patients treated, 63% of patients achieved a complete hematologic response (CHR) with or without peripheral blood recovery (neutrophils >1.0×10^9L and platelets > 100×10^9/L). Fourteen percent achieved a complete cytogenetic response *(72)*. Again, these results were achieved without substantial toxicity, though, not surprisingly, up to 20% of patients experienced grade 3 to 4 myelosuppression in this study. Nevertheless, only 2% of patients developed febrile neutropenia. Of 260 myeloid blast crisis patients treated, 64% had some form of response, with 26% clearing their marrows to less than 5% blasts *(73)*. Major and complete cytogenetic responses were seen in 15 and 6% of patients, respectively. Median survival was 6.8 months (8.6 months in patients with no prior therapy for blast crisis), and 30% of patients are projected to be still alive at 14 mo. Historically, patients treated with chemotherapy for myeloid blast crisis have had a median survival of approx. 3 mo. Toxicity was comparable to that seen in the accelerated phase study.

4.2.3.3. Dose Selection. From the Phase I study, complete hematologic responses occurred in almost all patients treated at doses of 300 mg and above, and cytogenetic responses were seen once this dose level was reached. In addition, pharmacokinetic data showed that this dose level achieved in vivo concentrations approaching the predicted in vitro IC50 for cellular proliferation of 1 μM *(70)*. Finally, an analysis of responses in white blood counts and platelets over time suggested that doses of 400 to 600 mg were on the plateau of a dose-response curve, indicating that this dose range would be an efficacious dose for phase II testing. However, in the dose escalation study, an MTD of STI571 was never reached *(68)*. While traditional drug development has involved dose escalation until an MTD is established, with molecularly targeted therapies, this may not be an appropriate endpoint. A more appropriate endpoint may be the optimal effective dose that achieves the desired pharmacologic effect of molecular target inhibition. Therefore, in the case of STI571 and CML, an optimal effective dose should approximate that which achieves maximal Bcr-Abl kinase inhibition. An analysis of Bcr-Abl kinase inhibition, assaying for decreases in phosphorylation of the Bcr-Abl substrate, Crkl, has shown that a plateau in inhibition is seen above 250 mg *(68)*.

Additional experiments are being conducted to determine the percentage of kinase activity that is being inhibited at these dose levels *(74)*. CML lends itself to this kind of molecular monitoring, in that tumor cells are easily accessible and that the kinase itself or its substrates can be monitored for inhibition. These types of assays will clearly be more problematic for solid tumors, but will be necessary to determine the penetration of these types of agents into solid tumors. In the absence of specific assays, even information about intracellular drug levels in tumor samples would be a useful surrogate. This type of data, regarding maximal kinase inhibition, could be particularly useful in explaining response variability and could also be useful in individualizing therapy.

4.2.3.4. Future Directions in Therapy of CML. The clinical data presented here demonstrate that STI571 is employed to optimum effect when used early, prior to progression. An ongoing phase III randomized study is comparing STI571 with interferon-α plus ara-C in newly diagnosed patients. The results of this study when combined with more mature data from the phase II studies will help determine the place of STI571 in future CML treatment algorithms. It is tempting to speculate that as Bcr-Abl may be the sole oncogenic abnormality driving proliferation in early stage disease, STI571 alone may be sufficient therapy in some patients with CML. However, as additional genetic abnormalities accumulate with disease progression, CML cells may no longer be dependent on Bcr-Abl for survival. Thus, in blast crisis patients, therapy with STI571 alone is clearly insufficient for most patients.

4.2.3.5. The Problem of Resistance and the Rationale for Combination Therapy. Despite the high initial response rates in blast crisis patients, many patients relapse. That resistance to STI571 can develop is obvious, and the reasons for this are under intense scrutiny. Resistance may be multifactorial and can be divided into mechanisms associated with persistent inhibition of Bcr-Abl kinase activity and mechanisms associated with reactivation of Bcr-Abl kinase activity at relapse. Patients with persistent inhibition of Bcr-Abl kinase activity would be predicted to have additional oncogenic abnormalities, allowing Bcr-Abl-independent proliferation. Patients with reactivation of Bcr-Abl kinase activity would be expected to have resistance mechanisms that either prevent STI571 from reaching the target or render the target insensitive to STI571. The former includes protein binding of STI571 and drug efflux, while the latter includes *bcr-abl* gene amplification or mutations involving the kinase domain of *bcr-abl* *(75–78)*. It is possible, using phosphotyrosine assays (as described above) to distinguish these two broad classes of resistance and monitor in vivo drug efficacy. In a recent report, reactivation of Bcr-Abl kinase activity, as assessed by Crkl phosphorylation, was seen in 11 out of 11 blast crisis patients who developed resistance to STI571 *(79)*. Ex vivo, these cells remained sensitive to STI571, though requiring much higher doses of the inhibitor. In 3 out of 11 resistant cases, gene amplification of *bcr-abl* was shown to have occurred. This confirms several reports of Bcr-Abl gene amplification as a mechanism of resistance in CML cell lines *(75–77)*. Interestingly, *bcr-abl* gene amplification appears to reverse once the selective pressure, i.e., STI571, has been removed, suggesting that following an interruption in therapy, patients could potentially become sensitive once again to the drug. Other relapsed patients had point mutations in the kinase domain of Bcr-Abl that rendered the kinase insensitive to STI571 *(79)*. Interestingly, this point mutation occurred at a predicted contact point between STI571 and the kinase domain, based on the crystal structure of the Abl kinase co-crystallized with STI571 *(80)*. However, evaluation of larger patient numbers will be required to determine the frequency of Bcr-Abl amplification and mutation in patients resistant to STI571. Lastly, there has been a suggestion from animal studies that protein binding of STI571 could be responsible for relapse *(78)*. However, samples from relapsed patients have decreased cellular sensitivity to STI571, suggesting that intrinsic cellular resistance and not protein binding are responsible *(79)*.

To circumvent resistance, the combination of STI571 with other active antileukemic agents would seem desirable. We have shown that inhibition of Bcr-Abl by STI571 can reverse the intrinsic drug resistance seen in CML cells and that combinations with drugs such as daunorubicin, ara-C, and interferon-α are associated with additive or even synergistic effects in vitro, providing a strong rationale for combination studies *(81)*. Similar studies have been performed with etoposide and ara-C *(82)*. Combination studies with low dose interferon and ara-C are currently underway for chronic phase patients, while combinations of STI571 with high dose chemotherapy regimens (vincristine, daunorubicin, and prednisone and high dose ara-C) are planned for lymphoid and myeloid blast crisis patients, respectively. Potentially, other promising small molecular weight signal transduction inhibitors, such as farnesyl transferase inhibitors, may be useful either alone (in STI571 failures) or in combination with STI571 to prevent the emergence of resistance in patients with advanced disease *(83)*.

5. TRANSLATING THE SUCCESS OF STI571 TO OTHER MOLECULAR TARGETS

The clinical trials with STI571 are a dramatic demonstration of the potential of targeting molecular pathogenetic events in a malignancy. In applying this paradigm to other malignancies, it is important to realize that Bcr-Abl and CML have several features that were critical to the success of this agent. As previously noted, Bcr-Abl tyrosine kinase activity has clearly been demonstrated to be critical to the pathogenesis of CML. Thus, not only was the target of STI571 known, but is was directed against a critical event in the development of CML. Another important feature is that the results demonstrate, as with most malignancies, treatment of early stage disease yields better results. Specifically, the rate and durability of responses has been notably superior in chronic phase as opposed to blast phase patients. Therefore, to reproduce the success of STI571 in other malignancies, it is imperative to identify the critical early events in malignant progression. It is equally important that selection for clinical trials is limited to those patients whose malignancies express the appropriate target. In clinical trials using STI571, this was clearly feasible, as patients with activation of Bcr-Abl were easily identifiable by the presence of the Ph chromosome. In this regard, as reagents to analyze molecular endpoints are developed, these same reagents should be useful in identifying appropriate candidates for treatment with a specific agent. With the combination of a critical pathogenetic target that is easily identifiable early in the course of the disease and an agent that targets this abnormality, remarkable results can be achieved. The obvious goal is to identify these early pathogenetic events in each malignancy and to develop agents that specifically target these abnormalities.

REFERENCES

1. Nowell PC, Hungerford DA. A minute chromosome in human chronic granulocytic leukemia. *Science* 1960; 132:1497–1501.
2. Rowley JD. The role of chromosome translocations in leukemogenesis. *Semin Hematol* 1999;36:59–72.
3. Tsujimoto Y, Finger LR, Yunis J, Nowell PC, Croce CM. Cloning of the chromosome breakpoint of neoplastic B cells with the t(14;18) chromosome translocation. *Science* 1984; 226:1097–1099.

4. Reed JC, Tsujimoto Y, Epstein SF, Cuddy M, Slabiak T, Nowell PC, et al. Regulation of bcl-2 gene expression in lymphoid cell lines containing normal #18 or t(14;18) chromosomes. *Oncogene Res* 1989; 4:271–282.

5. Dalla-Favera R, Bregni M, Erikson J, Patterson D, Gallo RC, Croce CM. Human c-myc onc gene is located on the region of chromosome 8 that is translocated in Burkitt lymphoma cells. *Proc Natl Acad Sci USA* 1982; 79:7824–7827.

6. Adams JM, Gerondakis S, Webb E, Corcoran LM, Cory S.Cellular myc oncogene is altered by chromosome translocation to an immunoglobulin locus in murine. plasmacytomas and is rearranged similarly in human Burkitt lymphomas. *Proc Natl Acad Sci USA* 1983; 80:1982–1986.

7. Bosch F, Jares P, Campo E, Lopez-Guillermo A, Piris MA, Villamor N, et al. PRAD-1/cyclin D1 gene overexpression in chronic lymphoproliferative disorders: a highly specific marker of mantle cell lymphoma. *Blood* 1994; 84:2726–2732.

8. Guidez F, Ivins S, Zhu J, Soderstrom M, Waxman S, Zelent A. Reduced retinoic acid-sensitivities of nuclear receptor corepressor binding to PML- and PLZF-RARalpha underlie molecular pathogenesis and treatment of acute promyelocytic leukemia. *Blood* 1998; 91:2634–2642.

9. Collins SJ. Acute promyelocytic leukemia: relieving repression induces remission. *Blood* 1998; 91:2631–2633.

10. Lin RJ, Nagy L, Inoue S, Shao W, Miller WH Jr, Evans RM. Role of the histone deacetylase complex in acute promyelocytic leukaemia. *Nature* 1998; 391:811–814.

11. He LZ, Guidez F, Tribioli C, Peruzzi D, Ruthardt M, Zelent A, et al. Distinct interactions of PML-RARalpha and PLZF-RARalpha with co-repressors determine differential responses to RA in APL. *Nat Genet* 1998; 18:126–135.

12. Yoshida H, Kitamura K, Tanaka K, Omura S, Miyazaki T, Hachiya T, et al. Accelerated degradation of PML-retinoic acid receptor alpha (PML-RARA) oncoprotein by all-trans-retinoic acid in acute promyelocytic leukemia: possible role of the proteasome pathway. *Cancer Res* 1996; 56:2945–2948.

13. Huang ME, Ye YC, Chen SR, Chai JR, Lu JX, Zhoa L, et al. Use of all-trans retinoic acid in the treatment of acute promyelocytic leukemia. *Blood* 1988; 72:567–572.

14. Fenaux P, Chastang C, Chevret S, Sanz M, Dombret H, Archimbaud E, et al. A randomized comparison of all transretinoic acid (ATRA) followed by chemotherapy and ATRA plus chemotherapy and the role of maintenance therapy in newly diagnosed acute promyelocytic leukemia. The European APL Group. *Blood* 1999; 94:1192–1200.

15. Soignet SL, Maslak P, Wang ZG, Jhanwar S, Calleja E, Dardashti LJ, et al. Complete remission after treatment of acute promyelocytic leukemia with arsenic trioxide. *N Engl J Med* 1998; 339:1341–1348.

16. Liu P, Tarle SA, Hajra A, Claxton DF, Marlton P, Freedman M, et al. Fusion between transcription factor CBF beta/PEBP2 beta and a myosin heavy chain in acute myeloid leukemia. *Science* 1993; 261:1041–1044.

17. Langabeer SE, Walker H, Rogers JR, Burnett AK, Wheatley K, Swirsky D, et al. Incidence of AML1/ETO fusion transcripts in patients entered into the MRC AML trials. MRC Adult Leukaemia Working Party. *Br J Haematol* 1997; 99:925–928.

18. Downing JR, Higuchi M, Lenny N, Yeoh AE. Alterations of the AML1 transcription factor in human leukemia. *Semin Cell Dev Biol* 2000; 11:347–360.

19. Wang J,Hoshino T, Redner RL, Kajigaya S, Liu JM. ETO, fusion partner in t(8;21) acute myeloid leukemia, represses transcription by interaction with the human N- CoR/mSin3/HDAC1 complex. *Proc Natl Acad Sci USA* 1998; 95:10860–10865.

20. Lutterbach B, Hou Y, Durst KL, Hiebert SW. The inv(16) encodes an acute myeloid leukemia 1 transcriptional corepressor. *Proc Natl Acad Sci USA* 1999;96:12822–12827.

21. Langabeer SE, Walker H, Gale RE, Wheatley K, Burnett AK, Goldstone AH, et al. Frequency of CBF beta/MYH11 fusion transcripts in patients entered into the U.K.MRC AML trials. The MRC Adult Leukaemia Working Party. *Br J Haematol* 1997; 96:736–739

22. Guidez F, Petrie K, Ford AM, Lu H, Bennett CA, MacGregor A, et al. Recruitment of the nuclear receptor corepressor N-CoR by the TEL moiety of the childhood leukemia-associated TEL-AML1 oncoprotein. *Blood* 2000; 96:2557–2561.

23. Rowley JD. Letter: a new consistent chromosomal abnormality in chronic myelogenous leukemia identified by quinacrine fluorescence and Giemsa staining. *Nature* 1973; 243:290–293.

24. Shtivelman E, Lifshitz B, Gale RP, Canaani E.Fused transcript of abl and bcr genes in chronic myelogenous leukaemia. *Nature* 1985; 315:550–554.

25. Lugo TG, Pendergast AM, Muller AJ, Witte ON. Tyrosine kinase activity and transformation potency of bcr-abl oncogene products. *Science* 1990; 247:1079–1082.

26. Golub TR, Barker GF, Lovett M, Gilliland DG. Fusion of PDGF receptor beta to a novel ets-like gene, tel, in chronic myelomonocytic leukemia with t(5;12) chromosomal translocation. *Cell* 1994; 77:307–316.

27. Morris SW, Kirstein MN, Valentine MB, Dittmer KG, Shapiro DN, Saltman DL, et al. Fusion of a kinase gene, ALK, to a nucleolar protein gene, NPM, in non-Hodgkin's lymphoma. *Science* 1994; 263:1281–1284.

28. Nakao M, Yokota S, Iwai T, Kaneko H, Horiike S, Kashima K, et al. Internal tandem duplication of the flt3 gene found in acute myeloid leukemia. *Leukemia* 1996; 10:1911–1918

29. Rombouts WJ, Blokland I, Lowenberg B, Ploemacher RE. Biological characteristics and prognosis of adult acute myeloid leukemia with internal tandem duplications in the Flt3 gene. *Leukemia* 2000; 14:675–683.

30. Abu-Duhier FM, Goodeve AC, Wilson GA, Gari MA, Peake IR, Rees DC, et al. FLT3 internal tandem duplication mutations in adult acute myeloid leukaemia define a high-risk group. *Br J Haematol* 2000; 111:190–195.

31. Meshinchi S, Woods WG, Stirewalt DL, Sweetser DA, Buckley JD, Tjoa TK, et al. Prevalence and prognostic significance of Flt3 internal tandem duplication in pediatric acute myeloid leukemia. *Blood* 2001; 97:89–94.

32. Yamamoto Y, Kiyoi H, Nakano Y, Suzuki R, Kodera Y, Miyawaki S, et al. Activating mutation of D835 within the activation loop of FLT3 in human hematologic malignancies. *Blood* 2001; 97:2434–2439.

33. Gari M, Goodeve A, Wilson G, Winship P, Langabeer S, Linch D, et al. c-kit proto-oncogene exon 8 in-frame deletion plus insertion mutations in acute myeloid leukaemia. Br *J Haematol* 1999; 105:894–900.

34. Beghini A, Peterlongo P, Ripamonti CB, Larizza L, Cairoli R, Morra E, et al. C-kit mutations in core binding factor leukemias. *Blood* 2000; 95:726–727.

35. Daley GQ, Van Etten RA, Baltimore D.Induction of chronic myelogenous leukemia in mice by the P210bcr/abl gene of the Philadelphia chromosome. *Science* 1990; 247:824–830.

36. Heisterkamp N, Jenster G, ten Hoeve J, Zovich D, Pattengale PK, Groffen J. Acute leukaemia in bcr/abl transgenic mice. *Nature* 1990; 344:251–253.

37. Kuefer MU, Look AT, Pulford K, Behm FG, Pattengale PK, Mason DY, et al. Retrovirus-mediated gene transfer of NPM-ALK causes lymphoid malignancy in mice. *Blood* 1997; 90:2901–2910.

38. Mizuki M, Fenski R, Halfter H, Matsumura I, Schmidt R, Muller C, et al. Flt3 mutations from patients with acute myeloid leukemia induce transformation of 32D cells mediated by the Ras and STAT5 pathways. *Blood* 2000; 96:3907–3914.

39. Merghoub T, Gurrieri C, Piazza F, Pandolfi PP. Modeling acute promyelocytic leukemia in the mouse: new insights in the pathogenesis of human leukemias. *Blood Cells Mol Dis* 2001; 27:231–248.

40. Okuda T, Cai Z, Yang S, Lenny N, Lyu CJ, van Deursen JM, et al. Expression of a knocked-in AML1-ETO leukemia gene inhibits the establishment of normal definitive hematopoiesis and directly generates dysplastic hematopoietic progenitors. *Blood* 1998; 91:3134–3143.

41. Rhoades KL, Hetherington CJ, Harakawa N, Yergeau DA, Zhou L, Liu LQ, et al. Analysis of the role of AML1-ETO in leukemogenesis, using an inducible transgenic mouse model. *Blood* 2000; 96:2108–2115.

42. Higuchi M, O'Brien D, Lenny N, Yang S, Cai Z, Downing JR. Expression of AML1-ETO immortalizes myeloid progenitors and cooperates with secondary mutations to induce granulocytic sarcoma/acute myeloid leukemia. *Blood* 2000; 96:222a.

43. Castilla LH, Garrett L, Adya N, Orlic D, Dutra A, Anderson S, et al. The fusion gene Cbfb-MYH11 blocks myeloid differentiation and predisposes mice to acute myelomonocytic leukaemia. *Nat Genet* 1999; 23:144–146.

44. Adams JM, Harris AW, Pinkert CA, Corcoran LM, Alexander WS, Cory S, et al. The c-myc oncogene driven by immunoglobulin enhancers induces lymphoid malignancy in transgenic mice. *Nature* 1985; 318:533–538.

45. Ramqvist T, Magnusson KP, Wang Y, Szekely L, Klein G, Wiman KG. Wild-type p53 induces apoptosis in a Burkitt lymphoma (BL) line that carries mutant p53. *Oncogene* 1993; 8:1495–1500.

46. Milner AE, Grand RJ, Waters CM, Gregory CD. Apoptosis in Burkitt lymphoma cells is driven by c-myc. Oncogene 1993; 8:3385–3391.

47. Gavioli R, Frisan T, Vertuani S, Bornkamm GW, Masucci MG. c-myc overexpression activates alternative pathways for intracellular proteolysis in lymphoma cells. *Nat Cell Biol* 2001; 3:283–288.

48. Zwiebel JA. New agents for acute myelogenous leukemia. *Leukemia* 2000; 14:488–490.

49. Warrell RP Jr, He LZ, Richon V, Calleja E, Pandolfi PP. Therapeutic targeting of transcription in acute promyelocytic leukemia by use of an inhibitor of histone deacetylase. *J Natl Cancer Inst* 1998; 90:1621–1625.

50. Wang J, Saunthararajah Y, Redner RL, Liu JM. Inhibitors of histone deacetylase relieve ETO-medi-ated repression and induce differentiation of AML1-ETO leukemia cells. *Cancer Res* 1999; 59:2766–2769.

51. Kosugi H, Towatari M, Hatano S, Kitamura K, Kiyoi H, Kinoshita T, et al. Histone deacetylase inhibitors are the potent inducer/enhancer of differentiation in acute myeloid leukemia: a new approach to anti-leukemia therapy. *Leukemia* 1999; 13:1316–1324.

52. Yu KH, Weng LJ, Fu S, Piantadosi S, Gore SD. Augmentation of phenylbutyrate-induced differentia-tion of myeloid leukemia cells using all-trans retinoic acid. *Leukemia* 1999; 13:1258–1265.

53. Maeda T, Towatari M, Kosugi H, Saito H. Up-regulation of costimulatory/adhesion molecules by his-tone deacetylase inhibitors in acute myeloid leukemia cells. *Blood* 2000; 96:3847–3856.

54. O'Dwyer ME, Druker BJ. Chronic myelogenous leukaemia—new therapeutic principles. *J Intern Med* 2001; 250:3–9.

55. Silver RT, Woolf SH, Hehlmann R, Appelbaum FR, Anderson J, Bennett C, et al. An evidence-based analysis of the effect of busulfan, hydroxyurea, interferon, and allogeneic bone marrow transplantation in treating the chronic phase of chronic phase of chronic myeloid leukemia: developed for the Ameri-can Society of Hematology. *Blood* 1999; 94:1517–1536.

56. Interferon alfa versus chemotherapy for chronic myeloid leukemia: a meta-analysis of seven random-ized trials: Chronic Myeloid Leukemia Trialists' Collaborative Group. *J Natl Cancer Inst* 1997; 89:1616–1620.

57. Guilhot F, Chastang C, Michallet M, Guerci A, Harousseau JL, Maloisel F, et al. Interferon alfa-2b combined with cytarabine versus interferon alone in chronic myelogenous leukemia. French Chronic Myeloid Leukemia Study Group. *N Engl J Med* 1997; 337:223–229.

58. Deininger MW, Goldman JM, Melo JV. The molecular biology of chronic myeloid leukemia. *Blood* 2000; 96:3343–3356.

59. Tybulewicz VL, Crawford CE, Jackson PK, Bronson RT, Mulligan RC. Neonatal lethality and lym-phopenia in mice with a homozygous disruption of the c-abl proto-oncogene. *Cell* 1991; 65:1153–1163.

60. Yaish P, Gazit A, Gilon C, Levitzki A. Blocking of EGF-dependent cell proliferation by EGF receptor kinase inhibitors. *Science* 1988; 242:933–935.

61. Druker BJ, Lydon NB. Lessons learned from the development of an abl tyrosine kinase inhibitor for chronic myelogenous leukemia. *J Clin Invest* 2000; 105:3–7.

62. Druker BJ, Tamura S, Buchdunger E, Ohno S, Segal GM, Fanning S, et al. Effects of a selective inhibitor of the Abl tyrosine kinase on the growth of Bcr-Abl positive cells. *Nat Med* 1996; 2:561–566.

63. Deininger JM, Lydon N, Melo JV. The tyrosine kinase inhibitor CGP57148B selectively inhibits the growth of BCR-ABL-positive cells. *Blood* 1997; 90:3691–3698.

64. Kasper B, Fruehauf S, Schiedlmeier B, Buchdunger E, Ho AD, Zeller WJ. Favorable therapeutic index of a p210(BCR-ABL)-specific tyrosine kinase inhibitor; activity on lineage-committed and primitive chronic myelogenous leukemia progenitors. *Cancer Chemother Pharmacol* 1999; 44:433–438.

65. Carroll M, Ohno-Jones S, Tamura S, Buchdunger E, Zimmermann J, Lydon NB, et al. CGP 57148, a tyrosine kinase inhibitor, inhibits the growth of cells expressing BCR-ABL, TEL-ABL, and TEL-PDGFR fusion proteins. *Blood* 1997; 90:4947–4952.

66. Beran M, Cao X, Estrov Z, Jeha S, Jin G, O'Brien S, et al. Selective inhibition of cell proliferation and BCR-ABL phosphorylation in acute lymphoblastic leukemia cells expressing Mr 190,000 BCR-ABL protein by a tyrosine kinase inhibitor (CGP-57148). *Clin Cancer Res* 1998; 4:1661–1672.

67. le Coutre P, Mologni L, Cleris L, Marchesi E, Buchdunger E, Giardini R, et al. In vivo eradication of human BCR/ABL-positive leukemia cells with an ABL kinase inhibitor. *J Natl Cancer Inst* 1999; 91:163–168.

68. Druker BJ, Talpaz M, Resta DJ, Peng B, Buchdunger E, Ford JM, et al. Efficacy and safety of a spe-cific inhibitor of the BCR-ABL tyrosine kinase in chronic myeloid leukemia. *N Engl J Med* 2001; 344:1031–1037.

69. Deuker BJ, Sawyers CL, Kantarjian H, Resta DJ, Reese SF, Ford JM, et al. Activity of a specific inhibitor of the BCR-ABL tyrosine kinase in the blast crisis of chronic myeloid leukemia and acute lymphoblastic leukemia with the Philadelphia chromosome. *N Engl J Med* 2001; 344:1038–1042.

70. Peng B, Hayes M, Druker BJ, Talpaz M, Sawyers CL, Resta DJ, et al. Clinical pharmacokinetics and pharmacodynamics of STI571 in a phase I trial in chronic myelogenous leukemia (CML) patients. *Proc Am Assoc Cancer Res* 2000; 41: Abstr. no.3468.

71. Kantarjian H, Sawyers C, Hochhaus A, Guilhot F, Schiffer C, Resta D, et al. Phase II study of STI571, a tyrosine kinase inhibitor, in patients with resistant or refractory Philadelphia chromosome-positive chronic myeloid leukemia. *Blood* 2000; 96:470a.

72. Talpaz M, Silver RT, Druker B, Paquette R, Goldman JM, Reese SF, et al. A phase II study of STI571 in patients with Philadelphia chromosome-positive chronic myeloid leukemia in accelerated phase. *Blood* 2000; 96:469a.

73. Sawyers C, Hochhaus A, Feldman E, Goldman JM, Miller C, Ben-Am M, et al. A phase II study to determine the safety and anti-leukemic effects of STI571 in patients with Philadelphia chromosome-positive chronic myeloid leukemia in myeloid blast crisis. *Blood* 2000; 96:503a.

74. Karamlou K, Lucas L, Druker B. Identification of molecular endpoints as a guide for clinical decision making in STI571-treated chronic myelogenous leukemia patients. *Blood* 2000; 96:98a.

75. Mahon FX, Deininger MW, Schultheis B, Chabrol J, Reiffers J, Goldman JM, et al. Selection and characterization of BCR-ABL positive cell lines with differential sensitivity to the tyrosine kinase inhibitor STI571: diverse mechanisms of resistance. *Blood* 2000; 96:1070–1079.

76. le Coutre P, Tassi E, Varella-Garcia M, Barni R, Mologni L, Cabrita G, et al. Induction of resistance to the Abelson inhibitor STI571 in human leukemic cells through gene amplification. Blood 2000; 95:1758–1766.

77. Weisberg E, Griffin JD. Mechanism of resistance to the ABL tyrosine kinase inhibitor STI571 in BCR/ABL-transformed hematopoietic cell lines. *Blood* 2000; 95:3498–3505.

78. Gambacorti-Passerini C, Barni R, le Coutre P, Zucchetti M, Cabrita G, Cleris L, et al. Role of alpha1 acid glycoprotein in the in vivo resistance of human BCR-ABL(+) leukemic cells to the abl inhibitor STI571. *J Natl Cancer Inst* 2000; 92:1641–1650.

79. Gorre ME, Mohammed M, Ellwood K, Hsu N, Paquette R, Rao PN, et al. Clinical resistance to STI-571 cancer therapy caused by BCR-ABL gene mutation or amplification. *Science* 2001; 293:876–880.

80. Schindler T, Bornmann W, Pellicena P, Miller WT, Clarkson B, Kuriyan J. Structural mechanism for STI-571 inhibition of abelson tyrosine kinase. *Science* 2000; 289:1938–1942.

81. Thiesing JT, Ohno-Jones S, Kolibaba KS, Druker BJ. Efficacy of STI571, an abl tyrosine kinase inhibitor, in conjunction with other antileukemic agents against bcr-abl-positive cells. *Blood* 2000; 96:3195–3199.

82. Fang G, Kim CN, Perkins CL, Ramadevi N, Winton E, Wittmann S, et al. CGP57148B (STI-571) induces differentiation and apoptosis and sensitizes Bcr-Abl-positive human leukemia cells to apoptosis due to antileukemic drugs. *Blood* 2000; 96:2246–2253.

83. Peters DG, Hoover RR, Gerlach MJ, Koh EY, Zhang H, Choe K, et al. Activity of the farnesyl protein transferase inhibitor SCH66336 against BCR/ABL-induced murine leukemia and primary cells from patients with chronic myeloid leukemia. *Blood* 2001; 97:1404–1412.

15 Clinical Evaluation of Agents Targeting Epidermal Growth Factor Receptor (EGFR) in Cancer

Edward H. Lin, MD
and James L. Abbruzzese, MD

CONTENTS

INTRODUCTION
EGFR AND CANCER
CLINICAL EVALUATION OF EGFR ANTAGONISTS
FUTURE DIRECTIONS
ACKNOWLEDGMENT
REFERENCES

1. INTRODUCTION

Proteins encoded by oncogenes and tumor-suppressor genes are the essential signaling components of the complex cellular signaling networks *(1–3)*. Cancer arises from a multistep process promoted by the imbalanced growth signals as a consequence of gain of oncogene and/or loss of tumor suppressor genes *(4)*. The six essential cancer hallmarks include persistent cell growth signals, insensitivity to antigrowth signals, evasion of apoptosis, persistent angiogenesis, gain of cell immortality, and tumor invasion and metastasis *(5)*. As an oncogene, gain of epidermal growth factor receptor (EGFR) function is achieved through EGFR overexpression and has been shown to be associated with almost all the six essential hallmarks of cancer except the gain of cell immortality *(6,7)*. In various experimental models, EGFR inhibition leads to regression of tumor cell growth, inhibition of angiogenesis, induction of apoptosis, and inhibition of tumor invasion and metastasis *(7,8)*. Furthermore, overexpression of EGFR, frequently observed in a number of human cancers, is associated with poor overall prognosis, increased tumor recurrence, and decreased patient survival *(8)*. The hypothesis that EGFR might be a cancer therapeutic target was proposed by Mendelsohn *(6,7)* in the early 1980s; emerging only recently are the promising clinical trial results from a number of EGFR antagonists in different human cancers. This chapter will discuss the clinical developments and future directions of EGFR antagonists in cancer treatment.

From: *Oncogene-Directed Therapies*
Edited by: J. W. Rak © Humana Press Inc., Totowa, NJ

2. EGFR AND CANCER

Cell surface receptors are critical for a multicellular organism to transmit growth and differentiation signals as well as to mediate stress responses to external stimuli *(9)*. Evolved from a 20-member tyrosine kinase receptor superfamily, EGFR, a 170-kDa receptor tyrosine kinase glycoprotein, belongs to a 4-member HER receptor subfamily, which forms receptor heterodimers *(9)*. EGFR bears an extracellular ligand binding domain, a transmembrane lipophilic domain, a tyrosine kinase domain, and a tyrosine residues tail *(9,10)*. Naturally occurring ligands that bind to the EGFR include EGF, transforming growth factor (TGF)α, neuregulin, and amphiregulin. Upon ligand binding, EGFR undergoes receptor dimerization and autophosphorylation of the tyrosine residues tail by its intrinsic tyrosine kinase domain *(10)*. The phosphorylated EGFR activates the ras-dependent pathway via ras-raf-MEK mitogen-activated protein kinase (MAPK) and ras-rac-rho signaling cascades, respectively, and the ras-independent pathway via the src-shc signaling cascade *(9,10)*. These signaling cascades amplify the EGFR activation signals through a series of protein–protein interactions, leading to activation of nuclear transcription factors and expression of downstream effector genes *(5,10)*. The EGFR activation signals are fine-tuned by many positive and negative regulatory proteins *(11)*. The multitude of downstream effects of EGFR activation and complex receptor partnering with other cellular receptors such as integrin, bombesin receptor, etc., explain the versatile functions of EGFR as a cellular receptor and as an oncogene receptor when perturbed *(5,12-14)* (Fig. 1).

Persistent tumor growth is achieved through both EGFR overexpression and/or co-expression of TGFα, forming an autocrine loop shown to confer increased tumor growth and poor prognosis in a variety of human malignancies *(8,15)*. TGFα is a potent tumor growth signal as opposed to EGF. Upon TGFα binding, EGFR undergoes receptor activation, internalization, and receptor recycling without degradation, providing persistent tumor growth signals. In contrast, EGF-mediated EGFR activation results in receptor activation, internalization, and degradation, thus down-regulating the tumor growth signals *(8,15)*. Ras, a major effector of the EGFR signaling pathways, is frequently mutated in a wide variety of cancers and locks the EGFR signaling pathway in constitutive "on" state *(16)*. Ras also stimulates secretion of TGFα, further facilitating the tumor cell growth via the autocrine loop *(16)*. Mutations in TGFβ RII-SMAD4 pathways, a negative regulatory pathway counter balancing EGFR signaling, also contribute to uncontrolled tumor growth *(17)*.

PI3K-AKT, a key pathway of cellular apoptosis, interacts with EGFR pathway through insulin growth factor receptor (IGFR) and promotes evasion of apoptosis and

---

Fig. 1. Upon TGFα binding, EGFR undergoes receptor dimerization and autophosphorylation, and the phosphorylated EGFR activates the ras-dependent pathway via ras-raf-MEK-MAPK and ras-rac-rho signaling cascades through mediator proteins like Grb, SOS, and CdC42. The ras-independent pathway is mediated via the src-shc signaling cascade. Please note complex receptor partnering with integrin and protein kinase A (PKA) and bombesins and interconnectivity with other receptor pathways such as IGF-PI3K-PTEN and TGFβ/SMAD. EGFR activation signals are amplified through these signaling cascade, leading to activation of nuclear transcription factors and expression of downstream effector genes mediating tumor cell growth, insensitivity to antigrowth signals, evasion of apoptosis, cell motility and metastasis, and tumor angiogenesis. TGFα-EGFR autocrine loop is facilitated by EGFR recycling (not shown) and ras-mediated TGFα production.

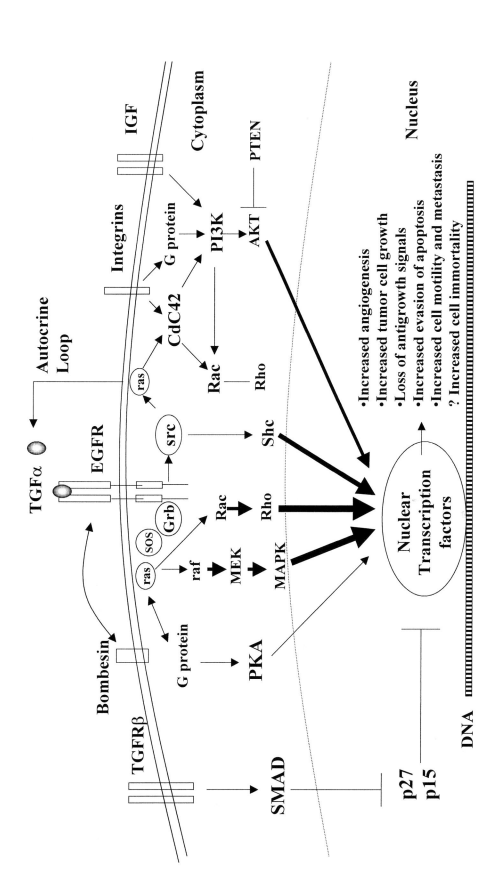

multidrug resistance phenotypes in cell line models *(18,19)*. PTEN, a tyrosine phosphatase that normally attenuates AKT, is lost in a number of epithelial cancers such as malignant glioma *(20)*. Liu and Karnes et al. showed that the inhibition of the EGFR with anti-EGFR monoclonal antibody C225 induced apoptosis in colon cancer cell lines through activation of caspase 3,9 and 10 *(21,22)*.

EGFR activation induces cyclin D1 expression required for progression through G1 phase. Conversely, EGFR inhibition with C225 leads to G1 arrest with reciprocal up-regulation of p27[(kipi)] and down-regulation of p21[(cipi)] in a colon cancer cell line mode *(23,24)*.

In addition to its roles in tumor cell growth and apoptosis, EGFR was also implicated in tumor cell motility, an important component of tumor invasion and metastasis *(13,25–28)*. Chen and Xie et al. reported that tumor cell motility and invasiveness are mediated by other mechanisms different from the mitogenic activity of EGFR *(25,26)*. Diel et al. studied the Panc-1 cell line and suggested that the Ras-raf-mek-MAPK pathway is required for EGFR directed cell proliferation, as well as cell migration *(27)*. The controversy pointed out an important issue, namely that assigning a particular pathway to a specific cancer phenotype represents gross oversimplification of the complex divergent EGFR signaling pathways and fails to underscore the importance of the dynamic receptor partnering and signaling cross-talk *(11–13)*. Transfection of full-length EGFR and a truncated EGFR into the DU145, a colon cell line, formed, respectively, invasive and noninvasive tumor phenotypes in vivo *(28)*. EGF and amphiregulin activation of EGFR preferentially mediates tumor cell motility and invasiveness as measured by cell motility and matrix degradation assays *(29–31)*. The increased tumor cell motility and invasiveness was due to the EGFR-mediated transcriptional activation of downstream effector genes such as metalloproteinase *(31)*, urokinase, and collagenase *(32)*.

Tumor angiogenesis is one of the most critical aspects of the host–tumor interaction, facilitating in vivo tumor cell growth, invasion, and metastasis *(33–35)*. Tumor angiogenesis occurs as a result of the abundance of angiogenic stimulators and/or shortage of angiogenic inhibitors *(33–35)*. Interestingly, TGFα acts as a more potent growth and more angiogenic ligand than EGF *(36)*. Neuregulin directly promotes angiogenesis through its binding to EGFR expressed on endothelial cells *(37)*. Angiogenic effects of TGFα may be due, in part, to its activation of AP-2, a transcription factor, to produce potent angiogenic factors such as interleukin (IL)-8 and vascular endothelial growth factor (VEGF) *(38)*. Furthermore, overexpression of EGFR and TGFα correlates with microvessel density, which is an independent prognostic factor in breast cancer *(39,40)*, lung cancer *(41,42)*, and prostate cancer *(43)*, etc. Although inhibition of EGFR alone or in combination with chemotherapy exerted only modest in vitro antitumor effects *(6)*, dramatic antitumor synergy was seen when EGFR inhibition was combined with chemotherapy or radiation in vivo *(7,44–48)*. This discrepancy in tumor response was explained, in part, by the anti-angiogenic properties of the EGFR antagonists *(44–48)*. Using a xenograft transitional cell bladder carcinoma mouse model, Perrotte et al. first showed that C225, a humanized monoclonal antibody against EGFR, inhibited in vivo tumor growth and metastasis by down-regulating VEGF, IL-8, and fibroblast growth factor (FGF), followed by induction of endothelial cell apoptosis and reduction of tumor microvessel density *(44)*. C225 in combination with radiation also dramatically improved the efficacy of radiation on local tumor control by a factor of 1.59 with a single dose of C225 and by a factor of 3.62 with three doses of C225, as compared with radiation alone *(45)*. Significant tumor necrosis and tumor vessel thrombosis were noted in tumors treated with C225 plus radiation compared with radiation alone *(45)*. Additional evidence of enhanced antitumor synergy through inhibition of tumor angiogenesis was provided through a xenograft pancreatic cancer mouse model using Lp26.1 pancreatic cell line exploring C225 *(46)* or protein kinase inhibitor (PKI)-166 *(47)* plus/minus gemcitabine. Induction of endothelial cell apoptosis was noted with either C225 or PKI-166 alone or with gemcitabine, but not placebo or gemcitabine alone *(46,47)*. Almost identical finding of endothelial apoptosis was seen with ZD1839, another EGFR-tyrosine kinase inhibitors (TKI), in a xenograft colon cancer model using the GEO cell line *(48)*.

EGFR overexpression is uniformly noted in a wide variety of human epithelial malignancies; however, a great deal of heterogeneity of EGFR exists even among malignancies derived from same organ site *(8)*. Head and neck cancer *(49,50)* and meningioma *(51)* are among the highest EGFR-expressing tumors, followed by cancers of the pancreas *(52,53)*, lung *(54–57)*, colon *(58,59)*, esophagus *(60)*, kidney *(61)*, and papillary thyroid gland *(62)*. Liver cancer is considered an EGFR-negative tumor *(63–65)*, while cancers of the breast *(66,67)*, ovary *(68–71)*, endometrium *(72–75)*, cervix *(76,77)*, prostate *(78,79)*, bladder *(80,81)*, biliary tract *(82)*, stomach *(83)*, and malignant gliomas *(84)* are considered low to moderate EGFR expressing tumors. The variations in EGFR overexpression across different tumor types or even within the same tumor specimens are largely due to the inherent biological heterogeneity in EGFR and its ligands, plus differences in tumor grade, histology types, study design and detection techniques, sample size, sources, and quality of tumor specimens *(8)*. EGFR overexpression is associated with poor patient prognosis, decreased overall survival, and increased tumor stage and metastasis in cancers of the head and neck *(49,50)*, pancreas *(52,53)*, lung *(54–57)*, colorectum *(58,59)*, esophagus *(60)*, papillary thyroid *(62)*, breast *(66,67)*, ovary *(68–70)*, and bladder *(80,81)* and malignant gliomas *(85)*. The association of EGFR overexpression with poor prognosis is controversial in cancers of the cervix and endometrium. In prostate cancer, an association of EGFR overexpression with hormonal refractory status was suggested only in one study *(78,79)*. No associations of EGFR overexpression with poor prognosis or decreased survival were shown in meningioma *(51)*, and in cancers of the kidney *(63)*, liver *(63–65)*, prostate *(78,79)*, thyroid follicular type *(83)*, and stomach *(84,86)*. However, studies continued to evolve in this arena, and a recent study showed that MAPK was strongly associated with EGFR activation in intestinal-type gastric cancer *(86)* (Table 1).

3. CLINICAL EVALUATION OF EGFR ANTAGONISTS

To develop potent EGFR antagonists, pharmaceutical companies had utilized two major methods, with the first one involving the use of humanized monoclonal antibody technology targeting the ligand-binding domain of the EGFR. C225 (Cetuximab™; Imclone, Somerville, NJ, USA) *(6,7)*, ABX-EGF (Abgenix, Fremont, CA, USA) *(88)*, and h-R3 (Center of Molecular Immunology, Havana, Cuba) *(89)* are monoclonal antibody-based EGFR antagonists. The second method utilizes sophisticated conventional drug design technology to develop small molecules that can inhibit the phosphorylation of EGFR through reversible competition with ATP, the substrate of the tyrosine kinase domain of the EGFR. ZD1839 (Iressa™; AstraZeneca), OSI-774 (Tarceva™; OSI Pharmaceuticals, previously also known as CP-358,774; Pfizer), CI-1033 (pan erb

Table 1
Percentage of EGFR Expression by Tumor Site and Its Prognostic Significance

Tumor organ sites	% of Tumor EGFR (+)	Overall prognosis	Overall survival (OS)	Tumor stage and metastasis	References
Colorectal	25–77	Poor	Decreased	Increased	58,59
Esophageal	35–88	Poor	Decreased	Increased	8,60
Gastric	8–40	—	—	—	85,86
Pancreas	43–80	Poor	Decreased	Increased	52,53
Hepatocellular	0–10	—	—	—	63–65
Biliary tract	67–86	NA	NA	NA	82
Head and neck	85–100	Poor	Decreased	Increased	49,50
Lung	40–80	Poor	Decreased	Increased	54–57
Breast	14–91	Poor	Decreased	Increased	66,67
Endometrial	56	?	?	?	72,75
Cervical	20–74	—	No	—	76,77
Ovarian	12–70	Poor	Decreased	Increased	68,70
Prostate	65	—	No	?	78,79
Renal	50–90	—	No	—	62
Bladder	40–86	Poor	Decreased	Increased	80,81
Meningioma	68–100	—	No	—	51
Malignant gliomas	10–50	Poor	Decreased	Increased	87
Thyroid: papillary	78	Poor	Decreased	Increased	62
Thyroid: follicular	33	NA	NA	NA	83

NA, not available; —, no impact; ?, controversial results.

TKI; Pfizer), and PKI166 (Norvartis, Basel, Switzerland) are quinazoline class compounds that act as reversible EGFR-TKIs active against a variety of EGFR-positive tumor cell lines in vitro and in xenograft tumor models either alone *(90-91)* or with chemotherapy such as cisplatin *(92)* and irinotecan *(93)*. C225, ZD1839, and OSI-774 are leading the development and have entered phase III clinical trials. The active EGFR antagonists have a narrow IC50 ranging from 0.2 to 2 nM explaining why these agents have similar target potencies in vitro and in vivo (Table 2). Second generation irreversible EGFR-TKIs are being developed using high-throughput drug development technology *(94,95)*.

3.1. C225

Baselga et al. reported a phase I multicenter safety study of C225 given as a single intravenous dose, weekly for 4 wk, and weekly with intravenous cisplatin in 53 patients with refractory cancer *(96)*. The most frequent side effects of C225 were grade 1 and 2 skin rash, nausea, asthenia, flu-like syndromes, and transient liver transaminase elevations. Seven skin toxicities were relatively uncommon, including four cases of skin flushing, one case of seborrheic dermatitis, and one case of acneiform eruptions. Grade 3 or 4 toxicities were extremely rare at 1.6% (5 of 317 treatment courses) and included one case each for aseptic meningitis, diarrhea, epiglottis, dyspnea, and anaphylactoid reactions, respectively. Three of these five serious reactions occurred when C225 was combined with intravenous cisplatin *(96)*. Weekly C225 showed nonlinear pharmacokinetics in the dose range of 200–400 mg/m^2, associated with complete saturation of the sys-

Table 2
EGFR Antagonists in Clinical Development

Drug no.	Trade name	Nature of compound	IC50	Clinical phase
C225	Cetuximab	Monoclonal Antibody	0.2 nM	Phase III
ZD1839	Iressa	Quinazoline-TKI	2 nM	Phase III
OSI-774	Tarceva	Quinazoline-TKI	2 nM	Phase III
PKI166	NA	Quinazoline-TKI	1.5 nM	Phase I
CI-1033	NA	Quinazoline-TKI	—	Phase I
ABX-EGF	NA	Monoclonal Antibody	0.5 nM	Phase I
H-R3	NA	Monoclonal antibody	—	Phase I

temic clearance *(96)*. C225 clearance did not change with the repeated administration or with the co-administration of the cisplatin *(96)*. Despite the fact that this was a phase I study, increased tumor stabilization rates were observed with a single dose of C225 (54%, 7 of 13 patients) and with repeated dosing (69%, 11 of 16 patients), with half of the latter 16 patients experiencing durable disease stabilization. Two patients with head and neck tumors treated at the dose level of 200 mg/m^2 and 400 mg/m^2 achieved partial responses. Overall, 69% of the patients treated with C225 at a dose greater than 50 mg/m^2 achieved stable disease and completed 12 wk, of therapy *(96)*. Mendelsohn, Shin and colleagues reported the results of a phase I pharmacodynamic study of C225 by assessing EGFR activation and receptor saturation via direct tumor sampling. No detectable EGFR activation was observed in patients treated with C225 at the 100 mg/m^2 dose level (100 mg/m^2 bolus followed by weekly doses of 100 mg/m^2). Greater than 70% EGFR saturation was observed with C225 given at 400 mg/m^2 bolus followed by weekly at 250 mg/m^2 *(97)*. Given these pharmacokinetic and pharmcodynamic findings, the optimal C225 schedule was felt to be 400 mg/m^2 loading followed by weekly doses of 250 mg/m^2 given intravenously.

Given the encouraging results observed in preclinical models with C225 *(45)*, a phase I clinical trial exploring C225 in combination with radiation in locally advanced squamous cell carcinoma of head and neck (SCCHN) was launched (N = 15 patients). In this trial, 13 of the 15 (87%) patients experienced durable complete remissions (CR) and compared favorably with the expected historical CR rates of 31–46% *(98)*. In another trial, Hong et al. selected patients with recurrent SCCHN with either progressive or stable disease to receive C225 plus cisplatin after receiving two cycles of cisplatin alone. The prior dose and schedule of cisplatin were maintained along with standard weekly C225 dosing. Only the results from patients with stable disease following cisplatin induction were reported and among 38 patients, 1(2%), 7(18%), and 22 (58%) achieved complete remission, partial response, and stable disease respectively *(99)*. Commonly observed adverse reactions related to C225 were again folliculitis/acne and allergic reaction.

With a similar study design, Saltz et al. *(100)* conducted a phase II trial exploring C225 plus irinotecan in patients with metastatic colorectal cancer who failed first-line irinotecan-based therapy. One hundred and twenty-one patients were enrolled into this study after meeting the entry criteria, which required the presence of measurable disease, documented disease progression with irinotecan, EGFR expression (approx 70% of the patients are EGFR positive), performance status, adequate organ function, and no intercurrent chemotherapy between irinotecan failure and protocol entry for at least 4 wk. Patients then received standard weekly C225 dosing plus the same prior irinotecan dose and schedule. The treatment was well tolerated with only modest grade 3 toxicities, including diarrhea (17%), nausea (9%), neutropenia (8%), acneiform rash (8%), fatigue (6%), and allergic reaction (3%). Grade 1 to 2 acneiform rash was very common and was seen in 53% of the patients. Of the 121 patients enrolled in the study, 27 patients (22.5%) achieved a partial response with 32 (26%) of the patients experiencing stable disease *(100)*.

Based on the findings with the pancreatic xenograft model *(46)*, Abbruzzese et al. conducted a phase II multicenter trial of C225 in combination with gemcitabine in patients with advanced pancreatic cancer. Eighty-nine percent of the tumor specimens screened, expressed EGFR(+), using an immunohistochemistry technique. Of the 41 patients enrolled in the study, 5 (12%) patients achieved partial response, and 16 (39%) patients had stable disease or a minor response. Median time to tumor progression (TTP) was 16 wk (with 12 patients ongoing at the time of the report), which compared favorably to the historical median TTP of 9 wk achieved with gemcitabine alone. The most reported adverse events were acneiform rash (38%), folliculitis (16%), fatigue (41%), and grade 1 and 2 fever (38%) *(101)*.

A preliminary study from a phase II single-agent C225 study in renal cell carcinoma was also completed with observation of stable disease in this highly chemotherapy refractory tumor *(102)*.

3.2. ZD1839

Three phase I pharmacokinetics and pharmacodynamic studies of ZD1839 (Iressa) established the maximal tolerated and biologically effective dose range of 500–800 mg/d taken orally continuously *(103–106)*. About 12.5% (2 of 16) and 15% (4 of 25) of patients with non-small cell lung cancer (NSCLC) experienced partial responses in these two phase I studies *(103,104)*. Escalating doses of ZD1839 from 50 to 700 mg with 4–8 patients per dose cohort were given orally for 14 d, followed by 14 d of observation. Dose-limiting toxicity (DLT) was observed at the 700 mg dose level with grade 3 diarrheas occuring in two patients *(103,104)*. The incidence of DLT such as diarrhea, liver function abnormality, and skin rash was increased at the 1000 mg/d level *(103,104)*. Similar to the characteristic skin rash of C225, the skin rashes were follicular and acneiform, involving predominantly the face and trunk, occuring in a majority of the treated patients. The skin rash was mild to moderate in severity and, more often, was self-limiting without requiring discontinuation of therapy and gradually abated over time with supportive treatment. Skin biopsies showed increased apoptosis of dermis associated with dermal edema and lymphocyte infiltration at all dose levels of ZD1839 *(105)*. Skin biopsies performed before and after ZD1839 demonstrated decreased activated MAPK (p < 0.001) and decreased proliferative marker (Ki67) (p = 0.008), with a concomitant increase in the cyclin-dependent kinase (CDK) inhibitor p27^{kipi} and cytokeratin K6, a keratinocyte maturation marker (p = 0.0003), and phosphorylated STAT3 (p = 0.001) *(105)*. Tumor biopsies performed in another phase I study before and after 28 d with ZD1839 showed that the tyrosine kinase activity of the EGFR was inhibited by ZD1839 and Ki67, and the percentage of apoptosis appeared to correlate with the clinical outcome *(106)*. The maximal tolerated dose (MTD) was not reached in this study, since the ZD1839 was not escalated beyond 800 mg/d *(106)*.

A two-part phase I study exploring the combination of ZD1839 with the Mayo clinic 5FU and leucovorin regimen was conducted in patients with advanced colorectal cancer. Promising activity in colorectal cancer was observed without significant PK interactions with 5FU *(107)*. Miller et al. *(107)* recently reported the results of the pilot study of ZD1839 (Iressa) in combination with carboplatin and paclitaxel in patients with previously untreated advanced NSCLC. The study was conducted with either intermittent or continuous ZD1839 with carboplatin at AUC 6.0 and paclitaxel at 200 mg/m^2 every 3 wk. Of the 25 patients in this study, a partial response rate of 28% and a stable disease response rate of 40% were observed and neither cumulative toxicity nor significant drug–drug PK interactions were noted in this phase I study *(108)*.

3.3. OSI-774

Siu et al. and Karp et al. reported two separate phase I studies on CP-358,774 (now known as OSI-774) given on daily and weekly schedules respectively *(109,110)*. Both studies showed that CP-358, 774 was very well tolerated, with acneiform skin rash and diarrhea as the major DLT similar to that of ZD1839 and C225. The daily dosing schedule at 150 mg/d achieved target serum levels of 500 ng/mL correlating with the drug level required for antitumor effects observed in the preclinical models *(109)*. Rowinsky et al. evaluated pre- and post-treatment (d 28) effects of OSI-774 on p27, phosphorylated EGFR, and downstream effectors such as AKT and extracellular signal-regulated kinase (ERK) in malignant and normal tissue (skin) of the cancer patients (n = 10). Paired analysis showed significant decrement of activated p-ERK (p = 0.01) and increment of p27 (p = 0.004). One patient with rapidly progressive disease had an 80% increment in phosphorylated EGFR and phosphorylated AKT and a 30% increment in phosphorylated Erk *(110,112)*.

Three phase II studies were completed in refractory SCCHN, NSCLC, and ovarian cancer, respectively, with OSI-774 given at 150 mg daily. Senzer et al. reported the final results of a phase II evaluation of OSI-774 in patients with platinum refractory advanced squamous cell carcinoma of the head and neck (n = 125), which included both EGFR-positive (>90% of cases) and EGFR-negative tumors. The final update revealed that 11 of 125 (9%) and 13 of 125 (18%) of patients achieved partial response and stable disease respectively *(113,114)*. In the phase II trial in patients (n = 57) with refractory (failed two to three prior regimens) EGFR positive NSCLC, 1 of 57 (1.7%), 8 of 57 (14%), and 15 of 57 (26%) of the OSI-774-treated patients achieved complete response, partial response, and stable disease, respectively, with suggestion of benefits in time to tumor progression and survival *(115,116)*. In patients with platinum-refractory ovarian cancer (n = 34), 4 of 34 (12%) and 14 of 34 (41%) of the treated patients achieved partial response and stable disease, respectively *(117)*. Again, overall incidence of acneiform skin rash caused by OSI-774 occurred in 72% of the patients with mild, moderate, to severe skin rash occurring in 28%, 34%, and 8% of the patients, respectively. Similar to the finding with C225 and ZD1839, skin biopsies of the skin rash area revealed inflammatory neutrophilic infiltrations under the dermis. The diarrhea generally responded to dose reduction or treatment with loperamide *(109–117)*.

3.4. CI-1033

Shin et al, recently reported the results of a phase I trial on CI-1033, a pan erbB TKI in patients with solid tumors *(118)*. Nine dose levels of CI-1033 from 50–560 mg/d

Table 3
Clinical Evaluation of Agents Targeting EGFR in Solid Tumors

Clinical phase	No. of patients	Treatments	Cancer types	% Response rate			References
				CR	PR	SD	
I	13	C225 single dose	Solid tumors	—	—	54	96
I	16	C225 repeat doses	Solid tumors	—	—	69	96
I	16	C225 plus CDDP	Solid tumors	—	12	69	96
I	15	C225 plus XRT	SCCHN	87	13	—	98
II	38	C225 plus Cisplatin	SCCHN	2	18	58	99
II	121	C225 plus Irinotecan	Refractory colon Cancer	—	16	39	100
II	19	C225 plus Gemcitabine	Pancreatic Cancer	—	23	26	101
I	16	ZD1839 dose escalation	Refractory NSCLC	—	12	—	103
I	25	ZD1839 dose escalation	Refractory NSCLC	—	15	—	104
I	23	ZD1839+5FU/LV	Colorectal Cancer	4	17	—	107
I	25	ZD1839+CP	NSCLC	—	28	40	108
I	40	CP-358,774 Single dose	Healthy volunteer	—	—	—	NA
I	69	CP-358,774 escalation	Solid tumors	—	—	—	109
II	125	OSI-774 150 mg/d	Refractory SCCHN	—	9	18	114
II	57	OSI-774 150 mg/d	Refractory NSCLC	1.7	14	26	116
II	34	OSI774	Refractory Ovarian Cancer	—	12	41	117
I	37	CI-1033	Solid tumors	NA	NA	NA	118

XRT, radiation therapy; CP, carboplatin and paclitaxel; CDDP, cisplatin; NA, not available.

continuously were tested in 37 patients with chemotherapy refractory malignancies, and the MTD of CI-1033 had not been reached. The most common grade 1 and 2 toxicities beginning at the 50 mg/d dose level included acneiform rash, emesis, and diarrhea, consistent with the toxicity encountered with other EGFR antagonists. Three patients experienced reversible grade 3 thrombocytopenia (1 each at 50, 70, and 250mg levels), and 1 patient experienced reversible grade 3 hypersensitivity at 560mg dose level. On d 8 through serial tumor biopsy, cellular proliferative index Ki-67 was consistently down-regulated, and p27, a cell cycle inhibitory protein, was up-regulated (118). Preliminary antitumor activity was observed in this phase I study (118). Garrison et al, (119) studied CI-1033 given weekly and escalated through 100, 200, 400, 500, and 560 mg dose levels in 34 patients with solid tumors. Reversible DLT occurred in 2 of 3 patients at the 560 mg dose level. Similar side effects, such as diarrhea, emesis, and skin rash, were noted in this phase I study (119). The results of these phase I and II studies from C225, ZD1839, OSI-774, and CI-1033 are summarized in Table 3.

4. FUTURE DIRECTIONS

The above work represents at least two decades of concerted laboratory and clinical effort in pursuit of EGFR as a cancer therapeutic target. This effort will likely add the EGFR antagonists to the rapidly growing list of molecular-targeted anticancer agents along with Herceptin, Rituximab, and Gleevec, approved for breast cancer

Table 4
Ongoing/Planned Pivotal Phase III Trials with EGFR Antagonists

	C225	ZD1839	OSI-774
SCCHN	XRT/C225 vs XRT CDDP/C225 vs CDDP	—	
NSCLC	CP/C225 vs CP	CP plus ZD1839 vs CP	CP plus OSI774 vs CP
Colon Cancer	planned	—	—
Pancreatic Cancer	Gemcitabine+C225 vs Gemcitabine	—	Gemcitabine+OSI774 vs Gemcitabine

CDDP, cisplatin; CP, carboplatin and paclitaxel; XRT, radiation; IFL, irinotecan; 5FU, leucovorin.

(120), Non-Hodgkin's lymphoma *(121),* and chronic myelogenous leukemia (CMI) *(122,123),* respectively.

Randomized phase III studies with C225 plus chemotherapy have been launched in locally advanced SCCHN and metastatic NSCLC, with studies planned for metastatic colorectal cancer and pancreatic cancer. Randomized phase III clinical trials have also been launched, respectively, with ZD1839 and OSI-774 in combination with chemotherapy vs chemotherapy in metastatic NSCLC, with plans to study other cancers as well (Table 4).

While these pivotal phase III randomized clinical studies are essential steps for drug development, it is imperative that we expand both basic research endeavors in EGFR and clinical research repertoires with these EGFR antagonists in cancer treatment, as well as in cancer prevention. It is also essential to design and conduct future "translational" studies of the EGFR antagonists, which integrate surrogate assays such as skin biopsy, tumor biopsy, and novel imaging, as these translational studies will ultimately serve as a two-way bridge for this widely recognized knowledge gap between the bench and clinic and will provide critical clues for novel combination treatment strategies.

We are transitioning from an era of cytotoxic chemotherapy to an era of rationally designed molecular-targeted cancer therapy, which holds great future promise, as identification and testing of the critical anticancer targets has led to the successful development of a number of molecular-targeted agents *(120–123)* and will likely add the EGFR antagonists and many others in the future. Unlike conventional cytotoxic therapy, the rationally designed molecular-targeted therapies enjoy the therapeutic advantage of targeting the tumor cells, while potentially sparing nontarget normal tissues based on the difference in target expression between normal tissue and tumor. Molecular-targeted therapy not only enables clinicians to design surrogate clinical endpoints based on tumor targets *(97,111,112),* but also potentially permits profiling the tumor for the appropriate target(s), thereby facilitating highly individualized cancer therapy.

To fulfill the great promise of molecular-targeted cancer therapies, many important questions pertaining to the clinical development of the EGFR antagonists remain and are also applicable to the whole class of molecular-targeted agents: What are the molecular mechanisms of synergy when an EGFR antagonist is combined with chemotherapy or radiotherapy? What would be the best way to combine the EGFR antagonist with standard chemotherapy or radiation—concurrent (most commonly used design), intermittent, or sequential? What are the effects of EGFR antagonist on tumor angiogenesis in patients, and how to best assess in vivo angiogenesis in patients? What are the impacts of EGFR antagonist on minimal residue disease or in the adjuvant setting with or without chemotherapy? Most importantly, could we gradually phase out the chemotherapy backbone in the treatment of cancer through the combination with other molecular-targeted agents? Evidence of such combination-targeted therapy is beginning to emerge in animal models when EGFR antagonist (either Iressa or C225) are combined with interferon (IFN)α *(124)*, Herceptin *(125)*, and inhibitor of VEGFR *(126)*. This strategy may potentially further narrow the spectrum of systemic toxicity without compromising overall antitumor efficacy. Cancer chemoprevention trials are also adopting similar strategies of combining EGFR antagonist with molecular-targeted agents such as Cox-2 inhibitors *(127)*.

Given the heightened optimism surrounding molecular-targeted therapy, it is also appropriate to acknowledge the limitations and many potential hurdles that molecular-targeted therapy must overcome as redundancies of targets, signaling cross-talk, and genomic instabilities that exist in practically all solid tumors and in leukemias. For example, Gleevec is not as effective in CML-blast crisis as in early stage CML. This is due at least in part, to the genomic instability and bcr-abl oncogene amplifications in CML blast crisis *(122,123)*. It should be emphasized that molecular-targeted therapy can also produce unique toxicity, as opposed to the typical toxicity profile of cytotoxic agents. In some cases, this is due the expression of target within the normal tissues.

Albeit rarely requiring stopping therapy, the commonly observed skin rash associated with EGFR antagonists can be quite distressing to a small number of patients, and the management of this toxic effect may be further complicated by the concurrent use of chemotherapy, such as cisplatin and gemcitabine *(96,101)*. Even though it is feasible to predict side effects based upon the target distribution (EGFR is expressed in the skin and gut) and the target agent specificity, all clinical investigations of novel agents, either alone or in combination, should draw from the lessons learned from the unexpected 19% congestive heart failure rate associated with the use of Herceptin plus doxorubicin in the treatment of metastatic breast cancer *(120)*.

To validate the target response, clinical evaluations of molecular-targeted therapy are increasingly relying on the development of surrogate markers through direct target tissue sampling and functional imaging techniques *(128)*. Functional and molecular imaging techniques have added a new dimension to the conventional radiographic images based on anatomic evaluation of tumor size in patients. Regardless of the technologies used to assess tumor response, overall survival still remains the irreplaceable " gold standard endpoint" determined through phase III randomized clinical trials to receive drug registration and approval. Clinical response, TTP, and surrogate marker response should continue to serve as useful clinical endpoints in phase I and II clinical studies.

We have entered an era of a rationally designed molecular-targeted therapy. Recent successful treatment of gastro intestinal stromal tumors (GIST) by Gleevec, a specific TKI that targets c-kit, which is a critical oncogene in GIST, provides greater optimism and impetus for molecular-targeted therapy *(129,130)*. cDNA microarray *(131)* and proteinomics chips *(132,133)* will be increasingly used to identify and analyze the critical potential candidate anticancer targets among thousands of genes and proteins of the complex cellular signaling networks *(134,135)*. Despite these technological advances, many challenges lie ahead. However, highly individualized molecular-targeted therapy will continue to evolve to benefit an increasing number of our cancer patients.

ACKNOWLEDGMENT

The authors would like to thank Elaine White for her expert assistance in editing the manuscript and Jennette Craig for her assistance in manuscript preparation.

REFERENCES

1. Varmus H. A historical overview of oncogenes. In: Weinberg RA, ed. *Oncogenes and the Molecular Origin of Cancer.* CSH Laboratory Press, Cold Spring Harbor, NY, 1989; pp. 3–44.
2. Krontiris TG. Oncogenes. *N Eng J Med* 1995; 333:303–306.
3. Weinberg RA. Tumor suppressor genes. *Science* 1991; 254:1138–1142.
4. Fearon ER, Vogelstein B. A genetic model for colorectal tumorigenesis. *Cell* 1990; 61:759–764.
5. Hanahan D, Weinberg RA. The hallmarks of cancer. *Cell* 2000; 100:57–70.
6. Mendelsohn J. Epidermal growth factor receptor inhibition by a monoclonal antibody as anticancer therapy. *Clin Cancer Res* 1997; 3:2703–2707.
7. Mendelsohn J. Blockade of epidermal growth factor receptor: an anticancer therapy—The Fourth Annual Joseph Burchenal American Association of Cancer Research Clinical Research Award Lecture. *Clin Cancer Res* 2000; 6:747–753.
8. Salomon DS, Brandt R, Ciardiello F, Normannon N. Epidermal growth factor-related peptides and their receptors in human malignancies. *Crit Rev Oncol Hematol* 1995; 19:183–232.
9. Wells A. EGF receptor. *Int J Biochem Cell Biol* 1999; 31:637–643.
10. Klambt C. EGF receptor signaling: the importance of presentation. *Curr Biol* 2000; 10:388–391.
11. Moghal N, Sternberg PW. Multiple positive and negative regulators of signaling by the EGF-receptor. *Curr Opin Cell Biol* 1999; 11:190–196.
12. Daly RJ. Take your partners please—signal diversification by the erbB family of receptor tyrosine kinases. *Growth Factors* 1999; 16:255–263.
13. Carpenter G.Employment of the epidermal growth factor receptor in growth factor-independent signaling pathways. *J Cell Biol* 1999; 146:697–702.
14. Hackel PO, Zwick E, Prenzel N, et al. Epidermal growth factor receptor: critical mediators of multiple receptor pathways. *Curr Opin Cell Biol* 1999; 11:184–189.
15. Reddy CC, Wells A, Lauffenburger DA. Differential EGFR trafficking influences relative mitogenic potencies of epidermal growth factor and transforming growth factor α. *J Cell Physiol* 1996; 166:512–522.
16. Rowinsky EK, Windle JJ, Von Hoff DD. Ras protein farnesyltransferase: a strategic target for anticancer therapeutic development. *J Clin Oncol* 1999; 17:3631–3652.
17. Zhou S, Kinzler KW, Vogelstein B. Going mad with SMADS. *N Engl J Med* 1999; 341–1144.
18. Kulik G, Klippel A, Weber MJ. Antiapoptotic signaling by IGF like I receptor, Pl3K and Akt. *Mol Cell Biol* 1997; 17:1595–1606.
19. Wu X, Fan Z, Hasui H, et al. Apoptosis induced by an anti-epidermal growth factor receptor monoclonal antibody in a human colorectal carcinoma cell line and its delay by insulin. *J Clin Invest* 1995; 95:1897–1905.
20. Thomas CY, Stallings-Mann M, Wharen R. Mutation of the PTEN tumor suppressor gene contributes to deregulation of the AKT pathway and activation of overexpressed epidermal growth factor receptors (EGFR) in glioblastoma (GBM). *Proc Am Soc Clin Oncol* 2000; 19:9(abstr 2562).
21. Liu B, Fang M, Schmidt M, et al. Induction of apoptosis and activation of the caspase cascade by anti-EGF receptor monoclonal antibody in DiFi human colon cancer cells do not involve the c-jun N-terminal kinase activity. *Br J Cancer* 2000; 82:1991–1999.
22. Karnes WE Jr, Weller SG, Adjei RN, et al. Inhibition of epidermal growth factor receptor tyrosine kinase induces protease dependent apoptosis in human colon cancer cells. *Gastroenterology* 1998; 114:930–993.
23. Wu X, Rubin M, Fan Z, et al. Involvement of p27kipi in G1 arrest mediated by an anti-epidermal growth factor receptor monoclonal antibody. *Oncogene* 1996; 12:1397–1403.

24. Fan Z, Shang BY, Lu Y, et al. Reciprocal changes in p27(Kip1) and p21(Cip1) in growth inhibition mediated by blockade or overstimulation of epidermal growth factor receptors. *Clin Cancer Res* 1997; 3:1943–1948.

25. Chen P, Gupta K, Wells A. Cell movement elicited by EGFR requires kinase and autophosphorylation but is separable from mitogenesis. *J Cell Biol* 1994; 124:547–555.

26. Xie H, Turner T, Wang MH, et al. In vitro invasiveness of the DU145 human prostate carcinoma is modulated by EGFR mediated signals. *Clin Exp Metastasis* 1995; 13:407–419.

27. Giehl K, Skripezynski B, Mansard A, et al. Growth factor-dependent activation of the Ras-raf-MEK-MAPK pathway in the human pancreatic carcinoma cell line PANC-1 carrying activated K-ras: implications for cell proliferation and cell migration. *Oncogene* 2000; 19:2930–2942.

28. Turner T, Che P, Goodly L, Wells A. EGFR signaling enhances in vivo invasiveness of the DU145 human prostate carcinoma cells. *Clin Exp Metastasis* 1997; 14:409–418.

29. Price JT, Wilson HM, Haites NE. Epidermal growth factor increase the in vitro invasion and motility and adhesion interactions of the primary renal cell carcinoma line A704. *Eur J Cancer* 1996; 32A:1977–1982.

30. Shibata T, Kwano T, Nagyasu H, et al. Enhancing effects of epidermal growth factor on human squamous cell carcinoma motility and matrix degradation but not growth. *Tumor Biol* 1996; 17:168–175.

31. Konapaka SB, Fridman R, Reddy KB. Epidermal growth factor and amphiregulatin upregulate matrix metalloprotease-9 in human breast cancer cells. *Int J Cancer* 1997; 70:722–726.

32. Watabe T, Yoshida K, Shindoh M, et al. Ets1 and Ets2 transcription factors activate and promote tumor invasion associated urokinase and collagenase genes in response to epidermal growth factor. *Int J Cancer* 1998; 77:128–137.

33. Folkman J, Klagburn M. Angiogenic factors. *Science* 1987; 235:442–447.

34. Fidler IJ. Molecular biology of cancer: invasion and metastasis. In: De Vita JR, Hellman S, Rosenberg SA, eds. *Cancer Principles and Practice of Oncology (ed5)*. Lippincott, Philadelphia, 1997, pp. 135–152.

35. Folkman J. Angiogenesis in cancer, vascular, rheumatoid and other diseases. *Nat Med* 1995; 1:27–31.

36. Scheriber AB, Winkler ME, Derynck R. Transforming growth factor-alpha: a more potent angiogenic mediator than epidermal growth factor. *Science* 1986; 232:1250–1253.

37. Russell KS, Stern DF, Polverini PJ, Bender JR. Neuregulin activation of ErbB receptors in vascular endothelium leads to angiogenesis. *Am J Physiol* 1999; 277:H2205–H2211.

38. Gille J, Swerlick RA, Caughman SW. Transforming growth factor alpha induced transcriptional activation of the vascular permeability factor (VPF/VEGF) gene requires AP-2 dependent DNA binding and transactivation. *EMBO J* 1997; 16:75–79.

39. Del Jong JS, van Diest PJ, van der Valk P, Baak JP. Expression of growth factors, growth inhibiting factors and their receptors in invasive breast cancer. II. Correlations with proliferation of and angiogenesis. *J Pathol* 2000; 184:53–57.

40. Smith K, Fox SB, Whitehouse R, et al. Upregulation of basic fibroblast growth factor in breast carcinoma and its relationship to vascular density, oestrogen receptor, epidermal growth factor receptor and survival. *Ann Oncol* 1999; 10:707–713.

41. Pastorino U, Andreola S, Tagliabue E, et al. Immunocytochemical markers in stage I lung cancer: relevance to prognosis. *J Clin Oncol* 1999; 15:2858–2865.

42. Giatromanolaki A, Koukourakis MI, Kakolyris S, et al. Vascular endothelial growth factor, wild-type p53, and angiogenesis in early operable non-small cell lung cancer. *Clin Cancer Res* 1998; 4:3017–3024.

43. Strohmeyer D, Rossing C, Strauss F, et al. Tumor angiogenesis is associated with progression after radical prostatectomy in pT2 and pT3 prostate cancer. *Prostate* 2000; 42:26–33.

44. Perrotte P, Matsumoto T, Inoue K, et al. Anti-epidermal growth factor receptor antibody C225 inhibits angiogenesis in human transitional cell carcinoma growing orthotopically in nude mice. *Clin Cancer Res* 1999; 5:257–265.

45. Milas L, Mason K, Hunter N, et al. In vivo enhancement of tumor radioresponse by C225 antiepidermal growth factor receptor antibody. *Clin Cancer Res* 2000; 6:701–708.

46. Bruns CJ, Harbison MT, Davis DW, et al. Epidermal growth factor receptor blockade with C225 plus gemcitabine results in regression of human pancreatic carcinoma growing orthotopically in nude mice by antiangiogenic mechanisms. *Clin Cancer Res* 2000; 6:1936–1948.

47. Bruns CJ, Solorzano CC, Harbison MT, et al. Blockade of the epidermal growth factor receptor signaling by a novel tyrosine kinase inhibitor leads to apoptosis of endothelial cells and therapy of human pancreatic carcinoma. *Cancer Res* 2000; 60:2926–2935.

48. Ciardiello F, Captuto R, Pomatoico G, et al. Inhibition of growth factor production and angiogenesis in human cancer cell lines by ZD1839 (Iressa™), an EGFR selective tyrosine kinase inhibitor. *Clin Cancer Res* 2000; 6:4542 (abstr 376).

49. Grandis JR, Melhem MF, Gooding WE, et al. Levels of TGF-alpha and EGFR protein in head and neck squamous cell carcinoma and patient survival. *J Natl Cancer Inst* 1998; 90:824–832.

50. Maurizi M, Almadori G, Ferrandina G, et al. Prognostic significance of epidermal growth factor receptor in laryngeal squamous cell carcinoma. *Br J Cancer* 1996; 74:1253–1257.

51. Torp SH, Helseth E, Dalen A, et al. Expression of epidermal growth factor receptor in human meningiomas and meningeal tissue. *Am Path Sur* 1992; 100:797–802.

52. Dong M, Nio Y, Gui KJ, et al. Epidermal growth factor and its receptor as prognostic indicators in Chinese patients with pancreatic cancer. *Anticancer Res* 1998; 18:4613–4619.

53. Yamanaka Y, Friess H, Kobrin MS, et al. Coexpression of epidermal growth factor receptor and ligands in human pancreatic cancer is associated with enhanced tumor aggressiveness. *Anticancer Res* 1993; 13:565–569.

54. Volm M, Rittgen W, Drings P. Prognostic value of ERBB-1, VEGF, cyclin A, FOS, JUN and MYC in patients with squamous cell lung carcinomas. *Br J Cancer* 1998; 77:663–669.

55. Veale D, Kerr N, Givson GJ, et al. The relationship of quantitative epidermal growth factor receptor expression in non-small cell lung cancer to long-term survival. *Br J Cancer* 1993; 68:162–165.

56. Ohsaki Y, Tanno S, Fujita Y, et al. Epidermal growth factor receptor expression correlates with poor prognosis in non-small cell lung cancer patients with p53 overexpression. *Oncol Rep* 2000; 7:603–607.

57. Pavelic K, Banjac Z, Pavelic J, et al. Evidence for a role of EGF receptor in the progression of human lung carcinoma. *Anticancer Res* 1993; 13:1133–1137.

58. Mayer A, Takimoto M, Fritz E, et al. The prognostic significance of proliferating cell nuclear antigen, epidermal growth factor receptor, and mdr gene expression in colorectal cancer. *Cancer* 1993; 71:2454–2460.

59. Hemming AW, Davis NL, Kluftinger A, et al. Prognostic markers of colorectal cancer: an evaluation of DNA content, epidermal growth factor receptor, and Ki-67. *J Surg Oncol* 1992; 51:147–152.

60. Iihara K, Shiozaki H, Tahara E, et al. Prognostic significance of transforming growth factor-alpha in human esophageal carcinoma. *Cancer* 1993; 171:2902–2909.

61. Hofmockel G, Riess S, Bassukas ID, et al. Epidermal growth factor family and renal cell carcinoma: expression and prognostic impact. *Eur Urol* 1997; 31:478–484.

62. Haugen DRF, Akslen LA, Varhaug JE, et al. Prognostic impact of EGFR in papillary thyroid carcinoma. *Br J Cancer* 1993; 68:808–812.

63. Harada K, Shiota G, Kawasaki H. Transforming growth factor-alpha and epidermal growth factor receptor in chronic liver disease and hepatocellular carcinoma. *Liver* 1999; 19:318–325.

64. Kiss A, Wang NJ, Xie JP, et al. Analysis of transforming growth factor (TGF)-alpha/epidermal growth factor receptor, hepatocyte growth factor/c-met, TGF-beta receptor type II, and p53 expression in human hepatocellular carcinomas. *Clin Cancer Res* 1997; 3:1059–1066.

65. Hamazaki K, Yunoki Y, Tagashira H, et al. Epidermal growth factor receptor in human hepatocellular carcinoma. *Cancer Detect Prev* 1997; 21:355–360.

66. Sainsbury JR, Malcolm AJ, Appleton DR, et al. Presence of epidermal growth factor receptor as an indicator of poor prognosis in patients with breast cancer. *J Clin Pathol* 1985; 38:1225–1228.

67. Gullick WJ. The role of the epidermal growth factor receptor and the c-erbB-2 protein in breast cancer. *Int J Cancer Suppl* 1990; 5:55–61.

68. Bartlett JM, Langdon SP, Simpson BJ, et al. The prognostic value of epidermal growth factor receptor mRNA expression in primary ovarian cancer. *Br J Cancer* 1996; 73:301–306.

69. Scambia G, Benedetti-Panici P, Ferrandina G, et al. Epidermal growth factor, oestrogen and progesterone receptor expression in primary ovarian cancer: correlation with clinical outcome and response to chemotherapy. *Br J Cancer* 1995; 72:361–366.

70. van Dam PA, Vergote IB, Lowe DG, et al. Expression of c-erbB-2, c-myc, and c-ras oncoproteins, insulin-like growth factor receptor I and epidermal growth factor receptor in ovarian carcinoma. *J Clin Pathol* 1994; 47:914–919.

71. Berchuck A, Rodriguez GC, Kamel A, et al. Epidermal growth factor receptor expression in normal ovarian epithelium and ovarian cancer. I. Correlation of receptor expression with prognostic factors in patients with ovarian cancer. *Am J Obstet Gynecol* 1991; 164:669–674.

72. Nagai N, Oshita T, Fujii T, et al. Prospective analysis of DNA ploidy, proliferative index and epidermal growth factor receptor as prognostic factors for pretreated uterine cancer. *Oncol Reports* 2000; 7:551–559.

73. Khalifa MA, Abdoh AA, Mannel RS, et al. Prognostic utility of epidermal growth factor receptor overexpression in endometrial adenocarcinoma. *Cancer* 1994; 73:370–376.

74. Reinartz JJ, George E, Lindgren BR, et al. Expression of p53, transforming growth factor alpha, epidermal growth factor receptor, and c-erbB-2 in endometrial carcinoma and correlation with survival and known predictors of survival. *Hum Pathol* 1994; 25:1075–1083.

75. Nagai N, Oshita T, Fujii T, et al. Prospective analysis of DNA ploidy, proliferative index and epidermal growth factor receptor as prognostic factors for pretreated uterine cancer. *Oncol Reports* 2000; 7:551–559.

76. Skomedal H, Kristensen GB, Lie AK, et al. Aberrant expression of the cell cycle associated proteins TP53, MDM2, p21, p27, cdk4, cyclin D1, RB, and EGFR in cervical carcinomas. *Gynecol Oncol* 1999; 73:223–228.

77. Scambia G, Ferrandina G, Distefano M, et al. Epidermal growth factor receptor (EGFR) is not related to the prognosis of cervical cancer. *Cancer Lett* 1998; 123:135–139.

78. Mellon K, Thompson S, Charlton RG, et al. p53, c-erbB-2 and the epidermal growth factor receptor in the benign and malignant prostate. *J Urol* 1992; 147:496–499.

79. Visakorpi T, Kallioniemi OP, Koivula T, et al. Expression of epidermal growth factor receptor and ERBB2 (HER-2/Neu) oncoprotein in prostate carcinomas. *Mod Pathol* 1992; 5:643–648.

80. Neal DE, Marsh C, Bennett MK, et al. Epidermal-growth-factor receptors in human bladder cancer: comparison of invasive and superficial tumors. *Lancet* 1985; 1:366–368.

81. Ravery V, Colombel M, Popov Z, et al. Prognostic value of epidermal growth factor-receptor, T138 and T43 expression in bladder cancer. *Br J Cancer* 1995; 71:196–200.

82. Lee CS, Pirdas A. Epidermal growth factor receptor immunoreactivity in gallbladder and extrahepatic biliary tract tumors. *Pathol Res Pract* 1995; 191:1087–1091.

83. Lemoine NR, Hughes CM, Gullick, et al. Abnormalities of the EGFR system in human thyroid neoplasia. *Int J Cancer* 1991; 49:558–561.

84. Lemonine NR, Jain S, Silvestre F, et al. Expression of epidermal growth factor receptor and c-erbB2 proto-oncogenes in human stomach cancer. *Br J Cancer* 1991; 64:79–83.

85. Yasui W, Sumiyoshi H, Hata J, et al. Expression of epidermal growth factor receptor in human gastric and colonic carcinomas. *Cancer Res* 1988; 48:137–141.

86. Rojo F, Albanell J, Sauleda S, et al. Characterization of epidermal growth factor receptor and transforming growth factor alpha expression in gastric cancer and its association with activation of mitogen activated protein kinases. *Proc Am Soc Clin Oncol* 2001; 20:430a (abstr 1717).

87. Fuller GN, Bigner SH. Amplified cellular oncogenes in neoplasms of the human central nervous system. *Mutat Res* 1992; 276:299–306.

88. Figlin RA, Belldegrun A, and Lohner E, et al. ABX-EGF: a fully human anti EGF receptor antibody in patients with advanced cancer. *Proc Am Soc Clin Oncol* 2001; 20:276a (abstr 1102).

89. Crombet-Ramos T, Torres L, Solano ME, et al. Pharmacological and clinical evaluation of the humanized anti-EGFR monoclonal antibody h-R3, in patients with advanced epithelial carcinomas. *Proc Am Soc Clin Oncol* 2001; 20:85a (abstr 1012).

90. Moulder SL, Yakes M, Bianco R, et al. Small molecule EGF receptor tyrosine kinase inhibitor ZD1839 (Iressa) inhibits Her2/Neu (erb-2) overexpressing breast tumor cells. *Proc Am Soc Clin Oncol* 2001; 20:3a (abstr 8).

91. Heimberger AB, Archer GE, McLendon RE, et al. Oral administration of specific EGFR TKI (ZD1839 Iressa TM), is active against EGFR-overexpressing intracranial tumors. *Clin Cancer Res* 2000; 6:4542 (abstr 379).

92. Al Hazaa A, Birchall MA, Bowen ID, et al. ZD1839 (Iressa TM), an EGFR-TKI, and cisplatin have an additive effect on programmed cell death, in human head and neck carcinoma cell *in vitro*. *Clin Cancer Res* 2000; 6:4542 (abstr 377).

93. Houghton PJ, Cheshire PJ, Harwood FC, et al. Evaluation of ZD 1839 (Iressa TM) alone and in combination with irinotecan (CPT11) against pediatric solid tumor xenografts. *Clin Cancer Res* 2000; 6:4542 (abstr 379).

94. Fry DW. Site-directed irreversible inhibitors of the erbB family of receptor tyrosine kinases as novel chemotherapeutic agents for cancer. *Anticancer Drug Des* 2000; 15:3–16.

95. Blaudschun R, Brenneisen P, Wlaschek M, et al. The rationale and strategy used to develop a series of highly potent, irreversible, inhibitors of the epidermal growth factor receptor family of tyrosine kinases. *Curr Med Chem* 1999; 6:825–843.

96. Baselga J, Pfister D, Cooper MR, et al. Phase I studies of anti-epidermal growth factor receptor chimeric antibody C225 alone and in combination with cisplatin. *J Clin Oncol* 2000; 18:904–914.

97. Mendelsohn J, Shin DM, Donato N, et al. A phase I study of chimerized anti-epidermal growth factor receptor (EGFr) monoclonal antibody, C225 in combination with cisplatin in patients with recurrent head and neck squamous cell carcinoma. *Proc Am Soc Clin Oncol* 2000; 18:389a (abstr 1502).

98. Boner JA, Ezekeil MP, Robert F, et al. Continued response following treatment with IMC-C225, an EGFr MoAb, combined with RT in advanced head and neck malignancies. *Proc Am Soc Clin Oncol* 2000; 18:388a (abstr 5F).

99. Hong WK, Arquette M, Nabell L, et al. Efficacy and safety of the antiepidermal growth factor antibody (EGFR) IMC-225, in combination with cisplatin in patients with recurrent squamous cell carcinoma of the head and neck (SCCHN) refractory to cisplatin containing chemotherapy. *Proc Am Soc Clin Oncol* 2001; 20:224a (abstr 895).

100. Saltz L, Rubin M, Hochster H, et al. Cetuximab (IMC-225) plus irinotecan (CPT11) is active in CPT11-refractory colorectal cancer (CRC) that express epidermal growth factor receptor (EGFR). *Proc Am Soc Clin Oncol* 2001; 20:3a (abstr 7).

101. Abbruzzese JL, Rosenberg A, Xiong Q, et al. Phase II study of antiepidermal growth factor receptor (EGFR) antibody cetuximab (C225) in combination with gemcitabine in patients with advanced pancreatic cancer. *Proc Am Soc Clin Oncol* 2001; 20:130a (abstr 518).

102. Gunnett K, Motzer R, Amato R, et al. Phase II study of antiepidermal growth factor receptor (EGFr) antibody C225 alone in patients with metastatic renal cell carcinoma. (RCC). *Proc Am Soc Clin Oncol* 2000; 18:341a (abstr 1309).

103. Hammond L, Ranso M, Ferry D, et al. ZD1839, an oral epidermal growth factor receptor (EGFr) tyrosine kinase inhibitor: first phase I pharmacokinetic (PK) results in patients. *Proc Am Soc Clin Oncol* 2000; 18:388 (abstr 1500).

104. Baselga J, Herbst R, LoRusso P, et al. Continuous administration of ZD1839 (Iressa), a novel oral epidermal growth factor receptor tyrosine kinase inhibitor (EGFR-TKI), in patients with five selected tumor types: evidence of activity and good tolerability. *Proc Am Soc Clin Oncol* 2000; 18:389 (abstr 686).

105. Albanell J, Rojo F, Cervant H, et al. Pharmacodynamic effects of Iressa, an oral epidermal growth factor tyrosine kinase inhibitor in skin biopsies from cancer patients participating in a phase I trials. *Clin Cancer Res Suppl* 2000; 6:4543 (abstr 383).

106. Goss GF, Hirte H, Lorimer I, et al. Final results of the dose escalation phase of a phase I pharmacokinetics (PK), pharmacodynamic (PD) and biologic activity study of ZD 1839: NCIC CTG IND. 122 *Proc Am Soc Clin Oncol* 2001; 20:85a (abstr 335).

107. Miller VA, Johnson D, Heelan RT, et al. A pilot trial demonstrates the safety of ZD1839 (Iressa), an oral epidermal growth factor receptor tyrosine kinase inhibitor (EGFR-TKI), in combination with carboplatin (c) and paclitaxel (P) in previously untreated advanced nonsmall cell lung cancer (NSCLCA). *Proc Am Soc Clin Oncol* 2001; 20:85a (abstr 1301).

108. Hammond LA, Figueroa J, Schwartzberg L, et al. Feasibility and pharmacokinetic (PK) trial of ZD1839 (IressaTM), an epidermal growth factor receptor tyrosine kinase inhibitor (EGFR-TKI), in combination with 5 fluorouracil (5FU) and leucovorin (LV) in patients with advanced colorectal cancer. *Proc Am Soc Clin Oncol* 2001; 20:137a (abstr 554).

109. Siu LL, Soulieres D, Senzer N, et al. Dose and schedule escalation of epidermal growth factor receptor (EGFR) tyrosine kinase inhibitor (TK), CP-358,774. A phase I study. *Proc Am Soc Clin Oncol* 2000; 18:388a (abstr 1498).

110. Karp DD, Silberman SL, Csudae R, et al. Phase I dose escalation study of epidermal growth factor receptor (EGFR) tyrosine kinase (TK) inhibitor CP358, 774 in patients with advanced solid tumors. *Proc Am Soc Clin Oncol* 1999; 18:388a (abstr 1499).

111. Rowinsky EK, Hammond L, Siu L, et al. Dose schedule finding, pharmacokinetic (PK), biologic, and functional imaging studies of OSI-774, a selective epidermal growth factor receptor (EGFR) tyrosine kinase inhibitor. *Proc Am Soc Clin Oncol* 2001; 20:2a (abstr 5).

112. Hidalgo M, Liu LL, Neumunaitis J, et al. A phase I and pharmacologic study of OSI-774, an epidermal growth factor receptor-tyrosine kinase inhibitor in patients with advanced solid malignancies. *J Clin Oncol* 2001; 19:3267–3279.

113. Siu LL, Soulieres D, Senzer N, et al. A Phase II trial of the epidermal growth factor receptor (EGFR) tyrosine kinase inhibitor (TK), CP-358,774, following plastinum-based chemotherapy in patients with head and neck (SCCHN). *Clin Cancer Res Suppl* 2000; 6:4544 (abstr 387).

114. Senzer NN, Soulieres D, Siu L, et al. Phase II evaluation of OSI-774, a potent oral antagonist of the EGFR-TK in patients with advanced squamous cell carcinoma of the head and neck. *Proc Am Soc Clin Oncol* 2001; 20:3a (abstr 6).

115. Bonomi P, Perez-Soler R, Chachoua A, et al. A Phase II trial of the epidermal growth factor receptor (EGFR) tyrosine kinase inhibitor (TK), CP-358,774, following platinum-based chemotherapy in patients with advanced non-small cell lung cancer (NSCLC). *Clin Cancer Res Suppl* 2000; 6:4544 (abstr 386).

116. Perez-Soler R, Chachousa A, Huberman M, et al. A phase II trial of the epidermal growth factor receptor (EGFR) tyrosine kinase inhibitor OSI-774, following platinum based chemotherapy, in patients with advanced EGFR- expressing, non small cell lung cancer (NSCLCA). *Proc Am Soc Clin Onco* 2001; 20:310a (abstr 1325).

117. Finkler N, Gordon A, Crazier M, et al. Phase 2 evaluation of OSI-774, a potent oral antagonist of the EGFR-TK in patients with advanced ovarian carcinoma. *Proc Am Soc Clin Oncol* 2001; 20:208a (abstr 831).

118. Shin DM, Nemunaitis J, Zinner, et al. A phase I clinical biomarker study of CI-1033, a novel pan-erbB tyrosine kinase inhibitor in patients with solid tumors. *Proc Am Soc Clin Oncol* 2001; 20:82a (abstr 324).

119. Garrison MA, Tolcher A, McCreenry H, et al. A phase I and pharmacokinetic study of CI-1033, a Pan-ErbB tyrosine kinase inhibitor, given orally on day 1, 8, 15 every 28 days to patients with solid tumors. *Proc Am Soc Clin Oncol* 2001; 20:72a (abstr 283).

120. Cobleigh MA, Vogel CL, Tripahty D, et al. Multinational study of the efficacy and safety of humanized anti-Her2 monoclonal antibody in women who have Her2-overexpressing metastatic breast cancer that has progressed after chemotherapy for metastatic disease. *J Clin Oncol* 1999; 17:2639–2648.

121. McLaughlin P, Gillo-Lopez AJ, Link BK, et al. Rituximab chimeric anti CD20 monoclonal antibody therapy for relapsed indolent lymphoma: half of patients respond to a four dose treatment program. *J Clin Oncol* 1998; 16:2825–2833.

122. Druker BJ, Talpaz M, Resta DJ, et al. Efficacy and safety of a specific inhibitor of the BCR-ABL tyrosine kinase in chronic myeloid leukemia. *N Engl J Med* 2001; 344:1031–1037.

123. Druker BJ, Sawyers CL, Kantarjian H, et al. Activity of a specific inhibitor of the BCR-ABL tyrosine kinase in the blast crisis of chronic myeloid leukemia and acute lymphoblastic leukemia with the Philadelphia chromosome. *N Engl J Med* 2001; 344:1038–1042.

124. Budillon A, Di Gennaro E, Bruzzese F, et al. Synergistic antitumor activity of IFNα in combination with ZD1839 (Iressa TM), an EGFR tyrosine kinase inhibitor, in HNSCC and melanoma cell lines. *Clin Cancer Res* 2000; 6:4542 (abstr 378).

125. Ye D, Mendelsohn J, Fan Z. Augmentation of a humanized anti-HER2 mAb 4D5 induced growth inhibition by a human-mouse chimeric anti-EGF receptor mAb C225. *Oncogene* 1999; 18:731–738.

126. Ciardiello F, Bianco R, Damiano V, et al. Antiangiogenic and antitumor activity of anti-epidermal growth factor receptor C225 monoclonal antibody in combination with vascular endothelial growth factor antisense oligonucleotide in human GEO colon cancer cells. *Clin Cancer Res* 2000; 6:3739–3747.

127. Gupta RA, DuBois RN. Combinations for cancer prevention. *Nat Med* 2000; 6:974–975.

128. Ramos-Suzarte M, Rodriguez N, Oliva JP, et al. 99mTc-labeled antihuman epidermal growth factor receptor antibody in patients with tumors of epithelial origin: Part III. Clinical trials safety and diagnostic efficacy. *J Nuclear Med* 1999; 40:768–775.

129. Blanke CD, von Mehren M, Joensuu H, et al. Evaluation of the safety and efficacy of an orally molecularly targeted, STI-571 in patients with unresectable or metastatic gastrointestinal stromal tumors (GISTS) expressing c-Kit (CD117). *Proc Am Soc Clin Oncol* 2001; 20:1a (abstr 1).

130. Van Oosterom AT, Juson I, Verweij J, et al. STI571, an active drug in metastatic gastrointestinal stroma tumors (GISTS), an EORTC phase I study. *Proc Am Soc Clin Oncol* 2001; 20:1a (abstr 2).

131. Alizadeh AA, Eisen MB, Davis RE, et al. Distinct types of diffuse large B-cell lymphoma identified by gene expression profiling. *Nature* 2000; 403:503–511.

132. Jain KK. Application of proteomics in oncology. *Pharmacogenomics* 2000; 1:385–393

133. Fung ET, Thulasiraman V, Weinberger SR, et al. Protein biochips for differential profiling. *Curr Opin Biotechnol* 2001; 12:65–69.

134. Lopez-Crapez E, Livache T, Marchand J, et al. K-ras mutation detection by hybridization to a polypyrrole DNA chip. *Clin Chem* 2001; 47:186–194.

135. von Eggeling F, Davies H, Lomas L, et al. Tissue-specific microdissection coupled with ProteinChip array technologies: applications in cancer research. *BioTechniques* 2000; 29:1066–1070.

16 Inhibition of the HER-2/neu Oncogene

A Translational Research Model for the Development of Future Targeted Therapies

Gottfried E. Konecny, MD, Jane Arboleda, PhD, Dennis J. Slamon, MD, PhD, and Mark Pegram, MD

CONTENTS

1. INTRODUCTION

The HER-2/neu gene encodes a 185-kilodalton (kDa) transmembrane protein that is a member of the type I receptor tyrosine kinase family, whose other members include the epidermal growth factor receptor (EGFR), HER-3, and HER-4 *(1)*. The HER-2/neu receptor protein is expressed in a wide variety of tissues, including the breast, ovary, endometrium, lung, liver, gastrointestinal tract, kidney, and central nervous system, and HER-2/neu is believed to play an important signaling role in cellular proliferation and differentiation in these tissues *(2–7)*.

From: *Oncogene-Directed Therapies*
Edited by: J. W. Rak © Humana Press Inc., Totowa, NJ

A role for HER-2/neu as an oncogene was first recognized in rodent systems. The activated form of the rodent homolog of the HER-2/neu gene, c-*neu*, was initially identified as an extremely potent transforming oncogene in DNA isolated from rats treated with ethylnitrosourea *(8)*. This form of the *neu* oncogene contains a point mutation in the transmembrane domain that led to the neu protein existing in a constitutively activated state. Its normal cellular counterpart was subsequently isolated from rat and human cDNA libraries *(9–13)*.

The molecular alteration that occurs in human tumors is amplification of the normal gene on chromosome 17q;21, resulting in overexpression of the normal gene product. Soon after the human HER-2/neu gene was cloned *(9)*, compelling clinical data were generated demonstrating that HER-2/neu gene amplification occurs in 25–30% of human breast, and in a lesser percentage of ovarian cancers *(2,14,15)*. This molecular alteration is an independent predictor of both relapse-free and overall survival in both diseases *(2,14–20)*. Initially, this finding was controversial, with many published studies failing to demonstrate an association between HER-2/neu amplification overexpression and clinical outcome. However, in retrospect, it is clear that most of these contradicting studies failed to demonstrate an association between HER-2/neu status and prognosis, due to methodological limitations, such as underpowered sample sizes, clinical follow-ups that were too short, or insensitive methods for detection of the HER-2/neu alteration, such as immunohistochemistry on formalin-fixed paraffin-embedded tissue *(21,22)*. It is now clear from large cohorts with long follow-up and suitable reagents that HER-2/neu amplification overexpression is an independent prognostic factor for both node-positive *(16,17,20)* and node-negative breast cancer *(18,19)*. In an attempt to differentiate between HER-2/neu overexpression simply being a prognostic epiphenomenon associated with a poor prognosis and it having a direct causal role in aggressive biological behavior, we engineered a series of human breast cancer cell lines to overexpress the gene at levels similar to those seen in cancers with HER-2/neu gene amplification and compared them to their nonoverexpressing parental controls. Introduction of this alteration into HER-2/neu-nonoverexpressing breast cancer cells resulted in marked increases of DNA synthesis, anchorage-dependent, and anchorage-independent growth, tumorigenicity, and metastatic potential *(23–26)*. Other investigators have conducted similar experiments, in which HER-2/neu transfection resulted in transformation of both NIH3T3 and human breast cells, confirming that this alteration plays a pathogenic role in tumorigenesis *(27,28)*.

2. TARGETING HER-2/neu-OVEREXPRESSING CANCERS

Following the observation that HER-2/neu overexpression plays an active role in pathogenesis of breast cancer, efforts were made to identify and characterize inhibitors of HER-2/neu. One approach was to generate antibodies that inhibit the growth of cells that possess activated HER-2/neu receptors *(29)*. A murine monoclonal antibody, 4D5, was found to have significant and dose-dependent antiproliferative activity specifically against HER-2/neu-overexpressing cells, while having no effect on cells expressing physiologic levels of HER-2/neu *(30)*. This antibody recognizes an extracellular epitope in the cysteine-rich II domain that resides very close to the transmembrane region of p185[HER-2]. New breakthroughs in biotechnology have made it possible to humanize murine monoclonal antibodies by identifying the minimum sequences of amino acid residues in the complementary determining region (CDR) of the murine antibody required for antigen specificity and to substitute these regions for the CDRs of a consensus human IgG molecule *(31)*. This recombinant humanized monoclonal antibody directed against HER-2/neu, now known as trastuzumab (Herceptin®), allows chronic human administration without development of human anti-mouse antibodies (HAMAs), which can otherwise rapidly neutralize therapeutic murine antibodies *(32–34)*.

Preclinical studies conducted at UCLA demonstrated that the antiproliferative effects of 4D5 and the dose-dependent antitumor efficacy against HER-2/neu-overexpressing xenografts in athymic mice were maintained following antibody humanization *(35)*. Furthermore, solution-phase binding studies determined that trastuzumab binds to the HER-2/neu extracellular domain with an affinity (Kd) of 0.1 nmol/L, which is 3-fold greater than that of 4D5 *(31)*.

Trastuzumab is based on an IgG_1 consensus sequence, thus allowing for the possibility of antibody-dependent cellular cytotoxicity (ADCC) against tumor target cells by immune effector cells expressing the Fcγ receptors *(36,37)*. ADCC requires the presence of activation Fcγ receptors on effector cells such as natural killer (NK) cells, monocytes and macrophages. NK cells express the activation Fcγ receptor, Fcγ RIII, but do not express the inhibitory counterpart, Fcγ RIIB *(37)*. Interestingly, monocytes and macrophages express both activation FcγRIII and inhibitory FcγRIIB receptors. The development of an orthotopic nude mouse model with effector cells lacking the activation FcγRIII receptor has recently been described *(37)*, which serves as a suitable model to determine the contribution of ADCC to the in vivo activity of trastuzumab. Knock-out mice deficient of the common Fcγ receptor, FcγRIII, were mated with athymic nuce mice (nu/nu) to generate FCγRIII–/– (nu/nu) mice for use in xenograft human tumor models *(37)*. In FcγRIII+/+ athymic nude mice, trastuzumab treatment resulted in nearly complete tumor inhibition (96%), with only a small fraction of mice developing palpable tumors. However, in FcγRIII–/– mice, tumor mass was merely reduced by 44%, and palpable tumors developed in nearly all of the animals *(37)*. Similar to these preclinical experiments, an additional orthotopic nude mouse model lacking the inhibition FcγRII receptors in effector cells, such as monocytes or macrophages, was developed using the same strategy. Trastuzumab was more effective in FcγRIIB–/– at arresting tumor cell growth in this nude mouse model. Taken together, these results clearly demonstrate the involvement of both an activation and inhibitory Fcγ receptor pathway in effector cell-mediated cytotoxicity of trastuzumab in vivo.

To further validate these findings, a mutant 4D5 HER-2/neu antibody was constructed that contained alanine instead of aspartate at residue 265 of the 4D5 IgG_1 heavy chain, a region critical for FCγ receptor binding. This mutation did not disrupt antibody-antigen interactions, as it retained the wild-type characteristics of p185HER-2/neu receptor blockage. However, the in vitro and in vivo ADCC capacity of the antibody was lost as a consequence of its reduced affinity for FcγRIII on effector cells. Similarly, the mutated 4D5 antibody had less growth inhibitory activity compared to wild-type 4D5 in the breast cancer xenograft model, confirming the contribution of Fcγ receptor-mediated cellular cytotoxicity to the activity of trastuzumab or 4D5 in vivo *(37)*.

3. HER-2/neu SIGNAL TRANSDUCTION PATHWAYS

HER-2/neu forms hetero-oligomers with other members of the type I receptor tyrosine kinase family (such as EGFR, HER-3, and HER-4) in response to specific ligands

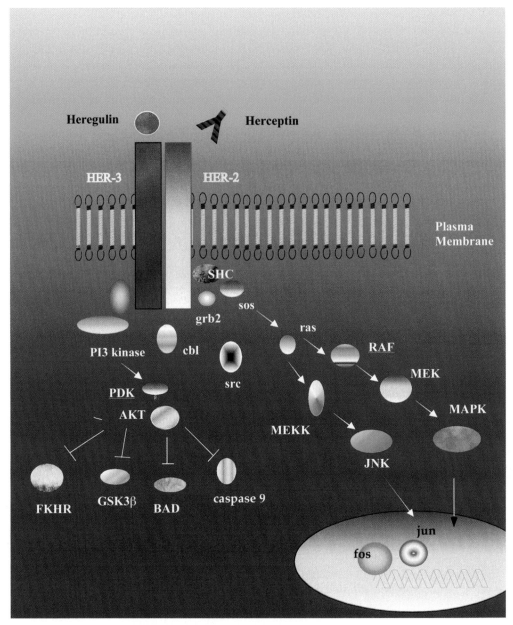

Fig. 1. HER-2/neu signal transduction pathways.

called neuregulins/heregulins *(38–41)*. Thus, HER-2/neu is an essential component of these receptor complexes, although no ligand that interacts with HER-2/neu alone has yet been characterized. However, when HER-2/neu is amplified and expressed at abnormally high levels, the kinase activity becomes constitutively activated, possibly due to autoactivation caused by crowding of adjacent HER-2/neu receptor molecules within the cell membrane *(42)*. This leads to ligand-independent activation of the HER-2/neu protein, resulting in an increase in mitogenic signaling and increased cell proliferation (Fig. 1). Important downstream substrates of HER-2/neu include members of the mitogen-activated protein (MAP) kinase cascade (43). Initially, HER-2/neu tyrosine phosphorlyation creates a binding site for the adaptor proteins, Grb2 and Shc. Association of Grb2 with activated HER-2/neu localizes Sos to the plasma membrane, where it is able to interact with Ras proteins. These Ras proteins are anchored to the inner leaflet of the plasma membrane. In its active GTP-bound form, Ras interacts with effector proteins, including the Raf protein-serine/threonine kinase. Activated Raf initiates a protein kinase cascade (MAP kinase), leading to extracellular regulated kinase (ERK) activation, which translocates to the nucleus, where it regulates transcription factors by phosphorylation (44). Importantly, ligand-dependent activation of HER-2/neu can also occur through formation of hetero-oligomer complexes with HER-3 receptors. HER-3, however, plays a distinct role, as it lacks a functional tyrosine kinase domain and preferentially forms oligomeric complexes in the absence of ligands (45). The HER-3 receptor itself can, therefore, only signal downstream by forming hetero-oligomers consisting of HER-2/neu and HER-3 molecules (39,40,46). Heregulins, which are natural ligands for the HER-3 and HER-4 receptors, can interfere with the oligomeric HER-3 complexes, thus releasing vacant HER-3 molecules from a preferred complex, allowing subsequent formation of new membrane receptor complexes consisting of HER-3 and adjacent HER-2 molecules (40,45).

An important signaling molecule downstream of this HER-2/HER-3 complex is phosphatidylinositol 3-kinase (PI3-kinase) (43). Although HER-2/neu has no PI3-kinase binding site, it may associate with PI3-kinase through heterodimerization with HER-3 (37,47,48). PI3-kinase plays a very important role in the cell signaling pathway. Its functions include cell survival (49), differentiation (50,51) and cytoskeletal structure regulation (52). Stimulation of PI3-kinase activates the family of AKT serine and threonine kinases (AKT1, AKT2, AKT3), which are cellular homologues of the viral oncogene, v-akt (53). Active AKT proteins have been shown to phosphorylate and inactivate members of the forkhead family (FH) of transcription factors (FKHR, FKHR1, and AFX), thereby inhibiting apoptosis. They have also been shown to induce cell survival by inactivation of BAD and caspase 9, which is consistent with the observation that growth factors in several systems can promote cell survival. AKT also appears to be a signaling intermediate upstream of survival gene expression, which is dependent on the transcription factor, NF-κB (54). Thus, the PI3-kinase/AKT pathway is essential for inhibition of apoptosis in response to growth factor activation (55,56). Furthermore, we were able to demonstrate that activation of AKT2, induced by heregulin through activation of P13-kinase, increased invasive capabilities of breast cancer cells overexpressing the HER-2/neu receptor in vitro, while expression of dominant-negative AKT2 blocked invasion of HER-2-overexpressing cells (57). Importantly, trastuzumab was similarly able to block invasion of HER-2 cells via down-regulation of AKTs in HER-2-overexpressing cells (58).

Consistent with these observations, it has also recently been demonstrated that heregulin B1 can trigger a rapid stimulation of p21-activated kinase 1 (PAK) and its redistribution into the leading edges of motile cells, thus promoting cell migration (59,60). Recent studies also suggest that AKT regulates insulin-like growth factor I receptor (IGF-IR) expression (61). Overexpression of AKT (AKT1 or AKT2) resulted in elevated IGF-IR expression, and inhibition of AKT activity down-regulated IGF-IR expression. Since IGF-IR is frequently overexpressed in several types of human malignancies, this study supports the hypothesis that active AKT promotes invasiveness of cancer cells, also through up-regulation of IGF-IR expression *(61)*.

A recent study reports up-regulation of vascular endothelial growth factor (VEGF) by heregulin in cancer cells *(62)*. Cancer cells engineered to stably overexpress HER-2/neu demonstrated induction of the basal level of VEGF, and exposure to heregulin further enhanced VEGF secretion *(62)*. These findings indicate a positive association between HER-2/neu and VEGF expression and are consistent with recently published data, using the mutated *neu* gene in NIH 3T3 cells *(63)*, which similarly demonstrated a correlation between HER-2/neu and VEGF expression in vitro. We were able to confirm up-regulation of VEGF by HER-2/neu at the RNA and protein levels in a number of breast cancer cell lines that had been stably transfected with the HER-2/neu gene (Epstein and Slamon, unpublished data). Other investigators were able to down-regulate VEGF expression and, thus, attenuate the angiogenic potential of HER-2/neu-overexpressing cells by using inhibitory HER-2/neu antibodies *(63)*.

In summary, the primary response to HER-2/neu activation is rapid transcriptional induction of a large family of genes called immediate early genes. Many of these immediate early genes themselves encode transcription factors, so their induction in response to growth factor stimulation leads to altered expression of an even larger number of other downstream genes, thereby establishing new patterns of gene expression associated with increased cell proliferation, tumorigenicity, and invasiveness of tumor cells. Since these changes are associated with aggressive biological behavior in tumor cells, HER-2/neu represents a suitable target for therapeutic interventions by antibodies or other molecules that can oppose the effects of the HER-2/neu kinase on cell signal transduction.

4. IN VITRO EFFECTS OF MONOCLONAL ANTI-HER-2/neu ANTIBODIES

Both the murine 4D5 and humanized antibody form, trastuzumab, reduce the percentage of HER-2/neu-positive cells undergoing S phase and increase the percentages of cells in the G_0/G_1 phase in a dose-dependent manner *(64,65)*. Treatment of HER-2/neu-overexpressing cells with 4D5 resulted in a marked induction of the CDK2 kinase inhibitor, $p27^{KIP1}$, which is consistent with the observation that treatment of HER-2/neu-overexpressing cells with trastuzumab results in a cytostatic inhibition of cell cycle progression *(25,47,65)*. Treatment with 4D5 resulted in accumulation of $p27^{KIP1}$, but inactivation of the CDK2 complex can also occur without increasing expression of $p27^{KIP1}$, as redirection of $p27^{KIP1}$ onto CDK2 is sufficient to inactivate cyclin activity and block the cell cycle *(65)*. Similar data have been reported for the EGFR, in which inhibition of the EGFR kinase in receptor-overexpressing cells resulted in up-regulation of $p27^{KIP1}$. Tumor cells did not enter S phase when $p27^{KIP1}$ levels were increased, resulting in G_1 arrest and growth inhibition of the cells *(66)*.

Early reports have suggested that binding of 4D5 to HER-2/neu results in activation of the HER-2/neu receptor, as monitored by an increase in tyrosine autophosphorylation *(67,68)*. When SK-BR-3 cells, which overexpress HER-2/neu, are growth-inhibited by trastuzumab treatment, a modest but reproducible increase in tyrosine phosphorylation content is seen *(47)*. Data derived from these experiments clearly show that while trastuzumab may cause modest autophosphorylation of HER-2, the intensity of this signal is significantly lower compared to that of heregulin in experimental models with HER-2/neu-overexpressing cells *(47)*. A recent investigation suggests that HER-2/neu antibodies achieve inhibition of signal transduction through their ability to interfere with receptor oligomer formation of HER-2/neu with other type I receptor tyrosine kinase family members and that this effect was due to acceleration of ligand dissociation *(69)*.

Furthermore, down-modulation of receptor-ligand complexes is thought to be a major attenuation mechanism for receptor-induced signaling; however, it has recently been shown that HER-2, HER-3, and HER-4 are impaired relative to EGFR with regards to their ability to undergo ligand-mediated endocytosis *(70)*. Nevertheless, although the rate of down-modulation appears to be slower than that observed for EGFR, significant removal of HER-2/neu receptors from cell membranes has been described *(71,72)*. Down-regulation of active ligand-bound growth factor receptors is caused by receptor-mediated endocytosis. Following formation of clathrin coated pits and early endosomes, a sorting process takes place, for which the molecular details are not yet precisely known. This leads either to lysosomal degradation of the ligand–receptor complexes or recycling of the receptor back to the cell membrane *(73,74)*.

Adaptor proteins suggested to be involved in the ligand-induced down-regulation of EGFR, resulting in lysosomal degradation, are members of the Cbl family. In support of endosomal sorting, defective Cbl proteins enhance recycling of EGFR molecules *(75)*. In HER-2/neu-overexpressing cells, a mutant Cbl receptor displayed retarded antibody-induced down-regulation and lysosomal degradation, suggesting that tumor inhibitory antibodies utilize the Cbl pathway, at least in part, to degrade HER-2/neu *(76)*. Thus, the therapeutic potential of certain antibodies may be due to their ability to direct HER-2/neu receptors to a Cbl-regulated proteolytic pathway.

In summary, both the effects of trastuzumab on HER-2/neu-mediated signaling and/or its effect on down-regulation of HER-2/neu expression levels are complex, and their exact contributions to the clinical activity of this therapeutic antibody remain to be defined.

5. PHASE I CLINICAL TRIALS

Based on the demonstration of preclinical efficacy, both the murine monoclonal and humanized forms of the HER-2/neu antibody were initially administered to human subjects in a series of single- and multi-dose phase I clinical trials conducted at UCLA. Toxicology and pharmacokinetics of single- and multi-dose antibody administered intravenously to patients with HER-2/neu-positive refractory metastatic breast cancer were studied. Trastuzumab demonstrated a favorable pharmacokinetic profile, achieving trough serum concentrations higher than those required for maximal antiproliferative effects in vitro. It also had a favorable toxicological profile, with the most commonly reported side effects during phase I being occasional fever during the first infusion and pain at the sites of metastasis. Importantly, these symptoms were described as mild or moderate. Furthermore, there was no evidence of human anti-humanized antibodies against trastuzumab. This was in contrast to a phase I trial conducted with murine 4D5 antibody, in which HAMAs developed rapidly, as expected, in treated patients *(26)*.

6. COMBINING TRASTUZUMAB WITH CHEMOTHERAPY

Trastuzumab alone is not cytotoxic in vitro, at least during short-term exposure. One popular method of rendering antibodies cytotoxic, envisioned by researchers in the

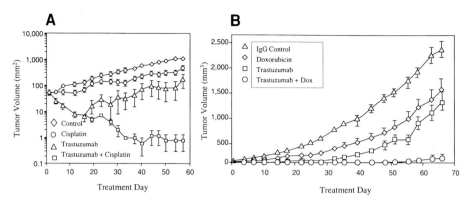

Fig. 2. Effect of therapy with cisplatin **(a)** or doxorubicin **(b)** and trastuzumab on growth of MCF-7/HER-2 breast tumor xenografts in nude mice. Cells were cultivated in estrogen-primed female nude mice for 7 d, then randomized to four treatment groups: 1) human IgG; 2) IgG and cisplatin **(a)** or doxorubicin **(b)**; 3) trastuzumab; and 4) cisplatin **(a)** or doxorubicin **(b)** combined with trastuzumab *(36).*

anticancer antibody field, was to covalently link cytotoxic drugs to therapeutic monoclonal antibodies. In one such effort, antibodies against EGFR were coupled to cisplatin and tested against EGFR-expressing xenografts in vivo *(77).* As controls for this experiment, the investigators also tested uncoupled free anti-EGFR antibodies administered concomitantly with free cisplatin. The results were surprising, in that this combination of uncoupled agents had more antitumor activity than the covalently linked species, and much more than either drug alone.

Because of the close homology between EGFR and HER-2/neu, we and others have conducted similar experiments with anti-HER-2/neu antibodies (Fig. 2) and have observed cytotoxic effects that appear to be more than additive when combining anti-HER-2/neu antibodies with cisplatin *(24,78–80).* A well-characterized mechanism of the synergistic interaction between anti-receptor antibodies and platinum salts is that antibody treatment inhibits repair of drug-induced DNA damage *(24).* This reversal of DNA repair results in accumulation of platinum-DNA adducts in the nucleus and concomitant enhanced cytotoxicity of cisplatin *(24).* We have termed this effect "receptor-enhanced chemosensitivity (REC)". To more extensively study the nature of the interaction(s) between trastuzumab and cisplatin, we employed the combination index/isobologram method described by Chou and Talalay *(81)* to classify drug interactions. We found the combination of trastuzumab and cisplatin to be highly synergistic. We have now expanded upon our antibody/drug interaction studies to include combinations of trastuzumab with alkylating agents, taxanes, topoisomerase II inhibitors, vinka alkaloids, and anthracyclines. Of these, the platinum analogs, docetaxel, vinorelbine, etoposide, thiotepa, cyclophosphamide, and ionizing radiation were found to have synergistic cytotoxicity when combined with trastuzumab *(82,83).*

7. PHASE II TRASTUZUMAB CLINICAL TRIALS

Four phase II clinical trials of single-agent trastuzumab, or trastuzumab in combination with cisplatin, have been conducted. In a pilot phase II study of single-agent trastuzumab for patients with HER-2/neu-overexpressing breast cancer who failed prior chemotherapy for metastatic disease, an 11% response rate was observed *(84)*. In an expanded phase II study of trastuzumab as a single agent for patients who failed one or two prior chemotherapeutic regimens for metastatic disease, a 14% response rate was noted *(85)*. More recently, results from single-agent trastuzumab given as first-line therapy for HER-2/neu-positive metastatic breast cancer were reported *(86)*. In this study, a higher response rate of about 25% was observed, suggesting that single-agent trastuzumab may be more effective in patients less heavily pretreated with chemotherapy. In addition, this study randomized patients to two different dose levels of trastuzumab. The first dose level was the standard 4 mg/kg loading dose, followed by 2 mg/kg/wk, and the second dose was double the standard dose (8 mg/kg load plus 4 mg/kg/wk). No apparent difference in response rates was seen at the higher dose level, and this dose appeared to cause more frequent side effects *(86)*. A significant contribution from all of these studies is a better understanding of the toxicology of trastuzumab. For the most part, trastuzumab is very well tolerated when administered as a single agent. Approximately 30–40% of patients experienced mild fevers and/or chills during the initial loading dose (4 mg/kg). Other commonly reported side effects included nausea/vomiting, pain at the site of tumor, asthenia, diarrhea, and headaches. These reactions can usually be managed by administration of acetaminophen (paracetamol), diphenhydramine hydrocloride, or meperidine hydrocloride, or even by slowing the rate of infusion.

The first trial of the combination of trastuzumab with chemotherapy in a clinical setting was performed at UCLA in 1992 *(80)*. A unique feature of this phase II trial was that to gain entry into the study, all patients were required to have chemoresistant breast cancer, as defined by objective evidence of disease progression during active chemotherapy treatment. The study population consisted of extensively pretreated advanced breast cancer patients with HER-2/neu overexpression. Patients were treated with a loading dose of 250 mg intravenous trastuzumab, followed by weekly doses of 100 mg intravenously for 9 wk. Chemotherapy consisted of cisplatin (75 mg/m^2) on d 1, 29, and 57. Clinical response data in this study were confirmed by an independent, blinded response evaluation committee. Objective partial clinical responses were seen in 24% of patients, and an additional 24% had either minor response or disease stabilization. This compares extremely favorably with both single-agent cisplatin (a reported response rate from five separate clinical trials of approx 7%, 95% confidence limits 2–11%) and single-agent trastuzumab (a response rate of about 12% in pretreated patients with metastatic disease) *(80,84)*.

8. FIRST-LINE CHEMOTHERAPY PLUS TRASTUZUMAB FOR HER-2/neu-OVEREXPRESSING METASTATIC BREAST CANCER

A large prospective randomized controlled trial of standard chemotherapy with trastuzumab (Herceptin) has been completed *(87)*. The trial was conducted in 469 patients with HER-2/neu-overexpressing metastatic breast cancer who had not previously been treated with chemotherapy for metastatic disease. Standard chemotherapy consisted of doxorubicin (60 mg/m^2) or epirubicin (75 mg/m^2) plus cyclophosphamide (600 mg/m^2) intravenously every 21 d for anthracycline-naïve patients (281 patients), or paclitaxel (175 mg/m^2) intravenously over 3 h for those patients who had previously been treated with an anthracycline in the adjuvant setting (188 patients). A feature of the patient characteristics for this cohort was that the patients in the paclitaxel arm had worse prognostic features at diagnosis, as might be anticipated, given their prior adjuvant

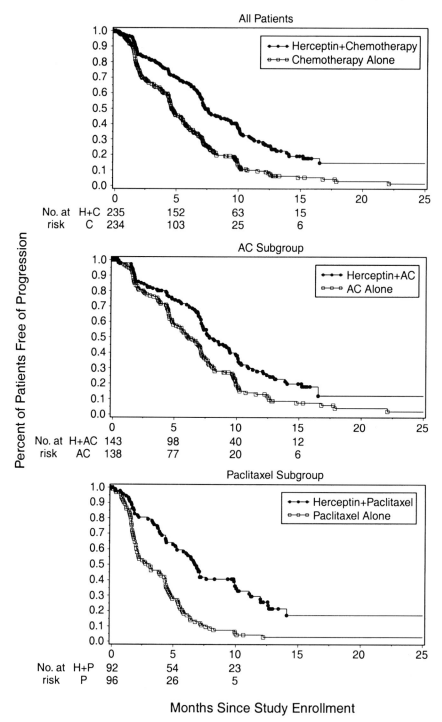

Fig. 3. Kaplan-Meier estimates of progression-free survival of patients with metastatic breast cancer, according to whether patients were randomly assigned to first-line chemotherapy (an anthracycline and cyclophosphamide or paclitaxel) plus trastuzumab or chemotherapy alone. H, Herceptin; AC, doxorubicin or epirubicin and cyclophosphamide; P, paclitaxel; C, chemotherapy. (Reproduced with permission from Ref. 87). Copyright 2001, Massachusetts Medical Society; all rights reserved.

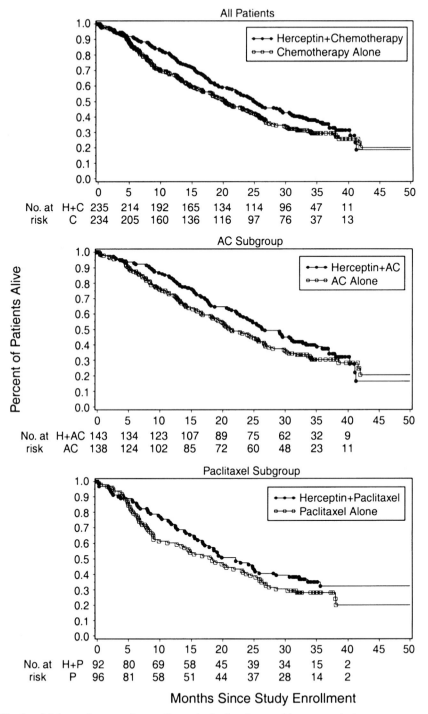

Fig. 4. Kaplan-Meier estimates of overall survival of patients with metastatic breast cancer, according to whether patients were randomly assigned to first-line chemotherapy (an anthracycline and cyclophosphamide or paclitaxel) plus trastuzumab or chemotherapy alone. (Reproduced with permission from Ref. 87). Copyright 2001, Massachusetts Medical Society; all rights reserved.

Table 1
Effect of Herceptin® on the Activity of an Anthracycline and Cyclophosphamide
or Paclitaxel as First-Line Therapy for Patients with Metastatic Breast Cancer

	CTX	CTX + H	AC	AC + H	P	P + H
Number of patients	234	235	138	143	96	92
Progression-free	4.6	7.4	6.1	7.8	3.0	6.9
survival (months)	$p < 0.001$		$p < 0.001$		$p < 0.001$	
Response rates (%)	32	50	42	56	17	41
	$p < 0.001$		$p = 0.02$		$p < 0.001$	
Median duration of	6.1	9.1	6.7	9.1	4.5	10.5
response (months)	$p < 0.001$		$p = 0.005$		$p < 0.01$	
Median survival	20.3	25.1	21.4	26.8	18.4	22.1
(months)	$p = 0.046$		$p = 0.16$		$p = 0.17$	

CTX, chemotherapy; H, Herceptin; AC, doxorubicin (60 mg/m^2) or epirubicin (75 mg/m^2) and cyclophosphamide (600 mg/m^2) q3W; and P, paclitaxel (175 mg/m^2) q3W.

treatment with an anthracycline. Patients on the paclitaxel arm were more likely to be premenopausal, have estrogen/progesterone receptor-negative tumors, more positive lymph nodes, and a higher incidence of prior radiation treatment. About 20% of these patients had been treated with myeloablative chemotherapy, followed by peripheral blood-derived or bone marrow-derived hematopoietic stem cells. These patients also had a shorter time from diagnosis to relapse compared with patients treated on the doxorubicin/cyclophosphamide arm. Based on these pretreatment characteristics, one might expect that the response to treatment in the paclitaxel group would be lower than the response in the doxorubicin/cyclophosphamide-treated group in this study. However, even with this caveat, the response rate in the paclitaxel group was somewhat of a surprise, in that the response rate for first-line single-agent paclitaxel was only 15%, compared with 38% for the doxorubicin-containing arm. Patients randomized to receive trastuzumab in combination with conventional chemotherapy had a higher overall response rate, a longer median response duration, a significantly longer time to disease progression, and an increased median survival (Figs 3 and 4) (Table 1) *(87)*. With a median follow-up of 35 mo, trastuzumab combined with either chemotherapy regimen decreased the relative risk of death by 24% and increased the median survival from 20.3 mo to 25.1 mo *(87)*. This is particularly noteworthy, given the fact that two-thirds of the women on the chemotherapy-alone arms subsequently received trastuzumab at the time of disease progression on a companion study protocol, following initial protocol treatment. It is also noteworthy that trastuzumab, the first biologic agent to be approved by the FDA for breast cancer treatment, prolongs the survival of metastatic breast cancer patients.

9. INCREASED RISK OF CARDIOTOXICITY

Along with the clinical success of trastuzumab came an unexpected toxicity; namely, cardiac dysfunction, especially in those patients who received concomitant trastuzumab and doxorubicin. Expression of HER-2/neu in adult myocardium had not been previously well-characterized, although it was presumed to be very low, on the basis of low-level HER-2/neu expression, as seen by immunohistochemical analysis or low levels of transcript expression detectable by reverse transcription polymerase chain reaction (RT-PCR). Cardiac dysfunction, as defined by the New York Heart Association (NYHA) classes I through IV, occurred in 39 out of 143 (27%) patients receiving trastuzumab plus doxorubicin/cyclophosphamide (AC) vs 8% receiving AC alone. However, NYHA I–IV also occurred in 12 out of 91 (13%) patients receiving trastuzumab plus paclitaxel vs 1% receiving paclitaxel alone. The incidence of severe cardiac dysfunction (NYHA class III and IV) was highest among patients receiving trastuzumab plus AC, with a 16% vs 3% incidence in those receiving AC alone and was 2% in those treated with trastuzumab plus paclitaxel vs 1% receiving paclitaxel alone *(87)*.

Doxorubicin is known to selectively reduce the expression of genes important for the structural integrity and enzymatic function of cardiac myocytes *(88)*. It has recently been reported that a transcriptional factor, STAT3, downstream of the transmembrane cytokine receptor, gp130, can induce protective signals against doxorubicin-induced cardiomyopathy that inhibit the doxorubicin-related reduction of cardioprotective genes *(89)*. Recent experimental data obtained in vitro, as well as in transgenic animals, suggest an important role for gp130-dependent signaling in cardiac myocyte survival *(90,91)*. The recent discovery of HER-2/gp130 heterodimer formation *(92)* suggests that HER-2/neu can directly promote cardiac myocyte survival via this heterodimer formation. Furthermore, heregulins can directly promote cardiac myocyte survival in vitro via HER-2/HER-4 heterodimer formation *(93)*. This heterodimer-activated pathway appears to be required to maintain cardiac myocyte viability under normal conditions and during cardiogenesis *(91)*. However, the gp130-dependent pathway appears to play an important role in the stress-induced survival pathway, which is not required under normal physiologic conditions *(91)*. It is likely that inhibition of HER-2/neu by antibodies can reduce activation of gp130, thus abrogating the protective function of this molecule, and thereby possibly making myocytes susceptible to doxorubicin-induced cardiomyopathy.

Further studies will, therefore, require careful design to avoid the cardiotoxicity issues associated with the use of trastuzumab/anthracycline administration. With recognition of the cardiotoxicity potential, we have proposed a non-anthracycline trastuzumab/chemotherapy regimen consisting of a docetaxel/platinum combination, which avoids the anthracycline-associated cardiotoxicity issues. More importantly, this approach will take advantage of the observed synergy between trastuzumab and these agents *(82,83)*.

10. HER-2/neu DETECTION IN CLINICAL SAMPLES

The need for accurate detection of the HER-2/neu alteration has now become even more important, because therapeutic decisions for patients are dependent upon this information. Optimal use of trastuzumab therapy requires accurate determination of HER-2/neu status, as this is presently the strongest predictor of response to trastuzumab treatment.

Numerous different approaches have been used to detect HER-2/neu amplification at the DNA level (slot blot or Southern blot, fluorescence *in situ* hybridization [FISH], PCR-based techniques), at the transcriptional level (Northern analysis, RT-PCR), or at the protein level (Western blot, immunohistochemistry [IHC], enzyme-linked immunosorbent assay [ELISA]). It is clear that all of the solid matrix blotting techniques suffer from

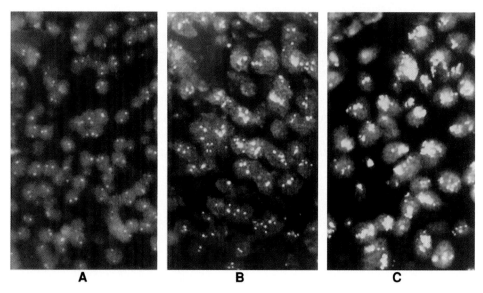

Fig. 5. Representative photomicrographs of breast tumor tissue sections after FISH with a spectrum orange-labeled HER-2/neu probe. A single band pass filter combination has been used in all photomicrographs. **(A)** HER-2/neu gene single-copy status (1000X); **(B)** Low-level amplification; **(C)** High-level amplification (1000X). (Interphase cytogenetics of the HER-2/neu oncogene in breast cancer, Giovanni Pauletti and Dennis Slamon in introduction to fluorescence in situ hybridization principles and clinical application. Edited by M. Andreeff and D. Pinkel. Copyright 1999; reprint permission by Wiley-Liss, Inc., a subsidiary of John Wiley & Sons, Inc.)

potential dilutional artifacts resulting from admixture of normal stromal, inflammatory, and vascular cells in clinical tumor samples *(14,94)*. Techniques involving *in situ* detection are generally more sensitive in identifying gene amplification or protein overexpression. The most widely used technique for detection of HER-2/neu overexpression at the protein level is IHC; however, the drawback of this technique is that multiple primary antibodies are currently in clinical use, each of which has differing sensitivity and specificity, as well as different cut-off values to distinguish overexpressing from nonoverexpressing tumors *(21)*. It is, therefore, difficult to know whether a sample scored as HER-2/neu-positive in one laboratory will be confirmed by another laboratory. Another concern is that the degree of IHC staining for HER-2/neu is subjective and qualitative. It is clear that formalin fixation of tumor samples and storage in paraffin results in epitope degradation, so that sensitivity is lost over time in archival clinical material *(14,21)*.

The most accurate technique currently available for detection of HER-2 gene alteration is DNA FISH (Fig. 5) *(94,95)*. In this assay, a fluorescent-labeled genomic DNA probe containing the HER-2/neu gene and its flanking sequence is allowed to hybridize to tumor cell DNA within a standard paraffin-embedded tumor section mounted on a microscope slide. A second DNA probe, specific for chromosome 17 and labeled with a different color than the HER-2/neu probe, is used to distinguish true HER-2/neu gene amplification from chromosome 17 ploidy. Using this technique, a quantitative copy number of HER-2/neu genes per chromosome 17 centromere can be ascertained. One theoretical disadvantage of this assay is the inability to detect so-called single-copy overexpressors. In such cases, the HER-2/neu protein is overexpressed in the absence of HER-2/neu amplification *(94)*. However, the frequency of single-copy HER-2/neu

Table 2
Discordance of the IHC and FISH Results Among 529 Patients Entered into
the Pivotal Clinical Trials of Herceptin as First- or Second/Third-Line Single
Agent or in Combination with Chemotherapy

	IHC			
	0	*1+*	*2+*	*3+*
FISH-negative	207	28	67	21
FISH-positive	7	2	21	176

overexpression in breast cancers is estimated to be less than 5% of all overexpressing tumors. Moreover, these cases do not appear to have the poor prognosis of the amplified/overexpressors *(20)*. Therefore, the advantages of FISH in terms of sensitivity and specificity far outweigh this disadvantage in terms of diagnostic accuracy *(22,94)*.

Three pivotal clinical trials led to Food and Drug Administration (FDA) approval of Herceptin (first-line single-agent therapy, second- or third-line single-agent therapy, and combination therapy of trastuzumab and chemotherapy in first-line treatment of breast cancer). In a retrospective subgroup analysis, the tumor samples of most of the patients included in these studies were analyzed by FISH *(96–98)*. The findings of this analysis indicate that the response to trastuzumab, either as a single agent or in combination with chemotherapy, was greater among those patients whose tumors demonstrated HER-2/neu gene amplification detected by FISH compared to those patients who were classified as HER-2/neu-positive solely by IHC, using the clinical trials kit (CB11 and 4D5 HER-2/neu antibodies) on paraffin-embedded formalin-fixed tissue. FISH results were available from 540 (67%) of the 805 patients entered into the three pivotal clinical trials. The discordance between FISH and IHC in defining HER-2/neu-positive breast cancer patients is displayed in Table 2. Importantly, 21 (11%) of 197 patients scored as IHC 3+ were classified as negative for HER-2/neu gene amplification, and 67 (76%) of 88 patients scored as IHC 2+ were classified as negative for amplification of HER-2/neu. Among the patients classified as HER-2/neu-positive by FISH, 21 out of 105 (20%) and 17 out of 41 (41%) responded to second/third-line therapy and first-line therapy, respectively, and 130 out of 240 (54%) of patients responded to the trastuzumab chemotherapy combination. Comparison of the results of this subgroup analysis with the response rates reported earlier for patients classified as HER-2/neu-positive by IHC *(85–87)* suggest that FISH is superior in determining the probability of response to trastuzumab as a single agent or in combination with chemotherapy compared to IHC.

11. FUTURE DEVELOPMENTS

Defining safe well-tolerated and effective clinical regimens incorporating trastuzumab remains an important priority. As described above, preclinical data suggest that there are synergistic interactions between some chemotherapeutic agents such as platinum-based regimens, docetaxel, or navelbine *(64,82,83)*. Phase II studies with these combination partners have been initiated, and preliminary results are encouraging, with high response rates and favorable toxicity profiles *(99,100)*. Importantly, these combination partners have not been associated with cardiac toxicity and, therefore, have demonstrated a low risk of cardiotoxicity in combination with trastuzumab.

Furthermore, the use of adjuvant trastuzumab for HER-2/neu-positive early stage breast cancer is a very attractive treatment approach, as trastuzumab is a therapeutic with a high molecular weight (148 kDa), for which penetration into bulky tumors is unfavorable. Therefore, the efficacy of trastuzumab would theoretically be maximal in a micrometastatic disease situation, where intratumoral pharmacokinetic boundaries are not present. Most of the adjuvant studies will administer 1 yr of trastuzumab, but the decision for this duration, though reasonable, is empiric. Regarding potential cardiotoxicity of trasuzumab, we have initiated a non-anthracycline adjuvant chemotherapy/trastuzumab regimen consisting of a docetaxel/carboplatin combination that will avoid anthracycline-associated cardiotoxicity issues in the adjuvant setting, in which many women may be cured as a result of their initial surgery and radiation. Most importantly, this combination will take advantage of the synergistic interactions between these agents when given concomitantly.

Many clinical issues regarding HER-2/neu amplification/overexpression have not yet been resolved. Its use as a target for future drug development provides a wealth of opportunities for future basic and clinical research. The fact that trastuzumab prolongs the survival of patients with metastatic breast cancer is not only clinically significant for breast cancer therapy, but is also the ultimate experimental proof from a scientific perspective that HER-2/neu does play an important role in the pathophysiology of breast cancer. The HER-2/neu paradigm of targeted cancer therapy is now an important model for drug discovery and drug development in the biotechnology and pharmaceutical industries. Identification of new therapeutic targets will result in significant therapeutic benefits for patients suffering, not only from breast cancer, but from many other human cancers.

ACKNOWLEDGMENTS

This work was supported by the Revlon/UCLA Women's Cancer Research Program. The authors thank Wendy Aft for her excellent preparation of this manuscript.

REFERENCES

1. Rajkumar T, Gullick WJ. The type I growth factor receptors in human breast cancer. *Breast Cancer Res Treat* 1994; 29:3–9.
2. Slamon DJ, Clark GM, Wong SG, Levin WJ, Ullrich A, McGuire WL. Human breast cancer: correlation of relapse and survival with amplification on HER-2/*neu* oncogene. *Science* 1987; 235:177–182.
3. Bigsby RM, Li AX, Bomalaski J, Stehman FB, Look KY, Sutton GP. Immunohistochemical study of HER-2/neu, epidermal growth factor receptor, and steroid receptor expression in normal and malignant endometrium. *Obstet Gynecol* 1992; 79:95–100.
4. Rotter M, Block T, Busch R, Thanner S, Hofler H. Expression of HER-2/neu in renal-cell carcinoma. Correlation with histologic subtypes and differentiation. *Int J Cancer* 1992; 52:213–217.
5. Press MF, Pike MC, Hung G, Zhou JY, Ma Y, George J, et al. Amplification and overexpression of HER-2/neu in carcinomas of the salivary gland: correlation with poor prognosis. *Cancer Res* 1994; 54:5675–5682.
6. Osako T, Miyahara M, Uchino S, Inomata M, Kitano S, Kobayashi M. Immunohistochemical study of c-erbB-2 protein in colorectal cancer and the correlation with patient survival. *Oncology* 1998; 55:548–555.
7. Martin-Lacave I, Utrilla JC. Expression of a neu/c-erbB-2-like product in neuroendocrine cells of mammals. *Histol Histopathol* 2000; 15:1027–1033.

8. Shih C, Padhy LC, Murray M, Weinberg RA. Transforming genes of carcinomas and neuroblastomas introduced into mouse fibroblasts. *Nature* 1981; 290:261–264.

9. Coussens L, Yang-Feng TL, Liao YC, Chen E, Gray A, McGrath J, et al. Tyrosine kinase receptor with extensive homology to EGF receptor shares chromosomal location with neu oncogene. *Science* 1985; 230:1132–1139.

10. Semba K, Kamata N, Toyoshima K, Yamamoto T. A v-erbB-related protooncogene, c-erbB-2, is distinct from the c-erbB-1/epidermal growth factor-receptor gene and is amplified in a human salivary gland adenocarcinoma. *Proc Natl Acad Sci USA* 1985; 82:6497–6501.

11. Bargmann CI, Hung MC, Weinberg RA. The neu oncogene encodes an epidermal growth factor receptor-related protein. *Nature* 1986; 319:226–230.

12. Hung MC, Schechter AL, Chevray PY, Stern DF, Weinberg RA. Molecular cloning of the neu gene: absence of gross structural alteration in oncogenic alleles. *Proc Natl Acad Sci USA* 1986; 83:261–264.

13. Yamamoto T. Ikawa S, Akiyama T, Semba K, Nomura N, Miyajima N, et al. Similarity of protein encoded by the human c-erb-B-2 gene to epidermal growth factor receptor. *Nature* 1986; 319:230–234.

14. Slamon DJ, Godolphin W, Jones LA, Holt JA, Wong SG, Keith DE, et al. Studies of the HER-2/neu proto-oncogene in human breast and ovarian cancer. *Science* 1989; 244:707–712.

15. Berchuck A, Kamel AS, Whitaker R, Kerns B, Olt G, Kinney R, et al. Overexpression of HER-2/neu is associated with poor survival in advanced epithelial ovarian cancer. *Cancer Res* 1990; 50:4087–4091.

16. Toikkanen S, Helin H, Isola J, Joensus H. Prognostic significance of HER-2 oncoprotein expression in breast cancer: a 30-year follow-up. *J Clin Oncol* 1992; 10:1044–1048.

17. Seshadri R, Firgaira FA, Horsfall DJ, McCaul K, Setlur V, Kitchen P. Clinical significance of HER-2/neu oncogene amplification in primary breast cancer. The South Australian Breast Cancer Study Group. *J Clin Oncol* 1993; 11:1936–1942.

18. Quenel N, Wafflart J, Bonichon F, de Mascarel I, Trojani M, Durand M, et al. The prognostic value of c-erbB2 in primary breast carcinomas: a study on 942 cases. *Breast Cancer Res Treat* 1995 35:283–291.

19. Andrulis IL, Bull SB, Blackstein ME, Sutherland D, Mak C, Sidlofsky S, et al. neu/erbB-2 amplification identifies a poor-prognosis group of women with node-negative breast cancer. Toronto Breast Cancer Study Group. *J Clin Oncol* 1998 16:1340–1349.

20. Pauletti G, Dandekar S, Rong H, Ramos L, Peng H, Seshadri R, et al. Assessment of methods for tissue-based detection of the HER-2/neu alteration in human breast cancer: a direct comparison of fluorescence in situ hybridization and immunohistochemistry. *J Clin Oncol* 2000; 18:3651–3664.

21. Press MF, Hung G, Godolphin W, Slamon DJ. Sensitivity of HER-2/neu antibodies in archival tissue samples: potential source of error in immunohistochemical studies of oncogene expression. *Cancer Res* 1994; 54:2771–2777.

22. Pegram MD, Pauletti G, Slamon DJ. HER-2/neu as a predictive marker of response to breast cancer therapy. *Breast Cancer Res Treat* 1998; 52:65–77.

23. Chazin VR, Kaleko M, Miller AD, Slamon DJ. Transformation mediated by the human HER-2 gene independent of the epidermal growth factor receptor. *Oncogene* 1992; 7:1859–1866.

24. Pietras RJ, Fendly B, Chazin VR, Pegram MD, Howell SB, Slamon DJ. Antibody to HER-2/neu receptor blocks DNA repair after cisplatin in human breast and ovarian carcinoma cells. *Oncogene* 1994; 9:1829–1838.

25. Pegram MD, Finn RS, Arzoo K, Beryt M, Pietras RJ, Slamon DJ. The effect of HER-2/neu overexpression on chemotherapeutic drug sensitivity in human breast and ovarian cancer cells. *Oncogene* 1997; 15:537–547.

26. Pegram M, Slamon D. Biological rationale for HER2/neu (c-erbB2) as a target for monoclonal antibody therapy. *Semin Oncol* 2000; 27:13–19.

27. Hudziak RM, Schlessinger J, Ullrich A. Increased expression of the putative growth factor receptor p185HER2 causes transformation and tumorigenesis of NIH 3T3 cells. *Proc Natl Acad Sci USA* 1987; 84:7159–7163.

28. Pierce JH, Arnstein P, DiMarco E, Artrip J, Kraus MH, Lonardo F, et al. Oncogenic potential of erbB-2 in human mammary epithelial cells. *Oncogene* 1991; 6:1189–1194.

29. Drebin JA, Link VC, Stern DF, Weinberg RA, Greene MI. Down-modulation of an oncogene protein product and reversion of the transformed phenotype by monoclonal antibodies. *Cell* 1985; 41:697–706.

30. Fendly BM, Winget M, Hudziak RM, Lipari MT, Napier MA, Ullrich A. Characterization of murine monoclonal antibodies reactive to either the human epidermal growth factor receptor or HER2/neu gene product. *Cancer Res* 1990; 50:1550–1158.

31. Carter P, Presta L, Gorman CM, Ridgway JB, Henner D, Wong WL, et al. Humanization of an anti-p185HER2 antibody for human cancer therapy. *Proc Natl Acad Sci USA* 1992; 89:4285–4289.

32. Losman MJ, DeJager RL, Monestier M, Sharkey RM, Goldenberg DM. Human immune response to anti-carcinoembryonic antigen murine monoclonal antibodies. *Cancer Res* 1990; 50:1055s–1058s.

33. Tjandra JJ, Ramadi L, McKenzie IF. Development of human anti-murine antibody (HAMA) response in patients. *Immunol Cell Biol* 1990; 68:367–376.

34. Avner B, Swindell L, Sharp E, Liao SK, Ogden JR, Avner BP, et al. Evaluation and clinical relevance of patient immune responses to intravenous therapy with murine monoclonal antibodies conjugated to adriamycin. *Mol Biother* 1991; 3:14–21.

35. Pietras RJ, Pegram MD, Finn RS, Maneval DA, Slamon DJ. Remission of human breast cancer xenografts on therapy with humanized monoclonal antibody to HER-2 receptor and DNA-reactive drugs. *Oncogene* 1998; 17:2235–2249.

36. Pegram M, Baly D, Wirth C, Gilkerson E, Slamon DJ, Sliwkowski MX. Antibody-dependent cell-mediated cytotoxicity in breast cancer patients in phase III clinical trials of a humanized anti-HER2 antibody. *Proc Am Assoc Cancer Res* 1997; 38:602. (Abstr. 4044)

37. Clynes RA, Towers TL, Presta LG, Ravetch JV. Inhibitory Fc receptors modulate in vivo cytoxicity against tumor targets. *Nature Med* 2000; 6:443–446.

38. Plowman GD, Green JM, Culouscou JM, Carlton GW, Rothwell VM, Buckley S. Heregulin induces tyrosine phosphorylation of HER4/p180erbB4. *Nature* 1993; 366:473–475.

39. Carraway KL III, Cantley LC. A neu acquaintance for erbB3 and erbB4: a role for receptor heterodimerization in growth signaling. *Cell* 1994; 78:5–8.

40. Sliwkowski MX, Schaefer G, Akita RW, Lofgren JA, Fitzpatrick VD, Nuijens A, et al. Coexpression of erbB2 and erbB3 proteins reconstitutes a high affinity receptor for heregulin. *J Biol Chem* 1994; 269:14661–14665.

41. Klapper LN, Glathe S, Vaisman N, Hynes NE, Andrews GC, Sela M, et al. The ErbB-2/HER2 oncoprotein of human carcinomas may function solely as a shared coreceptor for multiple stroma-derived growth factors. *Proc Natl Acad Sci USA* 1999; 96:4995–5000.

42. Reese DM, Slamon DJ. HER-2/neu signal transduction in human breast and ovarian cancer. *Stem Cells* 1997; 15:1–8.

43. Amundadottir LT, Leder P. Signal transduction pathways activated and required for mammary carcinogenesis in response to specific oncogenes. *Oncogene* 1998; 16:737–746.

44. Mansour SJ, Matten WT, Hermann AS, Candia JM, Rong S, Fukasawa K, et al. Transformation of mammalian cells by constitutively active MAP kinase kinase. *Science* 1994; 265:966–970.

45. Landgraf R, Eisenberg D. Heregulin reverses the oligomerization of HER3. *Biochemistry* 39:8502–8511.

46. Pinkas-Kramarski R, Shelly M, Glathe S, Ratzkin BJ, Yarden Y. Neu differentiation factor/neuregulin isoforms activate distinct receptor combinations. *J Biol Chem* 1996; 271:19029–19032.

47. Sliwkowski MX, Lofgren JA, Lewis GD, Hotaling TE, Fendly BM, Fox JA. Nonclinical studies addressing the mechanism of action of trastuzumab (Herceptin). *Semin Oncol* 1999; 26:60–70.

48. Schaefer G, Akita RW, Sliwkowski MX. A discrete three-amino acid segment (LVI) at the C-terminal end of kinase-impaired ErbB3 is required for transactivation of ErbB2. *J Biol Chem* 1999; 274:859–866.

49. Yao R, Cooper GM. Requirement for phosphatidylinositol-3 kinase in the prevention of apoptosis by nerve growth factor. *Science* 1995; 267:2003–2006.

50. Ohmichi M, Decker SJ, Saltiel AR. Activation of phosphatidylinostiol-3 kinase by nerve growth factor involves indirect coupling of the trk proto-oncogene with src homology 2 domains. *Neuron* 1992; 9:769–777.

51. Soltoff SP, Rabin SL, Cantley LC, Kaplan DR. Nerve growth factor promotes the activation of phosphatidylinositol 3-kinase and its association with the trk tyrosine kinase. *J Biol Chem* 1992; 267:17472–17477.

52. Nobes CD, Hawkins P, Stephens L, Hall A. Activation of the small GTP-binding proteins rho and rac by growth factor receptors. *J Cell Sci* 1995; 108: 225–233.

53. Stall SP. Molecular cloning of the akt oncogene and its human homologues AKT1 an AKT2: amplification of AKT1 in a primary human gastric adenocarcinoma. *Proc Natl Acad Sci USA* 1987; 84:5034–5037.

54. Datta SR, Brunet A, Greenberg ME. Cellular survival: a play in three Akts. *Genes Dev* 1999; 13:2905–2927.

55. Biggs WH III, Meisenhelder J, Hunter T, Cavenee WK, Arden KC. Protein kinase B/Akt-mediated phosphorylation promotes nuclear exclusion of the winged helix transcription factor FKHR1. *Proc Natl Acad Sci USA* 1999; 96:7421–7426.

56. Jackson JG, Kreisberg JI, Koterba AP, Yee D, Brattain MG. Phosphorylation and nuclear exclusion of the forkhead transcription factor FKHR after epidermal growth factor treatment in human breast cancer cells. *Oncogene* 2000; 19:4574–4581.

57. Arboleda J, Lyons JF, Kabbinavar FF, Bray MR, Snow BE, Ayala R, et al. Overexpression of AKT2/PKBβ leads to upregulation of collagen IV binding receptors, increased invasion and metastasis of human breast and ovarian cancer cells, *submitted.*

58. Arboleda J, Slamon DJ. Heregulin induced cell invasion of HER-2/neu transfected breast cancer cell line is mediated through activation of the phosphatidylinositol 3-kinase/AKT2 pathway. Abstract for Cold Spring Harbor Laboratory Meeting on Tyrosine Phosphorylation and Cell Signaling, 1999; p 11.

59. Adam L, Vadlamudi R, Kondapaka SB, Chernoff J, Mendelsohn J, Kumar R. Heregulin regulates cytoskeletal reorganization and cell migration through the p21-activated kinase-1 via phosphatidylinositol-3 kinase. *J Biol Chem* 1998; 273:28238–28246.

60. Chausovsky A, Waterman H, Elbaum M, Yarden Y, Geiger B, Bershadsky AD. Molecular requirements for the effect of neuregulin on cell spreading, motility and colony organization. *Oncogene* 2000; 19:878–888.

61. Tanno S, Tanno S, Mitsuuchi Y, Altomare DA, Xiao GH, Testa JR. AKT activation up-regulates insulin-like growth factor I receptor expression and promotes invasiveness of human pancreatic cancer. *Cancer Res* 2001; 61:589–593.

62. Yen L, You XL, Al Moustafa AE, Batist G, Hynes NE, Mader S, et al. Heregulin selectively upregulates vascular endothelial growth factor secretion in cancer cells and stimulates angiogenesis. *Oncogene* 2000; 19:3460–2369.

63. Petit AM, Rak J, Hung MC, Rockwell P, Goldstein N, Fendly B, et al. Neutralizing antibodies against epidermal growth factor and ErbB-2/neu receptor tyrosine kinases down-regulate vascular endothelial growth factor production by tumor cells in vitro and in vivo: angiogenic implications for signal transduction therapy of solids tumors. *Am J Pathol* 1997; 151:1523–1530.

64. Pegram MD, Slamon DJ. Combination therapy with trastuzumab (Herceptin) and cisplatin for chemoresistant metastatic breast cancer: evidence for receptor-enchanced chemosensitivity. *Semin Oncol* 1999; 26:89–95.

65. Lane HA, Beuvink I, Motoyama AB, Daly JM, Neve RM, Hynes NE. ErbB2 potentiates breast tumor proliferation through modulation of p27(Kip1)-Cdk2 complex formation: receptor overexpression does not determine growth dependency. *Mol Cell Biol* 2000; 20:3210–3223.

66. Busse D, Doughty RS, Ramsey TT, Russell WE, Price JO, Flanagan WM, Reversible G(1) arrest induced by inhibition of the epidermal growth factor receptor tyrosine kinase requires up-regulation of p27(KIP1) independent of MAPK activity. *J Biol Chem* 2000; 275:6987–6995.

67. Kumar R, Shepard HM, Mendelsohn J. Regulation of phosphorylation of the c-erbB-2/HER2 gene product by a monoclonal antibody and serum growth factor(s) in human mammary carcinoma cells. *Mol Cell Biol* 1991; 11:979–986.

68. Sarup JC, Johnson RM, King KL, Fendly BM, Lipari MT, Napier MA, et al. Characterization of an anti-p185HER2 monoclonal antibody that stimulates receptor function and inhibits tumor cell growth. *Growth Reg* 1991; 1:72–82.

69. Klapper LN, Vaisman N, Hurwitz E, Pinkas-Kramarski R, Yarden Y, Sela M. A subclass of tumor-inhibitory monoclonal antibodies to ErbB-2/HER2 blocks crosstalk with growth factor receptors. *Oncogene* 1997; 14:2099–2109.

70. Baulida J, Kraus MH, Alimandi M, Di Fiore PP, Carpenter G. All ErbB receptors other than the epidermal growth factor receptor are endocytosis impaired. *J Biol Chem* 1996; 271:5251–5257.

71. Hudziak RM, Lewis GD, Winget M, Fendly BM, Shepard HM, Ullrich A. p185HER2 monoclonal antibody has antiproliferative effects in vitro and sensitizes human breast tumor cells to tumor necrosis factor. *Mol Cell Biol* 1989; 9:1165–1172.

72. De Santes K, Slamon D, Anderson SK, Shepard M, Fendly B, Maneval D, et al. Radiolabeled antibody targeting of the HER-2/neu oncoprotein. *Cancer Res* 1992; 52:1916–1923.

73. Maier LA, Xu FJ, Hester S, Boyer CM, McKenzie S, Bruskin AM, et al. Requirements for the internalization of a murine monoclonal antibody directed against the HER-2/neu gene product c-erbB-2. *Cancer Res* 1991; 51:5361–5369.

74. Waterman H, Yarden Y. Molecular mechanisms underlying endocytosis and sorting of ErbB receptor tyrosine kinases. *FEBS Lett* 2001; 490:142–152.

75. Waterman H, Levkowitz G, Alroy I, Yarden Y. The RING finger of c-Cbl mediates desensitization of the epidermal growth factor receptor. *J Biol Chem* 1999; 274:22151–22154.

76. Klapper LN, Waterman H, Sela M, Yarden Y. Tumor-inhibitory antibodies to HER-2/ErbB-2 may act by recruiting c-Cbl and enhancing ubiquitination of HER-2. *Cancer Res* 2001; 60:3384–3388.

77. Aboud-Pirak E, Hurwitz E, Pirak ME, Bellot F, Schlessinger J, Sela M. Efficacy of antibodies to epidermal growth factor receptor against KB carcinoma in vitro and in nude mice. *J Natl Cancer Inst* 1988; 80:1605–1611.

78. Hancock MC, Langton BC, Chan T, Toy P, Monahan JJ, Mischak RP, et al. A monoclonal antibody against the c-erbB-2 protein enhances the cytotoxicity of cis-diamminedichloroplatinum against human breast and ovarian tumor cell lines. *Cancer Res* 1991; 51:4574–4580.

79. Arteaga CL, Winnier AR, Poirier MC, Lopez-Larraza DM, Shawver LK, Hurd SD, et al. p185c-erbB-2 signal enhances cisplatin-induced cytotoxicity in human breast carcinoma cells: association between an oncogenic receptor tyrosine kinase and drug-induced DNA repair. *Cancer Res* 1994; 54:3758–3765.

80. Pegram MD, Lipton A, Hayes DF, Weber BL, Baselga JM, Tripathy D, et al. Phase II study of receptor-enhanced chemosensitivity using recombinant humanized anti-p185 HER2/neu monoclonal antibody plus cisplatin in patients with HER-2/neu-overexpressing metastatic breast cancer refractory to chemotherapy treatment. *J Clin Oncol* 1998; 16:2659–2671.

81. Chou TC, Talalay P. Quantitative analysis of dose-effect relationships: the combined effects of multiple drugs or enzyme inhibitors. *Adv Enzyme Regul* 1984; 22:27–55.

82. Konecny G, Pegram M, Beryt M, Untch M, Slamon DJ. Therapeutic advantage of chemotherapy durgs in combination withe Herceptin against human breast cancer cells with HER-2/*neu* overexpression. *Breast Cancer Res Treat* 1999; 57:114 (abstr 467).

83. Pegram M, Hsu S, Lewis G, Pietras R, Beryt M, Sliwkowski M, et al. Inhibitory effects of combinations of HER-2/neu antibody and chemotherapeutic agents used for treatment of human breast cancers. *Oncogene* 1999; 18:2241–2251.

84. Baselga J, Tripathy D, Mendelsohn J, Baughman S, Benz CC, Dantis L, et al. Phase II study of weekly intravenous recombinant humanized anti-p185HER2 monoclonal antibody in patients with HER2/neu-overexpressing metastatic breast cancer. *J Clin Oncol* 1996; 14:737–744.

85. Cobleigh MA, Vogel CL, Tripathy D, Robert NJ, Scholl S, Fehrenbacher L, et al. Multinational study of the efficacy and safety of humanized anti-HER2 monoclonal antibody in women who have HER2-overexpressing metastatic breast cancer that has progressed after chemotherapy for metastatic disease. *J Clin Oncol* 1999; 17(9):2639–2648.

86. Vogel CL, Cobleigh MA, Tripathy D, Gutheil JC, Harris LN, Fehrenbacher L, et al. Efficacy and safety of trastuzumab as a single agent in first-line treatment of HER2-overexpressing metastatic breast cancer. *J Clin Oncol* 2002; 20(3):719–726.

87. Slamon DJ, Leyland-Jones B, Shak S, Fuchs H, Paton V, Bajamonde A, et al. Use of chemotherapy plus a monoclonal antibody against HER2 for metastatic breast cancer that overexpresses HER2. *N Engl J Med* 2001; 344:783–792.

88. Ito H, Miller SC, Billingham ME, Akimoto H, Torti SV, Wade R, et al. Doxorubicin selectively inhibits muscle gene expression in cardiac muscle cells in vivo and in vitro. *Proc Nalt Acad Sci USA* 1990; 87:4275–4279.

89. Kunisada K, Tone E, Fujio Y, Matsui H, Yamauchi-Takihara K, Kishimoto T. Activation of gp130 transduces hypertrophic signals via STAT3 in cardiac myocytes. *Circulation* 1998; 98:346–352.

90. Hunter JJ, Chien KR. Signaling pathways for cardiac hypertrophy and failure *N Engl J Med* 1999; 341:1276–1283.

91. Chien KR. Myocyte survival pathways and cardiomyopathy:implications for trastuzumab cardiotoxicity. *Semin Oncol* 2000; 27:9–14.

92. Qiu Y, Ravi L, Kung HJ. Requirement of ErbB2 for signalling by interleukin-6 in prostate carcinoma cells. *Nature* 1998; 393:83–85.

93. Zhao YY, Sawyer DR, Baliga RR, Opel DJ, Han X, Marchionni MA, et al. Neuregulins promote survival and growth of cardiac myocytes. Persistence of ErbB2 and ErbB4 expression in neonatal and adult ventricular myocytes. *J Biol Chem* 1998; 273:10261–10269.

94. Pauletti G, Godolphin W, Press MF, Slamon DJ. Detection and quantitation of HER-2/neu gene amplification in human breast cancer archival material using fluorescence in situ hybridization. *Oncogene* 1996; 13:63–72.

95. Kallioniemi OP, Kallioniemi A, Kurisu W, Thor A, Chen LC, Smith HS, et al. ERBB2 amplification in breast cancer analyzed by fluorescence in situ hybridizaiton. *Proc Natl Acad Sci USA* 1992; 89:5321–5325.

96. Mass RD, Sanders C, Charlene K, Johnson L, Everett T, Anderson S. The concordance between the clinical trials assay (CTA) and fluorescence in situ hybridization (FISH) in the Herceptin pivotal trials. *Proc Am Soc Clin Oncol* 2000; 19:291 (abstr).

97. Mass RD, Press M, Anderson S, Murphy M, Slamon D. Improved survival benefit from Herceptin (Trastuzumab) in patients selected by fluorescence in site hybridization (FISH). *Proc Am Soc Clin Oncol* 2001; 20:22a (abstra 85).

98. Vogel C, Cobleigh M, Tripathy D, Mass R, Murphy M, Stewart SJ. Superior outcomes with Herceptin (trastuzumab) (H) in fluorescence in situ hybridization (FISH)-selected patients. *Proc Am Soc Clin Oncol* 2001; 20:22a (abstra 86).

99. Burstein HJ, Kuter I, Campos SM, Gelman RS, Tribou L, Parker LM, et al. Clinical activity of trastuzumab and vinorelbine in women with HER2-overexpressing metastatic breast cancer. *J Clin Oncol* 2001; 19(10):2722–2730.

100. Slamon DJ, Patel R, Northfelt R, Pegram M, Rubin J, Sebastian G, et al. Phase II pilot study of herceptin combined with taxotere and carboplatin (TCH) in metastatic breast cancer (MBC) patients overexpressing the HER2-neu proto-oncogene: a pilot study of the UCLA network. *Proc Am Soc Clin Oncol* 2001; 20:49a (abstr 193).

17 Farnesyltransferase Inhibitors as Anticancer Agents

Adrienne D. Cox, PhD

CONTENTS

1. INTRODUCTION

The long awaited molecular age of cancer diagnostics and pharmaceuticals is arriving at last, and it is fitting that drugs designed to interfere in the function of Ras, the first oncogenic protein found in human tumors, are leading the way. One class of such drugs, farnesyltransferase inhibitors (FTIs), illustrate both the promise and the cautions that accompany such molecularly targeted therapies. On one hand, FTIs represent a class of rationally designed drugs targeting the farnesyltransferase (FTase) enzyme that posttranslationally modifes Ras and other farnesylated proteins, and they have shown some efficacy in clinical trials as anticancer agents. On the other hand, several surprises have accompanied the development of FTIs, the most important of which is that FTIs do not inhibit Ras function primarily; indeed, the ultimate downstream targets of FTase inhibition are yet to be identified. This review describes the development of FTIs as anti-Ras and anticancer treatments, from both a basic and a translational science perspective, ending with a discussion of present understanding and future prospects for this novel class of therapeutic agents.

2. Ras ONCOGENES AS TARGETS FOR ANTICANCER THERAPY

The Ras family of small GTPases normally act as biological on/off switches to regulate diverse cellular functions including proliferation, differentiation, and death *(1)*. Regulated themselves by binding either to GTP (in the "on" state) or to GDP (in the "off" state), Ras proteins are part of a complex molecular circuitry in which multiple pathways interact to relay signals from cell surface to nucleus and ultimately alter the

From: *Oncogene-Directed Therapies*
Edited by: J. W. Rak © Humana Press Inc., Totowa, NJ

expression profile of the numerous genes whose promoters contain Ras-responsive elements. In more than 30% of all human cancers, the Ras signaling circuitry is up-regulated, either by mutations (typically at codons 12, 13, or 61) that cause Ras to assume a constitutively active GTP-bound conformation, or by amplification or overexpression of normal Ras that also results in excess Ras-GTP activity *(2)*. Elegant studies have shown that the loss of such aberrant Ras activity impairs maintenance of the tumorigenic phenotype in a variety of systems, including in human tumor cell lines that lack their activated K-ras (13D) allele due to homologous recombination *(3)* or their activated N-ras (61K) allele due to chromosomal transfer *(4)*, and in a mouse melanoma model genetically engineered to express a tetracycline-inducible H-Ras (12V) mutant *(5)*. Such studies, in which genetic loss of oncogenic Ras function impairs tumorigenicity even in the continued presence of other genetic mutations, provide support for the idea that pharmacological targeting of Ras as anticancer therapy can have a real impact on human disease.

3. TARGETING Ras POSTTRANSLATIONAL PROCESSING WITH FTIS

To be localized correctly within the cell and to be biologically active, Ras proteins must be modified posttranslationally in a series of steps beginning with a farnesyl isoprenoid lipid modification at a carboxy-terminal cysteine that is part of the CAAX motif, where C = cysteine, A = aliphatic, and X = any amino acid *(6–8)*. Farnesol is an obligate intermediate in the cholesterol biosynthetic pathway, and the attachment of the farnesyl group to Ras proteins is the obligate initial step in Ras processing *(9–11)*; subsequent steps include endoproteolytic cleavage of the AAX residues, followed by carboxymethylation of the now-terminal farnesylated cysteine, and then by palmitoylation of the upstream cysteine(s) of H-Ras, N-Ras, or K-Ras4A. K-Ras4B has a stretch of six contiguous lysines upstream of the CAAX motif instead of the palmitoylatable cysteines. Following the completion of each of these steps, Ras proteins localize to the inner surface of the plasma membrane where they can be activated by their upstream regulators and where they can, in turn, signal to downstream effector target molecules.

The farnesyl modification is carried out by the enzyme FTase *(12,13)*, which transfers the farnesyl moiety from farnesyl pyrophosphate (FPP) to substrate proteins containing CAAX motifs terminating in specific amino acids, especially S, M, Q, A, and T (in H-Ras, X = S; in N- and K-Ras, X = M). Even before it was shown that the newly identified FTase enzyme could be inhibited by tetrapeptides mimicking the Ras CAAX motif *(13)*, FTase became a target for a tremendous effort in rational drug design of FTase inhibitors (FTIs) *(14,15)*.

Many FTIs have been discovered and/or synthesized from natural fungal and plant products to combinatorial libraries to rationally designed peptide mimetics to nonpeptidic nonthiol-containing compounds that are competitive with respect to FPP, to the CAAX motif, or even bisubstrate compounds containing different portions of the molecule, each of which is competitive with respect to FPP or CAAX. The development of these compounds has been reviewed thoroughly *(2,16–19)*. Initially, FTIs were tested for their ability to block Ras processing and biological activity in signaling and transformation assays including MAPK activation, transcriptional transactivation, proliferation, focus formation, soft agar colony formation, and tumorigenicity of Ras-transformed rodent model cell lines. Now, such compounds are conventionally screened first for their ability to inhibit FTase attachment of FPP to an H-Ras substrate in vitro, then for their ability to inhibit the growth of human tumor cell lines in monolayer culture and in soft agar colony forming assays. If the compounds demonstrate selectivity for inhibition of FTase compared to the related enzyme geranylgeranyltransferase I (GGTase I), which recognizes CAAX motifs where X = L, as well as for inhibition of tumor cells vs normal cells, then the next step is screening in nude mouse or transgenic mouse tumorigenicity assays. Several FTIs that inhibit Ras processing and decrease tumor growth in animals with little toxicity have been brought to clinical trials; some of these trials have progressed recently as far as phase II/III efficacy studies, as will be discussed below. However, it is critical to remember that, despite the original intent of their design and of their ability to inhibit Ras farnesylation and biological activity, FTIs are not actually anti-Ras drugs; instead, they are anti-FTase drugs. This distinction has important implications for the ways in which FTIs may be used as anticancer therapy.

3.1. Ras, RhoB, and Other Targets of FTIs

Because FTIs were initially designed and thought of as anti-Ras drugs, it was a great surprise when studies showed that *(i)* *ras* mutation status was not correlated with FTI sensitivity *(20); (ii)* the time course of phenotypic reversion following FTI treatment was often too short to be explained by the mere cessation of processing of newly synthesized Ras proteins that have an approx 24-h half-life *(21,22);* and *(iii)* FTI treatment resulted in a loss of processing of H-Ras but not of K-Ras proteins *(23).* The latter findings were explained by work demonstrating that K-Ras and N-Ras (CAAX X = M), but not H-Ras (CAAX X = S), could become substrates for alternative prenylation by the enzyme GGTase I when FTase was inhibited by FTIs *(24–26).* This alternative prenylation thus allowed K- and N-Ras to escape the loss of processing that H-Ras underwent upon FTI treatment, and possibly explained some of the surprising lack of FTI toxicity to normal cells, by permitting the continued function of endogenous normal K- and N-Ras *(27).* Nevertheless, these results forced the recognition that the loss of Ras farnesylation might not be the explanation for the ability of FTIs to inhibit tumor growth in cells transformed by oncogenes other than H-Ras itself. It seems clear that tumor cells containing oncogenically mutated H-Ras and wild-type p53 tumor suppressor protein are quite susceptible to FTI treatment *(28,29),* and there are other reports of FTI sensitivity paralleling Ras mutation *(30)* or activity *(31),* but in many cases the role of Ras is not so clear. Instead, additional farnesylated protein substrates of FTase must provide biologically relevant targets of FTIs. The search for such target(s) is still underway as of this writing, although a compelling case has been made for the Ras-related protein, RhoB, as one possibility that can explain some, but not all, consequences of FTI treatment *(32).*

RhoB, a member of the Rho family of Ras-related GTPases, is an immediate early protein with a short half-life (T1/2 2 to 3 h) *(33)* and an unusual carboxylterminal sequence (CCKVL) *(34).* It has the distinctive property of being the only prenylated protein known to contain populations that are either farnesylated (F) or geranylgeranylated (GG) *(34,35).* Evidence that RhoB may mediate some of the biological consequences of FTI treatment includes the ability of RhoB-GG to reverse morphological transformation and to inhibit growth of Ras-transformed, but not normal, Rat-1 fibroblasts *(36,37).* Further, cells from RhoB knock-out mice are resistant to FTI-mediated apopotosis *(37)*. On the other hand, there is also evidence to suggest that RhoB cannot be the only physiologically relevant target of FTIs. For example, one study *(38)* showed that both F and GG forms of RhoB are growth inhibitory in human tumor cells, implying that FTI treatment, which causes an increase in the amount of RhoB-GG (via alternative prenylation following inhibition of farnesylation), would not, thereby, switch RhoB from a tumorigenic or neutral phenotype to a growth inhibitory phenotype. In RhoB knock-out mice, FTI treatment was still able to mediate inhibition of anchorage-independent growth *(37)*, indicating that the presence of RhoB is not necessary for this response to FTIs. Therefore, at least one target in addition to or instead of Ras and RhoB must be important for mediating FTI responsiveness.

3.2. Effect of FTIs on Cell Cycle

FTIs have been reported to have a variable effect on the cell cycle, but most often cause arrest in the G2/M phase *(39,40)*. This led to speculation that the loss of function of the farnesylated centromere binding proteins CENP-E and CENP-F could be responsible for cellular sensitivity to FTIs *(41)*. Other evidence has emerged from a study of A549 and Calu-1 human lung carcinoma cell lines to suggest that the FTI-2153 blocks bipolar spindle formation and chromosome alignment, thereby preventing cells from progressing from prophase to metaphase *(42)*. In addition, human tumor cell lines bearing H-RAS mutations and wild-type p53 accumulate in G1, presumably due to the induction of p53 and the cyclin-dependent kinase (CDK) inhibitor p21$^{Waf/Cip}$, which resulted from FTI treatment with L-744,832 or SCH 66336 *(28,29,43)*. Thus, multiple effects of FTIs on cell cycle progression are possible and appear to be cell context-dependent.

3.3. Effect of FTIs on Cell Survival

Because FTIs prevent the processing of newly synthesized proteins, but do not cause the removal of prenyl groups from proteins already processed, it was assumed that they would be cytostatic, but not cytotoxic, drugs. Indeed, when used as single agents, FTIs do not cause apoptosis under most conditions. However, loss of anchorage causes cells in culture to become susceptible to induction of apoptosis by FTIs *(44)*, as does removal of growth factors by serum deprivation *(45)*. Disrupting the PI3-K/Akt survival pathway with LY294002 enhances FTI-induced apoptosis *(45–48)*, whereas constitutively active Akt2 can rescue it *(47)*. Further, cell cycle inhibitors such as roscovitine and olomoucine, which inhibit CDKs, synergize with FTIs to promote apoptosis in transformed cells including leukemic (HL-60, CEM) and prostate cancer (LNCaP) cell lines *(48)*; the increase in release of mitochrondrial cytochrome c results in caspase-3 activation and apoptosis. Interestingly, FTase itself has been shown to be a target of caspase-3 cleavage during apoptosis *(49)*, although this effect is shared with GGTase I, as it is the α subunit shared by FTase and GGTase I that is the caspase-3 substrate.

Finally, although the mechanistic explanation is unknown, in general FTIs are cytostatic in vivo when tested in nude mouse tumorigenicity studies, but can be cytotoxic when tested in transgenic mice. Dramatic and rapid regression was seen in H-RAS transgenic mice where the H-RAS transgene was driven by a mouse mammary tumor virus (MMTV) promoter or by the whey acidic protein (Wap) promoter *(43,50,51)*; less dramatic results were seen in N-Ras *(52)* and K-Ras transgenics *(53)*, presumably due to less efficient inhibition of Ras processing in these Ras-driven tumor models. A critical question for clinical trials and ultimate clinical utility is whether humans are more like nude mice or transgenic mice in this respect.

3.4. FTI Inhibition of Other Aspects of the Transformed Phenotype

In addition to deregulation of proliferation and cell survival, the development and maintenance of the malignant state include such characteristics as increased angiogenesis and decreased oxygenation in the tumor bed. When FTIs were regarded primarily as anti-Ras drugs, it was reasonably assumed that of course they should also block angiogenesis, which can be induced by Ras-mediated increases in vascular endothelial growth factor (VEGF) *(54,55);* however, if FTIs act via other, non-Ras targets, then their anti-angiogenic properties might be more difficult to predict. Although few studies have addressed this question specifically, the FTI A-170634 did reduce VEGF-induced angiogenesis in a corneal neovascularization model *(56).* Further, the FTI L744,832 reduced EGFRvIII-mediated VEGF secretion in astrocytoma cells *(57,58),* as well as tumor hypoxia in T24-tumor bearing nude mice *(59).* These studies support the notion that the overall effects of FTIs in cancer treatment may not be limited to effects on proliferation or survival, and instead may come ultimately from inhibition of multiple aspects of the transformed phenotype.

4. UTILITY OF FTIS IN CANCER TREATMENT

FTIs have demonstrated activity against a wide variety of human tumor cell lines in vitro in soft agar colony forming assays, including those resistant to conventional cytotoxic anticancer agents such as doxorubicin, cisplatin, and paclitaxel *(60),* and, accordingly, the first large groups of phase I clinical trials world-wide with FTIs as single agents (R115777, SCH 66336, L778, 123, and BMS-214662) have been performed in a wide variety of human tumor types *(61).* Common toxicities have been reversible myelosuppression and fatigue, which are likely to be mechanism-related. Dose-limiting toxicity (DLT) for R115777 has been reported to be either neutropenia or neuropathy *(62)* depending on the trial, whereas gastrointestinal toxicity was the DLT for SCH 66336 *(63);* both of these drugs are orally bioavailable. L778,123 is no longer being put forward for trials due to structure-related cardiac toxicity, i.e., prolongation of the Q-T interval. This leaves most trials currently using the remaining three, with others under development. Interestingly, BMS-214662, which is currently given intravenously, appears to have an additional activity that allows it to be cytotoxic rather than simply cytostatic *(64),* and much effort is now being devoted to determining the characteristics of the compound causing this additional activity. Although initial phase I studies provided only hints of efficacy, with occasional partial responses reported, much effort is being devoted to optimizing the types of trials that will unmask the best ways in which to use this new class of drug. These trials are often accompanied by examination of a variety of surrogate markers, including measurement of inhibition of the FTase enzyme itself, as well as appearance of the unprocessed forms of H-Ras, the chaperone protein HDJ-2, and the nuclear structural protein lamin A *(65).*

4.1. Patient/Tumor Selection

In addition to the evidence cited above in Section 3.1. that FTIs may be particularly useful in tumors containing mutated H-Ras and wild-type p53, two other classes of tumors appear to be especially interesting targets for FTIs as a result of phase I/II clinical trials: hematopoietic malignancies, especially BCR/ABL positive leukemias *(66,67)*, and astrocytomas/gliomas. Although in general, FTIs did not demonstrate efficacy when used as single agents, reports of efficacy in phase I studies in the latter two tumor types have been encouraging. In particular, a very recent report indicated a 29% response rate in poor-risk acute leukemias, including two complete remissions *(68)*, although, oddly, no N-Ras mutations were found in any of the patient samples. Thus, although nearly all of the initial trials were naturally focused on those tumors in which Ras mutations were common (pancreas, colon, non-small cell lung cancer [NSCLC]), many of the more recent trials of FTIs as single agents are now focused on either tumors in which H-*ras* mutations are involved (head and neck) or tumors where FTIs have already demonstrated some signs of efficacy (leukemias, gliomas). It is also worth mentioning that preclinical studies have shown breast tumors to be particularly sensitive to FTIs, although in the absence of Ras mutations in this tumor type and a clear consensus on other biologically relevant targets of FTIs, it is not clear why this is the case. Most speculation centers on either Ras being important via its up-regulation downstream of enhanced activity of epidermal growth factor receptor (EGFR) family members or RhoB controlling other Rho family members.

4.2. FTIs in Combination Therapies

For the most part, FTIs are likely to be most useful when combined with other therapies. Indeed, combinations in vitro, as well as in vivo, in preclinical animal models of FTI and conventional cytotoxics have shown enhanced activity *(51,69,70)*. Synergy with taxanes is particularly impressive *(71–73)*, and recent clinical trials have been designed accordingly. An important consideration is that of sequencing: BMS-214662 has been shown to provide sequence-specific synergy with taxanes, such as paclitaxel, only when the FTI is administered (30 min) after the paclitaxel. Whether this sequence-specific synergy is due to the reported ability of paclitaxel to increase apoptosis when MEK is also inhibited *(74)* is unclear. Other combinations currently underway are with topoisomerase I inhibitors, such as irinotecan, and with topoisomerase II inhibitors, such as etoposide, to which ras mutation-positive tumors have been shown to be more sensitive than tumors lacking such mutations *(75)*. Finally, clinical trials are ongoing that combine FTIs with radiation therapy, as FTIs have been shown to be radiosensitizers, particularly where oncogenic H-Ras is present *(76–78)*. As the results of these trials become available, it is likely that both empirical and mechanistic advances in our understanding of FTI action will be obtained.

5. FUTURE PROSPECTS

Although no longer utilized as originally intended, i.e., strictly as anti-Ras drugs, FTIs are now being tested in the clinic for use as anticancer agents in a variety of tumor types. Their ultimate downstream targets have yet to be identified, and it is not yet clear which patient populations are the most suitable for treatment. The best schedules and combinations are currently being worked out empirically, and it is not yet known whether resistance will become a problem. Clearly these will be neither blockbuster drugs nor silver bullets. Nevertheless, the initial demonstrations of activity of FTIs in leukemias, gliomas, and breast cancer suggest that, despite the many surprises regarding mechanism that have been uncovered along the way, FTIs will ultimately become one of the first rationally designed anticancer agents to truly usher in the age of molecular medicine.

REFERENCES

1. Shields JM, Pruitt K, McFall A, Shaub A, Der CJ. Understanding Ras: 'it ain't over 'til it's over'. *Trends Cell Biol* 2000; 10:147–154.
2. Cox AD, Der CJ. Farnesyltransferase inhibitors and cancer treatment: targeting simply Ras? *Biochim Biophys Acta* 1997; 1333:F51–F71.
3. Shirasawa S, Furuse M, Yokoyama N, Sasazuki T. Altered growth of human colon cancer cell lines disrupted at activated Ki-ras. *Science* 1993; 260:85–88.
4. Plattner R, Anderson MJ, Sato KY, Fasching CL, Der CJ, Stanbridge EJ. Loss of oncogenic ras expression does not correlate with loss of tumorigenicity in human cells. *Proc Natl Acad Sci USA* 1996; 93:6665–6670.
5. Chin L, Pomerantz J, Polsky D, Jacobson M, Cohen C, Cordon-Cardo C, et al. Cooperative effects of INK4a and ras in melanoma susceptibility in vivo. *Genes Dev* 1997; 11:2822–2834.
6. Casey PJ, Solski PA, Der CJ, Buss JE. p21ras is modified by a farnesyl isoprenoid. *Proc Natl Acad Sci USA* 1989; 86:8323–8327.
7. Schafer WR, Kim R, Sterne R, Thorner J, Kim SH, Rine J. Genetic and pharmacological suppression of oncogenic mutations in ras genes of yeast and humans. *Science* 1989; 245:379–385.
8. Schaber MD, O'Hara MB, Garsky VM, Mosser SC, Bergstrom JD, Moores SL, et al. Polyisoprenylation of Ras in vitro by a farnesyl-protein transferase. *J Biol Chem* 1990; 265:14701–14704.
9. Glomset JA, Gelb MH, Farnsworth CC. Prenyl proteins in eukaryotic cells: a new type of membrane anchor. *Trends Biochem Sci* 1990; 15:139–142.
10. Maltese WA. Posttranslational modification of proteins by isoprenoids in mammalian cells. *Faseb J* 1990; 4:3319–3328.
11. Zhang FL, Casey PJ. Protein prenylation: molecular mechanisms and functional consequences. *Annu Rev Biochem* 1996; 65:241–269.
12. Manne V, Roberts D, Tobin A, O'Rourke E, De Virgilio M, Meyers C, et al. Identification and preliminary characterization of protein-cysteine farnesyltransferase. *Proc Natl Acad Sci USA* 1990; 87:7541–7545.
13. Reiss Y, Goldstein JL, Seabra MC, Casey PJ, Brown MS. Inhibition of purified p21ras farnesyl:protein transferase by Cys-AAX tetrapeptides. *Cell* 1990; 62:81–88.
14. Gibbs JB. Ras C-terminal processing enzymes-new drug targets? *Cell* 1991; 65:1–4.
15. Gibbs JB, Oliff A, Kohl NE. Farnesyltransferase inhibitors: Ras research yields a potential cancer therapeutic. *Cell* 1994; 77:175–178.
16. Gelb MH, Scholten JD, Sebolt-Leopold JS. Protein prenylation: from discovery to prospects for cancer treatment. *Curr Opin Chem Biol* 1998; 2:40–48.
17. Rowinsky EK, Windle JJ, Von Hoff DD. Ras protein farnesyltransferase: a strategic target for anticancer therapeutic development. *J Clin Oncol* 1999; 17:3631–3652.
18. Oliff A. Farnesyltransferase inhibitors: targeting the molecular basis of cancer. *Biochim Biophys Acta* 1999; 1423:C19–C30.
19. Sebti SM, Hamilton AD. Farnesyltransferase and geranylgeranyltransferase I inhibitors in cancer therapy: important mechanistic and bench to bedside issues. *Expert Opin Investing Drugs* 2000; 9:2767–2782.
20. Sepp-Lorenzino L, Ma Z, Rands E, Kohl NE, Gibbs JB, Oliff A, et al. A peptidomimetic inhibitor of farnesyl:protein transferase blocks the anchorage-dependent and -independent growth of human tumor cell lines. *Cancer Res* 1995; 55:5302–5309.
21. Prendergast GC, Davide JP, deSolms SJ, Giuliani EA, Graham SL, Gibbs JB, et al. Farnesyltransferase inhibition causes morphological reversion of ras-transformed cells by a complex mechanism that involves regulation of the actin cytoskeleton. *Mol Cell Biol* 1994; 14:4193–4202.
22. Cox AD, Garcia AM, Westwick JK, Kowalczyk JJ, Lewis MD, Brenner DA, et al. The CAAX peptidomimetic compound B581 specifically blocks farnesylated, but not geranylgeranylated or myristylated, oncogenic ras signaling and transformation. *J Biol Chem* 1994; 269: 19203–19206.
23. Lerner EC, Zhang TT, Knowles DB, Qian Y, Hamilton AD, Sebti SM. Inhibition of the prenylation of K-Ras, but not H- or N-Ras, is highly resistant to CAAX peptidomimetics and requires both a farnesyltransferase and a geranylgeranyltransferase I inhibitor in human tumor cell lines. *Oncogene* 1997; 15:1283–1288.

24. Whyte DB, Kirschmeier P, Hockenberry TN, Nunez-Oliva I, James L, Catino JJ, et al. K- and N-Ras are geranylgeranylated in cells treated with farnesyl protein transferase inhibitors. *J Biol Chem* 1997; 272:14459–14464.

25. Zhang FL, Kirschmeier P, Carr D, James L, Bond RW, Wang L, et al. Characterization of Ha-ras, N-ras, Ki-Ras4A, and Ki-Ras4B as in vitro substrates for farnesyl protein transferase and geranylgeranyl protein transferase type I. *J Biol Chem* 1997; 272:10232–10239.

26. Rowell CA, Kowalczyk JJ, Lewis MD, Garcia AM. Direct demonstration of geranylgeranylation and farnesylation of Ki-Ras in vivo. *J Biol Chem* 1997; 272:14093–14097.

27. James G, Goldstein JL, Brown MS. Resistance of K-RasBV12 proteins to farnesyltransferase inhibitors in Rat1 cells. *Proc Natl Acad Sci USA* 1996; 93:4454–4458.

28. Sepp-Lorenzino L, Rosen N. A farnesyl-protein transferase inhibitor induces p21 expression and G1 block in p53 wild type tumor cells. *J Biol Chem* 1998; 273:20243–20251.

29. Ashar HR, James L, Gray K, Carr D, McGuirk M, Maxwell E, et al. The farnesyl transferase inhibitor SCH 66336 induces a G(2) → M or G(1) pause in sensitive human tumor cell lines. *Exp Cell Res* 2001; 262:17–27.

30. Nagasu T, Yoshimatsu K, Rowell C, Lewis MD, Garcia AM. Inhibition of human tumor xenograft growth by treatment with the farnesyl transferase inhibitor B956. *Cancer Res* 1995; 55:5310–5314.

31. Feldkamp MM, Lau N, Roncari L, Guha A. Isotype-specific Ras. GTP-levels predict the efficacy of farnesyl transferase inhibitors against human astrocytomas regardless of Ras mutational status. *Cancer Res* 2001; 61:4425–4431.

32. Lebowitz PF, Prendergast GC. Non-Ras targets of farnesyltransferase inhibitors: focus on Rho. *Oncogene* 1998; 17:1439–1445.

33. Jahner D, Hunter T. The ras-related gene rhoB is an immediate-early gene inducible by v-Fps, epidermal growth factor, and platelet-derived growth factor in rat fibroblasts. *Mol Cell Biol* 1991; 11:3682–3690.

34. Adamson P, Marshall CJ, Hall A, Tilbrook PA. Post-translational modifications of p21rho proteins. *J Biol Chem* 1992; 267:20033–20038.

35. Armstrong SA, Hannah VC, Goldstein JL, Brown MS. CAAX geranylgeranyl transferase transfers farnesyl as efficiently as geranylgeranyl to RhoB. *J Biol Chem* 1995; 270:7864–7868.

36. Du W, Prendergast GC. Geranylgeranylated RhoB mediates suppression of human tumor cell growth by farnesyltransferase inhibitors. *Cancer Res* 1999; 59:5492–5496.

37. Liu A, Du W, Liu JP, Jessell TM, Prendergast GC. RhoB alteration is necessary for apoptotic and antineoplastic responses to farnesyltransferase inhibitors. *Mol Cell Biol* 2000; 20:6105–6113.

38. Chen Z, Sun J, Pradines A, Favre G, Adnane J, Sebti SM. Both farnesylated and geranylgeranylated RhoB inhibit malignant transformation and suppress human tumor growth in nude mice. *J Biol Chem* 2000; 275:17974–17978.

39. Miquel K, Pradines A, Sun J, Qian Y, Hamilton AD, Sebti SM, et al. GGTI-298 induces G0-G1 block and apoptosis whereas FTI-277 causes G2-M enrichment in A549 cells. *Cancer Res* 1997; 57:1846–1850.

40. Song SY, Meszoely IM, Coffey RJ, Pietenpol JA, Leach SD. K-Ras-independent effects of the farnesyl transferase inhibitor L-744,832 on cyclin B1/Cdc2 kinase activity, G2/M cell cycle progression and apoptosis in human pancreatic ductal adenocarcinoma cells. *Neoplasia* 2000; 2:261–272.

41. Ashar HR, James L, Gray K, Carr D, Black S, Armstrong L, et al. Farnesyl transferase inhibitors block the farnesylation of CENP-E and CENP-F and alter the association of CENP-E with the microtubules. *J Biol Chem* 2000; 275:30451–30457.

42. Crespo NC, Ohkanda J, Yen TJ, Hamilton AD, Sebti SM. The farnesyltransferase inhibitor, FTI-2153, blocks bipolar spindle formation and chromosome alignment and causes prometaphase accumulation during mitosis of human lung cancer cells. *J Biol Chem* 2001; 276:16161–16167.

43. Barrington RE, Subler MA, Rands E, Omer CA, Miller PJ, Hundley JE, et al. A farnesyltransferase inhibitor induces tumor regression in transgenic mice harboring multiple oncogenic mutations by mediating alterations in both cell cycle control and apoptosis. *Mol Cell Biol* 1998; 18:85–92.

44. Lebowitz PF, Sakamuro D, Prendergast GC. Farnesyl transferase inhibitors induce apoptosis of Ras-transformed cells denied substratum attachment. *Cancer Res* 1997; 57:708–713.

45. Suzuki N, Urano J, Tamanoi F. Farnesyltransferase inhibitors induce cytochrome c release and caspase 3 activation preferentially in transformed cells. *Proc Natl Acad Sci USA* 1998; 95:15356–15361.

46. Du W, Liu A, Prendergast GC. Activation of the P13'K-AKT pathway masks the proapoptotic effects of farnesyltransferase inhibitors. *Cancer Res* 1999; 59:4208–4212.

47. Jiang K, Coppola D, Crespo NC, Nicosia SV, Hamilton AD, Sebti SM, et al. The phosphoinositide 3-OH kinase/AKT2 pathway as a critical target for farnesyltransferase inhibitor-induced apoptosis. *Mol Cell Biol* 2000; 20:139–148.

48. Edamatsu H, Gau CL, Nemoto T, Guo L, Tamanoi F. Cdk inhibitors, roscovitine and olomoucine, synergize with farnesyltransferase inhibitor (FTI) to induce efficient apoptosis of human cancer cell lines. *Oncogene* 2000; 19:3059-3068.

49. Kim KW, Chung HH, Chung CW, Kim IK, Miura M, Wang S, et al. Inactivation of farnesyltransferase and geranylgeranyltransferase I by caspase-3: cleavage of the common alpha subunit during apoptosis. *Oncogene* 2001; 20:358–366.

50. Kohl NE, Omer CA, Conner MW, Anthony NJ, Davide JP, deSolms SJ, et al. Inhibition of farnesyltransferase induces regression of mammary and salivary carcinomas in ras transgenic mice. *Nat Med* 1995; 1:792–797.

51. Liu M, Bryant MS, Chen J, Lee S, Yaremko B, Lipari P, et al. Antitumor activity of SCH 66336, an orally bioavailable tricyclic inhibitor of farnesyl protein transferase, in human tumor xenograft models and wap-ras transgenic mice. *Cancer Res* 1998; 58:4947–4956.

52. Mangues R, Corral T, Kohl NE, Symmans WF, Lu S, Malumbres M, et al. Antitumor effect of a farnesyl protein transferase inhibitor in mammary and lymphoid tumors overexpressing N-ras in transgenic mice. *Cancer Res* 1998; 58:1253–1259.

53. Omer CA, Chen Z, Diehl RE, Conner MW, Chen HY, Trumbauer ME, et al. Mouse mammary tumor virus-Ki-rasB transgenic mice develop mammary carcinomas that can be growth-inhibited by a farnesyl:protein transferase inhibitor. *Cancer Res* 2000; 60:2680–2688.

54. Charvat S, Duchesne M, Parvaz P, Chignol MC, Schmitt D, Serres M. The up-regulation of vascular endothelial growth factor in mutated Ha-ras HaCaT cell lines is reduced by a farnesyl transferase inhibitor. *Anticancer Res* 1999; 19:557–561.

55. Kerbel RS, Viloria-Petit A, Klement G, Rak J. 'Accidental' anti-angiogenic drugs. anti-oncogene directed signal transduction inhibitors and conventional chemotherapeutic agents as examples. *Eur J Cancer* 2000; 36:1248–1257.

56. Gu WZ, Tahir SK, Wang YC, Zhang HC, Cherian SP, O'Connor S, et al. Effect of novel CAAX peptidomimetic farnesyltransferase inhibitor on angiogenesis in vitro and in vivo. *Eur J Cancer* 1999; 35:1394–1401.

57. Feldkamp MM, Lau N, Rak J, Kerbel RS, Guha A. Normoxic and hypoxic regulation of vascular endothelial growth factor (VEGF) by astrocytoma cells is mediated by Ras. *Int J Cancer* 1999; 81:118–124.

58. Feldkamp MM, Lau N, Guha A. Growth inhibition of astrocytoma cells by farnesyl transferase inhibitors is mediated by a combination of anti-proliferative, pro-apoptotic and anti-angiogenic effects. *Oncogene* 1999; 18:7514–7526.

59. Cohen-Jonathan E, Evans SM, Koch CJ, Muschel RJ, McKenna WG, Wu J, et al. The farnesyltransferase inhibitor L744,832 reduces hypoxia in tumors expressing activated H-ras. *Cancer Res* 2001; 61:2289–2293.

60. Petit T, Izbicka E, Lawrence RA, Bishop WR, Weitman S, Von Hoff DD. Activity of SCH 66336, a tricyclic farnesyltransferase inhibitor, against human tumor colony-forming units. *Ann Oncol* 1999; 10:449–453.

61. Cox AD. Farnesyltransferase inhibitors: potential role in the treatment of cancer. *Drugs* 2001; 61:723–732.

62. Zujewski J, Horak ID, Bol CJ, Woestenborghs R, Bowden C, End DW, et al. Phase I and pharmacokinetic study of farnesyl protein transferase inhibitor R115777 in advanced cancer. *J Clin Oncol* 2000; 18:927–941.

63. Adjei AA, Erlichman C, Davis JN, Cutler DL, Sloan JA, Marks RS, et al. A Phase I trial of the farnesyl transferase inhibitor SCH66336: evidence for biological and clinical activity. *Cancer Res* 2000; 60:1871–1877.

64. Hunt JT, Ding CZ, Batorsky R, Bednarz M, Bhide R, Cho Y, et al. Discovery of (R)-7-cyano-2,3,4, 5-tetrahydro-1-(1H-imidazol-4-ylmethyl) - 3-(phenylmethyl)-4-(2-thienylsulfonyl)-1H-1,4-benzodiazepine (BMS-214662), a farnesyltransferase inhibitor with potent preclinical antitumor activity. *J Med Chem* 2000; 43:3587–3595.

65. Adjei AA, Davis JN, Erlichman C, Svingen PA, Kaufmann SH. Comparison of potential markers of farnesyltransferase inhibition. *Clin Cancer Res* 2000; 6:2318–2325.

66. Peters DG, Hoover RR, Gerlach MJ, Koh EY, Zhang H, Choe K, et al. Activity of the farnesyl protein transferase inhibitor SCH66336 against BCR/ABL-induced murine leukemia and primary cells from patients with chronic myeloid leukemia. *Blood* 2001; 97:1404–1412.

67. Karp JE. Farnesyl protein transferase inhibitors as targeted therapies for hematologic malignancies. *Semin Hematol* 2001; 38:16–23.
68. Karp JE, Lancet JE, Kaufmann SH, End DW, Wright JJ, Bol K, et al. Clinical and biologic activity of the farnesyltransferase inhibitor R115777 in adults with refractory and relapsed acute leukemias: a phase 1 clinical-laboratory correlative trial. *Blood* 2001; 97:3361–3369.
69. Sun J, Blaskovich MA, Knowles D, Qian Y, Ohkanda J, Bailey RD, et al. Antitumor efficacy of a novel class of non-thiol-containing peptidomimetic inhibitors of farnesyltransferase and geranylgeranyl-transferase I: combination therapy with the cytotoxic agents cisplatin, Taxol, and gemcitabine. *Cancer Res* 1999; 59:4919–4926.
70. Adjei AA, Davis JN, Bruzek LM, Erlichman C, Kaufmann SH. Synergy of the protein farnesyltrans-ferase inhibitor SCH66336 and cisplatin in human cancer cell lines. *Clin Cancer Res* 2001; 7:1438–1445.
71. Moasser MM, Sepp-Lorenzino L, Kohl NE, Oliff A, Balog A, Su DS, et al. Farnesyl transferase inhibitors cause enhanced mitotic sensitivity to taxol and epothilones. *Proc Natl Acad Sci USA* 1998; 95:1369–1374.
72. Shi B, Yaremko B, Hajian G, Terracina G, Bishop WR, Liu M, et al. The farnesyl protein transferase inhibitor SCH66336 synergizes with taxanes in vitro and enhances their antitumor activity in vivo. *Cancer Chemother Pharmacol* 2000; 46:387–393.
73. Yeung SC, Xu G, Pan J, Christgen M, Bamiagis A. Manumycin enhances the cytotoxic effect of pacli-taxel on anaplastic thyroid carcinoma cells. *Cancer Res* 2000; 60:650–656.
74. MacKeigan JP, Collins TS, Ting JP. MEK inhibition enhances paclitaxel-induced tumor apoptosis. *J Biol Chem* 2000; 275:38953–38956.
75. Koo HM, Gray-Goodrich M, Kohlhagen G, McWilliams MJ, Jeffers M, Vaigro-Wolff A, et al. The ras oncogene-mediated sensitization of human cells to topoisomerase II inhibitor-induced apoptosis. *J Natl Cancer Inst* 1999; 91:236–244.
76. Brown JM. Therapeutic targets in radiotherapy. *Int J Radiat Oncol Biol Phys* 2001; 49:319–326.
77. Cohen-Jonathan E, Muschel RJ, McKenna WG, Evans SM, Cerniglia G, Mick R, et al. Farnesyltrans-ferase inhibitors potentiate the antitumor effect of radiation on a human tumor xenograft expressing activated HRAS. *Radiat Res* 2000; 154:125–132.
78. Bernhard EJ, Kao G, Cox AD, Sebti SM, Hamilton AD, Muschel RJ, et al. The farnesyltransferase inhibitor FTI-277 radiosensitizes H-ras-transformed rat embryo fibroblasts. *Cancer Res* 1996; 56:1727–1730.

18 Targeting Oncogenic Signaling Pathways in Human Astrocytomas

Gelareh Zadeh, MD
and Abhijit Guha, MD, FRCSC, FACS

CONTENTS

1. INTRODUCTION

1.1. Epidemiology

Tumors of the central nervous system (CNS) can be categorized as primary or secondary. Metastatic or secondary tumors of the CNS are increasing in frequency, as we are better able to control local disease of common human cancers, resulting in longer life expectancy. Incidence of primary CNS tumors are also increasing for reasons that are currently unclear, with approximately 30,000 new cases diagnosed yearly in North America, according to the Central Brain Tumor Registry of the United States in 1998 *(1)*. This represents about 4% of all cancer-related deaths in adults, and the most common pediatric cancer, second only to leukemias. The types, location, and molecular pathogenesis of pediatric CNS tumors are for the most part different from those in adults, with this article restricting its comments to adult tumors. More than 50% of all primary CNS tumors arise from glial cells *(2,3)*, which are further characterized according to their presumed cell of origin, giving rise to astrocytomas, oligodendroglioma, ependymomas, and choroid plexus papillomas.

Among gliomas, astrocytomas are the most common by far, with the most malignant variety termed a glioblastoma multiforme (GBM), which, unfortunately, accounts for more than 50% of all gliomas in adults, with a mean age of onset of 62 yr *(1)*. There is a slight predominance of males in all three astrocytoma grades (male:female ratio 1.2–1.5:1), with no proven predisposing environmental factors. Co-relationships with

From: *Oncogene-Directed Therapies*
Edited by: J. W. Rak © Humana Press Inc., Totowa, NJ

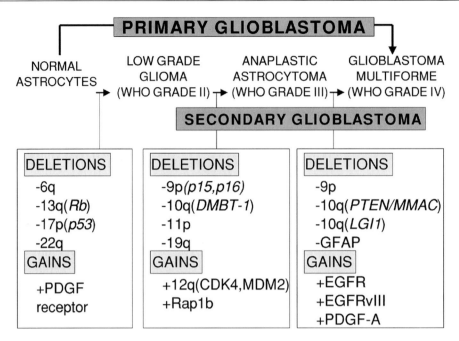

Fig. 1. Molecular pathogenesis of varying grades of human astrocytomas with associated gain and loss of function genetic alterations. At least two molecular progression profiles have been proposed to the most malignant grade IV of astrocytoma, also known as GBM. **(A)** Primary. Usually arising *de novo* in the elderly without presence of p53, Rb, and other genetic alterations. **(B)** Secondary. More prevalent in the younger adult with progression from lower grades of astrocytomas to a GBM. The hallmarks of a GBM, which is the most common grade, is loss of chromosome #10q (PTEN) and gain/amplification of chromosome #7p (wild-type and mutant EGFR).

trauma, radiation exposure, and cell phone use have been speculated. The vast majority of astrocytomas occur sporadically, with germline predisposing syndromes, such as neurofibromatosis-1 (NF-1), Li-Frauemeni, Turcott, and tuberous sclerosis, contributing to less than 5% of all newly diagnosed astrocytomas. However, these syndromes have helped to shed much light into the molecular pathogenesis of the more common sporadic astrocytomas.

1.2. Classification

Astrocytomas are graded according to the World Health Organization (WHO) into four increasing grades of malignancy, which usually progress from lower to higher grades *(4)* (Fig. 1). Pilocytic astrocytomas (WHO grade 1) are infiltrating tumors, usually found in children and young adults, and are characterized by a mild increase in the number of astrocytes and cellular atypia. They usually occur sporadically and are rarely associated with germline predisposition syndromes such as NF-1. Since these tumors usually have a long indolent behavior without progression to higher grades of malignancy, they often do not require any intervention other than close radiological follow-up after the diagnosis is made. Low grade astrocytomas (LGA; WHO grade II) are diffusely infiltrating tumors with moderate cellularity, mild nuclear atypia, and rare or absent mitotic figures. Anaplastic astrocytomas (AA; WHO grade III) are diffusely infiltrating tumors with increased cellularity, nuclear atypia, mitotic activity, and characteristic endothelial hyperproliferation. Finally, GBM (WHO grade IV) are characterized by all the microscopic features of AA, in addition to macroscopic and microscopic heterogeneity, glomeruloid microvascular proliferation, and regional and geographic necrosis *(4)*.

1.3. Current Treatment and Natural History

Grade is the most important prognosticator of astrocytomas *(5)*, with the mean life expectancy of patients with GBMs equal to 9–12 mo, AAs equal to 18 mo, and LGAs equal to 5 yr *(6)*. As mentioned, LGAs usually progress to a GBM, with a mean time to transformation of 4–8 yr *(7,8)*. Patients who present with LGA are typically 1 to 2 decades younger than those who at presentation harbor a GBM *(1,9)*. In addition to grade, other important positive prognosticators include younger age and a good functional state at the time of diagnosis (referred to as the Karnofsky Performance Score: KPS). Molecular and immunohistochemical (IHC) markers of proliferation, such as the Ki67 labeling index, which although increases with grade, has not proven to be an independent prognosticator beyond the main variables mentioned above. Recent evidence from our laboratory examining expression of mutant epidermal growth factor receptor (EGFRvIII) with reverse transcription polymerase chain reaction (RT-PCR), Western blots, and EGFRvIII-specific IHC expression, demonstrates that this common molecular aberration found in GBMs is an independent negative prognosticator, especially in patients less than 50 yr of age *(10)*.

Unfortunately, other than radiation, very little has altered the ultimate prognosis of astrocytomas, especially for GBMs. Aggressive surgical resection, while in certain cases improves the functional level of the patient and allows for a definitive diagnosis to be made, it does little to alter survival. External beam radiation, as evaluated in a landmark randomized controlled trial in 1978 *(11)*, has increased survival in GBMs from its historical levels of 4 mo to the current 9–12 mo *(12)*. Chemotherapy has added little to the median survival of GBM patients, which is most likely related to tumor cell resistance and heterogeneity. Chemotherapeutic agents that have been evaluated are many, including mithramycin *(13)* and BCNU (1,3-bis[2-chloroethyl]-1-nitrosurea; carmustine), with the latter nitrosurea family perhaps demonstrating little and unpredictable efficacy in combination with surgery and radiation in GBMs (36-wk median survival with BCNU vs 34.5 wk without BCNU) *(11)*. Recent attempts to utilize chemotherapy in GBMs include local delivery in the tumor bed after surgery to overcome the blood brain barrier (BBB) and systemic toxicity associated with slow release polymers *(14)*. In addition, a second-generation alkylating agent, temozolomide, has demonstrated some promise in early clinical trials and awaits larger clinical verification *(15,16)*. Compared to GBMs, patients with AAs often do respond to chemotherapy *(17)*, and therefore, they are recommended to receive chemotherapy in addition to surgery and external beam radiation. The discovery that loss of yet to be identified gene(s) on chromosomes #1p and #19q confers chemosensitivity and improved prognosis in oligodendrogliomas *(18)* represents a recent major positive change in the management of gliomas. Whether such chemosensitivity resides in a subpopulation of the much more common astrocytic lineage tumors is an exciting but yet unknown possibility.

2. MOLECULAR GENETICS OF ADULT ASTROCYTOMAS

2.1. Overall Molecular Pathogenesis

The most common adult astrocytoma is the GBM, which may develop *de novo* and are termed primary GBMs, or they may progress from lower grade astrocytomas and are termed secondary GBMs (Fig. 1). Whether all GBMs arise from progression, with the lower grade astrocytoma remaining clinically silent and, hence, presenting only as a primary GBMs, is of debate. However, molecular characterization suggests that these pathologically heterogenous tumors are also molecularly heterogenous, with at least two, if not more, molecular pathways leading to development of a GBM. Similar to other human malignancies, astrocytomas are characterized by the stepwise accumulation of gain-of-function mutations or amplification (oncogenes) and of loss-of-function mutations or deletions (tumor suppressor genes) *(19,20)*. The molecular signatures that seem to be more specific to GBMs, as compared to lower grade astrocytomas, are loss of parts or all of chromosome #10 and amplifications involving chromosome #7. On chromosome #10, loss of *PTEN/MMAC1* expression by mutations, loss of heterozygosity (LOH), and alternative mechanisms of gene silencing have been documented in most GBMs, with yet other tumor suppressor genes to be identified *(21,22)*. Amplifications of chromsome #7 involve *EGFR* in a third of GBM patients, with a large percentage harboring various mutations of *EGFR*, such as *EGFRvIII*, as described in further detail below *(23,24)*.

Additional common genetic alterations in astrocytomas include those that alter the *p53-MDM2-p19/ARF (25,26)* and the *Rb-p16-CDK4* cell cycle regulatory pathways *(27–29)* as discussed below. In addition to *EGFR*, other aberrantly regulated growth factors/receptors and signaling pathways are involved in promoting the proliferation of astrocytoma cells, recruitment of tumor vessels, invasion, apoptosis, etc. These include overexpression of platelet derived growth factor receptors *(PDGFR)* and their cognate ligands *(30–32)*, transforming growth factor *(TGF)*, insulin-like growth factor *(IGF)*, etc. *(33,34)*. Angiogenic-specific growth factors and their cognate receptors that are aberrantly regulated in high grade astrocytomas and contribute to the growth of these highly vascularized tumors, include vascular endothelial growth factor *(VEGF)* *(35,36)*, fibroblast growth factor *(FGF) (37,38)*, and *angiopoietins (39,40)*.

2.2. Aberrations in Cell Cycle Regulatory Pathway

Like a majority of human cancers, perturbations in both the *p53-* and *Rb*-regulated cell cycle regulatory pathways, are present in human astrocytomas. *p53* protein is a transcription factor that can inhibit cell cycle progression or induce apoptosis in response to stress or DNA damage, and inactivation of *p53* attenuates both of these cellular responses *(41,42)*. LOH of chromosome #17p is found in 30–40% of all astrocytomas grades *(44)*. Approximately one third of all astrocytomas with #17p loss have *p53* mutations, with 25% in GBMs, 34% in AA and 30% in LGAs *(45)*. Most mutations are missense mutations found on the conserved domains of exon 5–8, with no clear studies reporting brain-specific mutations, except one study that identified a preponderance of exon 4 mutations in GBMs *(46)*. There is good evidence that a second tumor suppressor gene on chromosome #17p13.3 exists, as a large number of tumors with *17p* LOH do not have corresponding *p53* mutations *(47)*. LOH of *17p* or *p53* mutations are rarely found in GBMS with EGFR amplification. This confirms the presence of two clinical categories of GBM: *(i)* primary or *de novo* GBM with *EGFR* amplification and no *p53* mutation; and *(ii)* secondary or progressive tumors with frequent *p53* mutation and no *EGFR* amplification *(48,49)*.

The *MDM2* oncogene is an important negative regulator of *p53*, which acts in a feedback loop to limit the action of *p53 (50)*, both by inhibiting its transactivating activity and by catalyzing its destruction *(51,52)*. Less than 5% of astrocytomas demonstrate *MDM2* amplification, and none of these tumors have *p53* mutations *(53)*. Furthermore, 50% of GBMs have overexpressed *MDM2* without gene amplification *(54)*. Although overexpressed in a large percentage of GBMs, the functional role of *MDM2* in glioma tumorigenesis remains unknown. Loss of *p19* expression is also prevalent in astrocytomas and seen in 30% of GBMs *(53)*. Since *p19* is a negative regulator of MDM2, this provides another mechanism of aberrant regulation of the *p53*-mediated cell cycle regulatory pathways in astrocytomas.

Similar to the *p53* pathway, loss of either *pRb* or other regulators of the *pRb*-mediated cell cycle regulatory pathway is also prevalent in the majority of astrocytomas. The *p16/cdk4/cyclinD/Rb* cell cycle regulatory pathway is integral in G1 to S phase transition. Inactivation of *p16* through homozygous deletion of *CDKN2A* gene occurs most commonly in 24% of AA and 33% of GBMs *(27,53)*. Rare point mutations of *CDKN2A* or transcriptional silencing due to *CDKN2A* promoter methylation may also inactivate or down-regulate *p16* in GBMs *(55,56)*. *p16* deletion is also associated with a high proliferative index as demonstrated by Ki67 staining *(57)*. LOH of *Rb* or point mutation of the *Rb* gene occurs in 30–40% of GBMs *(27)*, while amplification or overexpression of cdk4 is found in 10–20% of GBMs *(26)*. Primary GBMs demonstrate a higher rate of *p16* deletion compared to secondary GBMs, whereas *pRb* LOH and *CDK4* amplification occurs with similar frequency *(58)*.

2.3. Aberrations in Growth Factors and Growth Factor Receptors

Receptor protein tyrosine kinases (RPTKs) have clearly been linked to the pathogenesis of astrocytomas, with the two major classes being the PDGFR and the EGFR. Human astrocytomas express high amounts of both the *PDGF-A* and *-B* ligands, and together, with their cognate receptors, represent a paracrine and/or autocrine stimulatory action *(30)*. Amplification or mutation of either *PDGF* ligand or receptor genes is rare, though increased expression is common. *PDGFR-α* is overexpressed in 24% of human astrocytomas and probably is a fairly early event in the pathogenesis of astrocytomas, since it is expressed in all grades of astrocytomas compared to normal glial cells *(30)*. *PDGFR-β* is overexpressed in the higher astrocytoma grades and is often associated and postulated to be causally related to the characteristic florid tumor-associated vasculature *(30,59)*. Overexpression of ligands increases with AA and GBMs *(31,60)*, suggesting that the "closing" of the autocrine/paracrine loop is important in the pathogenesis of higher-grade astrocytomas. The functional relevance of these loops in the growth of astrocytomas has been tested with several approaches, including neutralizing antibodies, small molecule inhibitors, and dominant-negative mutants *(32)*. These encouraging preclinical data have led to clinical trials, targeting PDGF-mediated stimulation in astrocytomas, as discussed below.

EGFR, located on chromosome *7p11-p12 (61,62)*, is overexpressed late in the pathogenesis of astrocytomas *(63)*. Unlike *PDGFR*, overexpression of *EGFR* is as a result of gene amplification and/or rearrangement that produces both wild-type and several mutant types of *EGFR*, some of which are truncated and constitutively active. Amplification of *EGFR* is seen in only 3% of LGAs, 7% of AA, but 40–50% of GBMs *(53,63,64)*. The most common mutant *EGFR* in astrocytomas is the receptor variably known as *EGFRvIII* or *p140EGFR*, being expressed in at least 40% of GBMs that have *EGFR* amplification *(65,66)*. Although there are various intragenic deletions that occur in exons 2–7 of *EGFR*, which result in expression of *EGFRvIII*, coercive splicing results in an identical truncated protein in these cases. The mature coercively spliced mRNA encoding the mutant receptor lacks the 801 bases encoding amino acids #6–273 of the wild-type *EGFR*s extracellular domain *(24,66)*. The resulting *EGFRvIII*-truncated protein is constitutively phosphorylated *(66,67)* and confers an in vivo and in vitro growth advantage *(67)*. Our recent studies demonstrate that the cohort of GBMs, especially those patients younger than 50 yr of age, expressing *EGFRvIII* have a worse prognosis *(68)*. At a molecular level, this may be a result of the *EGFRvIII* conferring increased proliferative signals to the astrocytoma cells, along with recent results demonstrating increased protease activity and expression of angiogenic molecules such as *VEGF (69)*. Strategies to target *EGFR* and its mutants are of interest in treatment of GBMs, with early clinical trials initiated.

In addition to PDGF and EGF, other RPTKs have also been implicated in promoting the growth of astrocytomas. These include the *TGFβ* family, expressed in AAs and GBMs, but not in LGAs and normal brain *(70)*. In contrast to its usual physiological role of growth inhibition, *TGFβ* is mitogenic to astrocytoma cell lines *(71)*. This may be due to either an up-regulation of the TGFβ receptors, induction of other growth factors by TGFβ, or a dysregulation of the downstream signaling pathways in higher-grade astrocytomas. For example, both PDGF ligands are induced in astrocytoma cell lines by activation of TGFβ *(72)*, along with EGFR *(73)*, and other angiogenic factors such as VEGF and b-FGF *(74)*.

2.4. Regulators of Astrocytoma Tumor Angiogenesis

Malignant astrocytomas are one of the most vascularized of all human cancers. The tumor-induced vessels, in addition to being numerous, are also abnormal, in that they do not maintain the BBB, leading to peritumoral edema. In addition, they often lack a normal capillary bed, leading to shunting and often intratumoral hemorrhage. Like in other solid cancers, anti-angiogenic therapy, either alone or often in conjunction with radiation or chemotherapy, is an area of intense interest in astrocytomas. Several angiogenic cytokines have been implicated in the tumor-induced neo-angiogenesis, but most factors, such as PDGF, FGFs, and TGFβ have pleotropic effects in addition to their contribution to angiogenesis. However, VEGF and angiopoietins are two angiogenic-specific growth factor families, with aberrant expression in astrocytomas. *VEGF* is highly expressed by GBM cells and is principally induced by tumor hypoxia and aberrant cytokine expression by astrocytoma cells such as *PDGF, EGF*, etc. *(36,69)*. Expression of *VEGFR*s, especially *VEGFR2*, by the tumor endothelium is up-regulated secondary to the hypoxia and increased cytokines by astrocytoma cells. Antibodies against VEGF and VEGFRs, antisense strategies, and small molecule inhibitors have demonstrated encouraging preclinical activity, leading to early clinical trials targeting VEGF.

Similar to VEGF, angiopoietins are specific for angiogenesis in that their receptors are only fond in endothelial cells *(75,76)*. Tie2, the RPTK that is activated by Ang-1 and inhibited by Ang-2, is overexpressed and phosphorylated in GBMs *(39)*. Activation of Tie2 is however not an endothelial cell mitogen, unlike VEGFR2, but is postulated to be involved in vessel maturation. The functional role of angiopoietins in tumor angiogenesis and whether it does interact with VEGF and other angiogenic molecules are under current study in several tumor types, including astrocytomas. Much preclinical work is pending before therapeutic strategies, targeting angiopoietins and/or its receptors, come to the clinical arena.

2.5. Regulators of Astrocytoma Invasion and Cytoskeleton

One of the main reasons why malignant gliomas remain incurable by local therapies, such as surgery or radiation, is their highly infiltrative and invasive nature. The central process of invasion is degradation of the extracellular matrix (ECM) by proteolytic enzymes expressed by tumor cells. Matrix metalloproteases (MMPs), including collagenases, stromelysins, and gelatinases, and serine proteases (including urokinase-type plasminogen activator, uPA, and its receptor, uPAR) play a fundamental role in this process. An imbalance between expression and/or activity of MMPs and their endogenous tissue inhibitors (TIMPs) is, in part, responsible for tumor cell invasion. This is similar to the balance of pro-angiogenic factors and endogenous anti-angiogenic factors that regulate the "angiogenic switch" *(77)*. In fact, the factors that regulate invasion are an integral and vital part of the angiogenesis cascade.

There is a positive correlation between tumor malignancy and level of MMP-2, -9, and -12 expression in astrocytomas *(78,79,80)*. MMP-2 and -9 have created additional interest in GBMs due to their co-localization around proliferating blood vessels, suggesting a role in both angiogenesis and tumor invasion *(78,79)*. Angiogenic factors directly regulate MMP expression, such as VEGF-mediated induction of MMP-1, -3, and -9 in vascular smooth muscle cells *(81)*. This would be required to breakdown the ECM, allowing not only tumor cell invasion but also sprouting of new blood vessels. The endogenous negative tissue regulators of MMPs or TIMPs are also important regulators of astrocytoma invasion. The reports on TIMP-1 and TIMP-2 levels in astrocytomas remains inconclusive, with most of the earlier studies demonstrating a decreased level with increasing glioma grade, whereas recent studies have shown an increase in TIMP-1 in AAs and GBMs compared to LGA and normal brain *(79,82)*. Preclinical investigations with overexpression or underexpression of TIMPs, using cell culture and transgenic models, may be of use in helping decipher which of the TIMPs are of functional relevance in astrocytoma invasion. Exogenous inhibitors of MMPs, known as metalloprotease inhibitors, have shown promise in both preclinical and limited clinical trials in human malignant astrocytomas.

3. ABERRANT SIGNAL TRANSDUCTION PATHWAYS IN ASTROCYTOMA

3.1. p21-ras MAPK

Neuroectodermal-derived tumors, such as astrocytomas, do not harbor activating *p21-ras* mutations, the most common oncogene, which is found in 25–30% of all human cancers *(83)*. However, we have demonstrated that GBMs and their derived cell lines have high levels of p21-ras activation, which is functionally relevant in proliferation, angiogenesis, and radiation resistance *(69,84)*. Increased *p21-ras* activation was also a feature of LGAs, compared to normal brain, suggesting these tumors may also be candidates for agents targeting this pathway, such as farnesyl transferase inhibitors (FTIs), as discussed later. Activated Ras-GTP leads to stimulation of several downstream effector pathways; the most recognized of which is MAPKinase. Activated MAPK appears to follow a somewhat different profile across astrocytoma grades than

Ras-GTP. Although highest in GBMs, MAPK activity levels were not elevated in the LGAs, where Ras-GTP levels were elevated compared to normal brain *(85)*. This suggests that different downstream effector pathways of *p21-ras* are being employed in GBMs and LGAs. In addition to proliferation, MAPK signaling may also regulate angiogenic signals, as evidenced by our results on VEGF transcriptional regulation under normoxic and hypoxic conditions *(86)*. Although inhibition of MAPK activation by MEK (MAPKK) inhibitors do show antiproliferative effects on astrocytoma cells in vitro, their effects in vivo remains to be determined.

3.2. PI 3′ Kinase-Akt/PKB

The PI3′ Kinase (PI3′ K) pathway and its main downstream effector, Akt/PKB, is a major signaling pathway that can be activated in both a *p21-ras*-dependent and -independent manner. This pathway is of relevance in astrocytomas, since it is activated in astrocytoma cell lines (87–89). Additionally, *PTEN/MMAC1*, which is the most common tumor suppressor gene, whose expression is lost in GBMs, is a negative regulator of PI3′K activity. *PTEN* is located on chromosome #10q23, and its expression is lost in many human tumors, including GBMs *(21,22)*. *PTEN* functions as a dual specific protein and lipid phosphatase, with its lipid phosphatase function thought to be critical in its antitumorgenic effects. *PTEN* is an inositol phospholipid phosphatase, dephosphorylating the 3′ phosphate of two main PI3′K products, PtdInsP3 and PtdInsP2, thereby acting as a negative regulator of PI3′K activity *(88,90)*. Unchecked PI3′K activity by mutation, deletion, or gene inactivation of PTEN, results in the accumulation of a major downstream substrate of PI3′K, activated Akt/PKB. It, in turn, promotes cell survival, proliferation, and cytoskeletal organization *(91,92)*.

PTEN/MMAC1 mutations are absent in LGAs, rare in AAs, and detected in 25–30% of GBMs *(93)*. Secondary GBMs progressing from LGAs (Fig. 1) have a 4% frequency of *PTEN* mutations, compared to about a 32% mutational rate detected in the primary or *de novo* GBMs *(53)*. In GBMs, about 18% had both mutations of *PTEN* and amplification of *EGFR*, making these two the most tightly correlated molecular signatures of these tumors. *PTEN* protein expression is lost in over 70–95% of GBMs, suggesting that in addition to mutations and associated LOH, gene inactivation is also a major mechanism contributing to loss of *PTEN* function in these tumors *(88,94,95,96)*. The functional relevance of aberrant PI3′K-Akt/PKB activity and loss of *PTEN* in GBM cell lines has been demonstrated by reintroduction of wild-type *PTEN*, resulting in arrest of the GBM cells in G1 *(21,88,89)*. It should be noted that investigations to identify additional tumor suppressor genes on chromosome #10 in GBMs are ongoing, since multiple areas on both arms of the chromosome are known to be lost in GBMs are *(97)*. For example, *DMBT* is a putative gene on chromosome #10q25.3-26.1, which is homozygously deleted in a subset of GBMs and also in lower grade astrocytomas *(98)*.

3.3. PKC-Mediated Pathways

Protein kinase-C (PKC) is a large family of phospholipid-dependent serine/threonine kinases that are involved in a variety of signal transduction pathways. The various isoforms of PKC differ in their enzymatic properties, tissue expression, and intracellular localization, and consist of an N-terminal regulatory and a C-terminal kinase domain. PKC activation can be induced by increased intracellular calcium, anionic phospholipids, diacylglycerol (DAG), or tumor-promoting phorbol esters *(99)*. PKC is expressed at high levels in the fetal brain and is important in normal proliferation and differentiation of fetal, but not adult, glial cells *(100,101)*. Malignant astrocytomas express high levels of PKC compared to normal adult glial cells, and approach those of fetal astrocytes, perhaps as a result of de-differentiation *(102)*. Certain isozymes appear to be particularly overexpressed, such as α-PKC with antisense constructs directed against the α-PKC, resulting in reversion of the malignant phenotype *(103,104)*. However, it should be noted that the PKC isoforms that are relevant in astrocytomas, their functional role, and alterations with tumor grade is not fully clear, with one study demonstrating an inverse relation of PKC activity with astrocytoma grade *(105)*. Nevertheless, due to encouraging preclinical data with inhibitors of PKC, clinical trials with tamoxifen (a nonspecific PKC inhibitor, with a long track record in management of breast cancer, and known to cross the BBB) has been undertaken as discussed later. It is hoped that some of the encouraging results may be further exploited with more specific PKC isoform inhibitors in the future.

3.4. Apoptotic Pathways

The signaling pathways that regulate apoptosis are of relevance in astrocytomas, as in other tumors. Fas ligand and tumor necrosis factor can induce apoptosis through activation of death receptors such as Fas. Fas is highly expressed in astrocytoma cell lines and tumor specimens, with a direct correlation between levels and grade of tumor. There is also regional variation, with increased expression in areas of necrosis, leading to apoptotic bodies surrounding these regions in GBMs. Increased expression of *Bcl-2* has been reported in GBMs, but not in areas of necrosis. This would suggest that increased *Bcl-2* expression is to counterbalance the apoptotic effects of Fas and Fas ligand expression in GBMs *(106,107)*. It is hoped that our increased understanding of the regulation of these cell death pathways in astrocytomas will allow us to favorably manipulate the balance towards increased apoptosis in these tumors.

4. TARGETED ONCOGENIC SIGNALING PATHWAYS TARGETED IN ASTROCYTOMAS

4.1. Receptor Tyrosine Kinase Inhibitors

EGFRs and PDGFRs are of particular interest in astrocytomas, as discussed above. A variety of approaches have been taken to inhibit these RPTKs, including generation of neutralizing antibodies directed against the extracellular domain of full-length wild-type EGFR *(108)* and antisense therapy against the extracellular domain *(109)*. As astrocytoma cells expressing the truncated *EGFRvIII* confer a growth advantage, toxin-labeled antibodies directed against the novel glycine splice site of *EGFRvIII* may prove useful in blocking the mitogenic advantage conferred by this oncoprotein *(110)*. Additional trials in GBMs with antibody-dependent strategies targeting EGFRvIII is about to be initiated. However, the clinical utility of these approaches may depend in part on the cellular localization of EGFRvIII, as in certain cells, EGFRvIII appears to be primarily localized to a subcellular location, rather than being on the cell surface *(111)*. However, examination of GBM specimens does support that a significant portion of EGFRvIII is accessible to antibodies on the cell surface *(111)*.

Small molecule inhibitors of RPTKs and signaling pathways have the theoretical advantage of penetrating the BBB and reaching the infiltrating astrocytoma cells.

These two challenges may be a major obstacle of macromolecule therapies, such as antibodies and gene-based therapies. Naturally occurring fungal-derived tyrosine kinase inhibitors have shown promise, but have the major disadvantage of being non-specific *(112–114)*. Synthetic tyrosine kinase inhibitors or tyrphostins, based on combinatorial chemistry knowledge of signaling molecules and modifications of natural inhibitors, have shown remarkable specificity. For example, quinazolines such as AG-1478 and PD153035 are potent and specific inhibitors of EGFR, with an IC_{50} in the nanomolar range for PD153035 *(115)*. The quinoxaline AG-1296, on the other hand, is a specific inhibitor of PDGFR *(116)*. The 4,5-dianilinophthalimides are specific inhibitors of both EGFR and ErbB2, but do not inhibit PDGFR *(117)*. Similarly, SU-101 was developed from a drug screen and was shown to have efficacy and specificity against PDGFRs. Promising preclinical results in a variety of human tumor types in immunocompromised mice, including astrocytomas, led to a Phase1 *(118)* followed by a Phase2/3 trial, which has recently been completed, and unfortunately, no benefit was demonstrated. Other inhibitors against this RPTK family are currently undergoing preclinical evaluation. Although the specific mode of action of these tyrosine kinase inhibitors is not known in all cases, most appear to be competitive inhibitors of the ATP binding site on the RPTKs.

Early-generation tyrphostins were shown to inhibit EGF-tyrosine phosphorylation in astrocytoma cell lines in a dose-dependent fashion, which correlates with its potency as an antiproliferative agent in these cell lines *(119)*. The EGFR-specific tyrphostin AG-1478 has recently been evaluated on U87MG astrocytoma cells and U87MG cells transfected to express *EGFRvIII (120)*. Both cells were growth-inhibited by the agent, but U87:*EGFRvIII* cells were considerably more sensitive to the drug's effect. Despite such promising results in tissue culture, early results in nude mice injected with the human epidermoid cancer cell line A431 and treated with the tyrphostin PD153035 have not shown a significant beneficial effect *(121)*.

ZD-1839 (Iressa) is a quinazoline derivative that selectively inhibits the EGFR tyrosine kinase and is under clinical development in cancer patients. The antiproliferative activity of ZD-1839 alone or in combination with cytotoxic drugs differing in mechanism(s) of action, such as cisplatin, carboplatin, doxorubicin, etoposide, etc., was evaluated in vitro and demonstrated antiproliferative and apoptotic effects *(122)*. Also, the antitumor effect of ZD1839 is accompanied by inhibition in the production of autocrine and paracrine growth factors that sustain autonomous local growth and angiogenesis, therefore, this effect can be potentiated by the combined treatment with certain cytotoxic drugs, such as paclitaxel. Promising in vivo results provided a rationale for its clinical evaluation in combination with cytotoxic drugs. Presently, phase 3 clinical trials are being carried out in non-small cell lung cancer, and other tumor types are being considered, including phase 2 trials in astrocytomas *(122,123)*.

4.2. p21-ras *Pathway Inhibitors*

There has been great interest in developing pharmacological agents that inhibit *p21-ras*, since oncogenic mutations are seen in a wide variety of human cancers *(83)*. *p21-ras* pathway inhibition has focussed on FTIs, which blocks the posttranslational modification of *p21-ras*. This posttranslational modification is a 3- or 4-step process which is necessary for *p21-ras* to be recruited to the inner cell membrane and become activated (Fig. 2). The first and most critical step involves the addition of a 15-carbon

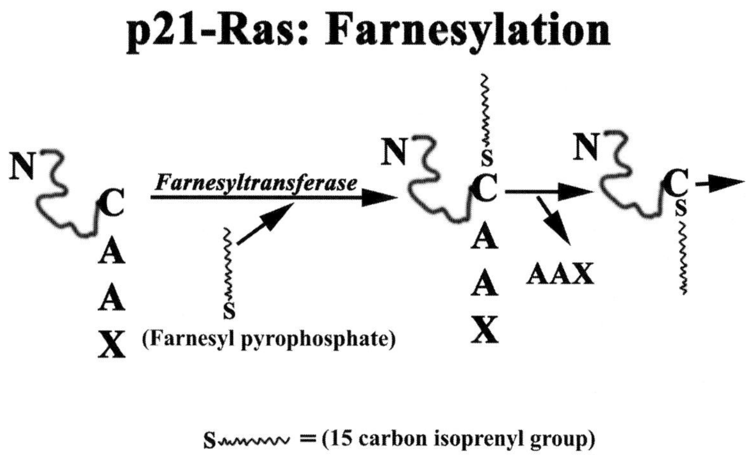

p21-Ras: Farnesylation

S⌇⌇⌇⌇⌇ = (15 carbon isoprenyl group)

Fig. 2. Processing of p21-Ras requires addition of isoprenyl moieties to the C-terminal CAAX box, allowing p21-Ras-GDP to bind to the inner cell membrane, where it can undergo guanine-nucleotide exchange by interaction with signaling molecules generated by activated receptors to become activated Ras-GTP. Ha-Ras is obligatorily farnesylated (15 carbon isoprenyl group added by farnesyl transferase from the donor farnesyl pyrophosphate) and, hence, most sensitive to FTIs K-Ras and, to a lesser extent, N-Ras, can be geranylated if farnesylation is inhibited and, hence, more resistant to FTIs. Astrocytomas, although not harboring oncogenic p21-Ras mutations, do have elevated Ras-GTP levels and are susceptible to growth inhibition by FTIs, which can be predicted by isoform-specific p21-Ras activity assay.

isoprenoid farnesyl pyrophosphate (FPP) through a thioesther bond at the cysteine residue of the CAAX (cysteine, aliphatic amino acid, aliphatic amino acid, other amino acid) box at the extreme C terminus of *p21-ras (124)*. It needs to be pointed out that 1 in 200 cellular proteins undergo farnesylation *(125)*, in addition to *p21-ras* and other members of the *Ras* superfamily, such as Rap2 proteins and RhoB *(106,126)*. Indeed, there is some evidence and debate that much of the antitumor effects of FTIs are not related to its action on *p21-ras* at all, but rather on the alteration of RhoB activity *(127)*. Nevertheless, over the last few years, there has been much interest in creating FTIs in order to target *p21-ras* signaling in human cancers. Developed agents include tetrapeptide analogs of the CAAX motif, benzodiazepine peptidomimetic CAAX inhibitors, FPP analogs, and bisubstrate analogs, which inhibit both FPP and the CAAX motif.

FTIs have been evaluated for their ability to inhibit the progression of a large number of human tumor cell lines. L-739,749 (Merck Pharmaceuticals West Point, PA, USA) was able to inhibit the proliferation of approx 70% of a wide variety of cell lines in anchorage-independent (soft agar) assays *(128-131)*. Our own experiments with the FTIs have demonstrated that the proliferation of a wide variety of GBM cell lines was inhibited in an anchorage-dependent growth assay in a dose-dependent manner *(131)*. At low doses, the effect was reversible with cessation of the drug, while at higher doses, it led to cell kill. Antiproliferative effects were a result of block at both the G1-S and G2-M checkpoints and increased apoptosis. In addition, GBM cell lines transfected to express the mutant *EGFRvIII* were more sensitive to the FTIs than the parental cells, suggesting that this subgroup of patients who have a poorer prognosis perhaps would benefit most from these agents. Furthermore, we have also demonstrated that FTIs also possess anti-angiogenic effects, by reducing the amount of *VEGF* secreted by astrocytoma cells, with the effect being most notable under hypoxic conditions *(132,133)*. Recently, we have demonstrated that indeed FTIs do have significant antitumorgenic effects in a GBM subcutaneous explant model in mice, with both antiproliferative and anti-angiogenic effects *(85)*. In addition, FTIs may be helpful in astrocytomas by radiosensitization of the tumors, since recent data from several laboratories demonstrate that *p21-ras* activity confers radioresistance *(134)*. With these and other preclinical data, demonstrating that GBMs may also be a rationale candidate for FTI therapy, though it does not have any oncogenic *p21-ras* mutations, a phase 1/2 clinical trial has been proposed and, hopefully, will start shortly.

Recognizing the large number of farnesylated proteins and potential side-effects, FTIs do not appear to demonstrate adverse effects on normal cells or in animals at doses that are potent inhibitors of tumor cell mitogenesis *(128)*. FTIs have, however, been shown to suffer from another common problem with conventional chemotherapy, namely that of drug resistance. It has become evident that these inhibitors are much more potent at inhibiting tumors with oncogenic H-Ras mutations than those tumors with K-Ras or N-Ras mutations *(135)*. Farnesylation occurs in all isoforms of *p21-ras*, though there is isoform specificity, with H-ras being fully dependent on it for proper activation. In contrast, K-Ras and, more specifically, K4B-Ras, which are the main oncogenic isoform mutations seen in human cancers, are relatively more resistant to FTIs *(136)*. The explanation for this differential sensitivity is that K-Ras and N-Ras (to a lesser extent), but not H-Ras, can undergo geranyl-geranylation, when farnesylation is inhibited *(136)*. We have recently been able to predict which GBMs would be more sensitive to FTIs, by measuring isoform-specific *p21-ras* activity in the cell lines and GBM explants *(85)*. This measurement can be undertaken on the operative specimens to select the most likely sensitive tumors, as part of future clinical trials.

4.3. Protein Kinase C Inhibitors

Pharmacological inhibitors of the PKC pathway have led to promising initial results in astrocytomas. A variety of nonspecific PKC inhibitors (polymyxin B and tamoxifen) and specific PKC inhibitors (staurosporine) have been shown to reduce astrocytoma cell proliferation *(137,138)*. Tamoxifen caused a dose-dependant inhibition of proliferation in astrocytoma cell lines through an estrogen receptor blockade mechanism *(139,140)*. Earlier clinical trials using the nonspecific PKC inhibitor tamoxifen have been disappointing; despite an established acceptable side-effect profile, this drug has shown only minor benefit in patients with astrocytomas *(141)*. However, more recent studies have reported that 25% of patients had a 50% decrease in tumor vol on magnetic resonance imaging, and 19% had stabilization of their disease *(142)*. 7-hydroxystaurosporine (UCN-01) is more selective for PKC inhibition and produces marked reduction in proliferation of in vitro astrocytoma cell lines and in vivo mouse models *(143)*. Phase 2 clinical trials of UCN-01 have been approved for adult recurrent malignant gliomas. One major hurdle in the use of these inhibitors involves the isozyme specificity of each agent. We are only now beginning to understand what roles the individual PKC isozymes play in individual cells, and it is likely that optimum pharmacological inhibition will depend on both an understanding of isozyme functions and on pharmacological agents that specifically inhibit certain isozymes while not inhibiting others.

4.4. Anti-Angiogenic Therapy

Anti-angiogenic therapy has certain appealing features outside of the fact that GBMs are highly vascularized tumors. These therapies have limited drug resistance, since endothelial cells do not posses the genetic heterogeneity or instability of cancer cells *(144)*. Anti-angiogenic agents employ a cytostatic strategy, and therefore, end points of therapy include progression-free survival and not tumor shrinkage, which may be highly desirable in a large percentage of astrocytomas, especially LGAs. In recent years, multiple molecular mediators and inhibitors of angiogenesis have emerged and have been tried in various clinical trials. VEGF inhibitors are identified as promising agents in glioma therapy, with various studies demonstrating in vitro and in vivo effects of targeting VEGF. Antisense VEGF constructs inhibit tumor formation in animal experiments of C6 rat gliomas and xenografts of malignant gliomas *(145,146)*. Dominant negative inhibition of VEGFR2 decreases vascularization and tumor growth of C6 rat glioma *(147)*. Small molecule inhibitors of VEGFR2, or related members of the split kinase RPTK family, are also of promise in a variety of cancers, though they have not been examined in GBMs. In addition to direct inhibition of *VEGF* or *VEGFR*, biological targets against mitogenic receptors or signaling pathways, such as *EGFR*, *PDGFR*, or *p21-ras*, in astrocytomas may have as a major component of their antitumor effects, an anti-angiogenic mechanism of inhibiting the *VEGF* pathway *(69)*.

Nonangiogenic receptor-mediated endothelial cell inhibitors are also a category of angiogenic therapies that have undergone clinical testing in astrocytomas. Thalidomide is best known in this category and well recognized through its teratogenic effects in humans. Thalidomide was assessed in phase 2 trials against malignant gliomas in a small group of patients and demonstrated minimal radiographic response (148–150). Efficacy of thalidomide together with radiation therapy is currently being studied. Angiostatin and endostatin are endogenous anti-angiogenic proteins that are also found in many solid tumors, including astrocytomas. Angiostatin has undergone preclinical studies in gliomas *(148,151)* and is currently being evaluated in a clinical trial on GBM patients. Endostatin is being studied against various solid tumors, but not yet in gliomas.

4.5. Anti-Invasion Therapies

MMPs break down the ECM, inducing invasion of gliomas and endothelial cells. Targeting this pathway theoretically inhibits tumorgenesis by preventing invasion and tumor vascularization. Endogenous MMP inhibitors or TIMPs, have limited tissue penetrance and poor oral absorption, hence they are not yet practical therapeutic strategies. Exogenous pharmaceutical compounds that inhibit MMPs are Marimastat and Prinomastat. Marimastat acts against all major classes of MMPs and is currently being studied in a double-blinded placebo-controlled trial in GBMs in patients receiving surgery and/or radiotherapy. In contrast, Prinomastat inhibits MMPs-2, -9, -13, and -14. In animal studies, it has shown promising results in gliomas and is currently being evaluated in clinical trials as a phase 1 trial for GBMs.

5. FUTURE DIRECTIONS

Delivery of biological therapies against relevant oncogenic signaling pathways in astrocytomas located in the brain poses unique challenges that are different from other organ sites. First, there is the consideration of toxicity, which can have devastating consequences, not only in focal but in more global neurological functions, such as intellect, emotion, and memory. The lessons learned from the consequence of whole brain radiation, especially in the developing nervous system, must be kept in mind. The second consideration is the heterogeneity, both at a molecular and pathological level, in astrocytomas, in which there are differences between and within a tumor. Therefore, it would be ideal, but not realistic, to have a molecular profile of each individual astrocytoma being treated, although we know regional variations may be an insurmountable barrier. Perhaps noninvasive imaging methods will allow us to determine the molecular profile of these tumors and thus guide our therapies in the future. The third consideration is the issue of the BBB, which, although broken in the vascularized and necrotic regions of GBMs, is still intact in the infiltrating edge where tumor recurrence occurs after conventional surgery and radiation. Local delivery with pumps and convection-based delivery systems, breaking the BBB with hyperosmolar or pharmaceutical strategies, intravascular delivery, or biodegradable slow-release wafers are just some of the innovative ideas being tried in astrocytomas to improve local delivery. These local delivery methods must balance the requirements for sufficient delivery of the biological compound to the infiltrating astrocytoma cells with long-term efficacy. Due to some of these challenges, which are related to the profile of astrocytomas and also attributed to growing in the brain, it is most unlikely that any of the novel biologicals will provide a significant cure by themselves. It is hoped that small incremental improvements in survival may be made by these biological therapies in combination with each other and with current conventional therapies, without increasing the morbidity to the patient.

REFERENCES

1. Central Brain Tumor Registry of the United States. 1997 Annual Report. CBTRUS, Chicago, 1998.
2. Schoenberg BS, Christine BW, Whisnant JP. The descriptive epidemiology of primary intracranial neoplasms: the Connecticut experience. *Am J Epidemiol* 1976; 104:499–510.
3. Zimmerman HM. The ten most common types of brain tumor. *Semin Roentgenol* 1971; 6:48–58.
4. Kleihues P, Cavenee WK. *World Health Organization Classification of Tumours: Pathology and Genetics of Tumours of the Nervous System.* IARC Press, Lyon, 2000.
5. Kleihues P, Burger P, Scheithauer B. *Histological Typing of Tumors of the Nervous System.* Springer-Verlag, Berlin, 1991.
6. Mahaley MS Jr., Mettlin C, Natarajan N, Laws ER Jr, Peace BB. National survey of patterns of care for brain-tumor patients. *J Neurosurg* 1989; 71:826–836.
7. Recht LD, Lew R, Smith TW. Suspected low-grade glioma: is deferring treatment safe? *Ann Neurol* 1992; 31:431–436.
8. Watanabe K, Sato K, Biernat W, et al. Incidence and timing of p53 mutations during astrocytoma progression in patients with multiple biopsies. *Clin Cancer Res* 1997; 3:523–530.
9. Davis FG, Freels S, Grutsch J, Barlas S, Brem S. Survival rates in patients with primary malignant brain tumors stratified by patient age and tumor histological type: an analysis based on surveillance, epidemiology, and end results (SEER) data, 1973–1991. *J Neurosurg* 1998; 88:1–10.
10. Feldkamp MM, Lala P, Lau N, Roncari L, Guha A. Expression of activated epidermal growth factor receptors, Ras-guanosine triphosphate, and mitogen-activated protein kinase in human glioblastoma multiforme specimens. *Neurosurgery* 1999; 45:1442–1453.
11. Walker MD, Hunt WE, MacCarty CS, et al. Evaluation of BCNU and/or radiotherapy in the treatment of anaplastic gliomas: a cooperative clinical trial. *J Neurosurg* 1978; 49:333–343.
12. Salcman M. Survival in glioblastoma: historical persepctive. *Neurosurgery* 1980; 7:435–439.
13. Jelsma R, Bucy PC. The treatment of glioblastoma multiforme of the brain. *J Neurosurg* 1967; 27:388–400.

14. Brem H, Piantadosi S, Burger PC, et al. Placebo-controlled trial of safety and efficacy of intraoperative controlled delivery by biodegradable polymers of chemotherapy for recurrent gliomas. The Polymer-brain Tumor Treatment Group. *Lancet* 1995; 345:1008–1012.

15. Janinis J, Efstathiou E, Panopoulos C, et al. Phase II study of temozolomide in patients with relapsing high grade glioma and poor performance status. *Med Oncol* 2000; 17:106–110.

16. Yung WK. Temozolomide in malignant gliomas. *Semin Oncol* 2000; 27:27–34.

17. Levin VA, Silver P, Hannigan J, et al. Superiority of post-radiotherapy adjuvant chemotherapy with CCNU, procarbazine, and vincristine (PCV) over BCNU for anaplastic gliomas: NCOG 6G61 final report. *Int J Radiat Oncol Biol Phys* 1990; 18:321–324.

18. Cairncross JG, Ueki K, Zlatescu MC, et al. Specific genetic predictors of chemotherapeutic response and survival in patients with anaplastic oligodendrogliomas. *J Natl Cancer Inst* 1998; 90:1473–1479.

19. Kleihues P. Subsets of glioblastoma: clinical and histological vs. genetic typing. *Brain Pathol* 1998; 8:667–668.

20. Louis DN, Gusella JF. A tiger behind many doors: multiple genetic pathways to malignant glioma. *Trends Genet* 1995; 11:412–415.

21. Li L, Ernsting BR, Wishart MJ, Lohse DL, Dixon JE. A family of putative tumor suppressors is structurally and functionally conserved in humans and yeast. *J Biol Chem* 1997; 272:29403–29406.

22. Steck PA, Pershouse MA, Jasser SA, et al. Identification of a candidate tumour suppressor gene, MMAC1, at chromosome 10q23.3 that is mutated in multiple advanced cancers. *Nat Genet* 1997; 15:356–362.

23. Libermann TA, Razon N, Bartal AD, Yarden Y, Schlessinger J, Soreq H. Expression of epidermal growth factor receptors in human brain tumors. *Cancer Res* 1984; 44:753–760.

24. Yamazaki H, Fukui Y, Ueyama Y, et al. Amplification of the structurally and functionally altered epidermal growth factor receptor gene (c-erbB) in human brain tumors. *Mol Cell Biol* 1988; 8:1816–1820.

25. Louis DN. The p53 gene and protein in human brain tumors. *J Neuropathol Exp Neurol* 1994; 53:11–21.

26. Reifenberger G, Reifenberger J, Ichimura K, Meltzer PS, Collins VP. Amplification of multiple genes from chromosomal region 12q13–14 in human malignant gliomas: preliminary mapping of the amplicons shows preferential involvement of CDK4, SAS, and MDM2. *Cancer Res* 1994; 54:4299–4303.

27. Ichimura K, Schmidt EE, Goike HM, Collins VP. Human glioblastomas with no alterations of the CDKN2A (p16INK4A, MTS1) and CDK4 genes have frequent mutations of the retinoblastoma gene. *Oncogene* 1996; 13:1065–1072.

28. Ueki K, Ono Y, Henson JW, Efird JT, von Deimling A, Louis DN. CDKN2/p16 or RB alterations occur in the majority of glioblastomas and are inversely correlated. *Cancer Res* 1996; 56:150–153.

29. Nishikawa R, Furnari FB, Lin H, et al. Loss of P16INK4 expression is frequent in high grade gliomas. *Cancer Res* 1995; 55:1941–1945.

30. Guha A, Dashner K, Black PM, Wagner JA, Stiles CD. Expression of PDGF and PDGF receptors in human astrocytoma operation specimens supports the existence of an autocrine loop. *Int J Cancer* 1995; 60:168–173.

31. Guha A, Glowacka D, Carroll R, Dashner K, Black PM, Stiles CD. Expression of platelet derived growth factor and platelet derived growth factor receptor mRNA in a glioblastoma from a patient with Li-Fraumeni syndrome. *J Neurol Neurosurg Psychiatry* 1995; 58:711–714.

32. Shamah SM, Stiles CD, Guha A. Dominant-negative mutants of platelet-derived growth factor revert the transformed phenotype of human astrocytoma cells. *Mol Cell Biol* 1993; 13:7203–7212.

33. Antoniades HN, Galanopoulos T, Neville-Golden J, Maxwell M. Expression of insulin-like growth factors I and II and their receptor mRNAs in primary human astrocytomas and meningiomas; in vivo studies using in situ hybridization and immunocytochemistry. *Int J Cancer* 1992; 50:215–222.

34. Trojan J, Johnson TR, Rudin SD, Ilan J, Tykocinski ML. Treatment and prevention of rat glioblastoma by immunogenic C6 cells expressing antisense insulin-like growth factor I RNA. *Science* 1993; 259:94–97.

35. Millauer B, Shawver LK, Plate KH, Risau W, Ullrich A. Glioblastoma growth inhibited in vivo by a dominant-negative Flk-1 mutant. *Nature* 1994; 367:576–579.

36. Plate KH, Breier G, Welch HA, Risau W. Vascular endothelial growth factor is a potential tumour angiogenesis factor in human gliomas in vivo. *Nature* 1992; 359:845–848.

37. Libermann TA, Friesel R, et al. An angiogenic growth factor is expressed in human glioma cells. *EMBO J* 1987; 6:1627–1632.

38. Morrison RS. Supression of basic fibroblastic growth factor by antisense oligodexynucleotides inhibits the growth of transformed human astrocytes. *J Biol Chem* 1991; 266:728–734.

39. Ding H, Roncari L, Wu X, et al. Expression and hypoxic regulation of angiopoietins in human astrocytomas. *J Neurooncol* 2001; 3:1–10.

40. Stratmann A, Risau W, Plate KH. Cell type-specific expression of angiopoietin-1 and angiopoietin-2 suggests a role in glioblastoma angiogenesis. *Am J Pathol* 1998; 153:1459–1466.

41. Ko LJ, Prives C. p53: puzzle and paradigm. *Genes Dev* 1996; 10:1054–1072.

42. Levine AJ. p53, the cellular gatekeeper for growth and division. *Cell* 1997; 88:323–331.

43. Giaccia AJ, Kastan MB. The complexity of p53 modulation: emerging patterns from divergent signals. *Genes Dev* 1998; 12:2973–2983.

44. el-Azouzi M, Chung RY, Farmer GE, et al. Loss of distinct regions on the short arm of chromosome 17 associated with tumorigenesis of human astrocytomas. *Proc Natl Acad Sci USA* 1989; 86:7186–7190.

45. Fulci G, Ishii N, Van Meir EG. p53 and brain tumors: from gene mutations to gene therapy. *Brain Pathol* 1998; 8:599–613.

46. Li Y, Millikan RC, Carozza S, et al. p53 mutations in malignant gliomas. *Cancer Epidemiol Biomarkers Prev* 1998; 7:303–308.

47. Chattopadhyay P, Rathore A, Mathur M, Sarkar C, Mahapatra AK, Sinha S. Loss of heterozygosity of a locus on 17p13.3, independent of p53, is associated with higher grades of astrocytic tumours. *Oncogene* 1997; 15:871–874.

48. Watanabe K, Tachibana O, Sata K, Yonekawa Y, Kleihues P, Ohgaki H. Overexpression of the EGF receptor and p53 mutations are mutually exclusive in the evolution of primary and secondary glioblastomas. *Brain Pathol* 1996; 6:217–223; discussion 23–24.

49. Louis DN. A molecular genetic model of astrocytoma histopathology. *Brain Pathol* 1997; 7:755–764.

50. Wu X, Bayle JH, Olson D, Levine AJ. The p53-mdm-2 autoregulatory feedback loop. *Genes Dev* 1993; 7:1126–1132.

51. Haupt Y, Maya R, Kazaz A, Oren M. Mdm2 promotes the rapid degradation of p53. *Nature* 1997; 387:296–299.

52. Kubbutat MH, Jones SN, Vousden KH. Regulation of p53 stability by Mdm2. *Nature* 1997; 387:299–303.

53. Rasheed BK, Wiltshire RN, Bigner SH, Bigner DD. Molecular pathogenesis of malignant gliomas. *Curr Opin Oncol* 1999; 11:162–167.

54. Newcomb EW, Cohen H, Lee SR, et al. Survival of patients with glioblastoma multiforme is not influenced by altered expression of p16, p53, EGFR, MDM2 or Bcl-2 genes [see comment]. *Brain Pathol* 1998; 8:655–667.

55. Costello JF, Berger MS, Huang HS, Cavenee WK. Silencing of p16/CDKN2 expression in human gliomas by methylation and chromatin condensation. *Cancer Res* 1996; 56:2405–2410.

56. Merlo A, Herman JG, Mao L, et al. 5' CpG island methylation is associated with transcriptional silencing of the tumour suppressor p16/CDKN2/MTS1 in human cancers. *Nat Med* 1995; 1:686–692.

57. Ono Y, Tamiya T, Ichikawa T, et al. Malignant astrocytomas with homozygous CDKN2/p16 gene deletions have higher Ki-67 proliferation indices. *J Neuropathol Exp Neurol* 1996; 55:1026–1031.

58. Biernat W, Tohma Y, Yonekawa Y, Kleihues P, Ohgaki H. Alterations of cell cycle regulatory genes in primary (de novo) and secondary glioblastomas. *Acta Neuropathol (Berl)* 1997; 94:303–309.

59. Hermansson M, Nister M, Betsholtz C, Heldin CH, Westermark B, Funa K. Endothelial cell hyperplasia in human glioblastoma: coexpression of mRNA for platelet-derived growth factor (PDGF) B chain and PDGF receptor suggests autocrine growth stimulation. *Proc Natl Acad Sci USA* 1988; 85:7748–7752.

60. Guha A. Platelet derived growth factor: a general review with emphasis on astrocytomas: *Pediatr Neurosurg* 1992; 17:14–20.

61. Haley J, Whittle N, Bennet P, Kinchington D, Ullrich A, Waterfield M. The human EGF receptor gene: structure of the 110 kb locus and identification of sequences regulating its transcription. *Oncogene Res* 1987; 1:375–396.

62. Kondo I, Shimizu N. Mapping of the human gene for epidermal growth factor receptor (EGFR) on the p13 leads to q22 region of chromosome 7. *Cytogenet Cell Genet* 1983; 35:9–14.

63. Louis DN, Gusella JF. A tiger behind many doors: multiple genetic pathways to malignant glioma. *Trends Genet* 1995; 11:412–415.

64. Wong AJ, Bigner SH, Bigner DD, Kinzler KW, Hamilton SR, Vogelstein B. Increased expression of the epidermal growth factor receptor gene in malignant gliomas is invariably associated with gene amplification. *Proc Natl Acad Sci USA* 1987; 84:6899–6903.

65. Steck PA, Lee P, Hung MC, Yung WK. Expression of an altered epidermal growth factor receptor by human glioblastoma cells. *Cancer Res* 1988; 48:5433–5439.

66. Ekstrand AJ, Longo N, Hamid ML, et al. Functional characterization of an EGF receptor with a truncated extracellular domain expressed in glioblastomas with EGFR gene amplification. *Oncogene* 1994; 9:2313–2320.

67. Nishikawa R, Ji XD, Harmon RC, et al. A mutant epidermal growth factor receptor common in human glioma confers enhanced tumorigenicity. *Proc Natl Acad Sci USA* 1994; 91:7727–7731.

68. Feldkamp MM, Lala P, Lau N, Roncari L, Guha A. Expression of activated epidermal growth factor receptors, Ras-guanosine triphosphate, and mitogen-activated protein kinase in human glioblastoma multiforme specimens. *Neurosurgery* 1999; 45:1442–1453.

69. Feldkamp MM, Lau N, Rak J, Kerbel RS, Guha A. Normoxic and hypoxic regulation of vascular endothelial growth factor (VEGF) by astrocytoma cells is mediated by Ras. *Int J Cancer* 1999; 81:118–124.

70. Yamada N, Kato M, Yamashita H, et al. Enhanced expression of transforming growth factor-beta and its type-I and type-II receptors in human glioblastoma. *Int J Cancer* 1995; 62:386–392.

71. Horst HA, Scheithauer BW, Kelly PJ, Kovach JS. Distribution of transforming growth factor-beta 1 in human astrocytomas. *Hum Pathol* 1992; 23:1284–1288.

72. Jennings MT, Hart CE, Commers PA, et al. Transforming growth factor beta as a potential tumor progression factor among hyperdiploid glioblastoma cultures: evidence for the role of platelet-derived growth factor. *J Neurooncol* 1997; 31:233–254.

73. Battegay EJ, Raines EW, Seifert RA, Bowen-Pope DF, Ross R. TGF-beta induces bimodal proliferation of connective tissue cells via complex control of an autocrine PDGF loop. *Cell* 1990; 63:515–524.

74. Mandriota SJ, Pepper MS. Vascular endothelial growth factor-induced in vitro angiogenesis and plasminogen activator expression are dependent on endogenous basic fibroblast growth factor. *J Cell Sci* 1997; 110:2293–2302.

75. Suri C, Jones PF, Patan S, et al. Requisite role of angiopoietin-1, a ligand for the TIE2 receptor, during embryonic angiogenesis. *Cell* 1996; 87:1171–1180.

76. Suri C, McClain J, Thurston G, et al. Increased vascularization in mice overexpressing angiopoietin-1. *Science* 1998; 282:468–471.

77. Folkman J. The role of angiogenesis in tumor growth. *Semin Cancer Biol* 1992; 3:65–71.

78. Forsyth PA, Wong H, Laing TD, et al. Gelatinase-A (MMP-2), gelatinase-B (MMP-9) and membrane type matrix metalloproteinase-1 (MT1-MMP) are involved in different aspects of the pathophysiology of malignant gliomas. *Br J Cancer* 1999; 79:1828–1835.

79. Kachra Z, Beaulieu E, Delbecchi L, et al. Expression of matrix metalloproteinases and their inhibitors in human brain tumors. *Clin Exp Metastasis* 1999; 17:555–566.

80. Wagner S, Stegen C, Bouterfa H, et al. Expression of matrix metalloproteinases in human glioma cell lines in the presence of IL-10. *J Neurooncol* 1998; 40:113–122.

81. Webb KE, Henney AM, Anglin S, Humphries SE, McEwan JR. Expression of matrix metalloproteinases and their inhibitor TIMP-1 in the rat carotid artery after ballon injury. *Arterioscler Thromb Vasc Biol* 1997; 17:1837–1844.

82. Lampert K, Machein U, Machein MR, Conca W, Peter HH, Volk B. Expression of matrix metalloproteinases and their tissue inhibitors in human brain tumors. *Am J Pathol* 1998; 153:429–437.

83. Bos JL. p21ras: an oncoprotein functioning in growth factor-induced signal transduction. *Eur J Cancer* 1995; 31A:1051–1054.

84. Guha A, Feldkamp MM, Lau N, Boss G, Pawson A. Proliferation of human malignant astrocytomas is dependent on Ras activation. *Oncogene* 1997; 15:2755–2765.

85. Feldkamp MM, Lau N, Roncari L, Guha A. Isotype-specific Ras. GTP-levels predict the efficacy of farnesyl transferase inhibitors against human astrocytomas regardless of Ras mutational status. *Cancer Res* 2001; 61:4425–4431.

86. Favata MF, Horiuchi KY, Manos EJ, et al. Identification of a novel inhibitor of mitogen-activated protein kinase kinase. *J Biol Chem* 1998; 273:18623–18632.

87. Haas-Kogan D, Shalev N, Wong M, Mills G, Yount G, Stokoe D. Protein kinase B (PKB/Akt) activity is elevated in glioblastoma cells due to mutation of the tumor suppressor PTEN/MMAC. *Curr Biol* 1998; 8:1195–1198.

88. Furnari FB, Lin H, Huang HS, Cavenee WK. Growth suppression of glioma cells by PTEN requires a functional phosphatase catalytic domain. *Proc Natl Acad Sci USA* 1997; 94:12479–12484.

89. Sun H, Lesche R, Li DM, et al. PTEN modulates cell cycle progression and cell survival by regulating phosphatidylinositol 3,4,5,-trisphosphate and Akt/protein kinase B signaling pathway. *Proc Natl Acad Sci USA* 1999; 96:6199–6204.

90. Cantley LC, Neel BG. New insights into tumor suppression: PTEN suppresses tumor formation by restraining the phosphoinositide 3-kinase/AKT pathway. *Proc Natl Acad Sci USA* 1999; 96:4240–4245.

91. Franke TF, Yang SI, Chan TO, et al. The protein kinase encoded by the Akt proto-oncogene is a target of the PDGF-activated phosphatidylinositol 3-kinase. *Cell* 1995; 81:727–736.

92. Stambolic V, Suzuki A, de la Pompa JL, et al. Negative regulation of PKB/Akt-dependent cell survival by the tumor suppressor PTEN. *Cell* 1998; 95:29–39.

93. Steck PA, Lin H, Langford LA, et al. Functional and molecular analyses of 10q deletions in human gliomas. *Genes Chromosom Cancer* 1999; 24:135–143.

94. Myers MP, Pass I, Batty IH, et al. The lipid phosphatase activity of PTEN is critical for its tumor supressor function. *Proc Natl Acad Sci USA* 1998; 95:13513–13518.

95. Maher EA, Furnari FB, Bachoo RM, et al. Malignant glioma: genetics and biology of a grave matter. *Genes Dev* 2001; 15:1311–1333.

96. von Deimling A, von Ammon K, Schoenfeld D, Wiestler OD, Seizinger BR, Louis DN. Subsets of glioblastoma multiforme defined by molecular genetic analysis. *Brain Pathol* 1993; 3:19–26.

97. Ichimura K, Schmidt EE, Miyakawa A, Goike HM, Collins VP. Distinct patterns of deletion on 10p and 10q suggest involvement of multiple tumor suppressor genes in the development of astrocytic gliomas of different malignancy grades. *Genes Chromosom Cancer* 1998; 22:9–15.

98. Mollenhauer J, Wiemann S, Scheurlen W, et al. DMBT1, a new member of the SRCR superfamily, on chromosome 10q25.3–26.1 is deleted in malignant brain tumours. *Nat Genet* 1997; 17:32–39.

99. Nishizuka Y. Intracellular signaling by hydrolysis of phopholipids and activation of protein kinase C. *Science* 1992; 258:607–614.

100. Honegger P. Protein kinase C-activating tumor promoters enhance the differentiation of astrocytes in aggregrating fetal brain cell cultures. *J Neurochem* 1986; 46:1561–1566.

101. Bhat NR. Role of protein kinase C in glial cell proliferation. *J Neurosci Res* 1989; 22:20–27.

102. Couldwell WT, Antel JP, Yong VW. Protein kinase C activity correlates with the growth rate of malignant gliomas: Part II. Effects of glioma mitogens and modulators of protein kinase C. *Neurosurgery* 1992; 31:717–724; discussion 724.

103. Xiao H, Goldthwait DA, Mapstone T. The identification of four protein kinase C isoforms in human glioblastoma cell lines: PKC alpha, gamma, epsilon, and zeta. *J Neurosurg* 1994; 81:734–740.

104. Ahmad S, Mineta T, Martuza RL, Glazer RI. Antisense expression of protein kinase C alpha inhibits the growth and tumorigenicity of human glioblastoma cells. *Neurosurgery* 1994; 35:904–908; discussion 908–909.

105. Benzil DL, Finkelstein SD, Epstein MH, Finch PW. Expression pattern of alpha-protein kinase C in human astrocytomas indicates a role in malignant progression. *Cancer Res* 1992; 52:2951–2956.

106. Weller M, Frei K, Groscurth P, Krammer PH, Yonekawa Y, Fontana A. Anti-Fas/APO-1 antibody-mediated apoptosis of cultured human glioma cells. Induction and modulation of sensitivity by cytokines. *J Clin Invest* 1994; 94:954–964.

107. Newcomb EW, Bhalla SK, Parrish CL, Hayes RL, Cohen H, Miller DC. bcl-2 protein expression in astrocytomas in relation to patient survival and p53 gene status. *Acta Neuropathol (Berl)* 1997; 94:369–375.

108. Jannot CB, Beerli RR, Mason S, Gullick WJ, Hynes NE. Intracellular expression of a single-chain antibody directed to the EGFR leads to growth inhibition of tumor cells. *Oncogene* 1996; 13:275–282.

109. De Giovanni C, Landuzzi L, Frabetti F, et al. Antisense epidermal growth factor receptor transfection impairs the proliferative ability of human rhabdomyosarcoma cells. *Cancer Res* 1996; 56:3898–3901.

110. Reist CJ, Archer GE, Kurpad SN, et al. Tumor-specific anti-epidermal growth factor receptor variant III monoclonal antibodies: use of the tyramine-cellobiose radioiodination method enhances cellular retention and uptake in tumor xenografts. *Cancer Res* 1995; 55:4375–4382.

111. Ekstrand AJ, Liu L, He J, et al. Altered subcellular location of an activated and tumour-associated epidermal growth factor receptor. *Oncogene* 1995; 10:1455–1460.

112. Graziani Y, Chayoth R, Karny N, Feldman B, Levy J. Regulation of protein kinases activity by quercetin in Ehrlich ascites tumor cells. *Biochim Biophys Acta* 1982; 714:415–421.

113. Akiyama T, Ishida J, Nakagawa S, et al. Genistein, a specific inhibitor of tyrosine-specific protein kinases. *J Biol Chem* 1987; 262:5592–5595.

114. Onoda T, Isshiki K, Takeuchi T, Tatsuta K, Umezawa K. Inhibition of tyrosine kinase and epidermal growth factor receptor internalization by lavendustin A methyl ester in cultured A431 cells. *Drugs Exp Clin Res* 1990; 16:249–253.

115. Fry DW, Kraker AJ, McMichael A, et al. A specific inhibitor of the epidermal growth factor tyrosine kinase. *Science* 1994; 265:1093–1095.

116. Levitzki A, Gazit A. Tyrosine kinase inhibition: an approach to drug development. *Science* 1995; 267:1782–1788.

117. Buchdunger E, Trinks U, Mett H, et al. 4,5-Dianilinophthalimide: a protein-tyrosine kinase inhibitor with selectivity for the epidermal growth factor receptor signal transduction pathway and potent in vivo antitumor activity. *Proc Natl Acad Sci USA* 1994; 91:2334–2338.

118. Mason W, Malkin M, Lieberman F, Cropp G, Hannah A. Pharmacokinetics of SU101, a novel signal transduction inhibitor, in patients with recurrent malignant glioma. *Proc Am Assoc Cancer Res* 1996; 37:166.

119. Miyaji K, Tani E, Shindo H, Nakano A, Tokunaga T. Effect of tyrphostin on cell growth and tyrosine kinase activity of epidermal growth factor receptor in human gliomas. *J Neurosurg* 1994; 81:411–419.

120. Han Y, Caday CG, Nanda A, Cavenee WK, Huang HJ. Tyrphostin AG 1478 preferentially inhibits human glioma cells expressing truncated rather than wild-type epidermal growth factor receptors. *Cancer Res* 1996; 56:3859–3861.

121. Hook KE, Kunkel MW, Elliott WL, Howard CT, Leopold WR. Epidermal growth factor receptor tyrosine kinase in A431 xenografts: inhibition by PD 153035 (3-(3-bromoanilino)-6, 7-dimethoxyquinazoline). *Proc Am Assoc Cancer Res* 1995; 36:434.

122. Sirotnak FM, Zakowski MF, Miller VA, Scher HI, Kris MG. Efficacy of cytotoxic agents against human tumor xenografts is markedly enhanced by coadministration of ZD1839 (Iressa), an inhibitor of EGFR tyrosine kinase. *Clin Cancer Res* 2000; 6:4885–4892.

123. Ciardiello F, Caputo R, Bianco R, et al. Inhibition of growth factor production and angiogenesis in human cancer cells by ZD1839 (Iressa), a selective epidermal growth factor receptor tyrosine kinase inhibitor. *Clin Cancer Res* 2001; 7:1459–1465.

124. Hancock JF, Magee AI, Childs JE, Marshall CJ. All ras proteins are polyisoprenylated but only some are palmitoylated. *Cell* 1989; 57:1167–1177.

125. Marshall CJ. Protein prenylation: a mediator of protein-protein interactions. *Science* 1993; 259:1865–1866.

126. Farrell FX, Yamamoto K, Lapetina EG. Prenyl group identification of rap2 proteins: a ras superfamily member other than ras that is farnesylated. *Biochem J* 1993; 289:349–355.

127. Lebowitz PF, Davide JP, Prendergast GC. Evidence that farnesyltransferase inhibitors suppress Ras transformation by interfering with Rho activity. *Mol Cell Biol* 1995; 15:6613–6622.

128. Yan N, Ricca C, Fletcher J, Glover T, Seizinger BR, Manne V. Farnesyltransferase inhibitors block the neurofibromatosis type I (NF1) malignant phenotype. *Cancer Res* 1995; 55:3569–3575.

129. Sepp-Lorenzino L, Ma Z, Rands E, et al. A peptidomimetic inhibitor of farnesyl:protein transferase blocks the anchorage-dependent and -independent growth of human tumor cell lines. *Cancer Res* 1995; 55:5302–5309.

130. Kohl NE, Omer CA, Conner MW, et al. Inhibition of farnesyltransferase induces regression of mammary and salivary carcinomas in ras transgenic mice. *Nat Med* 1995; 1:792–797.

131. Feldkamp MM, Lau N, Roncari L, Guha A. Isotype-specific Ras·GTP-levels predict the efficacy of farnesyl transferase inhibitors against human astrocytomas regardless of Ras mutational status, *Cancer Res.* 2001; 61:4425-4431.

132. Feldkamp MM, Lau N, Guha A. Growth inhibition of astrocytoma cells by farnesyl transferase inhibitors is mediated by a combination of anti-proliferative, pro-apoptotic, and anti-angiogenic effects. *Oncogene* 1999; 18:7514–7526.

133. Feldkamp MM, Lau N, Rak J, Kerbel RS, Guha A. Normoxic and hypoxic regulation of vascular endothelial growth factor (VEGF) by astrocytoma cells is mediated by Ras. *Int J Cancer* 1999; 81:118–124.

134. Kokunai T, Urui S, Tomita H, Tamaki N. Overcoming of radioresistance in human gliomas by p21WAF1/CIP1 antisense oligonucleotide. *J Neurooncol* 2001; 51:111–119.

135. James G, Goldstein JL, Brown MS. Resistance of K-RasBV12 proteins to farnesyltransferase inhibitors in Rat1 cells. *Proc Natl Acad Sci USA* 1996; 93:4454–4458.

136. Lerner EC, Qian Y, Blaskovich MA, et al. Ras CAAX peptidomimetic FTI-277 selectively blocks oncogenic Ras signaling by inducing cytoplasmic accumulation of inactive Ras-Raf complexes. *J Biol Chem* 1995; 270:26802–26806.

137. Pollack IF, Randall MS, Kristofik MP, Kelly RH, Selker RG, Vertosick FT Jr. Response of malignant glioma cell lines to activation and inhibition of protein kinase C-mediated pathways. *J Neurosurg* 1990; 73:98–105.

138. Couldwell WT, Hinton DR, Law RE. Protein kinase C and growth regulation in malignant gliomas. *Neurosurgery* 1994; 35:1184–1186.

139. Pollack IF, Randall MS, Kristofik MP, Kelly RH, Selker R, Vertosick FT Jr. Effect of tamoxifen on DNA synthesis and proliferation of human malignant glioma lines in vitro. *Cancer Res* 1990; 50:7134–7138.

140. Baltuch GH, Couldwell WT, Villemure J-G, Yong VW. Protein kinase C inhibitors suppress cell growth in established and low-passage glioma cell lines. A comparison between staurosporine and tamoxifen. *Neurosurgery* 1993; 33:495–501.

141. Couldwell WT, Weiss MH, DeGiorgio CM, et al. Clinical and radiographic response in a minority of patients with recurrent malignant gliomas treated with high-dose tamoxifen. *Neurosurgery* 1993; 32:485–489; discussion 489–490.

142. Couldwell WT, Hinton DR, Surnock AA, et al. Treatment of recurrent malignant gliomas with chronic oral high-dose tamoxifen. *Clin Cancer Res* 1996; 2:619–622.

143. Pollack IF, Kawecki S, Lazo JS. Blocking of glioma proliferation in vitro and in vivo and potentiating the effects of BCNU and cisplatin: UCN-01, a selective protein kinase C inhibitor. *J Neurosurg* 1996; 84:1024–1032.

144. Folkman J. Angiogenesis and angiogenesis inhibition: an overview. EXS 1997; 79:1–8.

145. Cheng SY, Huang HJ, Nagane M, et al. Suppression of glioblastoma angiogenicity and tumorigenicity by inhibition of endogenous expression of vascular endothelial growth factor. *Proc Natl Acad Sci USA* 1996; 93:8502–8507.

146. Saleh M, Stacker SA, Wilks AF. Inhibition of growth of C6 glioma cells in vivo by expression of antisense vascular endothelial growth factor sequence. *Cancer Res* 1996; 56:393–401.

147. Millauer B, Shawver LK, Plate KH, Risau W, Ullrich A. Glioblastoma growth inhibited in vivo by a dominant-negative Flk-1 mutant. *Nature* 1994; 367:576–579.

148. Puduvalli VK, Sawaya R. Antiangiogenesis — therapeutic strategies and clinical implications for brain tumors. *J Neurooncol* 2000; 50:189–200.

149. Fine HA, Figg WD, Jaeckle K, et al. Phase II trial of the antiangiogenic agent thalidomide in patients with recurrent high-grade gliomas. *J Clin Oncol* 2000; 18:708–715.

150. Cha S, Knopp EA, Johnson G, et al. Dynamic contrast-enhanced T2-weighted MR imaging of recurrent malignant gliomas treated with thalidomide and carboplatin. *AJNR Am J Neuroradiol* 2000; 21:881–890.

151. Meneses PI, Abrey LE, Hajjar KA, et al. Simplified production of a recombinant human angiostatin derivative that suppresses intracerebral glial tumor growth. *Clin Cancer Res* 1999; 5:3689–3694.

19 Targeting Oncogenes in Pediatric Malignancies

Giannoula Klement, MD,
and Robert S. Kerbel, PhD

CONTENTS

1. INTRODUCTION

Pediatric malignancies are markedly different from adult tumors, and the differences, along with a more concerted treatment network than typical for adult oncology, account for the significantly better survival rates and outcomes. The first reason is probably the different type of tumors which occurs in pediatrics. The solid malignancies of childhood are typically rapidly proliferating noncarcinomatous tumors, and the leukemias are clonal proliferation of early lymphoid progenitors. Both typically, harbor few if any genetic abnormalities. The slow-growing carcinomatous neoplasms, so characteristic of adulthood, are uncommon in pediatric oncology, and viruses, environmental toxins, and carcinogens appear, in general, to play a lesser role. Accordingly, when a child presents with a tumor where the accumulation of genetic changes rekindles a clonal carcinogenesis model reminiscent of adult carcinoma *(1),* the prognosis is usually very poor.

The second reason is that, either due to their immature nature, or, more likely, due to its genetics, pediatric tumors respond much better to chemotherapy. Since these are fact proliferating tumors, this genetic stability cannot be related to decreased number of doublings, but must be a consequence of an intact and fully functioning DNA repair system, which eliminates the mutations before they can become an integral part of the cancer genome. It also leaves the cell death machinery sufficiently intact to induce apoptosis in response to therapy and prevent the selection of a fast proliferating, chemoresistant clones. In tumors with complex genotype, such as is the case in neurob-

From: *Oncogene-Directed Therapies*
Edited by: J. W. Rak © Humana Press Inc., Totowa, NJ

lastoma of the older child, or anaplastic Willm's tumor, the development of therapeutic resistance is often linked to the sequential accumulation of mutations *(2)*. The development of drug resistance, as is the case in most adult carcinomas, correlates directly with poor survival.

Despite their differences in genetic make-up and in better therapeutic response, it would be erroneous to conclude, that oncogenes play a lesser role. Quite to the contrary, all common pediatric tumors such as neuroblastoma, rhabdomyosarcoma, Willm's tumor, and Ewing's sarcoma display subgroups in which the sequential accumulation of mutations results in poor prognosis phenotype, and which, despite aggressive therapy, continue to absorb most of our resources. The emotional and financial burden associated with the long-term morbidity in these children and their families is considerable, and concentrating our efforts on this exact population is of paramount importance.

The tools to identify this population are becoming increasingly more accurate. The molecular characterization of chromosomal aberrations and point mutations can now provide a guidance to the structure and function of genes involved in the growth and differentiation of a particular cell lineage and can be instrumental in directing our therapeutic strategies. The full implementation of a directed therapeutic strategy would require, however, a reevaluation of the present practice of mainly histopathological diagnosis in pediatric oncology. It would suggests that, in terms of cancer diagnosis, the histological phenotype of tumors carrying the same genetic alteration may be of less etiologic and therapeutic importance, and that the genes whose disruption contribute to malignant transformation should be the real focus of cancer classification and a guide in the choice of therapeutic targets. For example, when considering two children with soft tissue sarcoma, the presence or absence of reciprocal translocation between chromosomes 11 and 22 should take precedence over whether the histology is more consistent with Ewing's sarcoma, "atypical" Ewing's sarcoma or peripheral neuroectodermal tumor (PNET). The prognosis is altered very little based on their histological similarities.

An exhaustive review of all the genetic abnormalities associated with poor prognosis in pediatric oncology would clearly be beyond the scope of this chapter. Therefore, only a set of illustrative examples will be presented to provide the conceptual framework for the future clinical management of these patients. The goal of this review is to improve the understanding of the childhood malignancies, which were, in the not so distant past, thought to be very heterogenous in their clinical presentations, but which can now, with further insight into the function of genes that are altered, be explained on the basis of their genetic modification.

2. RETINOBLASTOMA

It was in this tumor that the importance of germinal alterations such as chromosomal deletions, translocations, amplifications, point mutations, or nondisjunctions, had been first realized 30 yr ago *(3–5)*. The now obvious genetic basis had been uncovered using clinical and epidemiological correlations, leading to a distinction between the hereditary and sporadic occurrences of this cancer. It was possible to identify, at least in 40% of the afflicted individuals, a clear hereditary component, leading to an increased frequency of bilateral tumors and an earlier age of onset. The findings led Knudson to propose the "two-hit" mechanism of carcinogenesis. The hypothesis has provided us with a conceptual explanation for the differences between the hereditary form, where tumor development is a result of a germinal genetic defect complimented by a "second hit" spontaneous genetic mutation, and the sporadic form where two spontaneous mutations must occur in one cell *(3)*.

The germinal genetic alteration was defined years later *(6)*, when a polymorphic heterozygous pattern on chromosome 13q14 was identified on the somatic unaffected tissues of patients with retinoblastoma, and lead to the successful cloning of the "recessive" oncogene RB-1. Since the first report *(7)*, more than 30 deletions have been described *(8,9)*; the common region of overlap is chromosome 13, band q14 *(10,11)*. These deletions could act as the first hit, and, if germinal, confer the risk of tumor formation as an autosomal dominant trait in families. The increasing resolution of cytogenetic technology and the use of DNA probes for loci in the immediate vicinity and within the RB-1 locus has also allowed the detection of previously undetected, subtle genomic rearrangements. Thus, we are finding that the autosomal dominant hereditary form of retinoblastoma, without a gross chromosomal deletion, often involves the same genetic locus as in cases showing large deletions of chromosome 13. The first step in the pathway toward tumorigenesis in retinoblastoma is usually a submicroscopic mutational event at the RB-1 locus at germinal or somatic level *(12)*. The second step in both heritable and nonhereditary retinoblastoma involves somatic alteration of the normal allele at the RB-1 locus in such a way that the mutant allele is unmasked.

Although the unmasking of predisposing mutations at the RB-1 locus occurs in mechanistically similar ways in sporadic and heritable retinoblastoma, only the latter carries the initial mutation in each cell. These patients are, because of this mutation, at a greatly increased risk for the development of second primary tumors, particularly osteogenic sarcoma *(13)*. The association of these two otherwise rare tumors was determined by the analysis of restriction fragment length polymorphism (RFLP) of the constitutional retinoblastoma and osteosarcoma genotypes on chromosome 13. The data indicated that osteosarcomas arising in patients with retinoblastoma had become homozygous specifically around the chromosomal region carrying the RB1 locus *(14)*. Interestingly, the same constitutional heterozygosity was observed in sporadic osteosarcomas, suggesting a similar genetic pathogenesis.

The molecular isolation of the *RB-1* gene identified a unique sequence probe, termed *H3-8*, localized to the region *13q14.1*, and displaying hybridization patterns consistent with homozygous deletion *(15)*. These deletions were shown to arise either germinally or somatically in bilateral or unilateral disease *(15)*, and their causality is implied from the finding that the reintroduction of the wild-type gene into retinoblastoma (the WERI-Rb27 line) or osteosarcoma (the SaOS-2 line), through recombinant retroviral vector transfer, can restore the alterations in morphology, growth rate, and tumorigenic capability *(16)*.

The sequence analysis of a cDNA clone provided some information about the nature and features of the RB1 protein product *(6,17)*. Using purified anti-RB1 antibodies, the protein was shown to be 110,000–114,000 D, unglycosylated, nuclear phosphoprotein associated with DNA binding activity *(18)*. A posttranslational modification of the RB protein is involved phase-specific phosphorylation and dephosphorylation of the RB protein during the cell cycle *(19)*. This phosphorylation of the RB protein overrides growth suppression and allows cell division to take place. In vitro immunoprecipitation experiments have shown binding of such proteins as E2F, a transcription factor, and cyclin A, a cell cycle regulator, to the unphosphorylated RB protein at the G1 stage of the cell cycle. The RB/E2F/cyclin A complex inhibits the functional roles of other promoter elements, causing transcription to cease. In contrast, the phosphorylated RB protein at the G1/S boundary, release transcriptional factors, which then become positive transcriptional elements and activating kinases moving the cell through the M and G2 phases of the cell cycle. Thus, positive and negative regulation of transcription, and thus cell proliferation, are linked to the phosphorylation cycle of the RB suppressor gene. In tumors in which RB protein is mutated or absent, these intracellular transcriptional elements are constitutively dissociated promoting uncontrolled progression through the cell cycle, a behavior characteristic of a malignant phenotype.

Unfortunately, the identification of the gene and the description of its function has led to lamentably few modifications in the clinical management of these patients. With the realization of the heightened sensitivity of these children to radiation, and the appreciation of the pleiotropic effect of the gene that results in the development of osteosarcoma even outside the radiation port (20), we have tried to maximize other therapeutic modalities, such as surgery and chemotherapy, before irradiating a tumor, but few people are exploring alternative avenues in this patient population. Hopefully, with the advent of biological modifiers, it will be possible to avoid radiation and aggressive chemotherapy in these children altogether.

3. WILM'S TUMOR

The genes involved in the development and progression of Wilm's tumor (malignant nephroblastoma) are much less defined (21). The first genetic model for Wilm's tumor development was proposed in the early 1970s, and, similarly to retinoblastoma, was based on a statistical analysis of the age of onset of unilateral and bilateral tumors. It also predicts that all Wilm's tumors develop as a consequence of two mutational events. The first event can be either prezygotic (i.e., a constitutional or germline event) or postzygotic. If the first event is prezygotic, the tumor is potentially hereditary, and affected individuals are at risk of developing multiple tumors. By contrast, the nonhereditary or sporadic form results from two somatic mutations in a single cell. Because these two events are unlikely to occur independently in more than one cell, patients with nonhereditary Wilm's tumor are unlikely to develop more than one multiple tumor.

Pathological specimens from children who died of causes other than cancer, reveal a significant number of benign nephroblastoma nodules with no genetic abnormality. Willm's tumor originates from these pluripotent embryonic renal precursors, and it usually arises from persistent embryonic rests by the age of 5, although children with genetic predisposition may develop bilateral Wilm's tumor as early as 2 yr of age. The present clinical treatment of Wilm's tumor does not differentiate the genetically distinct subgroups. It involves surgical resection of the affected kidney, followed by chemotherapy, depending on the extent of the resection. Often, radiation is added in case of dissemination. This therapeutic approach achieves cure in approximately 80% of cases, relegating the other 20% to an aggressive, toxic, and minimally effective regimen. This so called anaplastic Wilm's remains refractory to treatment, and its refractoriness is most commonly linked to the frequency of *p53* mutations (22) and other genetic changes. At least three genes have been implicated in this subset of tumors. *WT-1* is inactivated in 15% of sporadic Willm's patients, β-catenin, a component of *Wnt* pathway, is observed in 15% of patients *(23)*, and insulin-like growth factor 2 (IGF2) is observed in 20% of patients *(24)*.

The present genetic model for Wilm's tumor progression was defined from the genetic analysis of the rare WAGR syndrome (a constellation of symptoms consisting of Wilm's tumor, aniridia, ambiguous genitalia, and mental retardation). The syndrome, and its associated neoplastic growth, correlates with constitutional deletion of part of chromosome 11, 11p13 *(25)*. A candidate Wilm's tumor susceptibility gene *WT-1*, has now been cloned from this region by three independent groups *(26–28)*. Whenever specific heterozygous dominant-negative mutations of *WT-1* are present in the germline, they are associated with severe abnormalities of renal and sexual differentiation, pointing to the role of *WT-1* in normal genitourinary development.

Even though the *WT-1* gene is now considered a major player in the tumorigenesis of nephroblastoma, the function and expression of the Wilm's tumor susceptibility gene must be much more complicated. Like retinoblastoma, and neuroblastoma, it was one of the pediatric cancers used by Knudson and Strong in modeling the number of rate-limiting genetic events required to initiate tumorigenesis *(4)*, but unlike the other two, familial Wilm's tumor is rare *(29)*. This may be a result of the lethality of this cancer prior to the advent of modern chemotherapy, suggesting these cases may become more common with the curative treatment of mutation carriers, or it may be associated with reduced fertility of these carriers due to the genitourinary malformations. The latter is more likely, since a fairly complete picture of familiar Wilm's tumor has been demonstrated in association with a germline mutation in a locus on chromosome 17, where no associated genitourinary malformations exist *(30)*.

In addition to the *WT-1* locus at chromosome 11p13 *(31–33)* and the imprinted locus, which is telomeric to it at 11p15 *(34,35)*, loss of heterozygosity (LOH) in sporadic Wilm's tumors has also been demonstrated at chromosomes *1p, 16q,* and *7p,* pointing to the presence of additional tumor suppressor genes yet to be identified *(36–38)*.

3.1. Constitutional Genetic Aberrations in Wilms

Numerous other genetic syndromes are associated with Wilm's tumor, and, again, not all of them manifest the typical chromosome 11p13 deletion. For example, children with Beckwith-Wiedemann syndrome (BWS) (macroglosia, somatic gigantism, neonatal hypoglycemia, omphalocele or abdominal wall defects, and visceromegaly) have constitutional duplications of the 11p15 region *(35,39)*. This second locus at 11p15 (telomeric to WT-1) has been designated *WT-2 (40)*. Whether the *BWS* gene and *WT-2* are identical is not clear. Complicating the analysis is the variable imprinting of this gene. In tumors with LOH, the maternal copy of chromosome 11p15 is lost due to genomic imprinting *(41)*, suggesting that the two copies of *WT-2* are not functionally equivalent. Furthermore, two known candidates for *WT-2* are now recognized. First is the *IGF-2* gene, an embryonic growth factor highly expressed in Wilm's tumors, whose expression is parent-specific (imprinted), such that *IGF-2* is only expressed from the paternal allele *(42)*. The second is an adjacent locus candidate, *H19*, which is also imprinted, but in the opposite direction, such that only the maternal allele is active *(24)*. In some Wilm's tumors, alterations of imprinting and consequently expression of both of the two loci have been reported, and what role *IGF2* or *H19* actually play in Wilm's tumorigenesis and whether additional loci that control the imprint may be involved, is presently the focus of intense investigation.

The tumor-specific LOH for DNA markers at chromosome 11p, found in 30–40% of tumors, is a higher than the expected incidence of tumor-specific LOH for other markers such as 1p (approx 12%) or 16q (approx 17%). Yet, it has been suggested, that 16q loss is associated with poorer prognosis *(43)*, suggesting the putative suppressor gene on 16q may be involved in tumor progression rather than tumor initiation. Notably, the association between outcome and loss of either chromosomal region was independent of either tumor stage or histopathologic features, implying that the underlying chromosomal loci may determine an adverse phenotype independently of these traditional parameters.

3.2. Genetic Syndromes in Wilms

A number of other genetic syndromes confer a predisposition for Wilm's tumor development on a child. To list a few, they are: Perlman Syndrome *(44)*, Sotos syndrome *(45)*, Denys-Drash (genitourinary defects, renal mesangial sclerosis, pseudohermaphroditism, and Wilm's) *(46,47)*, Frasier (genitourinary defects, focal glomerular sclerosis, intersex disorder, and Wilm's) *(48)*, and the genetic instability syndromes such as Bloom's *(49)* and Incontinentia pigmenti *(50)*. Not all of these have a single consistent genetic lesion confounding the difficulty identifying the causative mutation(s).

4. RHABDOMYOSARCOMA

4.1. Constitutional Genetic Aberrations in Rhabdomyosarcoma

Rhabdomyosarcoma (RMS) is the third most common extracranial solid tumor of childhood and is thought to arise from immature mesenchymal cells that are committed to skeletal muscle lineage. Its incidence is equal to or greater than that of all other forms of non-RMS soft tissue sarcoma (NRSTS) combined. Athough the overwhelming majority of cases of RMS occur sporadically and are cured with present therapeutic modalities such as surgery, chemotherapy, and radiation, the development of RMS can be associated with certain familial syndromes, such as neurofibromatosis and the Li-Fraumeni syndrome *(LFS)*. The later includes familial clustering of RMS and other soft tissue tumors in children, with adrenocortical carcinoma and early-onset breast carcinoma in adult relatives *(51,52)*, and has been associated with germline mutations of the *p53* tumor suppressor gene *(53)*. Unexpectedly, many of the "sporadic" RMS cases were found in a recent study to have germline mutations in their *p53* gene *(54)*, a finding which suggests that at least some of the very young children with seemingly sporadic RMS may have a hereditary predisposition to cancer. Even if this predisposition confers only an increased susceptibility to potentially toxic environmental agents, it raises the question whether genetics needs to be a more integral part of oncological diagnosis, and whether children with germline *p53* mutations should have their therapy altered to minimize or reduce their exposures to potentially carcinogenic interventions (e.g., ionizing radiation, alkylating agents, epipodophyllotoxins).

4.2. Genetic Syndromes in Rhabdomyosarcoma

Not all oncogenic transformation in RMS, however, are *p53*-dependent. The genetic abnormalities associated with syndromes such as BWS, a syndrome exhibiting a significant predisposition for sarcomas, are typically on 11p15, where the *IGF-2*, gene is located. Interestingly, many embryonal RMS without BWS have LOH at the 11p15 locus as well *(55,56)*. In these, the LOH involves loss of maternal genetic information and duplication of paternal genetic material at this locus *(57)*. Because only the paternal allele of IGF2 is transcriptionally active *(42)*, it is conceivable that, at least in this tumor LOH with paternal disomy leads to overexpression of *IGF-2*. However, it is also possible that LOH at 11p15 reflects a loss of a yet unidentified tumor suppressor activity, or that both activation of IGF2 and loss of tumor suppressor activity result from LOH at 11p15 in embryonal RMS. Both alveolar and embryonal RMS appear to overproduce *IGF-2*, a growth factor known to stimulate growth of tumor cells *(58,59)*, and blocking its effect by monoclonal antibodies directed against the receptor for *IGF-2* (type IIGF receptor) have been demonstrated to inhibit growth of RMS both in vitro and in vivo *(60,61)*. It is likely that *IGF-2* plays an important role in the unregulated growth of these tumors, but the mechanism that leads to overproduction of *IGF-2* in these tumors is unclear.

Many histologically identical RMS show very variable clinical presentation and, more often than not, we find clinically similar subtypes to share a common genetic aberration. The two major histologic subtypes of RMS, namely embryonal and alveolar, are characterized by genetic alterations that can be used to explain the clinical presentation of these tumors. Alveolar RMS has a characteristic translocation between the long arm of chromosome 2 and the long arm of chromosome 13, t(2;13)(q35;q14) *(62,63)*. This translocation has now been molecularly cloned and has been shown to involve the juxtaposition of the *PAX3* gene (or, rarely, the *PAX7* gene located at chromosome 1p36), believed to regulate transcription during early neuromuscular development and the *FKHR* gene, a member of the forkhead family of transcription factors *(55)*. The present contribute to the transformed phenotype, but the precise consequence of this tumor-specific translocation is unknown. A number of hypotheses have been proposed. It has been suggested that phosphatidylinositol 3-kinase (PI3K)/Akt and p70(S6K), act as crucial signaling molecules mediating the stimulatory effect of IGFs on myogenin expression and, thus, skeletal muscle differentiation. This is supported by the in vitro evidence that mutation within the myogenic promoter resulted in defective activation of the IGF/PI3K/Akt pathway and complete abolishment of the PI3K/Akt-induced myogenin expression in RMS-derived cell lines *(64)*. An alternative hypothesis has been presented by Margue at al., who proposed that one of the oncogenic functions of *PAX3* and *PAX3/FKHR* in RMS is protection from apoptosis *(65)*. The study established that BCL-XL, a prominent anti-apoptotic protein present in normal skeletal muscle and RMS cells, is transcriptionally modulated by PAX3 and PAX3/FKHR.

Finally, one of the most frequently observed oncogene abnormalities seen in RMS are *ras* mutations. Activated forms of both N-*ras* and K-*ras* have been isolated from both RMS cell lines as well as from tumor specimens *(66,67)*. A survey of embryonal RMS tumor specimens found a 35% incidence of either activated N-*ras* or K-*ras* *(68)*, but it is not known whether these alterations are primarily involved in the pathogenesis of these tumors or reflect secondary abnormalities that occur during progression.

5. NEUROBLASTOMA

The case of neuroblastoma probably presents one of the most complete picture of clinically relevant sequential activation of oncogenes and tumor suppressor genes in

Table 1
Genetic Basis of Three Clinically Distinct Subgroups of Neuroblastoma

	Age	N-myc	DNA ploidy	LOH/1p-	trkA	TrkB	VEGF	5-yr survival
Group 1	<1yr	Normal	Hyperdiploid or near triploid	<5%	High	Low	Normal	95%
Group 2	>1yr	Normal	Near diploid or near tetraploid	25–50%	Low	Low or nil	High	25–50%
Group 3	1–5yr	Amplified	Near diploid or near tetraploid	80–90%	Low or nil	High full-length low truncated	High	<5%

The past perception of neuroblastoma as a highly heterogeneous disorder with an unpredictable clinical course can be redefined on the basis of the genetic alterations leading to these clinical phenotypes. At least three genetically distinct subtypes of neuroblastoma can be identified, each correlating with discrete clinical counterpart. It appears that the downregulation of neurotropin receptors is, at least in this tumor, crucial for the development of a malignant phenotype.

pediatrics. In the past, neuroblastoma was thought to be a highly heterogeneous disorder with an unpredictable clinical course. Over the past 20 yr, however, tissue cytogenetic and molecular analysis has allowed for identification of at least three genetically and clinically distinct subtypes, with discrete clinical counterparts (69,70) (Table 1). The first, a hyperdiploid or triploid modal karyotype, with no 1p- or N-myc amplification, and high expression of trk-A, are usually infants with low stages of disease (stage 1, 2, or 4S by the International Neuroblastoma Staging System) and with a very favorable outcome (> 90% cure). The second group generally has a near diploid or tetraploid modal chromosome number or DNA content, 1p, 14q allelic loss or other structural changes, lacks N-myc amplification, and expresses trk-A in low levels. These patients are generally older with advanced stages of disease (stages 3 or 4), and have a slowly progressive course, with a cure rate of 25–50%. Finally, the third group is characterized by tumors with N-myc amplification, generally near diploid or tetraploid modal karyotype, 1p allelic loss, and low or absent trk-A expression. These patients are usually between 1 and 5 yr of age with advanced stages of disease and have a very poor prognosis (< 5%). While tumors in the good prognosis subset are thought to be genetically distinct, and, at least at present, not thought to evolve into the less favorable group with time, this may be related to lack of information about the genetic and molecular changes occurring with natural progression of the disease. If one were able to follow the natural course of malignant progression, it would likely resemble the sequence presented in Fig. 1.

While there are many instances where neuroblastomatous growths regress, the proliferative capacity makes them a susceptible premalignant lesion. In 1963, Beckwith and Perrin reported that as many as 60% of infants younger than 3 mo of age who died of causes other than cancer, show microscopic neuroblastic nodules, resembling neuroblastoma in situ. We know now, that these neuroblastic nodules occur uniformly in all fetuses studied, peak at 17–20 wk of gestation, and gradually regress by the time of birth (71,72). Considering the high percentage, it is likely that these neurob-

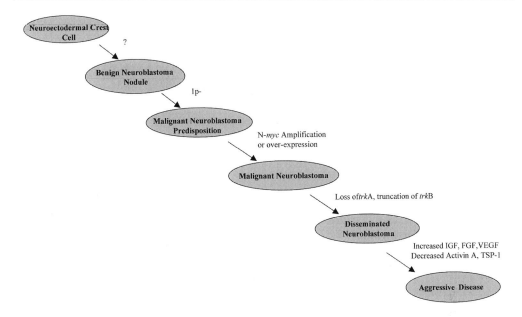

Fig. 1. A Genetic Model for Neuroblastoma Tumorigenesis. Benign neuroblastic nodules represent a normal stage of adrenal development. Their occurrence normally peaks at 17–20 wk of gestation, and they gradually regress by the time of birth. A loss of a tumor suppressor gene such as *p73* as a consequence of a 1p allelic loss, removes the normal sequence of pro-apoptotic signals during neuroectodermal differentiation. This can be further exacerbated by a subsequent N-*myc* oncogene activation, which disturbs the strict spatial and temporal activation growth fctors genes, and hinders normal tissue differentiation. The resulting unimpeded proliferation and powerful pro-angiogenenic drive lead to the development of aggressive disseminated neuroblastomas.

lastic cell rests represent a normal stage of adrenal development and as long as the strict spacial and temporal activation of the involved growth factor genes remains intact, the resulting differentiation of the tissues results in down-regulation of physiological growth and angiogenesis and subsequent regression. In contrast, it is quite likely these fast-proliferating cells may be the very cells from which aggressive adrenal neuroblastomas may develop whenever the gene activation/down-regulation is altered by, for example, loss of tumor supressor gene on chromosome 1 or N-*myc* amplification. Surprisingly, the mass screening studies in Japan and Quebec *(73–75)* suggest that only about half of all neuroblastomas detectable by screening actually regress, and that mass screening is ineffective in reducing the incidence of unfavorable advanced stage disease *(76)*.

The sequential activation of genes leading to neural crest differentiation and subsequent genetic stability involves neurotrophic factors and their receptors, but, at least at present, the specific role of each growth factor and its receptors in normal and aberrant growth is not clear. The difficulty may lie in the absence of appropriate models. Most neuroblastoma cell lines are neither dependent on, nor responsive to the presence of nerve growth factor (NGF) in vitro, probably reflecting more a prevalence of poor-prognosis cell lines in tissue culture studies than true in vivo state. Studies demonstrate multiple defects in the expression and function of the low-affinity NGF receptor (LNGFR) in neuroblastoma cell lines *(77,78)* and reveal that high *trk*-A expression in primary neuroblastoma cells would confer upon a cell the ability to differentiate in the presence of NGF *(79)*. The same cells die in the absence of NGF in vitro. The importance of an intact NGF/*trk*-A pathway is further underscored by clinical data showing that *trk*-A expression was inversely correlated with N-*myc* amplification *(80)*. It demonstrates quite convincingly that the combination of N-*myc* copy number and loss of *trk*-A expression provides prognostic information over either variable alone, and their exploration may provide important insights into the sequential oncogene activation/inactivation and the ultimate selection of an aggressive tumor clone.

The most common abnormality found in neuroblastoma is the deletions of the short arm of chromosome 1 (1p-), which is found in 70–80% of the near-diploid tumors *(81,82)*. Although near-diploid karyotypes with 1p deletions are commonly associated with advanced stages of disease, tumors from patients with lower stages are more likely to be hyperdiploid or triploid, with few structural rearrangements. The deletions of 1p vary in their proximal break points, but using DNA polymorphisms that reveal LOH, the region of consistent deletion is confined to subbands of 1p36, where at least two suppressor genes appear to be active *(83–85)*. Molecular studies have shown a strong correlation between 1p LOH and N-*myc* amplification *(86)*; since nearly all N-*myc* amplified tumors contain 1p deletion, but the reverse is not true, N-*myc* amplification is likely facilitated by the deletion of at least one tumor suppressor gene *(87)*. Finally, evidence indicates that allelic loss in neuroblastomas occurs with increased frequency on chromosomes 14 *(88)*, 11 *(89)*, 17 *(90)*, and other sites, pointing out the possible involvement of other suppressor genes in the pathogenesis of these tumors.

In most tumors, the histological evidence of gene amplifications, such as the extra-chromosomal double-minutes (d-mins) and chromosomally integrated heterogenously staining regions (HSRs) cannot be associated with the amplified gene. For neuroblastomas, however, the region amplified is virtually always derived from the distal short arm of chromosome 2, and contains the proto-oncogene N-*myc*. Brodeur and colleagues *(91,92)* demonstrated that N-*myc* amplification occurs in about 25% of primary neuroblastomas from untreated patients and that the amplification is associated with advanced stages of disease, rapid tumor progression, and a poor prognosis. N-*myc* amplification is usually present at the time of diagnosis, if it is going to occur, and this has been interpreted to mean that it is an intrinsic biologic property of a subset of aggressive tumors destined to have a poor outcome *(93)*. However, the close interplay that exists between the N-*myc* amplification and neurotropin expression, and the exact character of their activation/inhibition is only now being elucidated.

For one, despite the extensive information on neurotropins in normal brain development and maintenance, their role in the progression of neuroblastoma is only just emerging. The neurotrophin family includes NGF, brain-derived neurotrophic factor (BDNF), neurotrophin-3 (NT-3), and neurotrophin-4/5 (NT-4), and the genes *trk*-A, *trk*-B, and *trk*-C encode the respective primary receptors for NGF, BDNF, and NT-3 *(94–99)*. The primary receptor for NT-4 has not been described yet, but NT-4 appears to function through Trk-B *(100)*. The analysis of this family suggests that all neurotropins play a distinct role in tumor progression and maintenance, but the studies involving the association of *trk*-B and *trk*-C expression and prognosis are more limited than the *trk*-A association with good prognosis. The available information indicates that *trk*-B is expressed in approximately 36% of neuroblastomas, and its cognate ligand BDNF in 68% *(101)*. We know, that the truncated form of *trk*-B, which lacks the tyrosine kinase domain, is expressed predominantly in more differentiated tumors (ganglioneuroblastomas and ganglioneuromas), whereas the full-length *trk*-B transcript is co-expressed in tumors with N-*myc* amplification *(101)*. Thus, the *trk*-B/BDNF pathway may serve as an autocrine or paracrine pathway to promote survival in N-*myc* amplified tumors *(102)*. This pathway can, for example, rescue neuroblastoma cells from vinblastine toxicity, and render the cells chemoresistant *(103,104)* and enhance tumor cell proliferation *(105)*. Finally, there is early evidence emerging that it may be the specific constellation of these growth factors that confers an angiogenic phenotype on the neuroblastomas *(106)* and that tumor endothelial cell survival may be enhanced by these growth factors, whose activity was thought to be, at least in the past, specific to tissues of neuroectodermal origin *(107)*.

In contrast to *trk*-B, *trk*-C expression is found in 25% of neuroblastomas tested, and its pattern of expression resembles that of *trk*-A *(102,108)*. All tumors with *trk*-C expression also have high *trk*-A expression, and it does not add further prognostic significance *(109)*. It may, however, represent an alternate or additional pathway for neuronal differentiation in these tumors. With further knowledge about the factors that control growth and differentiation in neuroblastoma, it may be possible to direct the children with genetically unfavorable subtypes to alternative therapeutic options. At present, only the expression of N-*myc* and *trk*-A may have clinical utility for diagnosis and prognosis. In general, a negative correlation exists between the two *(110)*, and an N-*myc* amplified tumor with loss of *trk*-A expression should be treated differently than an nonamlified tumor with high *trk*-A expression. Some confusion still exists about the N-*myc* copy number and expression. Tumors with amplification generally express higher level of N-*myc*, but some heterogeneity exists in the level of expression among tumors with a single copy of N-*myc*. It is important to keep in mind that higher-expressing single-copy tumors do not appear to be an aggressive subset *(111)*. Expression of other oncogenes, such as H-*ras*, usually correlates with lower stages of disease and differentiated tumors *(112,113)*, but *ras* family genes are rarely activated by base pair mutations of critical codons in neuroblastomas *(114)*. Most importantly, the pattern of oncogene expression should be used to distinguish neuroblastomas of variable prognosis *(115)*, as well as to distinguish neuroblastoma from other histologically similar tumors, such as neuroepithelioma.

6. LEUKEMIAS

The evidence that genetic factors play a significant etiological role in acute leukemias, including acute lymphoblastic leukemia (ALL), was originally based on several observations, such as the association between various constitutional chromosomal abnormalities and childhood ALL, the occurrence of familial leukemia, and the high incidence of leukemia in identical twins. The frequency of leukemia is, indeed, much higher than would be expected in families of patients with leukemia *(116)*, and siblings of children with leukemia, including ALL, have an approx 2- to 4-fold greater risk of developing the disease than do unrelated children in the general population *(117)*. There is, however, some ambiguity as to the genetic basis for leukemic disposition in twins. While the concordance of acute leukemia in monozygotic twins is as high as 25% *(116)*, the risk is highest in infancy and diminishes with age, suggesting that a simultaneous exposure to a common pre- or postnatal leukemogenic event could produce the same frequencies. Similarly, a leukemogenic event occurring in utero in one twin could become the source of transplacental inoculation of malignant cells into the other *(118–120)*.

With the increase in the clinical utilization of molecular genetics, and the subsequent demonstration of specific karyotypic abnormalities in leukemic cells of children with the disease, a more complete picture is emerging. We are finding, that most of the constitutional chromosomal aberrations in childhood leukemias are different from the monosomic form of chromosomal aneuploidy discussed previously in the context of a two-hit model of carcinogenesis. Unlike the LOH model, which involves a genetic or epigenetic knock-out of a functional growth-affecting gene, the constitutional genetic aberration predisposing children to leukemias are usually trisomies. These may be, at least conceptually, harder to envision, because the impact of trisomy results in the addition of a copy of a particular gene or genes and not a LOH. Trisomies in the germline result in dramatic phenotypic variance from normal growth and development and are, for the most part, incompatible with life *(121)*. Only trisomies of chromosomes 13, 18, and 21 occur with any frequency in the germline in the general population *(122)*. Each is associated with a severe and well-defined clinical syndrome, but the biological basis of the syndrome development is unclear. It may be that the unbalanced number of chromosomes may, by itself, cause a problem during normal cell division, but if this is so, it would be difficult to explain the vigorous growth of these aneuploid cell lines in vitro. Likely, the presence of an extra chromosome poses a basic developmental problem due to a 50% increase in the dosage of a particular gene or genes, and disturbs the fine-tuning of growth factors and developmental pathways in higher organisms.

The classic constitutional aneuploidy demonstrating a predisposition to certain kinds of cancer is trisomy 21, also called Down's syndrome *(123)*. Clearly, it is the increase dosage of a gene or genes on chromosome 21 that confers the increased risk of leukemia on the Down's syndrome child, because in trisomy 21 mosaics, it is only the trisomic cell that is at risk for leukemic transformation, not the normal mosaic counterpart *(124)*. Furthermore, an acquired trisomy 21 is a relatively frequent chromosomal abnormality found in acute lymphocytic or nonlymphocytic leukemias *(125)*. While ALL and acute myeloid leukemia (AML) can occur in patients with Down's syndrome *(126)*, it is acute megakaryoblastic leukemia that is most commonly seen in these children *(127)*.

The predisposition to megakaryoblastic leukemia in trisomy 21 or trisomy 21 mosaicism is associated with hematopoietic disorders that are sufficiently characteristic as to imply common pathogenesis *(128)*. The so-called transient leukemoid reaction (TLR) is most common, but not restricted, to the Down's syndrome population. It classically manifests in newborns or early infancy as a myeloproliferative disorder that can include hepatosplenomegaly, leukocytosis, and circulating myeloblasts; the morphologic picture is consistent with congenital leukemia except that spontaneous remissions are common *(127,129)*. This condition is not, however, unequivocally benign, because 20–30% of Down's syndrome patients with TLR develop overt megakaryoblastic leukemia at 1–3 yr of age *(128)*.

Consistent with the Downs syndrome genetics, most of the RFLP analysis evidence identifies the extra chromosome as being of maternal origin (in approximately 95% of the cases), but some reports suggest that, in TLR or leukemia, an increased paternal contribution is seen *(130)*. If this observation is confirmed in additional studies, it will suggest that more complex genetic and epigenetic factors may influence the risk of leukemia or TLR among patients with trisomy 21. Interestingly, despite the completion of the human genome map, no growth-affecting gene(s) has been identified on chromosome 21. The genes residing on chromosome 21 are involved in chromatin structure, lymphocyte adhesion, interferon action, DNA transcription, and signal transduction, but none can be implicated in the constitutional phenotype or leukemogenic risk of patients with Down's syndrome *(131)*.

A number of additional genetic conditions that predispose children to leukemia should be considered here. Children with various congenital immunodeficiency diseases, including Wiskott-Aldrich syndrome, congenital hypogammaglobulinemia, ataxia-telangiectasia, and patients receiving chronic treatment with immunosuppressive drugs, all have an increased risk of developing lymphoid malignancies as well *(132)*. Since the majority of leukemias secondary to chronic immunosupression appear to be of mature B cell phenotypes (lymphoproliferative disorder), and the causative deregulation of the malignant growth may be posttranscriptional, there are identified genetic lesions in children with ataxia-telangiectasia and Fanconi's anemia. Both disorders are associated with an increased chromosomal fragility and result in frequent abnormalities of chromosomes 14 and 7, respectively.

In children with ataxia telangiectasia (A-T), the chromosome 14 rearrangement can be easily observed in peripheral T cells, and the resulting leukemia/lymphoma is mainly of T cell origin. The clonal progression ultimately evolves into a T cell prolymphocytic leukemia (T-PLL), which, in addition to the primary defect, also has a number of further genetic alterations. The primary translocations usually involves TCL-1 (at 14q32) or the c6.1B/MTCP1 A1 transcript (at-Xq28). A second gene, MTCP-1, which produces an alternative B1 transcript, has been also been described. The expression of TCL-1 occurs in the preleukemic clone cells of A-T patients in randomly selected A-T patients without large cytogenetic clones and without any evidence of leukemic changes *(133)*.

Fanconi anemia (FA) is an autosomal-recessive cancer susceptibility syndrome with seven complementation groups. Six of the FA genes have been cloned (corresponding to subtypes A, C, D2, E, F, and G) and the encoded proteins interact in a common pathway. There is wide range of mutations in the *FANCG* gene (splice, nonsense, and missense mutations), and, based on a mutational screen, a carboxy-terminal functional domain of the FANCG protein is required for complementation of FA-G cells and for normal assembly of the FANCA/FANCG/FANCC protein complex *(134)*.

Many somatic karyotypic abnormalities have now been described in childhood leukemias *(135,136)*, and a new clinical classification which would incorporate this emerging knowledge may be needed. The frequency of genetic alterations certainly supports that need, since we can identify a genetically abnormal clone in over 80% of children with new diagnosis of leukemia.

6.1. Acute Myeloid Leukemias

The original French-American-British Classification (FAB) divides these leukemias into those that are undiferentiated myeloblastic (M_0), myeloblastic without maturation (M_1), myeloblastic with maturation (M_2), hypergranular promyelocytic (M_3), myelomonocytic (M_4), monocytic (M_5), erythroid leukemia (M_6), and megacaryocytic leukemias (M_7). Interestingly, each of these subgroups created on the basis of their morphology at a time when the associated chromosomal changes were largely unknown, are affiliated with very distinct and typical genetic abnormalities. The fusion genes resulting from all these translocations, monosomies (losses), trisomies (gains), amplifications (HSRs) and deletions, not only fit the particular cell types and histological classifications, but often define the functional abnormalities described for the particular malig-

Table 2
Representative Examples of Genetic Alterations and Their Associated Clinically
Distinct Leukemic Phenotypes

Chromosome aberration	Gene	Protein	FAB class	Notes
t(8;21)(q22;q22)	AML1, ETO	Transcription factor	M2	Auer rods common myeloblastomas
t(17;19)(q22;p13)	HLF	Transcription factor		Pro-B ALL, hypercalcemia, disseminated intravascular coagulation
t(6;11)(q27;q23)	AF6, MLL	Homeobox	M4, M5	
t(11;17)(q23;q21)	PLZF, RARα	Transcription factor, hormone receptor	M3	
inv(16)(p13;q22) or t(16;16)(p13;q22)	SMMHC, CBFs	Muscle protein, transcription factor	M4Eo	
t(15;17)(q22;q21)	PML, RARα	Nuclear protein, hormone receptor	M3	Diseminated intravascular coagulation
t(6;9)(p23;q34)	DEK, CAN	Transcription factor, nuclear protein	M2, M4	
Monosomy 7 or del(7)(q22-q36)	?	?	All	Juvenile CML
t(9;22)(q34;q11)	BCR, ABL	Tyrosine kinase, serine-threonine kinase activity	M1, M2	
t(9;11)(p22;q23)	AF9, MLL	Homeobox	M4, M5	Infants, CNS leukemia, biphenotypic leukemia,
t(6;11)(q27;q23)	AF6, MLL	Homeobox	M4, M5	
Trisomy 8	?	?	All	Myelodysplastic syndromes
t(1;11)(q21;q23)	AF1q, MLL	Homeobox	M4, M5	
inv(3)(q21;q23) or t(3;3)(q21;q26)	EVIl	Transcription factor	M4, M7	Thrombocytosis and abnormal platelets
t(3;21)(q26;q22)	EVIl, EAP	Transcription factors	M2, AML1	Myelodysplastic syndromes
Monosomy 5 or del(5)(q11–q35)	?	?	All	Myelodysplastic syndromes and secondary leukemias
t(16;21)(p11;q22)	TLS, ERG	RNA-binding protein, transcription factor	All	
t(11;19)(q23;p13.1)	MLL, ELL	Homeobox	M4, M5	
t(12;22)(p13;q11)	TEL, MN1	Transcription factor	All	
Trisomy 11	MLL	Homeobox	M4, M5	
t(10;11)(p12;q23)	AF10, MLL	Homeobox	M4, M5	
t(1;22)(p13;q13)	?	?	M7	

Disruption of transcriptional control genes is a common mechanism by which many genetic rearranements may contribute to leukemogenesis. Two reasons account for the prevalence of transcriptional factor alterations. One, they bind to crucial regulatory elements in DNA, such as promoters and enhancers, and thus can stimulate or inhibit gene transcription, and two, their modular organization provides an ideal framework for their binding to DNA as multiple heterodimeric complexes. This later ability may also explain why the disrupted and newly rearranged transcriptional control gene can still produce a functional hybrid protein rather than inert peptide.

nancy in the past (*see* Table 2). Furthermore, the presence or absence of one or more of these genetic abnormalities is often of independent prognostic significance even when other factors such as age, FAB classification, and tumor burden at diagnosis are considered. Discussing the multiplicity of gene fusions present in leukemias is beyond the scope of this chapter and only few well-established examples will be used.

6.1.1. CHROMOSOME 8

Trisomy 8 is the most frequent genetic aberration in AML, but the leukemogenic gene whose increased expression produces the disease is unknown. One possibility is the *ETO* gene, because of its implication in another gene aberration, the t(8;21)(q22;q22). The t(8;21) translocation is among the best characterized of the AML-associated chromosomal abnormalities. It fuses the *AML*-1 gene (also known as *CBFA2*, *PEBP2αB*, and *RUNX1*) on chromosome 21 to the *ETO (MTG8)* gene on chromosome 8 *(137–139)*. The resulting fusion protein consists of the N terminus of AML1 fused to a nearly full-length ETO protein. The *AML*-1 gene encodes one of the DNA-binding subunits of the transcription factor complex core-binding factor (CBF). Native AML1 is able to form a heterodimer with the β subunit, CBFβ (PEBP2β), and thus regulate the transcription of target genes by binding to the DNA sequence TGT/cGGT through its *runt* homology domain *(140,141)*. The gene encoding CBFβ is also rearranged in AML of the M4Eo subtype, as a consequence of inv(16)(p13;q22) *(142)*. Knocking in the *AML1-ETO* fusion gene into the *Aml1* locus results in embryonic lethality and lack of definitive hematopoiesis in liver *(143,144)*. These effects are almost identical to the *AML1–/–* mice *(145)*, demonstrating that AML1-ETO is a dominant inhibitor of normal AML1/CBFβ function during hematopoietic lineage commitment.

The *AML*-1 gene is also involved in a *TEL/AML1* fusion in approximately 25% of all cases of childhood ALL, where, in contrast to the fusion product in myelogenous leukemia, it is associated with excellent prognosis *(146–149)*.

6.1.2. t(9;22)(q34;q11)

The t(9;22) or Philadelphia chromosome is perhaps the most extensively studied of the chromosomal translocations. The translocation results in fusion of the *BCR* gene on chromosome 22 to the *ABL* gene on chromosome 9. The t(9;22) is characteristic of chronic myeloid leukemia (CML), where almost all test *BCR/ABL*-positive. In childhood leukemias, only 3–5% of ALL are *BCR/ABL* positive, but these account for a large proportion of the mortality in this disorder. ABL is a predominantly nuclear protein with tyrosine kinase activity that is normally tightly regulated. Fusion of BCR to ABL results in constitutive activation of the ABL kinase and relocalization of the BCR/ABL fusion protein to the cytoskeleton *(150)*. The critical targets of the BCR/ABL kinase are not known, but it is likely that the fusion protein activates a number of signal transduction pathways, including the RAS pathway.

6.1.3. *E2A-HLF* FUSION GENE

E2A gene elements are involved in fusion events instigated by the t(17;19)(q22;p13) translocation, which juxtaposes the amino-terminal sequences of E2A (including the *trans*-activation domain) with the DNA binding and protein dimerization region of the protein encoded by the hepatic leukemia factor gene *(HLF)*. Recently assigned to a specific subfamily of the bZIP superfamily of transcription factors *(151,152)*, the HLF product is normally expressed only in the liver, brain, and kidney, but not in lymphoid cells. It bears significant homology to both DBP *(153)*, an albumin gene promoter D-box binding protein, and thyrotroph embryonic factor, which *trans*-activates thyroid-stimulating hormone β expression during anterior pituitary development *(154).*

Leukemias that express *E2A-HLF* share a number of clinical and biologic features: disease onset in early adolescence, pro-B immunophenotype, hypercalcemia, and disseminated intravascular coagulation. Although relatively rare, the *E2A-HLF*-associated leukemias have a poor prognosis, even when treated with intensive, multiagent chemotherapy.

6.1.4. MONOSOMY 5

Monosomy 5 and interstitial deletions of the long arm of chromosome 5 are one two of the earliest described chromosomal abnormalities in myeloid malignancies. They are observed, but not restricted to myelodysplastic syndromes, and a distinct subtype of myelodysplasia with 5q deletions is referred to as 5q minus syndrome *(155).* Because a chromosomal deletion associated with a malignancy often suggests a tumor suppressor gene that maps within the region, an intensive search for the 5q tumor suppressor gene is ongoing *(156),* but the critically deleted region of 5q is centered on chromosome bands 5q31–5q33, where genes encoding for hematopoietic growth factors such as granulocyte macrophage colony-stimulating factor (GM-CSF), M-CSF receptor, interleukin (IL)-3, IL-4, and IL-5 map as well, making the tumor supressor theory less likely.

7. FUTURE THERAPIES

While approximately half of children with AML can be cured with present therapeutic modalities, the remainder succumbs to the disease because of various forms of drug resistance. For this group, the hope lies in the recent advances in immunology, cytogenetics, and cellular and molecular biology, which have provided new insights into fundamental biological differences between leukemic myeloid blasts and their normal counterparts. Therapies such as: *(i)* antibody or small molecules directed against growth factors and their receptors on AML blasts; *(ii)* pharmacologic targeting of the pathologic t(15;17) translocation of acute promyelocytic leukemia with all-*trans* retinoic acid; *(iii)* pharmacologic and immunologic targeting of mutant *ras* oncogenes and related aberrant signaling in AML blast; and *(iv)* targeting of pathological signaling of the Bcr-Abl oncoprotein and c-kit tyrosine kinase in myeloid leukemias, herald an exciting new era of AML-specific therapies.

Even the most promising and highly targeted therapies such as STI-571 (Gleevec), used in the treatment of Philadelphia chromosome-positive CML, may be rapidly rendered ineffective by acquired drug resistance driven by the genetic instability of tumor cells *(157).* Moreover, while the initial chronic phase of CML, characterized by the expansion of terminally differentiated neutrophils due to a single *bcr/abl* genetic/oncogenic alteration, responds extremely well to this single-target therapy *(158,159),* the therapeutic efficiency is lost in the acute blast crisis phase. In this advanced disease state, further genetic abnormalities *(157)* and the reactivation of BCR-ABL signal transduction *(160)* result in unhindered progression of the disease in the face of continued therapy with STI-571. Despite the fundamental differences of this particular therapy with that of most conventional chemotherapies, which indiscriminately target dividing cancer cells, (i.e., STI-571 targets a specific mutant protein directly involved in cancer progression), acquired drug resistance occurs in a manner not dissimilar to traditional therapies.

Table 3
Effect of Oncogenes and Tumor Suppressor Genes on the Expression of Angiogenic Factors

Gene	Inhibitor decreased	Inducer increased	Reference
Tumor suppressor genes			
p53	TSP-1	VEGF	175,176
VHL		VEGF TGFβ	177,178
NF-1		Midkine	
PTEN	TSP-1	VEGF	179,180
Rb-1	Unknown		189
Oncogenes			
K-, H-, or N-*ras*	TSP-1	VEGF	161,181
H-*ras*	TIMP	MMP-9, MMP-2, MMP-14	181,182
N-*myc*	Activin A		183,184
v-*myc*	TSP-1		165
v-*myb*	TSP-2		185
c-*Jun*	TSP-1		186,187
v-*src*	TSP-1		180,188

Recent developments in the understanding of adult tumor progression may add a new dimension to the treatment of poor prognosis childhood tumors with multiple genetic abnormalities. It has been proposed that many oncogenes and tumor-suppressor genes are involved in the development of the angiogenic phenotype. Dominantly acting oncogenes such as *ras* and *raf* might be regarded as proangiogenic, because they are associated with overexpression of vascular endothelial growth factor (VEGF), a pro-angiogenic growth factor, and down-regulation of thrombospondin, a natural angiogenesis inhibitor *(161)*. Tumor-suppressor genes such as *p53*, on the other hand, exert the opposite effect down-regulating VEGF *(162)*, and up-regulating thrombospondin 1 *(163)*. Since the early reports of direct, *ras* oncogene-induced angiogenic drive *(161,164)*, many other oncogenes have been associated with induction of angiogenic factors or down-regulation inhibitors. *Myc* oncogene has been shown to induce angiogenic switch not only via down-modulation of thrombospondin-1 *(165)* or activin A *(166)*, but also by enabling cells to increase the availability of angiogenic factors such as VEGF *(167)*. For the numerous oncogenes and tumor suppressor genes associated with induction of angiogenesis in pediatric cancers see Table 3.

If so, anti-angiogenic treatment may provide a new approach to confronting the seemingly inevitable problem of acquired drug resistance. If the capacity of cancer cells to develop resistance is dependent on their "mutator" phenotype, then shifting the cellular target of therapy to a genetically stable cell, which the tumor depends on for growth and survival, may provide a possible means to evade, or delay, the problem of acquired drug resistance *(168)*. One such target for this strategy is the tumor-associated activated endothelial cell of a tumor's newly formed or forming microvasculature. The therapeutic targeting of the tumor vasculature is possible mainly because numerous molecular and functional differences have been identified that distinguish the tumor-associated "angiogenic" endothelium from its normal mature counterpart. For example, tumor-associated endothelial cells proliferate and migrate in response to tumor-induced stimuli, such as growth factors and cytokines, they proliferate much faster than their systemic counterpart *(169)*, and they express a large number of markers absent or poorly expressed in normal quiescent endothelial cells of mature vessels *(170)*.

The concept and potential of targeting the relatively genetically stable tumor-associated endothelial cell as a possible means of circumventing acquired drug resistance is supported by clinical observations. It has been known since the early days of chemotherapy, that the side-effects such as myelosuppression, gastrointestinal dysfunction, and hairloss, are rarely accompanied by any clinically meaningful host tolerance. Furthermore, the dose-limiting toxicities, exhibited on the genetically stable, diploid but rapidly proliferating cells of the skin, gastrointestinal mucosa, peripheral nervous system, and bone marrow, occur at doses much lower than those needed to cause tumor cell death. As recently shown *(171,172)*, these dose-limiting host toxicities can translate into a significant differential chemosensitivity of endothelial vs tumor cells, such that much lower doses of a drug can be used if the tumor endothelium is targeted, especially if the drug is given on a continuous low-dose basis. As pointed out by Browder et al. *(171)*, the one reason anti-angiogenic effects of chemotherapeutic drugs are not seen clinically, are due to the manner in which chemotherapeutic drugs are given. Using maximum tolerated doses (MTD) necessitates prolonged rest periods during which any collateral vascular damage on the tumor can be repaired, and unless these therapeutic breaks are shortened, or eliminated, no therapeutic advantage can be derived from the differential sensitivity between endothelial and tumor cells. Most importantly, this anti-vascular effect can be achieved with a diverse spectrum of chemotherapeutic agents such as vinblastine, adriamycin, cisplatinum, or taxol *(173)*, and these "metronomic dosing" regimens *(174)* can significantly minimize host toxicity.

There are currently no major efforts to clinically evaluate the efficacy of agents targeting genetic lesions in childhood neoplasia. In theory, such therapies may be effective as long as the process can be attributed to a defined oncogenic alterations or signaling pathways of abnormal differentiation. Until the feasibility of such therapies is more firmly defined, angiogenesis inhibition may provide an alternative therapy for children who are, because of the accumulation of numerous oncogenic changes, faced with poor prognosis and very taxing chemotherapeutic regimens. Undisputedly, significant progress has been achieved in pediatric oncology with therapeutic modalities, such as surgery, radiation, and chemotherapy, but the rise in survival rates experienced in the 1960s and 1970s has reached a plateau in the past two decades. The genomic plasticity of the tumor cell and its ability to adapt to an unfavourable environment and develop a drug-resistant clone is a major factor limiting the effectiveness of both old and new drugs directed against the tumor cell.

REFERENCES

1. Fearon ER, Vogelstein B. A genetic model for colorectal tumorigenesis. *Cell* 1990; 61:759–767.
2. Bader P, Schilling F, Schlaud M, Girgert R, Handgretinger R, Klingebiel T, et al. Expression analysis of multidrug resistance associated genes in neuroblastomas. *Oncol Rep* 1996; 6:1143–1146.
3. Knudson AG Jr. Mutation and cancer: statistical study of retinoblastoma. *Proc Natl Acad Sci USA* 1971; 68:820–823.

4. Knudson AG Jr, Strong LC. Mutation and cancer: a model for Wilm's tumor of the kidney. *J Natl Cancer Inst* 1972; 48:313–324.
5. Knudson AG Jr, Strong LC. Mutation and cancer: neuroblastoma and pheochromocytoma. *Am J Hum Genet* 1972; 24:514–532.
6. Lee WH, Bookstein R, Hong F, Young LJ, Shew JY, Lee EY. Human retinoblastoma susceptibility gene: cloning, identification, and sequence. *Science* 1987; 235:1394–1399.
7. Lele KP, Penrose LS, Stallard HB. Chromosome deletion in a case of retinoblastoma. *Ann Hum Genet* 1963; 27:171.
8. Chaum E, Ellsworth RM, Abramson DH, Haik BG, Kitchin FD, Chaganti RS. Cytogenetic analysis of retinoblastoma: evidence for multifocal origin and in vivo gene amplification. *Cytogenet Cell Genet* 1984; 38:82–91.
9. Squire J, Gallie BL, Phillips RA. A detailed analysis of chromosomal changes in heritable and non-heritable retinoblastoma. *Hum Genet* 1985; 70:291–301.
10. Francke U. Retinoblastoma and chromosome 13. *Cytogenet Cell Genet* 1976; 16:131–134.
11. Ward P, Packman S, Loughman W, Sparkes M, Sparkes R, McMahon A, et al. Location of the retinoblastoma susceptibility gene(s) and the human esterase D locus. *J Med Genet* 1984; 21:92–95.
12. Gallie BL, Campbell C, Devlin H, Duckett A, Squire JA. Developmental basis of retinal-specific induction of cancer by RB mutation. *Cancer Res* 1999; 59:1731s–1735s.
13. Abramson DH, Ellsworth RM, Kitchin FD, Tung G. Second nonocular tumors in retinoblastoma survivors. Are they radiationinduced? *Ophthalmology* 1984; 91:1351–1355.
14. Hansen MF, Koufos A, Gallie BL, Phillips RA, Fodstad O, Brogger A, et al. Osteosarcoma and retinoblastoma: a shared chromosomal mechanism revealing recessive predisposition. *Proc Natl Acad Sci USA* 1985; 82:6216–6220.
15. Dryja TP, Rapaport JM, Joyce JM, Petersen RA. Molecular detection of deletions involving band q14 of chromosome 13 in retinoblastomas. *Proc Natl Acad Sci USA* 1986; 83:7391–7394.
16. Huang HJ, Yee JK, Shew JY, Chen PL, Bookstein R, Friedmann T, et al. Suppression of the neoplastic phenotype by replacement of the RB gene in human cancer cells. *Science* 1988; 242:1563–1566.
17. Landschulz WH, Johnson PF, McKnight SL. The leucine zipper: a hypothetical structure common to a new class of DNA binding proteins. *Science* 1988; 240:1759–1764.
18. Lee WH, Shew JY, Hong FD, Sery TW, Donoso LA, Young LJ, et al. The retinoblastoma susceptibility gene encodes a nuclear phosphoprotein associated with DNA binding activity. *Nature* 1987; 329:642–645.
19. Buchkovich K, Duffy LA, Harlow E. The retinoblastoma protein is phosphorylated during specific phases of the cell cycle. *Cell* 1989; 58:1097–1105.
20. Kitchin FD, Ellsworth RM. Pleiotropic effects of the gene for retinoblastoma. *J Med Genet* 1974; 11:244–246.
21. Lee SB, Haber DA. Wilms tumor and the WT1 gene. *Exp Cell Res* 2001; 264:74–99.
22. Bardeesy N, Falkoff D, Petruzzi MJ, Nowak N, Zabel B, Adam M, et al. Anaplastic Wilm's tumour, a subtype displaying poor prognosis, harbours p53 gene mutations. *Nat Genet* 1994; 7:91–97.
23. Koesters R, Ridder R, Kopp-Schneider A, Betts D, Adams V, Niggli F, et al. Mutational activation of the beta-catenin proto-oncogene is a common event in the development of Wilm's tumors. *Cancer Res* 1999; 59:3880–3882.
24. Steenman MJ, Rainier S, Dobry CJ, Grundy P, Horon IL, Feinberg AP. Loss of imprinting of IGF2 is linked to reduced expression and abnormal methylation of H19 in Wilm's tumour. *Nat Genet* 1994; 7:433–439.
25. Riccardi VM, Sujansky E, Smith AC, Francke U. Chromosomal imbalance in the Aniridia-Wilm's tumor association: 11p interstitial deletion. *Pediatrics* 1978; 61:604–610.
26. Call KM, Glaser T, Ito CY, Buckler AJ, Pelletier J, Haber DA, et al. Isolation and characterization of a zinc finger polypeptide gene at the human chromosome 11 Wilm's tumor locus. *Cell* 1990; 60:509–520.
27. Gessler M, Poustka A, Cavenee W, Neve RL, Orkin SH, Bruns GA. Homozygous deletion in Wilms tumours of a zinc-finger gene identified by chromosome jumping. *Nature* 1990; 343:774–778.
28. Bonetta L, Kuehn SE, Huang A, Law DJ, Kalikin LM, Koi M, et al. Wilms tumor locus on 11p13 defined by multiple CpG island-associated transcripts. *Science* 1990; 250:994–997.
29. Diller L, Ghahremani M, Morgan J, Grundy P, Reeves C, Breslow N, et al. Constitutional WT1 mutations in Wilm's tumor patients. *J Clin Oncol* 1998; 16:3634–3640.

30. Rahman N, Arbour L, Tonin P, Renshaw J, Pelletier J, Baruchel S, et al. Evidence for a familial Wilm's tumour gene (FWT1) on chromosome 17q12-q21. *Nat Genet* 1996; 13:461–463.
31. Koufos A, Hansen MF, Lampkin BC, Workman ML, Copeland NG, Jenkins NA, et al. Loss of alleles at loci on human chromosome 11 during genesis of Wilm's tumour. *Nature* 1984; 309:170–172.
32. Orkin SH, Goldman DS, Sallan SE. Development of homozygosity for chromosome 11p markers in Wilm's tumour. *Nature* 1984; 309:172–174.
33. Fearon ER, Vogelstein B, Feinberg AP. Somatic deletion and duplication of genes on chromosome 11 in Wilm's tumours. *Nature* 1984; 309:176–178.
34. Henry I, Jeanpierre M, Couillin P, Barichard F, Serre JL, Journel H, et al. Molecular definition of the 11p15.5 region involved in Beckwith-Wiedemann syndrome and probably in predisposition to adrenocortical carcinoma. *Hum Genet* 1989; 81:273–277.
35. Reeve AE, Sih SA, Raizis AM, Feinberg AP. Loss of allelic heterozygosity at a second locus on chromosome 11 in sporadic Wilm's tumor cells. *Mol Cell Biol* 1989; 9:1799–1803.
36. Sheng WW, Soukup S, Bove K, Gotwals B, Lampkin B. Chromosome analysis of 31 Wilm's tumors. *Cancer Res* 1990; 50:2786–2793.
37. Maw MA, Grundy PE, Millow LJ, Eccles MR, Dunn RS, Smith PJ, et al. A third Wilm's tumor locus on chromosome 16q. *Cancer Res* 1992; 52:3094–3098.
38. Grundy RG, Pritchard J, Scambler P, Cowell JK. Loss of heterozygosity for the short arm of chromosome 7 in sporadic Wilms tumour. *Oncogene* 1998; 17:395–400.
39. Feinberg AP. The two-domain hypothesis in Beckwith-Wiedemann syndrome. *J Clin Invest* 2000; 106:739–740.
40. Junien C. Beckwith-Wiedemann syndrome, tumourigenesis and imprinting. *Curr Opin Genet Dev* 1992; 2:431–438.
41. Schroeder WT, Chao LY, Dao DD, Strong LC, Pathak S, Riccardi V, et al. Nonrandom loss of maternal chromosome 11 alleles in Wilms tumors. *Am J Hum Genet* 1987; 40:413–420.
42. Rainier S, Johnson LA, Dobry CJ, Ping AJ, Grundy PE, Feinberg AP. Relaxation of imprinted genes in human cancer. *Nature* 1993; 362:747–749.
43. Grundy PE, Telzerow PE, Breslow N, Moksness J, Huff V, Paterson MC. Loss of heterozygosity for chromosomes 16q and 1p in Wilm's tumors predicts an adverse outcome. *Cancer Res* 1994; 54:2331–2333.
44. Perlman M, Levin M, Wittels B. Syndrome of fetal gigantism, renal hamartomas, and nephroblastomatosis with Wilm's tumor. *Cancer* 1975; 35:1212–1217.
45. Hersh JH, Cole TR, Bloom AS, Bertolone SJ, Hughes HE. Risk of malignancy in Sotos syndrome. *J Pediatr* 1992; 120:572–574.
46. Patek CE, Little MH, Fleming S, Miles C, Charlieu JP, Clarke AR, et al. A zinc finger truncation of murine WT1 results in the characteristic urogenital abnormalities of Denys-Drash syndrome. *Proc Natl Acad Sci USA* 1999; 96:2931–2936.
47. Bardeesy N, Zabel B, Schmitt K, Pelletier J. WT1 mutations associated with incomplete Denys-Drash syndrome define a domain predicted to behave in a dominant-negative fashion. *Genomics* 1994; 21:663–664.
48. Barbaux S, Niaudet P, Gubler MC, Grunfeld JP, Jaubert F, Kuttenn F, et al. Donor splice-site mutations in WT1 are responsible for Frasier syndrome. *Nat Genet* 1997; 17:467–470.
49. Cairney AE, Andrews M, Greenberg M, Smith D, Weksberg R. Wilms tumor in three patients with Bloom syndrome. *J Pediatr* 1987; 111:414–416.
50. Roberts WM, Jenkins JJ, Moorhead EL, Douglass EC. Incontinentia pigmenti, a chromosomal instability syndrome, is associated with childhood malignancy. *Cancer* 1988; 62:2370–2372.
51. Li FP, Fraumeni JF Jr. Rhabdomyosarcoma in children: epidemiologic study and identification of a familial cancer syndrome. *J Natl Cancer Inst* 1969; 43:1365–1373.
52. Li FP, Fraumeni JF Jr. Soft-tissue sarcomas, breast cancer, and other neoplasms. A familial syndrome? *Ann Intern Med* 1969; 71:747–752.
53. Malkin D, Li FP, Strong LC, Fraumeni JF Jr, Nelson CE, Kim DH, et al. Germ line p53 mutations in a familial syndrome of breast cancer, sarcomas, and other neoplasms. *Science* 1990; 250:1233–1238.
54. Diller L, Sexsmith E, Gottlieb A, Li FP, Malkin D. Germline p53 mutations are frequently detected in young children with rhabdomyosarcoma. *J Clin Invest* 1995; 95:1606–1611.
55. Scrable HJ, Witte DP, Lampkin BC, Cavenee WK. Chromosomal localization of the human rhabdomyosarcoma locus by mitotic recombination mapping. *Nature* 1987; 329:645–647.
56. Scrable H, Witte D, Shimada H, Seemayer T, Sheng WW, Soukup S, et al. Molecular differential pathology of rhabdomyosarcoma. *Genes Chromosom Cancer* 1989; 1:23–35.

57. Scrable H, Cavenee W, Ghavimi F, Lovell M, Morgan K, Sapienza C. A model for embryonal rhab-domyosarcoma tumorigenesis that involves genome imprinting. *Proc Natl Acad Sci USA* 1989; 86:7480–7484.

58. El-Badry OM, Helman LJ, Chatten J, Steinberg SM, Evans AE, Israel MA. Insulin-like growth factor II-mediated proliferation of human neuroblastoma. *J Clin Invest* 1991; 87:648–657.

59. El-Badry OM, Romanus JA, Helman LJ, Cooper MJ, Rechler MM, Israel MA. Autonomous growth of a human neuroblastoma cell line is mediated by insulin-like growth factor II. *J Clin Invest* 1989; 84:829–839.

60. El Badry OM, Minniti C, Kohn EC, Houghton PJ, Daughaday WH, Helman LJ. Insulin-like growth factor II acts as an autocrine growth and motility factor in human rhabdomyosarcoma tumors. *Cell Growth Differ* 1990; 1:325–331.

61. Kalebic T, Tsokos M, Helman LJ. In vivo treatment with antibody against IGF-1 receptor suppresses growth of human rhabdomyosarcoma and down-regulates p34cdc2. *Cancer Res* 1994; 54:5531–5534.

62. Turc-Carel C, Lizard-Nacol S, Justrabo E, Favrot M, Philip T, Tabone E. Consistent chromosomal translocation in alveolar rhabdomyosarcoma. *Cancer Genet Cytogenet* 1986; 19:361–362.

63. Douglass EC, Valentine M, Etcubanas E, Parham D, Webber BL, Houghton PJ, et al. A specific chro-mosomal abnormality in rhabdomyosarcoma. *Cytogenet Cell Genet* 1987; 45:148–155.

64. Xu Q, Wu Z. The insulin-like growth factor-phosphatidylinositol 3-kinase-Akt signaling pathway regulates myogenin expression in normal myogenic cells but not in rhabdomyosarcoma-derived RD cells. *J Biol Chem* 2000; 275:36750–36757.

65. Margue CM, Bernasconi M, Barr FG, Schafer BW. Transcriptional modulation of the anti-apoptotic protein BCL-XL by the paired box transcription factors PAX3 and PAX3/FKHR. *Oncogene* 2000; 19:2921–2929.

66. Pulciani S, Santos E, Lauver AV, Long LK, Aaronson SA, Barbacid M. Oncogenes in solid human tumours. *Nature* 1982; 300:539–542.

67. Chardin P, Yeramian P, Madaule P, Tavitian A. N-ras gene activation in the RD human rhabdomyosar-coma cell line. *Int J Cancer* 1985; 35:647–652.

68. Stratton MR, Fisher C, Gusterson BA, Cooper CS. Detection of point mutations in N-ras and K-ras genes of human embryonal rhabdomyosarcomas using oligonucleotide probes and the polymerase chain reaction. *Cancer Res* 1989; 49:6324–6327.

69. Brodeur GM. Molecular basis for heterogeneity in human neuroblastomas. *Eur J Cancer* 1995; 31A:505–510.

70. Brodeur GM. Molecular pathology of human neuroblastomas. *Semin Diagn Pathol* 1994; 11:118–125.

71. Turkel SB, Itabashi HH. The natural history of neuroblastic cells in the fetal adrenal gland. *Am J Pathol* 1974; 76:225–244.

72. Ikeda Y, Lister J, Bouton JM, Buyukpamukcu M. Congenital neuroblastoma, neuroblastoma in situ, and the normal fetal development of the adrenal. *J Pediatr Surg* 1981; 16:636–644.

73. Bessho F, Hashizume K, Nakajo T, Kamoshita S. Mass screening in Japan increased the detection of infants with neuroblastoma without a decrease in cases in older children. *J Pediatr* 1991; 119:237–241.

74. Brodeur GM, Look AT, Shimada H, Hamilton VM, Maris JM, Hann HW, et al. Biological aspects of neuroblastomas identified by mass screening in Quebec. *Med Pediatr Oncol* 2001; 36:157–159.

75. Woods WG, Tuchman M, Bernstein ML, Leclerc JM, Brisson L, Look T, et al. Screening for neurob-lastoma in North America. 2-year results from the Quebec Project. *Am J Pediatr Hematol Oncol* 1992; 14:312–319.

76. Woods WG, Tuchman M, Robison LL, Bernstein M, Leclerc JM, Brisson LC, et al. Screening for neuroblastoma is ineffective in reducing the incidence of unfavourable advanced stage disease in older children. *Eur J Cancer* 1997; 33:2106–2112.

77. Baker DL, Reddy UR, Pleasure D, Thorpe CL, Evans AE, Cohen PS, et al. Analysis of nerve growth factor receptor expression in human neuroblastoma and neuroepithelioma cell lines. *Cancer Res* 1989; 49:4142–4146.

78. Azar C, Scavarda NJ, Reynolds CP, Brodeur GM. Multiple defects of the nerve growth factor recep-torin human neuroblastomas. *Prog Clin Biol Res* 1991; 366:219–226.

79. Azar CG, Scavarda NJ, Nakagawara A, Brodeur GM. Expression and function of the nerve growth factor receptor (TRK-A) in human neuroblastoma cell lines. *Prog Clin Biol Res* 1994; 385:169–175.

80. Nakagawara A, Arima-Nakagawara M, Scavarda NJ, Azar CG, Cantor AB, Brodeur GM. Association between high levels of expression of the TRK gene and favorable outcome in human neuroblastoma. *N Engl J Med* 1993; 328:847–854.

81. Brodeur GM, Green AA, Hayes FA, Williams KJ, Williams DL, Tsiatis AA. Cytogenetic features of human neuroblastomas and cell lines. *Cancer Res* 1981; 41:4678–4686.
82. Brodeur GM, Nakagawara A. Molecular basis of clinical heterogeneity in neuroblastoma. *Am J Pediatr Hematol Oncol* 1992; 14:111–116.
83. Cheng NC, van Roy N, Chan A, Beitsma M, Westerveld A, Speleman F, et al. Deletion mapping in neuroblastoma cell lines suggests two distinct tumor suppressor genes in the 1p35–36 region, only one of which is associated with N-myc amplification. *Oncogene* 1995; 10:291–297.
84. Takeda O, Homma C, Maseki N, Sakurai M, Kanda N, Schwab M, et al. There may be two tumor suppressor genes on chromosome arm 1p closely associated with biologically distinct subtypes of neuroblastoma. *Genes Chromosom Cancer* 1994; 10:30–39.
85. Schleiermacher G, Peter M, Michon J, Hugot JP, Vielh P, Zucker JM, et al. Two distinct deleted regions on the short arm of chromosome 1 in neuroblastoma. *Genes Chromosom Cancer* 1994; 10:275–281.
86. Fong CT, Dracopoli NC, White PS, Merrill PT, Griffith RC, Housman DE, et al. Loss of heterozygosity for the short arm of chromosome 1 in human neuroblastomas: correlation with N-myc amplification. *Proc Natl Acad Sci USA* 1989; 86:3753–3757.
87. Caron H, van SP, van HM, de KJ, Bras J, Slater R, et al. Allelic loss of chromosome 1p36 in neuroblastoma is of preferential maternal origin and correlates with N-myc amplification [comment] [see comments] [published erratum appears in Nat Genet 1993 Aug;4(4):431]. *Nat Genet* 1993; 4:187–190.
88. Fong CT, White PS, Peterson K, Sapienza C, Cavenee WK, Kern SE, et al. Loss of heterozygosity for chromosomes 1 or 14 defines subsets of advanced neuroblastomas. *Cancer Res* 1992; 52:1780–1785.
89. Srivatsan ES, Ying KL, Seeger RC. Deletion of chromosome 11 and of 14q sequences in neuroblastoma. *Genes Chromosom Cancer* 1993; 7:32–37.
90. Caron H. Allelic loss of chromosome 1 and additional chromosome 17 material are both unfavourable prognostic markers in neuroblastoma. *Med Pediatr Oncol* 1995; 24:215–221.
91. Katzenstein HM, Bowman LC, Brodeur GM, Thorner PS, Joshi VV, Smith EI, et al. Prognostic significance of age, MYCN oncogene amplification, tumor cell ploidy, and histology in 110 infants with stage D(S) neuroblastoma: the pediatric oncology group experience—a pediatric oncology group study. *J Clin Oncol* 1998; 16:2007–2017.
92. Komuro H, Valentine MB, Rowe ST, Kidd VJ, Makino S, Brodeur GM, et al. Fluorescence in situ hybridization analysis of chromosome 1p36 deletions in human MYCN amplified neuroblastoma. *J Pediatr Surg* 1998; 33:1695–1698.
93. Kong XT, Valentine VA, Rowe ST, Valentine MB, Ragsdale ST, Jones BG, et al. Lack of homozygously inactivated p73 in single-copy MYCN primary neuroblastomas and neuroblastoma cell lines. *Neoplasia* 1999; 1:80–89.
94. Hempstead BL, Martin-Zanca D, Kaplan DR, Parada LF, Chao MV. High-affinity NGF binding requires coexpression of the trk proto-oncogene and the low-affinity NGF receptor. *Nature* 1991; 350:678–683.
95. Kaplan DR, Hempstead BL, Martin-Zanca D, Chao MV, Parada LF. The trk proto-oncogene product: a signal transducing receptor for nerve growth factor. *Science* 1991; 252:554–558.
96. Klein R, Jing SQ, Nanduri V, O' Rourke E, Barbacid M. The trk proto-oncogene encodes a receptor for nerve growth factor. *Cell* 1991; 65:189–197.
97. Klein R, Nanduri V, Jing SA, Lamballe F, Tapley P, Bryant S, et al. The trkB tyrosine protein kinase is a receptor for brain-derived neurotrophic factor and neurotrophin-3. *Cell* 1991; 66:395–403.
98. Lamballe F, Klein R, Barbacid M. trkC, a new member of the trk family of tyrosine protein kinases, is a receptor for neurotrophin-3. *Cell* 1991; 66:967–979.
99. Squinto SP, Stitt TN, Aldrich TH, Davis S, Bianco SM, Radziejewski C, et al. trkB encodes a functional receptor for brain-derived neurotrophic factor and neurotrophin-3 but not nerve growth factor. *Cell* 1991; 65:885–893.
100. Klein R, Lamballe F, Bryant S, Barbacid M. The trkB tyrosine protein kinase is a receptor for neurotrophin-4.*Neuron* 1992; 8:947–956.
101. Nakagawara A, Azar CG, Scavarda NJ, Brodeur GM. Expression and function of TRK-B and BDNF in human neuroblastomas. *Mol Cell Biol* 1994; 14:759–767.
102. Brodeur GM, Nakagawara A, Yamashiro DJ, Ikegaki N, Liu XG, Azar CG, et al. Expression of TrkA, TrkB and TrkC in human neuroblastomas. *J Neurooncol* 1997; 31:49–55.
103. Scala S, Wosikowski K, Giannakakou P, Valle P, Biedler JL, Spengler BA, et al. Brain-derived neurotrophic factor protects neuroblastoma cells from vinblastine toxicity. *Cancer Res* 1996; 56:3737–3742.

104. Middlemas DS, Kihl BK, Zhou J, Zhu X. Brain Derived neurotropic factor promotes survival and chemoprotection of human neuroblastoma cells. *J Biol Chem* 1999; 274:16451–16460.

105. Lucarelli E, Kaplan D, Thiele CJ. Activation of trk-A but not trk-B signal transduction pathway inhibits growth of neuroblastoma cells. *Eur J Cancer* 1997; 33:2068–2070.

106. Eggert A, Ikegaki N, Kwiatkowski J, Zhao H, Brodeur GM, Himelstein BP. High-level expression of angiogenic factors is associated with advanced tumor stage in human neuroblastomas. *Clin Cancer Res* 2000; 6:1900–1908.

107. Donovan MJ, Lin MI, Wiegn P, Ringstedt T, Kraemer R, Hahn R, et al. Brain derived neurotrophic factor is an endothelial cell survival factor required for intramyocardial vessel stabilization. *Development* 2000; 127:4531–4540.

108. Yamashiro DJ, Nakagawara A, Ikegaki N, Liu XG, Brodeur GM. Expression of TrkC in favorable human neuroblastomas. *Oncogene* 1996; 12:37–41.

109. Svensson T, Ryden M, Schilling FH, Dominici C, Sehgal R, Ibanez CF, et al. Coexpression of mRNA for the full-length neurotrophin receptor trk-C and trk-A in favourable neuroblastoma. *Eur J Cancer* 1997; 33:2058–2063.

110. Nakagawara A, Arima M, Azar CG, Scavarda NJ, Brodeur GM. Inverse relationship between trk expression and N-myc amplification in human neuroblastomas. *Cancer Res* 1992; 52:1364–1368.

111. Seeger RC, Wada R, Brodeur GM, Moss TJ, Bjork RL, Sousa L, et al. Expression of N-myc by neuroblastomas with one or multiple copies of the oncogene. *Prog Clin Biol Res* 1988; 271:41–49.

112. Tanaka T, Slamon DJ, Shimoda H, Waki C, Kawaguchi Y, Tanaka Y, et al. Expression of Ha-ras oncogene products in human neuroblastomas and the significant correlation with a patient's prognosis. *Cancer Res* 1988; 48:1030–1034.

113. Tanaka T, Sugimoto T, Sawada T. Prognostic discrimination among neuroblastomas according to Ha-ras/trk A gene expression: a comparison of the profiles of neuroblastomas detected clinically and those detected through mass screening. *Cancer* 1998; 83:1626–1633.

114. Ballas K, Lyons J, Janssen JW, Bartram CR. Incidence of ras gene mutations in neuroblastoma. *Eur J Pediatr* 1988; 147:313–314.

115. Thiele CJ, McKeon C, Triche TJ, Ross RA, Reynolds CP, Israel MA. Differential protooncogene expression characterizes histopathologically indistinguishable tumors of the peripheral nervous system. *J Clin Invest* 1987; 80:804–811.

116. Miller RW. Deaths from childhood leukemia and solid tumors among twins and other sibs in the United States, 1960–67. *J Natl Cancer Inst* 1971; 46:203–209.

117. Draper GJ, Heaf MM, Kinnier Wilson LM. Occurrence of childhood cancers among sibs and estimation of familial risks. *J Med Genet* 1977; 14:81–90.

118. Hartley SE, Sainsbury C. Acute leukaemia and the same chromosome abnormality in monozygotic twins. *Hum Genet* 1981; 58:408–410.

119. Pombo de Oliveira MS, Awad el Seed FE, Foroni L, Matutes E, Morilla R, Luzzatto L, et al. Lymphoblastic leukaemia in Siamese twins: evidence for identity. *Lancet* 1986; 2:969–970.

120. Ford AM, Ridge SA, Cabrera ME, Mahmoud H, Steel CM, Chan LC, et al. In utero rearrangements in the trithorax-related oncogene in infant leukaemias. *Nature* 1993; 363:358–360.

121. Morton NE, Hassold TJ, Funkhouser J, McKenna PW, Lew R. Cytogenetic surveillance of spontaneous abortions. *Cytogenet Cell Genet* 1982; 33:232–239.

122. Hassold TJ, Jacobs PA. Trisomy in man. *Annu Rev Genet* 1984; 18:69–97.

123. Zipursky A. Susceptibility to leukemia and resistance to solid tumors in Down syndrome. *Pediatr Res* 2000; 47:704.

124. Ferster A, Verhest A, Vamos E, De Maertelaere E, Otten J. Leukemia in a trisomy 21 mosaic: specific involvement of the trisomic cells. *Cancer Genet Cytogenet* 1986; 20:109–113.

125. Robison LL, Nesbit ME Jr, Sather HN, Level C, Shahidi N, Kennedy A, et al. Down syndrome and acute leukemia in children: a 10-year retrospective survey from Childrens Cancer Study Group. *J Pediatr* 1984; 105:235–242.

126. Zipursky A, Poon A, Doyle J. Leukemia in Down syndrome: a review. *Pediatr Hematol Oncol* 1992; 9:139–149.

127. Zipursky A, Brown EJ, Christensen H, Doyle J. Transient myeloproliferative disorder (transient leukemia) and hematologic manifestations of Down syndrome. *Clin Lab Med* 1999; 19:157–167.

128. Doyle JJ, Thorner P, Poon A, Tanswell K, Kamel-Reid S, Zipursky A. Transient Leukemia followed by megakaryoblastic leukemia in a child with mosaic Down syndrome. *Leuk Lymphoma* 1995; 17:345–350.

129. Zipursky A, Doyle J. Leukemia in newborn infants with Down syndrome. *Leuk Res* 1993; 17:195.

130. Antonarakis SE. Parental origin of the extra chromosome in trisomy 21 as indicated by analysis of DNA polymorphisms. Down Syndrome Collaborative Group. *N Engl J Med* 1991; 324:872–876.

131. Sacchi N. Genes on chromosome 21 and cancer. In: Patterson D, Epstein CJ, eds. *Molecular Genetics of Chromosome 21 and Downs Syndrome.* Wiley-Liss, New York, 1990, pp.169.

132. Miller RW. Relation between cancer and congenital defects: an epidemiologic evaluation. *J Natl Cancer Inst* 1968; 40:1079–1085.

133. Thick J, Metcalfe JA, Mak YF, Beatty D, Minegishi M, Dyer MJ, et al. Expression of either the TCL1 oncogene, or transcripts from its homologue MTCP1/c6.1B, in leukaemic and non-leukaemic T cells from ataxia telangiectasia patients. *Oncogene* 1996; 12:379–386.

134. Nakanishi K, Moran A, Hays T, Kuang Y, Fox E, Garneau D, et al. Functional analysis of patient-derived mutations in the Fanconi anemia gene, FANCG/XRCC9. *Exp Hematol* 2001; 29:842–849.

135. Look AT. The cytogenetics of childhood leukemia: clinical and biologic implications. *Pediatr Clin North Am* 1988; 35:723–741.

136. Look AT, Downing JR. Molecular biology of leukemia and lymphoma. *Rev Invest Clin* 1994; Suppl:124–134.

137. Downing JR, Higuchi M, Lenny N, Yeoh AE. Alterations of the AML1 transcription factor in human leukemia. *Semin Cell Dev Biol* 2000; 11:347–360.

138. Nucifora G, Rowley JD. AML1 and the 8;21 and 3;21 translocations in acute and chronic myeloid leukemia. *Blood* 1995; 86:1–14.

139. Tighe JE, Daga A, Calabi F. Translocation breakpoints are clustered on both chromosome 8 and chromosome 21 in the t(8;21) of acute myeloid leukemia. *Blood* 1993; 81:592–596.

140. Meyers S, Lenny N, Hiebert SW. The t(8;21) fusion protein interferes with AML-1B-dependent transcriptional activation. *Mol Cell Biol* 1995; 15:1974–1982.

141. Frank R, Zhang J, Uchida H, Meyers S, Hiebert SW, Nimer SD. The AML1/ETO fusion protein blocks transactivation of the GM-CSF promoter by AML1B. *Oncogene* 1995; 11:2667–2674.

142. Liu P, Tarle SA, Hajra A, Claxton DF, Marlton P, Freedman M, et al. Fusion between transcription factor CBF beta/PEBP2 beta and a myosin heavy chain in acute myeloid leukemia. *Science* 1993; 261:1041–1044.

143. Yergeau DA, Hetherington CJ, Wang Q, Zhang P, Sharpe AH, Binder M, et al. Embryonic lethality and impairment of haematopoiesis in mice heterozygous for an AML1-ETO fusion gene. *Nat Genet* 1997; 15:303–306.

144. Okuda T, Cai Z, Yang S, Lenny N, Lyu CJ, van Deursen JM, et al. Expression of a knocked-in AML1-ETO leukemia gene inhibits the establishment of normal definitive hematopoiesis and directly generates dysplastic hematopoietic progenitors. *Blood* 1998; 91:3134–3143.

145. Okuda T, van Deursen J, Hiebert SW, Grosveld G, Downing JR. AML1, the target of multiple chromosomal translocations in human leukemia, is essential for normal fetal liver hematopoiesis. *Cell* 1996; 84:321–330.

146. Rubnitz JE, Downing JR, Pui CH, Shurtleff SA, Raimondi SC, Evans WE, et al. TEL gene rearrangement in acute lymphoblastic leukemia: a new genetic marker with prognostic significance. *J Clin Oncol* 1997; 15:1150–1157.

147. Shurtleff SA, Buijs A, Behm FG, Rubnitz JE, Raimondi SC, Hancock ML, et al. TEL/AML1 fusion resulting from a cryptic t(12;21) is the most common genetic lesion in pediatric ALL and defines a subgroup of patients with an excellent prognosis. *Leukemia* 1995; 9:1985–1989.

148. McLean TW, Ringold S, Neuberg D, Stegmaier K, Tantravahi R, Ritz J, et al. TEL/AML-1 dimerizes and is associated with a favorable outcome in childhood acute lymphoblastic leukemia. *Blood* 1996; 88:4252–4258.

149. Romana SP, Poirel H, Leconiat M, Flexor MA, Mauchauffe M, Jonveaux P, et al. High frequency of t(12;21) in childhood B-lineage acute lymphoblastic leukemia. *Blood* 1995; 86:4263–4269.

150. McWhirter JR, Wang JY. An actin-binding function contributes to transformation by the Bcr-Abl oncoprotein of Philadelphia chromosome-positive human leukemias. *EMBO J* 1993; 12:1533–1546.

151. Hunger SP, Ohyashiki K, Toyama K, Cleary ML. Hlf, a novel hepatic bZIP protein, shows altered DNA-binding properties following fusion to E2A in t(17;19) acute lymphoblastic leukemia. *Genes Dev* 1992; 6:1608–1620.

152. Inaba T, Roberts WM, Shapiro LH, Jolly KW, Raimondi SC, Smith SD, et al. Fusion of the leucine zipper gene HLF to the E2A gene in human acute B-lineage leukemia. *Science* 1992; 257:531–534.

153. Mueller CR, Maire P, Schibler U. DBP, a liver-enriched transcriptional activator, is expressed late in ontogeny and its tissue specificity is determined posttranscriptionally. *Cell* 1990; 61:279–291.

154. Drolet DW, Scully KM, Simmons DM, Wegner M, Chu KT, Swanson LW, et al. TEF, a transcription factor expressed specifically in the anterior pituitary during embryogenesis, defines a new class of leucine zipper proteins. *Genes Dev* 1991; 5:1739–1753.

155. Boultwood J, Lewis S, Wainscoat JS. The 5q-syndrome. *Blood* 1994; 84:3253–3260.

156. Fairman J, Chumakov I, Chinault AC, Nowell PC, Nagarajan L. Physical mapping of the minimal region of loss in 5q-chromosome. *Proc Natl Acad Sci USA* 1995; 92:7406–7410.

157. McCormick F. New-age drug meets resistance. *Nature* 2001; 412:281–282.

158. Druker BJ, Sawyers CL, Kantarjian H, Resta DJ, Reese SF, Ford JM, et al. Activity of a specific inhibitor of the BCR-ABL tyrosine kinase in the blast crisis of chronic myeloid leukemia and acute lymphoblastic leukemia with the Philadelphia chromosome. *N Engl J Med* 2001; 344:1038–1042.

159. Druker BJ, Talpaz M, Resta DJ, Peng B, Buchdunger E, Ford JM, et al. Efficacy and safety of a specific inhibitor of the BCR-ABL tyrosine kinase in chronic myeloid leukemia. *N Engl J Med* 2001; 344:1031–1037.

160. Gorre ME, Mohammed M, Ellwood K, Hsu N, Paquette R, Rao PN, et al. Clinical resistance to STI-571 cancer therapy caused by BCR-ABL gene mutation or amplification. *Science* 2001; 293:876–880.

161. Rak J, Mitsuhashi Y, Bayko L, Filmus J, Shirasawa S, Sasazuki T, et al. Mutant ras oncogenes upregulate VEGF/VPF expression: implications for induction and inhibition of tumor angiogenesis. *Cancer Res* 1995; 55:4575–4580.

162. Mukhopadhyay D, Tsiokas L, Sukhatme VP. Wild-type p53 and v-Src exert opposing influences on human vascular endothelial growth factor gene expression. *Cancer Res* 1995; 55:6161–6165.

163. Dameron KM, Volpert OV, Tainsky MA, Bouck N. Control of angiogenesis in fibroblasts by p53 regulation of thrombospondin-1. *Science* 1994; 265:1582–1584.

164. Rak J, Filmus J, Finkenzeller G, Grugel S, Marme D, Kerbel RS. Oncogenes as inducers of tumor angiogenesis. *Cancer Metastasis Rev* 1995; 14:263–277.

165. Janz A, Sevignani C, Kenyon K, Ngo CV, Thomas-Tikhonenko A. Activation of the myc oncoprotein leads to increased turnover of thrombospondin-1 mRNA. *Nucleic Acids Res* 2000; 28:2268–2275.

166. Breit S, Ashman K, Wilting J, Rossler J, Hatzi E, Fotsis T, et al. The N-myc oncogene in human neuroblastoma cells: down-regulation of an angiogenesis inhibitor identified as activin A. *Cancer Res* 2000; 60:4596–4601.

167. Ngo CV, Gee M, Akhtar N, Yu D, Volpert O, Auerbach R, et al. An in vivo function for the transforming Myc protein: elicitation of the angiogenic phenotype. *Cell Growth Differ* 2000; 11:201–210.

168. Kerbel RS. Inhibition of tumor angiogenesis as a strategy to circumvent acquired resistance to anticancer therapeutic agents. *BioEssays* 1991; 13:31–36.

169. Denekamp J. Vascular endothelium as the vulnerable element in tumours. *Acta Radiol Oncol* 1984; 23:217–225.

170. St Croix B, Rago C, Velculescu V, Traverso G, Romans KE, Montgomery E, et al. Genes expressed in human tumor endothelium. *Science* 2000; 289:1197–1202.

171. Browder T, Butterfield CE, Kraling BM, Marshall B, O'Reilly MS, Folkman J. Antiangiogenic scheduling of chemotherapy improves efficacy against experimental drug-resistant cancer. *Cancer Res* 2000; 60:1878–1886.

172. Klement G, Baruchel S, Rak J, Man S, Clark K, Hicklin DJ, et al. Continuous low-dose therapy with vinblastine and VEGF receptor-2 antibody induces sustained tumor regression without overt toxicity [see comments]. *J Clin Invest* 2000; 105:R15–R24.

173. Klement G, Huang P, Mayer B, Man S, Bohlen P, Hicklin DJ, et al. Differences in therapeutic indexes of combination metronomic chemotherapy and an anti-VEGFR-2 antibody in multidrug resistant human breast cancer xenografts. *Clin Cancer Res* 2002; 8:221–232.

174. Hanahan D, Bergers G, Bergsland E. Less is more, regularly: metronomic dosing of cytotoxic drugs can target tumor angiogenesis in mice. *J Clin Invest* 2000; 105:1045–1047.

175. Saito H, Tujitani S, Ikeguchi M, Maeta M, Kaibara N. Neoangiogenesis and relationship to nuclear p53 accumulation and vascular endothelial growth factor expression in advanced gastric carcinoma. *Oncology* 1999; 57:164–172.

176. Volpert OV, Dameron KM, Bouck N. Sequential development of an angiogenic phenotype by human fibroblasts progressing to tumorigenicity. *Oncogene* 1997; 14:1495–1502.

177. Siemeister G, Weindel K, Mohrs K, Barleon B, Martiny-Baron G, Marme D. Reversion of deregulated expression of vascular endothelial growth factor in human renal carcinoma cells by von Hippel-Lindau tumor suppressor protein. *Cancer Res* 1996; 56:2299–2301.

178. Ananth S, Knebelmann B, Gruning W, Dhanabal M, Walz G, Stillman IE, et al. Transforming growth factor betal is a target for the von Hippel-Lindau tumor suppressor and a critical growth factor for clear cell renal carcinoma. *Cancer Res* 1999; 59:2210–2216.

179. Zhong H, Chiles K, Feldser D, Laughner E, Hanrahan C, Georgescu MM, et al. Modulation of hypoxia-inducible factor 1alpha expression by the epidermal growth factor/phosphatidylinositol 3-kinase/PTEN/AKT/FRAP pathway in human prostate cancer cells: implications for tumor angiogenesis and therapeutics. *Cancer Res* 2000; 60:1541–1545.

180. Bouck N, Stellmach V, Hsu S. How tumors become angiogenic. In: Vande Woude JKG, ed. *Advances in Cancer Research.* Academic, New York, 1996, pp. 135–174.

181. Hanahan D, Christofori G, Naik P, Arbeit J. Transgenic mouse models of tumour angiogenesis: the angiogenic switch, its molecular controls, and prospects for preclinical therapeutic models. *Eur J Cancer* 1996; 32A:2386–2393.

182. Esparza J, Vilardell C, Calvo J, Juan M, Vives J, Urbano-Marquez A, et al. Fibronectin upregulates gelatinase B (MMP-9) and induces coordinated expression of gelatinase A (MMP-2) and its activator MT1-MMP (MMP-14) by human T lymphocyte cell lines. A process repressed through RAS/MAP kinase signaling pathways. *Blood* 1999; 94:2754–2766.

183. Hatzi E, Breit S, Zoephel A, Ashman K, Tontsch U, Ahorn H, et al. MYCN oncogene and angiogenesis: down-regulation of endothelial growth inhibitors in human neuroblastoma cells. Purification, structural, and functional characterization [in process citation]. *Adv Exp Med Biol* 2000; 476:239–248.

184. Fotsis T, Breit S, Lutz W, Rossler J, Hatzi E, Schwab M, et al. Down-regulation of endothelial cell growth inhibitors by enhanced MYCN oncogene expression in human neuroblastoma cells. *Eur J Biochem* 1999; 263:757–764.

185. Bein K, Ware JA, Simons M. Myb-dependent regulation of thrombospondin 2 expression. Role of mRNA stability. *J Biol Chem* 1998; 273:21423–21429.

186. Dejong V, Degeorgres A, Filleur S, Ait-Si-Ali S, Mettouchi A, Bornstein P, et al. The Wilm's tumor gene product represses the transcription of thrombospondin 1 in response to overexpression of c-Jun. *Oncogene* 1999; 18:3143–3151.

187. Kraemer M, Tournaire R, Dejong V, Montreau N, Briane D, Derbin C, et al. Rat embryo fibroblasts transformed by c-Jun display highly metastatic and angiogenic activities in vivo and deregulate gene expression of both angiogenic and antiangiogenic factors. *Cell Growth Differ* 1999; 10:193–200.

188. Bouck N. Tumor angiogenesis: the role of oncogenes and tumor suppressor genes. *Cancer Cells* 1990; 2:179–185.

189. Dawson DW, Volpert OV, Gillis P, Crawford SE, Xu H, Benedict W, et al. Pigment epithelium-derived fas a potent inhibitor of angiogenesis. *Science* 1999. 285(5425):245–248.

20 Inhibiting Signal Transduction as an Approach to Radiosensitizing Tumor Cells

Eric J. Bernhard, PhD, Anjali K. Gupta, MD,
Elizabeth Cohen-Jonathan, MD, PhD,
Ruth J. Muschel, MD, PhD,
Stephen M. Hahn, MD,
and W. Gillies McKenna, MD, PhD

CONTENTS

1. INTRODUCTION

Tumors and normal tissues vary widely in their sensitivity to radiation. A combination of the cellular signals that originate within a cell and those in response to environmental factors outside the cell interact to determine the relative resistance or sensitivity of cells to radiation. Either of these determinants of radiation sensitivity provides potential targets for enhancing radiation-induced tumor cell killing. Of particular interest are signaling pathways that differ in normal and tumor cells as a result of oncogenic activation. Such pathways present potentially useful targets for differential inactivation as an approach to radiosensitization.

From: *Oncogene-Directed Therapies*
Edited by: J. W. Rak © Humana Press Inc., Totowa, NJ

We have focused our studies on *ras* oncogene activation and its contribution to radiation resistance. However, RAS proteins are not the only signaling proteins implicated in conferring enhanced survival to tumor cells after irradiation. In this chapter, we discuss oncogene activation and its role in tumor radiation resistance. Potential points where oncogenic protein signaling can be interrupted and the strategies for reducing tumor cell radiation survival using this approach will be reviewed.

2. DIFFERENCES IN TUMOR RADIOSENSITIVITY AND ITS INFLUENCE ON RADIOTHERAPY RESPONSE

Early evidence of a role for radioresistance in tumor response to radiotherapy was provided by studies of head and neck tumor cell lines from tumors that had recurred after treatment. These cell lines were shown to be radioresistant when compared to human fibroblast cell lines *(1)*, and this was proposed to be a contributing factor in treatment failure. The effect of intrinsic radioresistance on the response of tumors to radiotherapy was further defined by the work of Malaise et al. These investigators examined the sensitivity of human tumor cells lines and demonstrated that the rank order of radiosensitivity of the different tumor types at clinically relevant radiation doses in vitro corresponded to their known clinical radioresponsiveness *(2–5)*. Since environmental factors that can influence tumor radiation sensitivity, such as hypoxia and tumor/normal tissue interactions, are not present when measuring in vitro radiosensitivity, the results obtained by these investigators provided evidence that the intrinsic radiosensitivity of tumor cells is a major determinant of in vivo radioresponsiveness. Malaise also extended this conclusion to differences within tumor types. He studied the distribution of radiosensitivity among cell lines of the same histology, showing that there was also wide variability in radiosensitivity in tumors of the same histology *(4)*. This work implied that the variability in sensitivity among tumors of similar histology could determine outcome. Some support for this conclusion came out of studies of head and neck tumor responses and radiosensitivity, which showed an association between in vitro radiosensitivity and clinical response. However, the results of these studies failed to achieve statistical significance *(6,7)*. This could be because the combined modality treatment for these tumors meant that surgery, as well as radiation, contributed to the observed responses. It should be noted that none of these studies addressed the role of the tumor microenvironment on radiation survival as they measured radiation clonogenic survival of single cells in vitro. Nonetheless, these studies did document differences in tumor cell intrinsic radiosensitivity and pointed to a role for this intrinsic radiosensitivity in the response of tumors to radiation therapy.

The clearest demonstration that differences in the radiosensitivity of tumors of similar histology could determine response is found in studies by West and her colleagues *(8,9)*. West prospectively studied the radiosensitivity of tumor cells in women with squamous cell carcinoma (SCC) of the cervix that were undergoing a course of radiotherapy alone with curative intent. In a series of studies, they showed that tumor radiosensitivity, determined before treatment using the Courtney-Mills soft agar clonogenic assay, predicted the outcome of treatment both in terms of local control and survival. There was no significant correlation between other parameters including patient age, tumor stage, or differentiation status and the outcome of radiotherapy. Larger tumors tended to be more radioresistant, but this correlation also failed to reach significance. West's results strongly support both the concept of intertumoral heterogeneity in

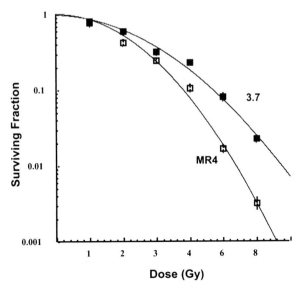

Fig. 1. Radiation survival of rat embryo fibroblasts transformed with H-ras and v-myc or immortalized with v-myc alone. Cells in log phase growth were plated and irradiated for clonogenic survival at the doses indicated. After 10–14 d, plates were stained and scored for colony formation. Surviving fraction at a given does is defined as (colonies formed in irradiated cultures/cells plated) × (colonies formed in nonirradiated cultures/cells plated).

intrinsic radiosensitivity and the conclusion that this heterogeneity contributes to treatment outcome.

3. INFLUENCE OF *RAS* ONCOGENES ON RADIOSENSITIVITY

Studies demonstrating the contribution of activated *ras* oncogenes to radiation resistance were begun at about the same time as the demonstration of intrinsic radiosensitivity differences in human tumors. Fitzgerald et al. were the first to report on enhanced radiation survival after transfection with activated N-*ras (10)*. Sklar subsequently showed that activated H- or K-*ras*, as well as N-*ras*, transfection yielded cells demonstrating increased radiation survival *(11)*. These findings have been replicated in a number of primary and immortalized rodent cell lines *(12–16)*. Transfection and overexpression of the unmutated H-*ras* proto-oncogene was also reported to increase radiation resistance in 3T3 cells *(17)*. Interactions between RAS and other oncoproteins in conferring radiation resistance have also been demonstrated. Transfection with oncogenes such as v-*myc* and adenovirus *Ela* can act synergistically with H-*ras* to confer radiation resistance (Fig. 1) *(12,18)*. Significant increases in radiation resistance were also seen in rat embryo fibroblasts co-transfected with H-*ras* and mutant p53 *(19)*. Ras-induced radiation resistance in rodent cells has been linked to decreased apoptosis *(20,21)* and prolonged G2 delay after irradiation *(22)*. Oncogenic RAS expression or overexpression of unmutated H-RAS has also been shown to impart radiation resistance in human cell lines. Miller et al. showed that transfection with normal H-*ras* increased radiation survival in human osteosarcoma cells in a manner that correlated with the level of H-RAS overexpression *(23,24)*. Increased radiation survival was also seen in cultured spheroids of breast cancer cells expressing

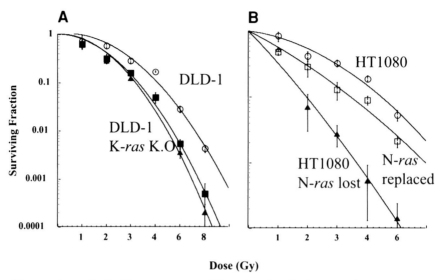

Fig. 2. Clonogenic survival of human tumor cell lines is reduced after loss of activated *ras*. Cells in log phase growth were plated and irradiated for clonogenic survival at the doses indicated. After 14–21 d, plates were stained and scored for colony formation. **(A)** (◯), DLD-1 cells expressing both activated and wild-type endogenous K-*ras* alleles; (▲) and (■), DLD-1 cells expressing only the wild-type endogenous K-*ras* allele. **(B)** (◯), HT1080 cells expressing both activated and wild-type endogenous N-*ras* alleles; (△), HT1080 expressing only the wild-type endogenous N-*ras* allele; (□), HT1080 expressing the wild-type endogenous N-*ras* allele and an activated N-ras introduced by transfection. Reproduced with permission from ref. *30.*

activated H-RAS *(25)*. In human fibroblast lines, transfection with H-*ras* alone resulted in neither transformation nor radioresistance. However, transfection with Simian virus 40 (SV40) large T increased radiation resistance in cells expressing H-RAS *(26)*. Human keratinocytes also showed little change in radiosensitivity at higher doses (D_O) after transfection with H-*ras,* however low dose radioresistance was modestly increased *(27)*. Increased radioresistance was not, however, seen in all cell types after *ras* transfection. Rat kidney epithelial cells were rendered more sensitive to radiation by transfection with K-*ras (28)*. Human mammary epithelial cells also showed no increase in radioresistance *(29)*, however the cells used in the latter study were highly radioresistant prior to *ras* transfection.

The results of survival determinations after oncogene transfection could be subject to artifacts resulting from the transfection itself. In order to circumvent this possibility and to address the role of oncogene activation in human cells on radiation survival directly, we used a genetic approach to demonstrate that the loss of activated N- or K-*ras* alleles from human tumor cell lines resulted in diminished radiation survival *(30)*. In these studies, the clonogenic survival of human DLD-1 colon carcinoma cells expressing one activated K-*ras* allele was compared to the survival of clones of this line having lost the active K-*ras* allele (Fig. 2A). Survival of HT1080 sarcoma cells expressing an activated N-*ras* allele was compared to HT1080 cells without this allele. (Fig. 2B). In both instances, loss of the mutant *ras* allele reduced radiation survival. Reintroduction of mutant N-*ras* into HT1080 partially restored radioresistance in these cells. These data demonstrate that the loss of an activated RAS oncogene signal reduces radiation survival

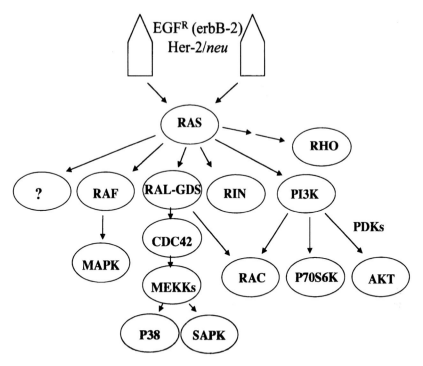

Fig. 3. Partipants in signaling, both upstream and downstream of RAS. Activators upstream of RAS, as well as signaling proteins that propagate signals from RAS, are illustrated. It should be noted that signaling between the different pathways leading from RAS in this diagram and the direction of signaling between certain participants is still an area of active investigation.

in two independent human cell lineages. Together, these data and the data obtained after *ras* oncogene transfection make a strong case for the contribution of RAS activity to the intrinsic radiation resistance of tumor cells and point to inhibition of H-, K-, and N-RAS as a potential means of reducing tumor radiation survival.

4. INHIBITING RAS EXPRESSION AND ACTIVITY

In normal cells, signaling in the RAS pathway is initiated when tyrosine kinase cell surface receptors bind growth factors. Binding of ligand causes autophosphorylation of the receptor. Receptor phosphorylation results in binding of the SH-2 domain containing GRB-2/SOS-1 complex. SOS in turn activates RAS by promoting the exchange of GTP for GDP. RAS-GTP triggers multiple signals that control gene transcription, cell survival, and stress responses (Fig. 3). RAS signaling ends with the hydrolysis of GTP to GDP. This hydrolysis is promoted by a RAS-GAP (GTPase activating protein). Activating mutations in RAS at amino acids 12, 13, or 61 greatly diminish GTP hydrolysis to GDP and RAS thus remains constitutively active. There has been no success reported in reconstituting mutant RAS GTPase activity. The remaining methods for inhibiting activated RAS have been to block RAS expression through the use of H-, K-, and N-*ras* antisense *(31–33)*, *ras*-specific ribozymes *(34–36)*, or transfection with vectors encoding recombinant antibody to ras *(37)*. The alternate approach that we have used has been to block RAS signaling by inhibiting the enzymes mediating post-translational maturation of this protein.

RAS proteins are processed in a series of reactions initiated by farnesylation of RAS at a cysteine residue in the fourth amino acid position from the C-terminal end (reviewed in ref. *38*). The enzyme farnesyltransferase recognizes the C-terminal sequence of RAS known as a CAAX recognition site, where C is the cysteine, X is methionine or serine, and A is isoleucine, leucine, or valine. Modification by the addition of the farnesyl chain is followed by proteolytic cleavage of the terminal 3 amino acids and finally methylation of the now farnesylated terminal cysteine *(39,40)*. The recognition sequences vary between H-, K-, and N-RAS *(41–43)*. The H-RAS recognition sequence is CVLS, while K-RAS A and B have the sequence CIIM or CVIM, respectively. The N-RAS recognition sequence is CVVM. K-RAS can also be modified by the addition of a geranylgeranyl group by geranylgeranyltransferase I when farnesylation is blocked *(43)*. Complete inhibition of K-RAS prenylation, therefore, requires inhibiting both farnesyltransferase and geranylgeranyltransferase I *(44–46)*. Farnesylation or geranylgeranylation are essential for the attachment of RAS to the inner surface of the plasma membrane *(47,48)*. Oncogenic RAS proteins lose their transforming activity when attachment to the plasma membrane is blocked *(49–52)*, making this modification an attractive target for inhibiting oncogenic ras effects.

Miller et al. *(23)* were the first to attempt to block RAS processing using the drug lovastatin. Since the synthesis of the poly-isoprenylated intermediates is part of the mevalonate pathway, inhibitors of the rate-limiting step of that pathway, the conversion of HMG-CoA into mevalonate by HMG-CoA reductase, reduces isoprenylation of ras. Lovastatin was used by Miller et al. *(23)* to reverse H-RAS-mediated radioresistance in human osteogenic sarcoma cells. Lovastatin, however, interferes with the biochemical pathways involved in cholesterol, heme, steroid, and other lipid metabolism within the cell, thus introducing the possibility of an effect that was not specific for RAS.

More recently, specific prenyltransferase inhibitors have been developed based on the structure of the RAS CAAX motif, the farnesyl isoprenyl group or isolated from pharmacologic screens for RAS inhibitory activity *(53,54)*. By inhibiting RAS posttranslational processing, farnesyltransferase inhibitors (FTIs) block oncogenic RAS activity with greater specificity for RAS and do not interfere with other aspects of cholesterol and lipid metabolism. However, despite their greater specificity, FTIs block the growth of both *ras* transformed cells *(55)* as well as tumor cells expressing wild-type *ras (56)*. These inhibitors have also been shown to slow the growth of experimental tumors in mice *(57–60)*. Because their effects are not limited to tumors expressing activated RAS, the possibility that inhibition of farnesylation of other proteins may mediate the antitumor effect of FTIs has been investigated. Prendergast et al. have shown that the prenylated protein Rho B is also an important target of FTIs in reversing RAS transformation *(61–64)*. Although FTIs are active against farnesyltransferase activity in both cells with mutant as well as wild-type *ras,* these drugs show little toxicity to nontransformed cells. Specific inhibitors of geranylgeranyltransferase I have also been developed and can be used with FTIs to block K-ras processing *(65–68)*.

The focus of our research has differed from studies of tumor growth inhibition, in that we have examined the effects of FTI on radiosensitivity rather than on growth inhibition. We have shown that FTI can reverse cellular resistance to radiation in mutant *ras*-containing rodent cell lines (Fig. 4) *(69)*. Radiosensitization has also been observed in human tumor cell lines containing acticated H- or K- *ras,* but not in cells

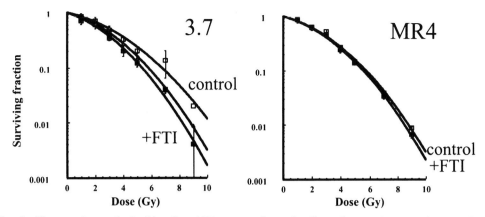

Fig. 4. Clonogenic survival of irradiated H-ras transformed cells and normal or myc immortalized REF after treatment with farnesyltransferase inhibitor. Clonogenic survival assays were performed after addition of FTI-277 at concentrations of 2.5 µM (3.7 cells) or 5 µM (MR4). The data points shown represent the mean of at least 3 dishes. The open symbol indicate the results from untreated cells, and the closed symbols indicate the results from cells treated with FTI-277. In the panel 3.7, the open triangles superimpose the result from untreated MR4 cells showing survival of cells expressing v-*myc* alone. Reproduced with permission from ref. *69.*

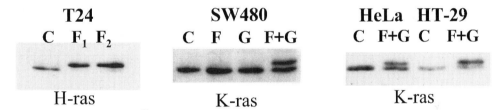

Fig. 5. Inhibition of H- and K-RAS processing by FTI or FTI plus GGTI. Log phase cultures of T24 cells were treated for 24 h with 5 µM FTI-277 (FI) or 2 µM L 744,832 (F2) samples were then harvested for Western blot analysis at 24 h. Western blots were probed with anti-H-RAS monoclonal antibody. Nonfarnesylated H-RAS migrates more slowly than the modified form. SW480, HeLa, and HT-29 cells were treated with 5 µM FTI-277 plus 8 µM GGTI 298 (F+G) or with carrier alone (C) for 24 h. SW 480 was also treated with either inhibitor alone. Cell lysates were obtained and analyzed by Western blotting with monoclonal antibody to K-RAS. Unprenylated K-RAS, like H-RAS, migrates more slowly.

with wild-type *ras* when RAS prenylation is inhibited (Fig. 5 and Table 1) *(70).* FTIs appear to be particularly effective as radiosensitizing agents in vivo. A study in mice bearing human T24 tumor xenografts demonstrated enhanced cytotoxicity from radiation in the presence of an FTI compared to non-FTI treated animals. Again, this effect was not seen in tumors expressing wild-type RAS (Fig. 6) *(71).* The effects of blocking RAS are not limited to alterations in the intrinsic radiosensitivity of tumor cells when these are grown as tumors in nude mice. We recently showed that FTI treatment of human tumor xenografts expressing mutant RAS also causes increased oxygenation of these tumors *(72).* This finding is surprising given the prediction that FTIs are anti-angiogenic *(73)* and points to the complex effects that are produced in tumors when

Table 1
Clonogenic Survival of Tumor Cells After 2 Gy Irradiation and
Prenyltransferase Inhibitor Treatment

Cell	Inhibitor treatment	SF_2 control	SF_2 treated
H-ras mutants:			
T24	FTI-277	0.86 (.04)[a]	0.50 (.02)
	L744,832	0.62 (.04)	0.37 (.02)
HS578T	FTI-277	0.79 (.07)	0.63 (.05)
K-ras mutants:			
	FTI-277	0.52 (.03)	0.54 (.03)
SW480	GGTI-298	0.46 (.03)	0.41 (.04)
		0.55 (.05)	0.45 (.04)
	FTI-277 + GGTI-298		
		0.51 (.05)[b]	0.36 (.08)[b]
A549	FTI-277 + GGTI-298	0.53 (.07)	0.15 (.02)
Wild-type ras:			
SKBr-3	FTI-277	0.47 (.06)	0.45 (.08)
	FTI-277 + GGTI-298	0.68 (.04)	0.66 (.06)
HeLa	FTI-277 + GGTI-298	0.54 (.05)	0.49 (.04)
		0.78 (.05)	0.82 (.07)
HT29	FTI-277		
		0.72 (.05)[b]	0.68 (.06)[b]

[a] SF_2 +/– (standard error). Cells were cultured in FTIs at 5 μM and GGTI-298 at 8 μM for irradiation. Inhibitors were diluted after 24 h as reported in ref. *70*.

[b] The data are derived from clonogenic survival curve data at the 2 Gy dose point. Clonogenic Surviving fraction of tumor clonogens after 2 Gy irradiation (SF_2) were derived from the linear regression analysis of limiting dilution assays. Values reflect corrections for the plating efficiency of nonirradiated cells. Table adapted with permission from ref. *70*.

Fig. 6. Radiosensitization of human tumor xenografts by FTI in vivo. (**A**) Survival of T24 tumor clonogens after treatment with FTI-276 and 8 Gy irradiation *in vivo*. After whole body irradiation, the mice were sacrificed, and the tumors were dissociated and plated for clonogenic survival determination. Colonies were stained and counted 14–21 d after irradiation. Each bar represents the mean plating efficiency obtained from replicate plating of a single tumor. (**B**) Mice with T24 tumor xenografts were treated for 7 d with L-744, 832 (40 mg/kg/d) or drug vehicle by subcutaneous (s.c.) micro-osmotic pump. After 3 d of treatment, the flank bearing the tumor was irradiated at a dose of 6 Gy or sham irradiated. Tumor measurements were made at the times indicated in three perpendicular dimensions (a, b, and c) and the vol was calculated as: Vol = $(\pi/6) \bullet a \bullet b \bullet c$. Mean tumor vol (N = 5 for each group) is shown. (**C**) Survival of HT-29 tumor clonogens isolated from mice treated with FTI-276 and 8 Gy irradiation. Each bar represents the mean plating efficiency obtained from a minimum of 3 tumors. (**D**) HT-29 tumor bearing mice were treated as described in panel B. The mean tumor vol (N = 4 for each group) is shown. Reproduced with permission from ref. *71*.

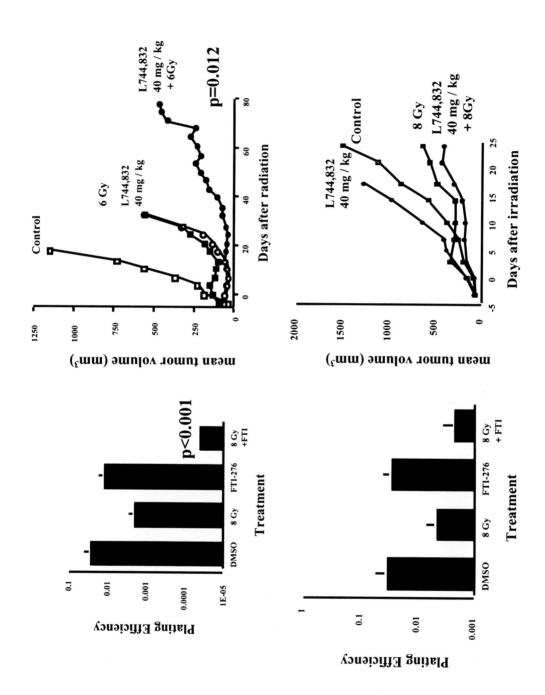

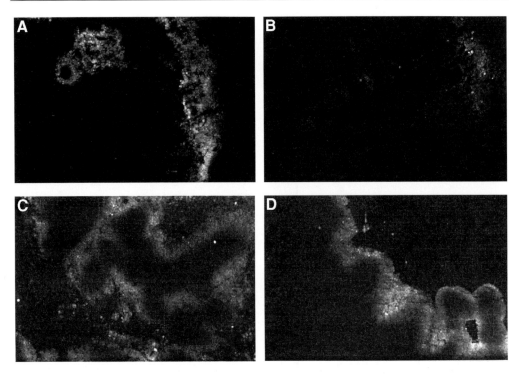

Fig. 7. Tumor oxygenation after FTI treatment of two bladder carcinoma xenografts. Tumor bearing nude mice were treated by continuous infusion with L778,123 at 20 mg/kg/d or with carrier for 13 d. Mice were then injected with the hypoxia detection marker EF5, sacrificed, and tumor sections processed as described in ref. *72*. Tumor sections were stained with Cy™ 3-conjugated ELK3-51, which is a mouse monoclonal antibody specific to EF5 *(140)*. Antibody binding was detected by epifluorescence microscopy, and images were captured using a change-coupled device (CCD) digital camera. Exposure times for EF5 photography were increased in tumors with faint EF5 binding. Exposure duration for each frame is as follows: T24, control, 0.67 s **(A)**; 13 d FTI-treated, 1.21 s **(B)**; RT-4, control, 3.61 s **(C)**; FTI-treated, 3.71 s **(D)**.

oncogenic signaling is disrupted. The enhancement of tumor oxygenation by FTIs may, however, contribute to the effectiveness of these agent in potentiating radiation killing of tumors, since oxygen is an important contributor to radiation killing *(74)*.

Thus, in the preclinical experimental setting, we have observed a clear association of FTI radiosensitization with expression of oncogenic *ras*. However, two factors lead to the possibility that FTI radiosensitization may occur in tumor cells lacking *ras* mutations. First, the exact determinants of FTI radiosensitization have not been determined, and prenylated proteins, other than RAS that may influence radiosensitivity, can be affected by FTIs *(61,63,64)*. Recent work by Prendergast and coworkers demonstrates that rhoB expression influences radiation-induced apoptosis and radiosensitivity in mouse fibroblasts *(75)*. There is now some indication that, clinically, radiosensitization with FTIs may not depend on the presence of oncogenic *ras* in tumors undergoing radiotherapy (see **Conclusions**). In addition, RAS activity is promoted by receptor tyrosine kinase activation. Thus, amplification or mutational activation of these receptors could lead to tumor radiation resistance in the absence of *ras* mutation. In this regard, both erbB-2 and Her-2/*neu* receptors have been implicated in radiation resis-

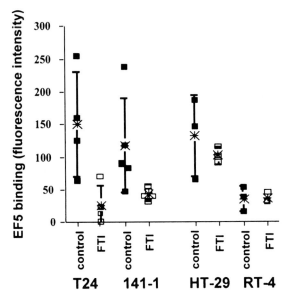

Fig. 8. Tumor oxygenation is increased in tumors with oncogenic H-ras. Tumor sections were stained, and images were captured as in Fig. 10 and as previously reported *(72)*. Images were analyed using Adobe® Photoshop® software. Mean EF5 staining intensity was quantitated in tumor regions staining with intensities 20 fluorescence channels above background. The mean fluorescence intensities of the positively staining regions in individual tumors is shown. Tumor-bearing mice were treated with L-744,832 40 mg/kg/d for 3–7 d (□), and control tumors were treated with carrier alone (■). The mean of values obtained in each group is indicated (*), as is the standard deviation (bars). Mann-Whitney analysis demonstrated statistical significance for the difference between FTI-treated and control T24 tumors (n = 4 each group; α[D] value of 0.05) and for the difference in FTI-treated and control 141-1 tumors (n = 5 each group; α[D] of 0.025).

tance, and antisense oligonucleotides to H-*ras* have been shown to radiosensitize cells overexpressing Her-2/*neu (76)*. In order to better define potential contributors to tumor radiation resistance, we have examined other proteins that are part of the RAS pathway, but that could promote radiation survival even in tumors where *ras* genes are not mutated.

5. PI3-KINASE AND RADIORESISTANCE

Phosphatidyl inositol 3-kinase (PI3K) activity is stimulated by RAS activation *(77)*. PI3K phosphorylates phosphatidylinositol (PtdIns) phosphates leading to the conversion of PtdIns 4,5-P2 to PtdIns 3,4,5-P3. PtdIns 3,4,5-P3 in turn causes membrane localization of protein kinase B (PKB/Akt) and the phosphoinositide-dependent kinases (PDK-1) *(78,79)*. PDK-1 phosphorylates one of two sites on PKB/Akt *(80)*, while a second PI3K activated kinase, ILK-1 phosphorylates a second site *(81)*, resulting in full activation of PKB/Akt *(82)*. PKB/Akt has been shown to act as an inhibitor of apoptosis *(83,84)*. One mechanism for the anti-apoptotic activity of PKB/Akt appears to be the phosphorylation and inactivation of the pro-apoptotic BAD protein, although multiple other proteins are also substrates for PKB/Akt phosphorylation *(85)*. These findings together implicate PKB/Akt as a possible regulator of cell survival

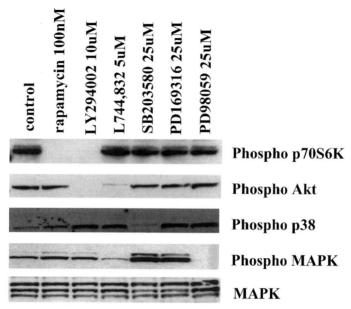

Fig. 9. Inhibitors of activating phosphorylation of proteins in the RAS signaling pathway. Cells were treated with inhibitors at the indicated concentrations and lysed without trypsinization in reducing Laemeli sample buffer. Samples containing equal amounts of protein were separated on a 12% sodium dodecyl sulfate (SDS) polyacrylamide gel and analyzed by Western blotting with polyclonal anti-phospho MAPK (Sigma, St. Louis, Mo, USA), polyclonal pan MAPK K-23 (Santa Cruz Biotechnology, Santa Cruz, CA, USA), polyclonal anti-phospho p38 MAPK, polyclonal anti-phospho p70S6K, polyclonal anti-phospho AKT, and polyclonal pan AKT (all from New England Biolabs, Beverly, MA, USA). Antibody binding was detected using the electrochemiluminescence (ECL™) chemiluminescence kit (Amersham Pharmacia Biotech, Piscatoway, NJ, USA). Reproduced with permission from ref. *90*.

downstream of PI3K. PI3K has other downstream effectors, including p70S6K, Rac, and GTP exchange factors. PI3K was initially implicated in radiation resistance in experiments that showed radiosensitization by the PI3K inhibitor wortmannin *(86,87)*. These results, though they implicated a PI3K-like kinase in radiation, could not unambiguously distinguish between inhibition of PI3K and the related ATM, ATR, and DNA-PK kinases, which are also targets of wortmannin *(86)*. It was, however, shown that wortmannin could sensitize cells lacking either DNA-PK or ATM *(87,88),* thus indicating that another member of this kinase family contributes to radiation resistance. In this regard, wortmannin was shown to inhibit PKB/Akt *(89).*

More recently, we examined a panel of pharmacological agents known to block various signaling proteins downstream of RAS (Fig. 3) and included the more specific PI3K inhibitor LY294002 *(90)*. The effects of this panel of inhibitors was first tested in the T24 bladder cancer cell line that expresses oncogenic H-RAS. As discussed above, we had evidence that RAS contributes to radiation resistance in this cell line, since the inhibition of RAS processing by FTIs radiosensitizes these cells *(70)*. The specificity of these inhibitors was verified by examining the inhibition of activating phosphorylation of proteins in the RAS pathway (Fig. 9). As expected in a cell line with endogenously activated H-RAS, T24 showed high basal levels of phosphorylated p70S6K,

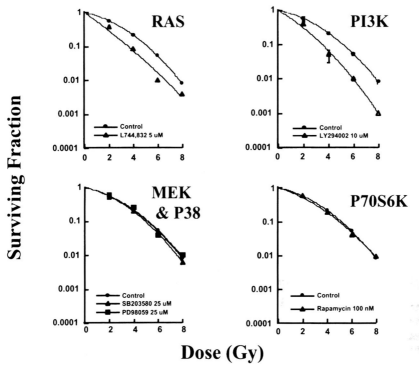

Fig. 10. Clonogenic radiation survival of T24 cells after inhibitor treatment. Cultures in log growth were treated with inhibitors at least 1 h prior to radiation. L744, 832 treatment was intiated 24 h prior to irradiation. Inhibitor treatment was continued for 24 h after irradiation, at which time drug-free media was added. Colonies were stained and counted 10–14 d after irradiation. Each point on the survival curve represents the mean surviving fraction from at least 3 dishes.

Akt, p38, and mitogen-activated protein kinase (MAPK). Inhibition of the Ras-Raf-MEK-MAPK pathway by the MEK inhibitor PD98059 blocked phosphorylation of MAPK, but had no effect on other RAS signaling effectors. SB203580 specifically inhibited p38 phosphorylation, while PD169316, another putative p38 inhibitor, showed no effect and was not used further. The PI3K inhibitor LY294002 inhibited the phosphorylation of both Akt and p70S6K, but not MAPK or p38. Rapamycin inhibited p70S6K phosphorylation and had no effect on Akt. Thus, these inhibitors could be used to probe differentially these components of RAS signaling. As demonstrated previously, inhibition of RAS farnesylation with FTI L744,832 radiosensitized T24 cells (Fig. 10a) *(70)* and decreased MAPK and Akt phosphorylation. Inhibition of PI3K by LY294002 radiosensitized T24 cells to the same extent as FTI treatment (Fig. 10b). In contrast, inhibition of p38, inhibition of MEK-MAPK, and inhibition of p70S6K had no effect on the radiosensitivity of T24 cells (Fig. 10c,d). These results implicate PI3K as an important contribution to RAS-mediated radiation survival in T24 cells. Further experiments demonstrated that inhibition of PI3K radiosensitized not only T24 cells, but also the DLD-1 human colon carcinoma line expressing activated K-*ras,* and the H-*ras*+ v-*myc*-transformed 3.7 rat embryo fibroblast line *(90)*. Other investigators have

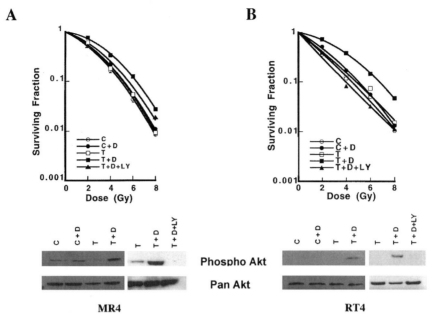

Fig. 11. Clonogenic radiation survival of RT-4 and MR4 cells after induction of costitutively activated PI3K Cells were transiently with the pGRE5/EBV dexamethasone-inducible plasmid vector with an insert encoding constitutively active PI3K. Cells were electroporated with a Gene pulser II System (Bio-Rad, Hercules, CA, USA) under conditions optimized for both the MR4 and RT4 cells. Cells were cultured for 48 h, and PI3K was induced by the addition of 1 µg/mL of dexamethasone. Cells were irradiated for clonogenic survival, and protein samples were harvested 24 h after the addition of dexamethasone. LY294002 10 µM was added 30 min prior to irradiation where indicated. C, control cultures; C+D, control cultures treated with dexamethasone; T, transfected cultures; T+D, transfected with dexamethasone to induce PI3K; T+D+LY, transfected cultures treated with dexamethasone to induce PI3K and then further treated with 10 µM LY294002. Western blots show PKB/Akt phosphorylation as an index of PI3K activation. PKB/Akt expression shows that loading is equal, and PKB/Akt levels are unchanged by these manipulations.

obtained similar results regarding the role of PI3K in radiation resistance using an H-*ras*-transformed rat intestinal epithelial cell model *(90a)*.

In order to confirm that PI3K was an important factor in radiation sensitivity, constitutively activated PI3K was transfected into cells lacking activated *ras*. Both MR4 myc-immortalized rat embryo fibroblasts and RT4 bladder carcinoma cells express wild-type RAS and are relatively radiation sensitive *(69,91)*. These cells were transfected with an inducible gene encoding active PI3K. When active PI3K was induced in the transfected cells, both cell lines showed increased phosphorylation of Akt, which we used as a marker for PI3K activity. This was accompanied by enhanced clonogenic survival after irradiation (Fig. 11). No alteration in survival was seen in control cells treated with the inducing agent dexamethasone or in transfectant cells in the absence of dexamethasone. Expression of the vector and exposure to dexamethasone did not alter the plating efficiency of the cells. Treatment of transfected cells expressing active PI3K in the presence of dexamethasone with LY294002 blocked Akt phosphorylation and sensitized these cells to radiation (Fig. 11).

These studies support the hypothesis that a pathway that includes RAS and PI3K contributes to radiation resistance in RAS-transformed cells. Both of these signaling molecules are thus attractive potential targets for inactivation in the context of radiotherapy. Similar studies by another group using chemical cytotoxins have shown sensitization of HL-60 leukemia cells that express an activated N-ras allele after blocking PI3K activity *(92)*. These results demonstrate that blocking PI3K may be a useful approach in the context of chemotherapy as well as radiotherapy. Studies examining the role of other signaling proteins that participate in this pathway may uncover other contributors to radiation resistance that could serve as targets for radio- or chemosensitization. Some of these proteins have already been studied as outlined in Subheadings 6–8.

6. RAF ONCOGENES AND RADIORESISTANCE

RAF is one protein that acts immediately downstream of RAS in signal transduction *(93)*, resulting in activation of the MAP kinase pathway *(94)*. RAF also binds 14-3-3 proteins, which are required for its activity *(95)*, as well as Cdc-25 phosphatase *(96)*, which is a regulator of cell cycle progression. RAF has also been shown to interact with bcl-2 *(97)*. Thus, RAF is implicated not only in mitogenic signaling, but also in cell cycle and apoptosis regulation. Activation of *raf* was first proposed to be involved in radiation resistance, by Kasid et al. in 1987, based on the isolation of *raf* in 3T3 cells transformed with DNA from a radiation-resistant cell line *(98)*. Interestingly, the raf-1 gene from this cell line showed no mutations in the coding sequence *(99)*. Further studies by this group have shown that radiation can influence RAF activity *(100,101)*. It is clear from these results that RAF activity is increased after exposure to radiation, but whether this activation augments radiation resistance is less well defined.

Overexpression of c-RAF has been correlated with resistance to radiation therapy in patients with head and neck tumors *(102)*. However, not all studies found an association between *raf* activation and radiation resistance. Britten et al. *(103)* reported an inverse correlation between radiation survival and RAF activity in cervical carcinoma cells, a finding that was echoed by Warenius et al. who examined c-*raf* expression and radiosensitivity *(104)*. Nevertheless, it was shown that both tumorigenicity *(105)* and radiation resistance *(105)* of *raf*-transformed 3T3 cells can be reduced by inhibiting RAF expression using antisense oligonucleotides against the *raf*-1 gene. Antisense oligonucleotides against *raf*-1 have also been used to reduce radiation resistance in human tumor cell lines overexpressing HER-2 or expressing oncogenic H-RAS *(76)*. Antisense oligonucleotides to *raf*-1 have also been used to radiosensitize tumors in vivo *(106)*. An obvious candidate for transmitting the signals from RAF, which mediates cellular radiation responses, is the MEK-MAP kinase cascade, which is activated through RAF signaling.

7. MAP KINASE AND RADIORESISTANCE

MAP kinase is part of a signaling cascade leading to gene transcription that is activated by RAS and RAF. MAP kinase is directly activated through phosphorylation by MEK kinase. The role of the MAP kinase pathway in radiation resistance is still controversial. Studies on the role of the MAP kinase cascade in radiation resistance have relied primarily on the MEK kinase inhibitor PD98059. Inhibition of MEK kinase with PD98059 has been reported to radiosensitize certain tumor cells *(107–109)*. However, other investigators found no effect of MEK kinase inhibition with PD98059 on apoptosis or clonogenic survival in three independent head and neck SCC lines with constitutively high levels of MAP kinase activity *(110)*. We examined the role of MAP kinase activity in the radiation resistance of T24 bladder tumor cells as outlined above (Fig. 10) and *(91)*. Our results showed that, although MAP kinase was active in T24 cells, inhibition of the MEK-MAP kinase pathway with PD98059 did not radiosensitize these cells. Thus it appears that MAP kinase activity is not critical to radiation resistance in a number of SCC lines nor in T24 cells that express activated H-RAS.

8. EGF RECEPTOR FAMILY AND RADIATION RESISTANCE

The epidermal growth factor receptor (EGFR) family consists of four closely related growth factor receptors, including EGFR or HER-1 (*erb*-B1), HER-2 (*erb*-B2), HER-3 (*erb*-B3), and HER-4 (*erb*-B4). EGFR (*erb*-B1) is recognized by EGF, transforming growth factor-α (TGF-α), and amphiregulins. Heregulins and neuregulins recognize *erb*-B3 and *erb*-B4. The last member of the family *erb*-B2 (HER-2/*neu* or p185^{neu}) does not directly blind any known ligand. Instead, it heterodimerizes with the three other family members and enhances ligand-binding affinity and reduces the rate of dissociation. These heterodimers also amplify the elicited signal through activation of the HER-2/*neu* intracellular kinase domain and auto-cross phosphorylation *(111)*. These receptors are transforming when overexpressed, and it is overexpression that is found in many human tumors. Activation by point mutation *(112)* and truncation *(113)* has also been seen in animal tumors. Through autophosphorylation of their intracellular domains *(114)*, these receptors initiate signaling via the grb-2/SOS complex and RAS activation. Two members of this family have been implicated in tumor resistance to ionizing radiation: the EGFR and Her-2/*neu*.

8.1. ErbB-1

Overexpression of the EGFR (or ErbB-1) has also been implicated in the radiation resistance of human tumors. A retrospective analysis showed that the number of EGFR positive cells was a significant predictive factor for overall survival and disease-free survival in patients' astrocytic tumors treated with definitive radiotherapy *(115)*. Similar results were also obtained in a study of head and neck cancers *(116)*. Experimentally, Milas et al. demonstrated enhanced tumor radiosensitivity after combined treatment of xenografts with C225 and radiation. In these studies, as in studies of FTIs, multiple effects were noted on tumors after combined treatment *(117)*. Other investigators have also shown radiosensitization after targeting the EGFR. Bonner et al. have shown that combining the anti-EGFR monoclonal C225 and radiation results in greater cell killing of SCCs than either treatment alone *(118)*. The expression of dominant negative EGFR has also been shown to reduce radiation resistance in mammary carcinoma cells *(119,120)*. These results of these studies have provided the basis for proceeding with clinical trials of the best characterized anti-EGFR strategy, the C225 anti-EGFR chimeric human-mouse monoclonal antibody *(121)*. Experimental studies combining C225 with radiation and a protein kinase A inhibitor have also shown a strong interaction between these agents in the killing of ovarian carcinoma cells *(122)*.

8.2. erbB-2 (Her-2/neu)

The Her-2/*neu* gene encodes a receptor (p185erbB-2) that is a member of the EGFR family. Overexpression has been documented in a number of malignancies including breast and ovarian cancers *(123,124)*, endometrial cancers *(125)*, and non-small cell lung cancer (NSCLC) *(126)*. Her-2/*neu* expression together with p53 status were the two molecular markers identified as predictive for poorer response in early stage breast cancer *(127)* and Her-2/*neu* expression by itself has been reported as predictive of poorer response *(124)* and metastasis *(128)*. Expression of Her-2/*neu* has been linked to radiation resistance in experiments with rodent cells *(76)*. Both in the clinic and in experimental systems, Her-2/*neu* appears to affect radiation response of human tumor cells. Radioresistant human gliomas and astrocytomas showed enhanced radiation-induced apoptosis and clonogenic survival after inhibition of Her-2/*neu* by transfection with a dominant negative Her-2/*neu* receptor or treatment with an exocyclic anti-HER2/neu peptide mimic *(129,130)*. Nakano et al. reported a significant difference in 5-yr survival after radiotherapy in cervical cancer patients stratified for erbB-2 expression *(131)*. Furthermore, the use of antibodies to p185erbB-2 has been reported in phase III clinical trials to increase time to recurrence and response rates to other modes of therapy in metastatic breast cancer *(132)*. Stackhouse et al. demonstrated that expression of an inducible single chain antibody to erbB-2 in SKOV3 tumor xenografts was able to radiosensitize these human ovarian cancer cells in vivo *(133)*. Interestingly, this radiosensitization was not observed in SKOV3 cells in vitro, implying that erbB-2 may either have a differential effect on the radiosensitivity of cells that are adherent, as opposed to growing in an anchorage-independent manner, or that erbB-2 overexpression may affect the tumor microenvironment. Another approach combined anti-p185 antibody with pseudomonas exotoxin or ricin A-chain. These chimeric molecules showed sensitization of cells both in vitro and in vivo to radiation *(134,135)*. Although of potential clinical benefit, the exact mechanism for this synergistic interaction when using this approach could be difficult to determine.

9. CONCLUSIONS

This review covered the role of pathways activated by mutation or overexpression of selected oncogenes in tumor radiation resistance. The oncogenes discussed included only those that have been intensively studied and for which strategies have been developed for blocking their activity. Several other oncogene products may also contribute to radiation survival including *abl (136)* and *src (137)*. Other proteins that have not been characterized, but are differentially expressed in radioresistant cells, may also play a role in mediating resistance to radiation *(138)*. Further study may demonstrate an important role for these other proteins and oncogenes in tumor cell radiation survival.

By far, the most closely studied oncogene pathways in radiation resistance are those involving RAS. Inhibiting the RAS pathway has been shown to reduce radiation survival in cultured cells and experimental tumors expressing activated *ras*. A Phase I trial of the FTI, L-778,123 in combination with standard radiotherapy was recently completed *(139)*. The combination of L-778,123 and radiotherapy was well-tolerated in NSCLC and head and neck cancer patients. No increase in acute normal tissue (mucosal) toxicities was noted. Of particular interest was the observation that objective responses were seen in 4 NSCLC patients who did not express a *ras* mutation. This observation is surprising given the results of preclinical studies where radiosensitization and tumor oxygenation were both linked to the presence of activated RAS. The results from this trial underline the need for a better understanding of both the factors that contribute to tumor radiation resistance in the context of whole organisms, and of the precise mechanism of interaction between radiation and farnesyltransferase inhibition. Further study of the signaling pathways blocked by FTIs and their role not only in intrinsic radiosensitivity, but also in determining tumor microenvironmental influences on the radiation response should provide a better understanding of tumor radiation resistance.

ACKNOWLEDGMENTS

The authors wish to thank Junmin Wu, George Cerniglia, and Vincent Bakanauskas for excellent technical assistance. This work was supported by grants: CA 75138 (W.G.M., R.J.M., and E.J.B.), DAMD17-98-1-8546 (E.J.B.), and CA 73820 (E.J.B.). Additional support was provided through a sponsored research agreement with Merck & Co. Inc. Dr. Cohen Jonathan is currently at the Institut Claudius Regaud, Toulouse France.

REFERENCES

1. Weichselbaum RR, Dahlberg W, Little JB. Inherently radioresistant cells exist in some human tumors. *Proc Natl Acad Sci USA* 1985; 82:4732–4735.
2. Fertil B, Malaise EP. Inherent cellular radiosensitivity as a basic concept for human tumor radiotherapy. *Int J Radiat Oncol Biol Phys* 1981; 7:621–629.
3. Fertil B, Malaise EP. Intrinsic radiosensitivity of human cell lines is correlated with radioresponsiveness of human tumors: analysis of 101 published survival curves. *Int J Radiat Oncol Biol Phys* 1985; 11:1699–1707.
4. Malaise EP, Fertil B, Chavaudra N, Guichard M. Distribution of radiation sensitivities for human tumor cells of specific histological types: comparison of in vitro to in vivo data. *Int J Radiat Oncol Biol Phys* 1986; 12:617–624.
5. Malaise EP, Fertil B, Deschavanne PJ, Chavaudra N, Brock WA. Initial slope of radiation survival curves is characteristic of the origin of primary and established cultures of human tumor cells and fibroblasts. *Radiat Res* 1987; 111:319–333.
6. Weichselbaum RR, Becket MA, Vijayakumar S, et al. Radiobiological characterization of head and neck and sarcoma cells derived from patients prior to radiotherapy. *Int J Radiat Oncol Biol Phys* 1990; 19:313–319.
7. Brock WA, Baker FL, Wike JL, Sivon SL, Peters LJ. Cellular radiosensitivity of primary head and neck squamous cell carcinomas and local tumor control. *Int J Radiat Oncol Biol Phys* 1990; 18:1283–1286.
8. West CM, Hendry JH, Scott D, Davidson SE, Hunter RD. 25th Patterson Symposium—is there a future for radiosensitivity testing. *Br J Cancer* 1991; 64:197–199.
9. West CM, Davidson SE, Burt PA, Hunter RD. The intrinsic radiosensitivity of cervical carcinoma: correlations with clinical data. *Int J Radiat Oncol* 1995; 31:841–846.
10. FitzGerald TJ, Daugherty C, Kase K, Rothstein LA, McKenna M, Greenberger JS. Activated human N-ras oncogene enhances x-irradiation repair of mammalian cells in vitro less effectively at low dose rate. *Am J Clin Oncol* 1985; 8:517–522.
11. Sklar MD. The ras oncogenes increnase the intrinsic resistance of NIH 3T3 cells to ionizing radiation. *Science* 1988; 239:645–647.
12. McKenna WG, Weiss MC, Endlich B, et al. Synergistic effect of the v-myc oncogene with H-ras on radioresistance. *Cancer Res* 1990; 50:97–102.
13. Ling CC, Endlich B. Radioresistance induced by oncogenic transformation. *Radiat Res* 1989; 120:267–279.

14. Hermens AF, Bentvelzen PA. Influence of the H-ras oncogene on radiation responses of a rat rhab-domyosarcoma cell line. *Cancer Res* 1992; 52:3073–3082.

15. Ong A, Li WX, Ling CC. Low-dose-rate irradiation of rat embryo cells containing the Ha-ras onco-gene. *Radiat Res* 1993; 134:251–255.

16. Minarik L, Hall E, Miller R. Tumorigenicity, oncogene transfection, and radiosensitivity. *Cancer J Sci Am* 1996; 2:351.

17. Samid D, Miller AC, Rimoldi D, Gafner J, Clark EP. Increased radiation resistance in transformed and nontransformed cells with elevated ras proto-oncogene expression. *Radiat Res* 1991; 126:244–250.

18. McKenna WG, Weiss MC, Bakanauskas VJ, et al. The role of the H-ras oncogene in radiation resis-tance and metastasis. *Int J Radiat Oncol Biol Phys* 1990; 18:849–859.

19. Bristow RG, Jang A, Peacock J, Chung S, Benchimol S, Hill RP. Mutant p53 increases radioresis-tance in rat embryo fibroblasts simultaneously transfected with HPV16-E7 and/or activated H-ras. *Oncogene* 1994; 9:1527–1536.

20. Chen CH, Zhang J, Ling CC. Transfected c-myc and c-Ha-ras modulate radiation-induced apoptosis in rat embryo cells. *Radiat Res* 1994; 139:307–315.

21. McKenna WG, Bernhard EJ, Markiewicz DA, Rudoltz MS, Maity A, Muschel RJ. Regulation of radi-ation-induced apoptosis in oncogene-transfected fibroblasts: influence of H-ras on the G2 delay. *Oncogene* 1996; 12:237–245.

22. McKenna WG, Iliakis G, Weiss MC, Bernhard EJ, Muschel RJ. Increased G_2 delay in radiation-resis-tant cells obtained by transformation of primary rat embryo cells with the oncogenes v-myc and H-ras. *Radiat Res* 1991; 125:283–287.

23. Miller AC, Kariko K, Myers CE, Clark EP, Samid D. Increased radioresistance of EJ*ras*-transformed human osteosarcoma cells and its modulation by lovastatin, an inhibitor of p21[ras] isoprenylation. *int J Cancer* 1993; 53:302–307.

24. Miller AC, Gafner J, Clark EP, Samid D. Differences in radiation-induced micronuclei yeilds of human cells: influence of ras gene expression and protein localization. *Int J Radiat Biol* 1993; 64:547–554.

25. Bruyneel EA, Storme GA, Schallier DC, Van den Berge DL, Hilgard P, Mareel MM. Evidence for abrogation of oncogene-induced radioresistance of mammary cancer cells by hexadecylphospho-choline in vitro. *Eur J Cancer* 1993; 29A1958–1963.

26. Su L-N, Little JB. Transformation and radiosensitivity of human diploid skin fibroblasts transfected with activated *RAS* oncogene and SV40 T-antigen. *Int J Radiat Biol* 1992; 62:201–210.

27. Mendonca MS, Boukamp P, Stanbridge EJ, Redpath JL. The radiosensitivity of human keratinocytes: influence of activated c-H-ras oncogene expression and tumorigenicity. *Int J Radiat Biol* 1991; 59:1195–206.

28. Harris JF, Chambers AF, Tam ASK. Some *ras*-transformed cells have increased radiosensitivity and decreased repair of sublethal readiation damage. *Somat Cell Mol Genet* 1990; 16:39–48.

29. Alapetite C, Baroche C, Remvikos Y, Goubin G, Moustacchi E. Studies on the influence of the pres-ence of an activated ras oncogene on the in vitro radiosensitivity of human mammary epithelial cells. *Int J Radiat Biol* 1991; 59:385–396.

30. Bernhard EJ, Stanbridge EJ, Gupta S, et al. Direct evidence for the contribution of activated N-ras and K-ras oncogenes to increased intrinsic radiation resistance in human tumor cell lines. *Cancer Res* 2000; 60:6597–6600.

31. Georges RN, Mukhopadhyay T, Zhang Y, Yen N, Roth JA. Prevention of orthotopic human lung can-cer growth by intratracheal instillation of a retroviral antisense K-ras construct. *Cancer Res* 1993; 53:1743–1746.

32. Gray GD, Hernandez OM, Hebel D, Root M, Pow-Sang JM, Wickstrom E. Antisense DNA inhibition of tumor growth induced by c-Ha-ras oncogene in nude mice. *Cancer Res* 1993; 53:577–580.

33. Jansen B, Schlagbauer-Wadl H, Eichler HG, et al. Activated N-ras contributes to the chemoresistance of human melanoma in severe combined immunodeficiency (SCID) mice by blocking apoptosis. *Cancer Res* 1997; 57:362–365.

34. Scherr M, Grez M, Ganser A, Engels JW. Specific hammerhead ribozyme-mediated cleavage of mutant N-ras mRNA in vitro and ex viv. Oligoribonucleotides as therapeutic agents. *J Biol Chem* 1997; 272:14304–14313.

35. Irie A, Anderegg B, Kashani-Sabet M, et al. Therapeutic efficacy of an adenovirus-mediated anti-H-ras ribozyme in experimental bladder cancer. *Antisense Nucleic Acid Drug Dev* 1999; 9:341–349.

36. Tokunaga T, Tsuchida T, Kijima H, et al. Ribozyme-mediated inactivation of mutant K-ras oncogene in a colon cencer cell line. *Br J Cancer* 2000; 83:833–839.

37. Russell J, Lang F, Huet T, et al. Radiosensitization of human tumor cell lines induced by the adenovirus-mediated expression of an anti-Ras single-chain antibody fragment. *Cancer Res* 1999; 59:5239–5244.

38. Glomset JA, Farnsworth CC. Role of protein modification reactions in programming interactions between ras-related GTPases and cell membranes. *Annu Rev Cell Biol* 1994; 10:181–205.

39. Farh L, Mitchell DA, Deschenes RJ. Farnesylation and proteolysis are sequential, but distinct steps in the CaaX box modification pathway. *Arch Biochem Biophys* 1995; 318:113–121.

40. Gutierrez L, Magee AI, Marshall CJ, Hancock JF. Post-translational processing of p21^{ras} is two-step and involves carboxyl-methylation and carboxy-terminal proteolysis. *EMBO J* 1989; 8:1093–1098.

41. Moores SL, Schaber MD, Mosser SD, et al. Sequence dependence of protein isoprenylation. *J Biol Chem* 1991; 266:14603–14610.

42. Reiss Y, Stradley SJ, Gierasch LM, Brown MS, Goldstein JL. Sequence requirements for peptide recognition by rat brain p21^{ras} protein farnesyltransferase. *Proc Natl Acad Sci USA* 1991; 88:732–736.

43. James G, Goldstein J, Brown M, Polylysine and CVIM sequences of K-rasB dictate specificity of prenylation and confer resistance to benzodiazepine peptidomimetic in vitro. *J Biol Chem* 1995; 270:6221–6226.

44. Sun J, Qian Y, Hamilton AD, Sebti SM. Both farnesyltransferase and geranylgeranyltransferase I inhibitors are required for inhibition of oncogenic K-ras prenylation but each alone is sufficient to supress human tumor growth in nude mouse xenografts. *Oncogene* 1998; 16:1467–1473.

45. Whyte DB, Kirschmeier P, Hockenberry TN, et al. K- and N-Ras are geranylgeranylated in cells treated with farnesyl protein transferase inhibitors. *J Biol Chem* 1997; 272:14459–14464.

46. Bernhard EJ, Muschel RJ, Cohen-Jonathan E, et al. Prenyltransferase inhibitors as radiosensitizers. In: Sebti SM, Hamilton AD ed. *Farnesyltransferase and geranylgeranyltransferase I: targets for Cancer and Cardiovascular Therapy.* Humana Press, Totowa, 2000.

47. Willumsen BM, Christensen A, Hubbert NL, Papageorge AG, Lowy DR. The p21 ras C-terminus is required for transformation and membrane association. *Nature* 1984; 310:583–586.

48. Jackson JH, Cockran CG, Bourne JR, Solski PA, Buss JE, Der C. Farnesol modification of Kirsten-ras exon 4B protein is essential for transformation. *Proc Natl Acad Sci USA* 1990; 87:3042–3046.

49. Buss JE, Soiski PA, Schaeffer JP, MacDonald MJ, Der CJ. Activation of the cellular proto-oncogene product p21ras by addition of a myristylation signal. *Science* 1989; 243:1600–1602.

50. Clarke S. Protein isoprenylation and methylation at carboxyl-terminal cysteine residues. *Ann Rev Biochem* 1992; 61:355–386.

51. Cox AD, Hisaka MM, Buss JE, Der CJ. Specific isoprenoid modification is required for function of normal, but not oncogenic, ras protein. *Mol Cell Biol* 1992; 12:2606–2615.

52. Kato K, Cox AD, Hisaka MM, Graham SM, Buss JE, Der CJ. Isoprenoid addition to ras protein is the critical modification for its membrane association and transforming activity. *Proc Natl Acad Sci USA* 1992; 89:6403–6407.

53. Gibbs J, Oliff A, Kohl N. Farnesyltransferase inhbitors: Ras research yields a potential cancer therapeutic. *Cell* 1994; 77:175–178.

54. Sebti 5, Hamilton A. Inhibition of ras prenylation: a novel approach to cancer chemotherapy. *Pharmacal Ther* 1997; 74:103–114.

55. Kohl NE, Mosser SD, deSolms SJ, et al. Selective inhibition of ras dependent transformation by a farnesyltransferase inhibitor. *Science* 1993; 260:1934–1936.

56. Sepp-Lorenzino L, Ma Z, Rands E, et al. A peptidomimetic inhibitor of Farnesyl:protein transferase blocks the anchorage-dependent and -independent growth of human tumor cell lines. *Cancer Res* 1995; 55:5302–5309.

57. Kohl N, Wilson F, Mosser S, et al. Protein farnesyl transferase inhibitors block the growth of ras-dependent tumors in nude mice. *Proc Natl Acad Sci USA* 1994; 91:9141–9251.

58. Kohl N, Omer C, Connor M, et al. Inhibition of farnesyltransferase induces regression of mammary and salivary carcinomas in ras transgenic mice. *Nat Med* 1995; 1:792–797.

59. Barrington RE, Subler MA, Rands E, et al. A farnesyltransferase inhibitor induces tumor regression in transgenic mice harboring multiple oncogenic mutations by mediating alterations in both cell cycle control and apoptosis. *Mol Cell Biol* 1998; 18:85–92.

60. Norgaard P, Law B, Joseph H, et al. Treatment with farnesyl-protein transferase inhibitor induces regression of mammary tumors in transforming growth factor (TGF) alpha and TGF alpha/neu transgenic mice by inhibition of mitogenic activity and induction of apoptosis. *Clin Cancer Res* 1999; 5:35–42,

61. Lebowitz PF, Davide JP, Prendergast GC. Evidence that farnesyltransferase inhibitors suppress Ras transformation by interfering with Rho activity. *Mol Cell Biol* 1995; 15:6613–6622.

62. Prendergast GC, Khosravi-Far R, Solski PA, Kurzawa H, Lebowitz PF, Der CJ. Critical role of Rho in cell transformation by oncogenic Ras. *Oncogene* 1995; 10:2289–2296.

63. Lebowitz PF, Du W, Prendergast GC. Prenylation of RhoB is required for its cell transforming function but not its ability to activate serum response element-dependent transcription. *J Biol Chem* 1997 272:16093–1609.

64. Lebowitz PF, Casey PJ, Prendergast GC, Thissen JA. Farnesyltransferase inhibitors alter the prenylation and growth-stimulating function of RhoB. *J Biol Chem* 1997; 272:15591–15594.

65. Lerner E, Qian Y, Hamilton A, Sebti S. Disruption of oncogenic K-ras4B processing and signaling by a potent geranylgeranyltransferase I inhibitor. *J Biol Chem* 1995; 270:26770–26773.

66. Macchia M, Jannitti N, Gervasi G, Danesi R. Geranylgeranyl diphosphate-based inhibitors of post-translational geranylgeranylation of cellular proteins. *J Med Chem* 1996; 39:1352–1356.

67. Sun J, Blaskovich MA, Knowles D, et al. Antitumor efficacy of a novel class of non-thiol-containing peptidomimetic inhibitors of farnesyltransferase and geranylgeranyltransferase I: combination therapy with the cytotoxic agents cisplatin, Taxol, and gemcitabine. *Cancer Res* 1999; 59:4919–4926.

68. Vasudevan A, Qian Y, Vogt A, et al. Potent, highly selective, and non-thiol inhibitors of protein geranylgeranyltransferase-I. *J Med Chem* 1999; 42: 1333–1340.

69. Bernhard EJ, Kao G, Cox AD, et al. The farnesyltransferase inhibitor FTI-277 radiosensitizes H-ras-transformed rat embryo fibroblasts. *Cancer Res* 1996; 56:1727–1730.

70. Bernhard EJ, McKenna WG, Hamilton AD, et al. Inhibiting ras prenylation increases the radiosensitivity of human tumor cell lines with activating mutations of *ras* oncogenes. *Cancer Res* 1998; 58:1754–1761.

71. Cohen-Jonathan E, Muschel RJ, Gillies McKenna W, et al. Farnesyltransferase inhibitors potentiate the antitumor effect of radiation on a human tumor xenograft expressing activated HRAS. *Radiat Res* 2000; 154:125–132.

72. Cohen-Jonathan E, Evans SM, Koch CJ, et al. The farnesyltransferase inhibitor L744,832 reduces hypoxia in tumors expressing activated H-ras. *Cancer Res* 2001; 61:2289–2293.

73. Rak J, Mitsuhashi Y, Bayko L, et al. Mutant ras oncogenes upregulate VEGF/VPF expression: implications for induction and inhibition of tumor angiogenesis. *Cancer Res* 1995; 55:4575–4580.

74. Molls M, Stadler P, Becker A, Feldmann HJ, Dunst J. Relevance of oxygen in radiation oncology. Mechanisms of action, correlation to low hemoglobin levels. *Strahlentherapie und Onkologie* 1998; 174:13–16.

75. Liu A, Cerniglia GJ, Bernhard EJ, Prendergast GC. RhoB is required to mediate apoptosis in neoplastically transformed cells following DNA damage. *Proc Natl Acad Sci USA,* 2001; 98:6192–6197.

76. Pirollo KF, Hao Z, Rait A, Ho CW, Chang EH. Evidence supporting a signal transduction pathway leading to the radiation-resistant phenotype in human tumor cells. *Biolchem Biophy Res Commun* 1997; 230:196–201.

77. Rodriguez-Viciana P, Warne PH, Dhand R, et al. Phosphatidylinositol-3-OH kinase as a direct target of Ras. *Nature* 1994; 370:527–532.

78. Carver DJ, Aman MJ, Ravichandran KS. SHIP inhibits Akt activation in B cells through regulation of Akt membrane localization. *Blood* 2000; 96: 1449–1456.

79. Kim S, Jee K, Kim D, Koh H, Chung J. Cyclic amp inhibits akt activity by blocking the membrane localization of pdk1. *J Biol Chem* 2001; 276:12864–12870.

80. Williams MR, Arthur JS, Balendran A, et al. The role of 3-phosphoinositide-dependent protein kinase 1 in activating AGC kinases defined in embryonic stem cells. *Curr Biol* 2000; 10:439–448.

81. Persad S, Attwell S, Gray V, et al. Regulation of protein kinase B/ Akt-serine-473 phosphorylation by integrin linked kinase (ILK): Critical roles for kinase activity and amino acids arginine-211 and serine-343. *J Biol Chem* 2001; 19:19.

82. Cho KS, Lee JH, Kim S, et al. Drosophila phosphoinositide-dependent kinase-1 regulates apoptosis and growth via the phosphoinositide 3-kinase-dependent signaling pathway. *Proc Natl Acad Sci USA* 2001; 98:6144–6149.

83. Kauffmann-Zeh A, Rodriguez-Viciana P, Ulrich E, et al. Suppression of c-Myc-induced apoptosis by Ras signalling through PI(3)K and PKB. *Nature* 1997; 385:544–548.

84. Kulik G, Klippel A, Weber MJ. Antiapoptotic signalling by the insulin-like growth factor I receptor, phosphatidylinositol 3-kinase, and Akt. *Mol Cell Biol* 1997; 17:1595–1606.

85. Coffer PJ, Jin J, Woodgett JR. Protein kinase B (c-Akt): a multifunctional mediator of phosphatidylinositol 3-kinase activation. *Biochem J* 1998; 335:1–13.

86. Sarkaria JN, Tibbetts RS, Busby EC, Kennedy AP, Hill DE, Abraham RT. Inhibition of phosphoinositide 3-kinase related kinases by the radiosensitizing agent wortmannin. *Cancer Res* 1998; 58:4375–4382.
87. Hosoi Y, Miyachi H, Matsumoto Y, et al. A phosphatidylinositol 3-kinase inhibitor wortmannin induces radioresistant DNA synthesis and sensitizes cells to bleomycin and ionizing radiation. *Int J Cancer* 1998; 78:642–647.
88. Rosenzweig KE, Youmell MB, Palayoor ST, Price BD. Radiosensitization of human tumor cells by the phosphatidylinositol3-kinase inhibitors wortmannin and LY294002 correlates with inhibition of DNA-dependent protein kinase and prolonged G2-M delay. *Clin Cancer Res* 1997; 3:1149–1156.
89. Burgering BM, Coffer PJ. Protein kinase B (c-Akt) in phosphatidylinositol-3-OH kinase signal transduction. *Nature* 1995; 376:599–602.
90. Gupta AK, Bakanauskas VJ, Cerniglia GJ, et al. The ras radiation resistance pathway. *Cancer Res* 2001; 6l:4278–4282.
90a. Grana TM, Rusyn EV, Zou H, Sartor CI, Cox AD. (2002) Ras mediates.radioresistance through both P13-K-dependent and Raf-dependent but MEK-independent signaling pathways. Cancer Res., in press (issue of July 15).
91. Gupta AK, Bernhard EJ, Bakanauskas VJ, Wu J, Musehel RJ, McKenna WG. RAS-Mediated radiation resistance is not linked to MAP kinase activation in two bladder carcinoma cell lines. *Radiat Res* 2000; 154:64–72.
92. O'Gorman DM, MeKenna SL, MeGahon AJ, Knox KA, Cotter TG. Sensitisation of HL6O human leukaemic cells to cytotoxic drug-induced apoptosis by inhibition of P13-kinase survival signals. *Leukemia* 2000; l4:602–611.
93. Zhang XE, Settleman J, Kyriakis JM, et al. Normal and oncogenic p21ras proteins bind to the amino-terminal regulatory domain of c-Raf-l. *Nature* 1993; 364:308–313.
94. Kyriakis JM, App H, Zhang XF, et al. Raf-1 activates MAP kinase-kinase. *Nature* 1992; 358:417–421.
95. Tzivion G, Luo Z, Avruch J. A dimeric 14-3-3 protein is an essential cofactor for Raf kinase activity. *Nature* 1998; 394:88–92.
96. Galaktionov K, Jessus C, Beach D. Raf1 interaction with Cdc25 phosphatase ties mitogenic signal transduction to cell cycle activation. *Genes Dev* 1995; 9:1046–1058.
97. Wang HG, Rapp UR, Reed JC. Bcl-2 targets the protein kinase Raf-1 to mitochondria [see comments]. *Cell* 1996; 87:629–638.
98. Kasid U, Pfeifer A, Weichselbaum RR, Dritschilo A, Mark GE. The raf oncogene is associated with a radiation-resistant human laryngeal cancer. *Science* 1987; 237:1039–1041.
99. Patel BK, Kasid U. Nucleotide sequence analysis of c-raf-1 cDNA and promoter from a radiation-resistant human squamous carcinoma cell line: deletion within exon 17. *Mol Carcinog* 1993; 8:7–12.
100. Kasid U, Suy S, Dent P, Ray S, Whiteside TL, Sturgill TW. Activation of Raf by ionizing radiation. *Nature* 1996; 382:813–816.
101. Suy S, Anderson WB, Dent P, Chang E, Kasid U. Association of Grb2 with Sos and Ras with Raf-1 upon gamma irradiation of breast cancer cells. *Oncogene* 1997; 15:53–61.
102. Riva C, Lavieille JP, Reyt E, Brambilla E, Lunardi J, Brambilla C. Differential c-myc, c-jun, c-raf and p53 expression in squamous cell carcinoma of the head and neck: implication in drug and radioresistance. *Eur J Cancer B Oral Oncol* 1995; 31B:384–391.
103. Britten RA, Klein K. Differential impact of Raf-1 kinase activity on tumor cell resistance to paclitaxel and docetaxel. *Anticancer Drugs* 2000; 11:439–443.
104. Warenius HM, Browning PG, Britten RA, Peacock JA, Rapp UR. C-raf-1 proto-oncogene expression relates to radiosensitivity rather than radioresistance. *Eur J Cancer* 1994; 30A:369–375.
105. Kasid U, Pfeifer A, Brennan T, et al. Effect of antisense c-raf-1 on tumorigenicity and radiation sensitivity of a human squamous carcinoma. *Science* 1989; 243:1354–1356.
106. Gokhale PC, McRae D, Monia BP, et al. Antisense raf oligodeoxyribonucleotide is a radiosensitizer in vivo. *Antisense Nucleic Acid Drug Dev* 1999; 9:191–201.
107. Carter S, Auer KL, Reardon DB, et al. Inhibition of the mitogen activated protein (MAP) kinase cascade potentiates cell killing by low dose ionizing radiation in A431 human squamous carcinoma cells. *Oncogene* 1998; 16:2787–2796.
108. Vrana JA, Grant S, Dent P. Inhibition of the MAPK pathway abrogates BCL2-mediated survival of leukemia cells after exposure to low-dose ionizing radiation. *Radiat Res* 1999; 151:559–569.
109. Cartee L, Vrana JA, Wang Z, et al. Inhibition of the mitogen activated protein kinase pathway potentiates radiation-induced cell killing via cell cycle arrest at the G2/M transition and independently of increased signaling by the JNK/c-Jun pathway. *Int J Oncol* 2000; 16:413–422.

110. Belka C, Knippers P, Rudner J, Faltin H, Bamberg M, Budach W. MEK1 and Erk1/2 kinases as targets for the modulation of radiation responses. *Anticancer Res* 2000; 20:3243–3249.

111. Klapper LN, Kirschbaum MH, Sela M, Yarden Y. Biochemical and clinical implications of the ErbB/HER signaling network of growth factor receptors. *Adv Cancer Res* 2000; 77:25–79.

112. Bargmann CI, Weinberg RA. Increased tyrosine kinase activity associated with the protein encoded by the activated neu oncogene. *Proc Natl Acad Sci USA* 1988; 85:5394–5398.

113. Downward J, Yarden Y, Mayes E, et al. Close similarity of epidermal growth factor receptor and v-erb-B oncogene protein sequences. *Nature* 1984; 307:521–527.

114. Downward J, Parker P, Waterfield MD. Autophosphorylation sites on the epidermal growth factor receptor. *Nature* 1984; 311:483–485.

115. Zhu A, Shaeffer J, Leslie S, Kolm P, El-Mahdi AM. Epidermal growth factor receptor: an independent predictor of survival in astrocytic tumors given definitive irradiation. *Int J Radiat Oncol Biol Phys* 1996; 34:809–815.

116. Maurizi M, Almadori G, Ferrandina G, et al. Prognostic significance of epidermal growth factor receptor in laryngeal squamous cell carcinoma. *Br J Cancer* 1996; 74:1253–1257.

117. Milas L, Mason K, Hunter N, et al. In vivo enhancement of tumor radioresponse by C225 antiepidermal growth factor receptor antibody. *Clin Cancer Res* 2000; 6:701–708.

118. Bonner JA, Raisch KP, Trummell HQ, et al. Enhanced apoptosis with combination C225/radiation treatment serves as the impetus for clinical investigation in head and neck cancers. *J Clin Oncol* 2000; 18:47S–53S.

119. Contessa JN, Reardon DB, Todd D, et al. The inducible expression of dominant-negative epidermal growth factor receptor-CD533 results in radiosensitization of human mammary carcinoma cells. *Clin Cancer Res* 1999; 5:405–411.

120. Reardon DB, Contessa JN, Mikkelsen RB, et al. Dominant negative EGFR-CD533 and inhibition of MAPK modify JNK1 activation and enhance radiation toxicity of human mammary carcinoma cells. *Oncogene* 1999; 18:4756–4766.

121. Harari PM, Huang SM. Head and neck cancer as a clinical model for molecular targeting of therapy: combining EGFR blockade with radiation. *Int J Radiat Oncol Biol Phys* 2001; 49:427–433.

122. Bianco C, Bianco R, Tortora G, et al. Antitumor activity of combined treatment of human cancer cells with ionizing radiation and anti-epidermal growth factor receptor monoclonal antibody C225 plus type I protein kinase. A antisense oligonucleotide. *Clin Cancer Res* 2000; 6:4343–4350.

123. Slamon DJ, Godolphin W, Jones LA, et al. Studies of the HER-2/neu proto-oncogene in human breast and ovarian cancer. *Science* 1989; 244:707–712.

124. Slamon DJ, Clark GM, Wong SG, Levin WJ, Ullrich A, McGuire WL. Human breast cancer: correlation of relapse and survival with amplification of the HER-2/neu oncogene. *Science* 1987; 235:177–182.

125. Saffari B, Jones LA, el-Naggar A, Felix JC, George J, Press MF. Amplification and overexpression of HER-2/neu (c-erbB2) in endometrial cancers: correlation with overall survival. *Cancer Res* 1995; 55:5693–5698.

126. Scheurle D, Jahanzeb M, Aronsohn RS, Watzek L, Narayanan R. HER-2/neu expression in archival non-small cell lung carcinomas using FDA-approved Hercep test. *Anticancer Res* 2000; 20:2091–2096.

127. Burke HB, Hoang A, Iglehart JD, Marks JR. Predicting response to adjuvant and radiation therapy in patients with early stage breast carcinoma. *Cancer* 1998; 82:874–877.

128. Braun S, Schlimok G, Heumos I, et al. ErbB2 overexpression on occult metastatic cells in bone marrow predicts poor clinical outcome of stage I-III breast cancer patients. *Cancer Res* 2001; 61:1890–1895.

129. Park BW, Zhang HT, Wu C, et al. Rationally designed anti-HER2/neu peptide mimetic disables P185HER2/neu tyrosine kinases in vitro and in vivo. *Nat Biotechnol* 2000; 18:194–198.

130. O'Rourke DM, Kao GD, Singh N, et al. Conversion of a radioresistant phenotype to a more sensitive one by disabling erbB receptor signaling in human cancer cells. *Proc Natl Acad Sci USA* 1998; 95:10842–10847.

131. Nakano T, Oka K, Ishikawa A, Morita S. Correlation of cervical carcinoma c-erb B-2 oncogene with cell proliferation parameters in patients treated with radiation therapy for cervical carcinoma. *Cancer* 1997; 79:513–520.

132. Ross JS, Fletcher JA. The HER-2/neu oncogene in breast cancer: prognostic factor, predictive factor, and target for therapy. *Oncologist* 1998; 3:237–252.

133. Stackhouse MA, Buchsbaum DJ, Grizzle WE, et al. Radiosensitization mediated by a transfected anti-erbB-2 single-chain antibody in vitro and in vivo. *Int J Radiat Oncol Biol Phys* 1998; 42:817–822.

134. Xu F, Leadon SA, Yu Y, et al. Synergistic interaction between anti-p185HER-2 ricin A chain immuno-toxins and radionuclide conjugates for inhibiting growth of ovarian and breast cancer cells that over-express HER-2. *Clin Cancer Res* 2000; 6:3334–3341.

135. Schmidt M, McWatters A, White RA, et al. Synergistic interaction between an anti-p185HER-2 pseudomonas exotoxin fusion protein [scFv(FRP5)-ETA] and ionizing radiation for inhibiting growth of ovarian cancer cells that overexpress HER-2. *Gynecol Oncol* 2001; 80:145–155.

136. FitzGerald TJ, Santucci MA, Das I, Kase K, Pierce JH, Greenberger JS. The v-abl, c-fms, or v-myc oncogene induces gamma radiation resistance of hematopoietic progenitor cell line 32d cl 3 at clinical low dose rate. *Int J Radiat Oncol Biol Phys* 1991; 21:1203–1210.

137. Shimm DS, Miller PR, Lin T, Moulinier PP, Hill AB. Effects of v-src oncogene activation on radiation sensitivity in drug-sensitive and in multidrug-resistant rat fibroblasts. *Radiat Res* 1992; 129:149–156.

138. Ramsamooj P, Kasid U, Dritschilo A. Differential expression of proteins in radioresistant and radiosensitive human squamous carcinoma cells. *J Natl Cancer Inst* 1992; 84:622–628.

139. Hahn SM, Bernhard EJ, Regine W, Mohiuddin M, Haller DG, Stevenson JP, Smith D, Pramanik B, Tepper J, DeLaney TF, Kiel KD, Morrison B, Deutsch P, Muschel RJ, and McKenna WG. A Phase I Trial of the Farnesyltransferase Inhibitor L-778,123 and Radiotherapy for locally advanced lung and head & neck cancer. *Clin Cancer Res* 2002;8:1065–1072.

140. Fenton BM, Paoni SF, Lee J, Koch CJ, Lord EM. Quantification of tumour vasculature and hypoxia by immunohistochemical staining and HbO2 saturation measurements. *Br J Cancer* 1999; 79:464–471.

21

Oncogenes as Targets for Cancer Vaccines

Samir N. Khleif, MD
and Joseph A. Lucci, III, MD

CONTENTS

1. INTRODUCTION

It has been long known that the immune system interacts with tumor cells *(1–12)* and scientists have long believed that tumors carry surface molecules, antigens, that are recognized by the immune system and can induce a protective immune response. Advances in molecular biology and immunology in the past two decades have provided concrete evidence for the presence of these antigens, which are called tumor-associated antigens (TAA) and also provided the tools for the potential development of immunologic approaches to target cells carrying these antigens.

The concept of Immunotherapy for cancer is over one hundred years old. The first reported cancer vaccine trial was by W.B. Coley in 1894 *(13)*. Coley's toxin, as it was called, was not so much a vaccine as a nonspecific immunostimulant. He used 13 different preparations of bacterial extracts, between 1892 and 1936, to treat patients with a variety of malignancies with surprising success *(14–19)*. He and others, including investigators at Mayo Clinic, reported over 50% durable responses in patient populations where 10–15% survival was historically expected. About the same time, in the early 1900s, Paul Ehrlich proposed the concept of immune surveillance *(20)*. Ehrlich suggested that tumors present unique antigens that could be recognized by the immune system, leading to continuous identification and removal of transformed cells. It was another 50 yr before his theory could be proven. In the 1950s, when inbred mouse strains became available, Ehrlich's theory was tested and proved the immunogenicity of tumors *(21,22)*. The tumor antigens were subsequently identified.

From: *Oncogene-Directed Therapies*
Edited by: J. W. Rak © Humana Press Inc., Totowa, NJ

The field of immunology has provided the knowledge of how internal and external proteins are processed by the cell and presented to the immune system as TAA as a requirement for antigen recognition, immune activation, and immune response. This chapter seeks to provide a basic understanding of these concepts and how they are applied to current tumor vaccine development. Also, we will discuss how oncogenes products serve as TAA and form some of the most ideal targets for the development of targeted vaccine therapy against cancer.

2. IMMUNOLOGY OF CANCER

The immune system has developed during evolution to acquire the capability of distinguishing self from foreign, for the purpose of differentiating cells carrying abnormal antigens from normal cells of the body. This occurs through two distinct arms of the immune system: the humoral arm and the cellular arm. The backbone of the humoral arm of the immune system is antibodies. Antibodies are synthesized by the B lymphocytes and target extracellular antigens. This is known as humoral immunity. The second arm of the immune system is the cell-mediated immunity, which is the function of T lymphocytes. The cell-mediated immune response is designed to recognize endogenously expressed antigens that are usually inaccessible to antibodies. These intracellular antigens are either altered native proteins or foreign proteins and are made accessible to the T cells by a mechanism called antigen processing and presentation, which will be discussed here. There are two types of T cells: CD4+, usually helper T cell, and CD8+, usually cytotoxic T lymphocytes (CTL). Both of these T cells recognize antigens through a direct interaction between the T cell receptor (TCR) and the antigen displayed by the major histocompatibility complex (MHC) on the surface of the target cells.

2.1. Antigen Processing and T Cell Interaction

Most proteins in nucleated cells, whether native, altered, or foreign, undergo degradation by ubiquitin-proteasome dependent mechanism (23). A selected group of the resultant peptides, 8–12 amino acid in length, are then transferred to the rough endoplasmic reticulum to bind with the MHC class I (MHC I) molecules. The now stable MHC I-antigen complex is the transported and displayed on the cell surface (24,25). Once on the cell surface, the MHC I-antigen complex can bind to the TCR. Thereby, nucleated cells make intracellular antigens available for T cell recognition by the TCR interaction with the MHC I-peptide complex. The CD8+ T cell is the T cell type that is responsible for recognizing these antigens in the context of MHC I molecules (26,27). This is a crucial step for the generation of immunologic responses against abnormal antigens, whether, foreign such as viral proteins or mutant protein, or abnormally expressed native proteins (28).

Another mechanism of antigen presentation to T cells is through MHC class II molecules (MHC II). MHC II are found on the surface of what is know as professional antigen presenting cells (APC), which include B cells, dendritic cells, and macrophages. Unlike antigens that are expressed on MHC I, antigens that are presented on MHC II are of extracellular origin. APCs ingest extracellular proteins, which originate from either extracellular organisms, or from soluble proteins released from dying cells, or by endocytosis. These proteins get processesed in endosome/liposomes after which they are transported to the Golgi apparatus. The resultant peptides are then packaged in MHC

Class II storage vesicles and get presented on the cell surface as 12–25 amino acids peptides in complexes with the MHC class II molecules. CD4+ T helper cells are the cells that are able to recognize antigens presented on MHC class II molecules. The binding of the CD4+ T cell receptor to be MHC II-peptides complex leads to the production of interleukin (IL)-2 and other cytokines, the activation of the IL-2 receptor gene, which leads to further proliferation of T helper cells, and the activation of antigen-specific cytotoxic T cells. CTLs, in turn, release mediators that can lyse or kill target cells *(29–32)*.

This process of T cell interaction with MHC-antigen complex, on the surface of cells, is known as immune surveillance. Immune surveillance is the process evolution has developed as a defense mechanism to identify and destroy infected cells, and thereby, eradicates cells expressing intracellular foreign or abnormal antigens *(30,33)*.

2.2. Oncogenes Products as Tumor-Associated Antigens (Antigenic Oncoproteins)

As outlined above, cancer possesses tumor-associated antigens (TAAs). Here, we will discuss how oncoproteins function as TAA, and how they could be targeted for vaccine therapy. Tumorigenesis is a complex multistep process involving sequential acquisition of genetic alterations in oncogenes and tumor suppressor genes. In this chapter, we will consider these two groups of genes, collectively, as oncogenes. Oncogenes are acquired either through the alteration of normal cellular genes or by the acquisition of a foreign transforming gene (exogenously acquired oncogene, e.g., viral oncogenes); The first mechanism, which is the alteration of endogenous genes, occurs in one of three forms: *(i)* open reading frame (ORF) mutation; *(ii)* gene amplification; or *(iii)* chromosomal rearrangement *(34)*. These result in either qualitatively or quantitatively novel protein products. ORF mutations or chromosomal rearrangements produce proteins with novel amino acid sequences, while gene amplification results in a higher copy number of the corresponding protein. The second mechanism by which oncogenes are acquired is through the acquisition of foreign genes from infectious agent-like tumor viruses. Whether the cancer is a result of the first or the second mechanism, when the resultant proteins are processed, they will produce novel peptides and, hence, new antigens on MHC molecules, which potentially form TAA. As will be discussed below, we currently know that many of these oncoproteins function as TAAs or antigenic oncoproteins (Table 1). Therefore, antigenic oncoproteins may be divided into two separate groups according to their origin. The first group consists of those antigens that have been generated endogenously (endogenous TAA), such as antigens which result from alterations in the cell's native endogenous molecules. The second group is the exogenous TAA, which are antigens that are acquired by the tumor cells from an exogenous source, such as oncogenic viruses or parasites.

1. Endogenous antigenic oncoproteins. These antigens are presented in three different forms according to the original genetic change: *(1)* Overexpressed proteins which result secondary to either oncogene amplification (e.g., *HER-2/neu*) *(35)* or posttranscriptional modification of a mutated protein, which leads to more stability and increase in the half-life of the protein (e.g., mutant p53) *(36–38)*. The higher level of the oncoprotein expression, which leads to higher level of peptide production, may overcome the immune tolerance produced by the normal low level expression of the wild-type proteins in normal tissue and hence, allows immune reconstitution. *(2)* Altered protein amino acid sequences, which may be due to a point mutation or a frame shift, both of

Table 1
A List of the Identified Antigenic Oncoproteins

Point mutation
— P53
— Ras
— P16
— β catenin, TPI, CDC27
Translocation
— BCR-ABL
— TEL-AML-1, EWS-FLI-1, EWS-ATF-1,
  EWS-WT-1, PAX-3-FKHR
Overexpressed
— P53
— Her-2-neu
Viral oncoproteins
— HPV E6 and E7
— EBV EBNA

which generate peptides with new amino acid sequences that are novel to the immune system. Examples of such mutated antigenic oncoproteins include the ras and p53 proteins *(39–41)*. P16 and β catenin are other oncoproteins that are found to be recognized by the T cell as TAA *(42–44)*. *(3)* Fusion proteins, which result from chromosomal translocation. The resultant fusion proteins contain a novel amino acid sequence at the break point, which, when degraded, result in novel peptides that flank the break point area and, hence, form potential TAAs *(45)*.

2. Exogenous antigenic oncoproteins. Many microorganisms have been implicated in malignant transformation of human tumors. Viruses, including both RNA and DNA viruses, are implicated in the development of some human cancers *(46,47)*. The viral genome gets integrated into the human chromosomal DNA leading to the endogenous expression of the viral protein in the tumor cell. These viral proteins undergo the same processing utilizing the same pathways used by self proteins, resulting in novel foreign peptides presented by the MHC class I molecule on the cell surface. The human papillomavirus (HPV), Epstein-Barr virus (EBV), hepatitis B virus (HBV), and hepatitis C virus (HCV) are some known examples of oncogenic viruses. Some of these will be discussed in more detail later in the chapter.

3. CANCER VACCINES

Vaccination against cancer aims to actively stimulate the immune system against antigenic targets that are expressed by the tumor. In general, vaccines are designed to stimulate the immune system to generate either humoral or cellular immune responses. Therefore, vaccines are classified into humoral or cell mediated vaccines. Since oncoproteins are intracellular antigens, vaccines that are directed against antigenic oncoproteins are usually designed to generate cellular immune responses to be able to recognize processed antigens in the context of MHC molecules.

In general, specific cell-mediated cancer vaccines are of two types. The first is a defined antigen vaccine, in which the vaccine aims to generate an immune response against specific antigenic targets. The second is a whole tumor undefined antigen vaccine that takes advantage of the fact that tumor cells carry all the tumor-specific antigens whether known or unknown. Since, in this chapter, we will be discussing vaccine development against specific oncoproteins, which are defined antigens, we will be mainly discussing the first type.

An ideal specific antigenic target for a cancer vaccine is a target that fulfils the following criteria:

1. Uniquely expressed in the cancer cell, either quantitatively or qualitatively, so that the resultant immune response would be able to distinguish tumor form normal cells and avoid the generation of autoimmune disease.
2. Important for the maintenance of the malignant phenotype; therefore, it will not be possible to be excluded or down-regulated in the tumor cell to avoid immune recognition.
3. Immunogenic, i.e., when given as a vaccine it would be capable of generating an immune response.
4. Expressed on the cell surface to be accessible and recognized by the immune system and in particular the T cell.

The following are the different vaccine approaches used to generate an immune response against specific antigenic targets:

1. Recombinant vaccine vectors. In this approach, the antigen will be administered as DNA genetic material to the host, in which genes encoding known antigenic proteins are inserted into a delivery expression vector. These delivery vectors are either live viral or naked DNA vectors. Vaccinia virus has been traditionally used as a vector for antigen vaccine delivery; however, other viral vectors are currently being introduced into clinical trials such as Fowl pox and Adenovirus. The second delivery system of the recombinant vaccine technology is the polynucleic acid/naked DNA vector. In this approach, genes of the targeted tumor antigen are inserted into a DNA vector under the control of an appropriate promotor that initiates gene expression, and the vector is injected directly into the host. Both of these methods are already being tested in clinical trials for advanced cancer using many TAA *(48–51)*. However, because of the inherent risk in administering an oncogene ORF into the host, this technology might not be widely accepted in the delivery of antigenic oncoproteins, fearing the possible integration of the oncogenic DNA sequences into the human genome with potential transforming effect. Therefore, utilizing a partial nontransforming fragment sequence of the oncogenes DNA (mini-gene) provides one solution to this issue *(52);* alternatively, other approaches for the delivery of these antigens that do not allow genetic integration should be used. These approaches will be discussed *below.*
2. Synthetic antigen vaccine. In this approach, the defined antigen will be synthesized in the form of a full protein, polypeptide, or synthetic peptide fragment. Full-length proteins and polypeptides would need to be taken up by APCs, processed, and represented on MHC molecules. The peptides may need to be taken up and represented by APCs or may lay down directly on MHC molecules. Many of these peptides have been recently identified or predicted and designed for vaccine therapy. These peptides are called immunodominant epitopes if they represent the dominant focus of an immunologic response. Vaccination with the synthetic antigens can be accomplished either by direct intradermal or subcutaneous injection or by administering the antigen(s) using antigen presenting cells such as dendritic cells (DC) as a delivery method. DC are mononuclear cells that can be generated from human peripheral blood cells in the presence of mixture of cytokines including granulocyte macrophage colony-stimulating factor (GM-CSF)

and IL-4 *(53)*. These DC have been shown to be powerful tools and capable of generating specific cytotoxic immune responses in both animals and humans *(54–57)*. In addition, vaccination with DC in human trials has shown efficacy in both immunological and clinical outcomes *(58)*. Direct injection of the synthetic antigens usually require the presence of an immune adjuvant, such as an oil emulsion-based adjuvant, CpG containing DNA sequences, or cytokines like GM-CSF, IL-2, or IL-12. Because of the concerns outlined above regarding administering antigenic oncoproteins with recombinant technologies, this might be more acceptable method of delivery. Indeed most of the clinical trials that are currently conducted utilizing oncoproteins as antigenic targets utilize this technology, as will be outlined *below.*

4. ONCOPROTEINS AS TARGETS FOR VACCINE THERAPY

Few oncogenes products have already been shown to function as antigenic oncoproteins or TAA. In this chapter, we will discuss how these oncogenes products form some of the most ideal molecules for the development of targeted vaccine therapy against cancer, focusing on some of the better known targets. These antigenic oncoproteins include point mutated proteins, such as ras and p53, overexpressed oncoproteins, such as p53 and Her2/nue, chromosomal translocation product, such as BCR-Abl fusion protein, and exogenous antigenic oncoprotein, such as HPV oncogenes products.

4.1. Ras

Ras proto-oncogenes are extensively characterized mutated genes in human cancers *(59,60)*. They encode a highly conserved family of 21 kDa proteins (p21), which is involved in signal transduction, regulating the cell cycle, and cell differentiation. A single amino acid substitution in the ras protein potentiates transformation and growth of human cells. Point mutated ras genes have been found with high frequency in a broad spectrum of human carcinomas. Our data indicate that ras is most commonly mutated in gastrointestinal and lung malignancies. It is mutated in 75% of pancreatic cancer, 45% of colorectal cancers, and 23% in adenocarcinoma of lung (unpublished data). More than 90% of ras mutations occur in codon 12, the rest occuring exclusively in codons 13 and 61. In our patient population, mutations in codon 12 are limited to a few substitutions. More than 80% of these changes are found to be the replacement of glycine with aspartic acid (asp), valine (val), or cystine (cys). These characteristics of a relatively limited number of mutations and the broad applicability to a wide variety of tumors have made ras an attractive target for vaccine development.

Many laboratories have generated convincing animal data to show that mutated ras is a suitable target for vaccine therapy. Peace et al. have demonstrated that vaccinating mice with peptides or a full protein containing a ras mutation, on either codon 12 or 61, were able to generate a specific immune response. The immune response was found to recognize tumor cells harboring the corresponding ras mutation, but not the wild-type ras *(39,61,62)*. These responses were found to be of either CD4+ or CD8+ subtypes *(39,61,62)*. Abrams et al. have also demonstrated that subcutaneous immunization of mice with 13-mer K-ras peptides spanning to different mutations at codon 12 induces specific T cell immune responses. These T cells were shown to be CD4+ with Th1 characteristics *(63–65)* and are MHC II restricted. Furthermore, they are found to be able to distinguish between targets presenting the corresponding mutation and the wild-type or other unrelated ras mutations *(63–65)*. Fenton and colleagues went on to demonstrate that K-ras vaccines were able to protect mice against tumor challenge with tumors harboring ras mutations *(66)*, and that this response was mediated through an MHC class I-restricted CTL response that was specific for the vaccine antigen. Skipper et al. have utilized a different immunization strategy by using a vaccinia virus containing the mutant ras expressing N-ras codon 61 mutation peptide. These investigators have also shown that this method of vaccination with the mutant ras is effective in generating CD8+ specific T cells *(67)*.

Moreover, human data have shown that specific immune responses could be generated in an in vitro system against the mutant ras. Fossum and colleagues have demonstrated that specific T cell responses, both CD4+ and CD8+, can be generated, in vitro, from patients with cancer that have a *K-ras* mutation on codon 13 *(68–71)*. The same group and others have also shown the in vitro generation of specific CTL against ras mutations on codon 12 and 61, and that some of these mutations are naturally processed and presented through different human lymphocyte antigen (HLA) class I and class II haplotypes *(72–75)*.

The above mentioned data demonstrated, in both animals and humans, that mutated ras protein can generate an immune response that is capable of distinguishing a single amino acid difference between the mutated ras in the tumor cell and the wild-type protein in the normal cell. Therefore, mutant ras protein, is a TAA or an antigenic oncoprotein that forms an ideal target for vaccine development. Accordingly, our group and others have conducted clinical trials to test the feasibility of ras vaccination in patients with tumors that harbor ras mutations.

In a phase I trial, we have subcutaneously immunized advanced adenocarcinoma patients with increasing doses of 13-mer mutant ras peptides, which correspond to the mutation that patients harbor in their tumors. We have found that the peptide vaccination was well tolerated with no significant systemic side effects. Furthermore, we have demonstrated that some vaccinated patients mount specific immunologic responses that are both CD4+ and CD8+ and are MHC class II- and I-restricted, respectively. These CTLs were capable of lysing tumor cells endogenously expressing the corresponding ras mutation, but not cells with the wild-type gene. Immunologic responses were generated against the three different mutations targeted on this trial Ras 12val, asp, or cys *(41,76,77)*. Similar results have been reported by Gjertsen and colleagues in a phase I/II trial using 17-mer ras peptides to vaccinate patients with pancreatic cancer *(78,79)*. In a follow-up study by the same group, the same mutated ras peptides were administered intradermally along with GM-CSF in patients with varying stages of pancreatic cancer. In this study, the investigators demonstrated that Ras-specific T cells were able to selectively accumulate in the tumor of one patient. In addition, patients with advanced cancer demonstrating an immune response to the peptide vaccine showed prolonged survival compared to nonresponders (median survival from start of treatment 148 d vs 61 d, respectively) *(80)*. These preliminary studies have shown that ras peptide vaccines is safe and can generate specific immune responses with some clinical results in patients with advanced disease. Currently, other clinical trials are currently being conducted to test the combination of different mutant ras peptides along with cytokines, such as GM-CSF, IL-2, and the combination of IL-2 and

GM-CSF. Also, studies are being designed to target patients with minimal disease, or on an adjuvant basis *(81)*.

4.2. p53

p53 is a tumor suppressor gene, and it is the most commonly mutated gene in human cancers. p53 protein is a nuclear transcription factor, which controls several downstream gene products implicated in cell cycle control *(82–85)*. Mutations of the *p53* gene have been detected in more than 50% of a wide variety of human cancers including colon, breast, ovary, and lung *(82,86–90)*.

The majority of the mutations in the p53 gene result in a missense substitution; less common mutation types include nonsense, deletions, or splicing *(91,92)*. More than 80% of mutations of the p53 protein contain a single amino acid substitution; therefore, this is one mechanism by which p53 may form an antigenic oncoprotein. However, unlike the ras protein, these mutations are distributed over a wide range of positions in the amino acid sequences. Hence, patients with a *p53* mutation will present with a wide range of different mutations, and therefore, different antigens will be required to make vaccines for different patients. This forms a limiting factor in developing a practical vaccine approach for mutant p53, since targeted vaccine therapy has to be customized for each mutation. Another form of antigenic presentation of p53 is an overexpressed protein. Mutations in p53 frequently stabilizes the protein leading to the increase in its half-life, and in turn, the overexpression of the protein *(93)*. Therefore, this protein could function as an antigen through two different mechanisms: *(i)* as a mutant foreign protein; and *(ii)* as an overexpressed self-protein. These factors make p53 an ideal target for vaccine trials for wide range of tumor types.

4.3. p53 Antigen as a Mutant Protein

Preliminary data suggesting that mutated p53 can act as a TAA was reported by Noguchi et al. *(94)*. These investigators have reported that antibodies to the p53 protein in lung cancer patients correlate with the presence of p53 mutations. Furthermore, the antibody titer is found to correlate with disease status *(52,95)*. These findings confirm that the human immune system can recognize and respond to p53 mutations.

In animal models, it has been shown that vaccinating mice with peptides spanning p53 point mutations can generate specific CD8+ CTL. These CD8+ T cells were able to recognize the mutant peptide sequences, but not the wild-type p53 peptides *(40)*. Other investigators have further demonstrated that specific CTLs generated in mice can recognize endogenously expressed mutant p53 *(95,96)*. Furthermore, immune responses that are generated against mutant p53 targets were also found to be able to protect mice against challenge with mutant p53 harboring tumors *(52,57,96,97)*. These data demonstrate that mutant p53 is processed and presented on the cell surface of tumor cells as a tumor antigen.

We have conducted a clinical trial in which patients with mutant *p53* were vaccinated with customized mutant p53 peptides, which matched the mutations that the patients harbor in their tumors. These peptides were also designed to carry flanking sequences that are predicted to bind to the patient's own HLA or long sequences that contain potential class I or II motifs. In this study, we found that we can generate specific-immune responses against the specific p53 mutation (Khleif et al., manuscript in preparation). Follow-up clinical trials in our institution are being conducted to further test the efficacy of this approach.

4.4. p53 Antigen as an Overexpressed Protein

As outlined above, p53 might present with many different mutations and, hence, many different antigens. This forms a limiting factor in developing a practical vaccine approach, since targeted vaccine therapy has to be customized for each mutation. As outlined above, mutations of the p53 protein also result in prolonged half-life and, therefore, the accumulation of high-level expression of the p53 protein in tumor cells. Due to the higher intracellular expression of the mutant p53 in tumor cells, wild-type epitopes may become immunogenic. Therefore, mutant p53 provides another mechanism by which the protein is presented as an antigen. Indeed, many studies in both mice and humans have proven that the wild-type amino acid sequences in the mutant p53 are processed and expressed on tumor cells and are antigenic. Investigators have shown that wild-type p53 epitopes can be recognized by CTLs on murine tumor cells *(98)* and that mice can be protected by wild-type p53 peptide vaccination against challenge with tumors expressing the p53 protein *(57)*. Roth et al. have also shown that vaccination of mice with recombinant wild-type p53 leads to a protective effect against challenge with tumors expressing high levels of mutant p53. In contrast, tumors with low level of p53 escaped immunologic rejection *(99)*.

Multiple p53 epitopes have been identified to bind to HLA-A2 molecules *(100–104)*. The p53: 264–272 peptide, which spans amino acids 264–272, is the most studied and has been shown by many investigators to have high affinity for HLA-A2 *(100–104)*. Recently, p53: 264–272 has been identified to be naturally processed and endogenously presented by HLA-A2 in different types of tumor cell lines *(37,38)*. These investigators have shown that specific CD8+ T cells generated from HLA-A2 donors against p53:264–272 peptide were able to lyse tumor cells overexpressing either the wild-type or the mutant p53 protein. On the other hand, these specific lymphocytes failed to lyse autologous cells derived from normal tissue *(36,105)*. Furthermore, other investigators, McCarty et al., have shown that human CTL generated against an HLA-A2 p53 epitope can protect severe combined immunodeficient (SCID) mice from human tumors overexpressing the p53 protein *(106)*. Few other epitopes have been already identified as potentials targets for vaccine therapy against overexpressed p53. As of now, we are conducting a clinical trial testing the vaccination of p53:264–272 peptides in HLA-A2 patients with minimal disease ovarian cancer or advanced breast cancer. Combinations of multiple peptides may form an attractive approach to use for this particular antigen.

4.5. BCR-ABL

BCR-ABL fusion protein is one of the most studied translocation gene products, which is known as Philadelphia chromosome. BCR-Abl is created by the translocation of chromosome 9 to 22, t(9:22)(q34;q11), which results in fusion of the c-abl oncogene to the break point cluster region within the ber gene *(107)*. The resultant gene encodes for a 210 kDa or a 190 kDa protein that possesses an enhanced tyrosine kinase activity with transforming capability *(107,108)*. The BCR-ABL gene product is found in over 90% of patients with chronic myelogenous leukemias (CML), less frequently in adult acute lymphocytic leukemias (ALL) (25%), 10% in pediatric ALL, and is also found in small a percentage of acute myelogenous leukemia (AML) *(109)*. A partial list of other antigenic oncoproteins that reuslt form a chromosomal translocation fusion appears in Table 1.

Since both BCR and ABL genes are fused in frame, the majority of the resultant BCR-ABL protein has normal amino acid sequence; hence, the majority of the resultant peptides are of self characteristics. Therefore, the peptides that potentially possess antigenic characteristics are those sequences that flank and contain the fusion site. Therefore, there are only few epitopes that would potentially form an antigenic product.

Chen et al. have shown that subcutaneous vaccination of animals with of peptides that span the fusion area of the BCR-ABL fusion protein results in responses of MHC class II-restricted CD4+ and MHC class I-restricted CD8+ T cells, which specifically recognize the fusion peptide *(110,111)*.

Human data have shown that peptides, spanning the fusion area of BCR-ABL, can generate specific immune responses by in vitro immunization of T cells. Bosch and colleagues demonstrated that a 17-mer peptide was able to generate an in vitro-specific MHC class II (DR-4)-restricted CD4+ T cell that can recognize leukemia cells expressing the fusion protein and the DR-4 class II molecule *(112)*. In another study, Bosch et al. have also shown that such CD4+ cells may also be HLA-DR2a-restricted *(113)*. This indicates that the protein is processed and expressed on the surface of the tumor cell in the proper HLA context, and it is expressed in the context of different HLA class II haplotypes *(112,113)*. MHC class I responses to BCR-ABL have also been investigated, with mixed results. Greco et al. reported that a 9-mer peptide spanning the BCR-ABL fusion could bind with HLA-A3 class I molecule. The investigators have demonstrated that a CTL response can be generated in vitro against the peptide and that the response could be enhanced by modifying the peptide to incorporate amino acid residues that increase the affinity of the peptide to HLA-A3 molecule *(114)*. Furthermore, Bocchia and colleagues have demonstrated that 9-mer and 11-mer peptides, which span the break point fusion site, can bind MHC class I with high affinity *(115)*. They have also found that these peptides are capable of eliciting a specific CTL response in 1 of 4 HLA-A3 healthy donors and 3 of 7 donors generated T cell proliferation, which was confined to the HLA-DRII haplotype. Therefore, these investigators have shown that in vitro T cell responses utilizing fusion peptides can be both HLA class I- and class II-restricted *(116)*.

Accordingly, clinical trials have commenced using BCR-ABL break point antigens. Pinilla-Ibarz and colleagues at Memorial Sloan Kettering Cancer Center *(117)* have reported a phase I/II clinical trial using a combination of multiple peptides spanning the break point. Escalating doses of peptides showed minimal toxicity. Delayed hypersensitivity and T cell proliferation responses were found in 3 patients at the 2 highest dose levels, but no CTL activity was found in any of 12 patients studied *(117)*. Although these findings are encouraging, further clinical studies are needed to explore the potentials of this antigen.

Other break point mutations that result in the production of antigenic fusion proteins are currently being studied, including EWS-FLI-1 and PAX3/FKHR *(118)* and others. The data from these antigenic oncoproteins are less developed than that with BCR-ABL, however, it looks promising, especially since it covers a different range of tumor types.

4.6. HER-2/neu

Her2/neu (c-erbB2) is a member of epidermal growth factor receptor (EGFR) family. It is an oncogene that encodes a 185 kDa protein with tyrosine kinase activity.

Her2/neu gene amplification is found in many epithelial cancers including colon, pancreas, genitourinary, and breast *(119–121)*. This leads to the overexpression of the Her2/neu protein. The overexpression of Her2/neu leads to the constitutive activation of the tyrosine kinase receptor; this in turn, increases mitogenic cell signaling, and hence, increases proliferation. The increase in the level of Her2/neu protein makes it a potential TAA and, hence, an antigenic oncoprotein target. Indeed, it has been shown that some patients that have advanced breast or ovarian cancers overexpressing Her2/neu have HER-2/neu-specific T cells or detectable HER-2/neu-specific IgG antibodies *(122)*.

In animal models, it has been found that vaccination with of Her2/neu antigens induce a protective effect against challenge with tumors overexpressing Her2/neu protein. This protection was found both CD4 and CD8 T cells-dependent *(123–126)*. Investigators have shown that immunization with either HER2/neu peptides or full-length protein prevents or delays the spontaneous development of mammary tumors overexpressing HER2/neu in a majority of mice transgenic for the rat Her-2/neu oncogene *(125,127)*.

Several Her2/neu HLA class I-restricted epitopes have been identified through elution or predictive techniques *(35,128–130)*. Ikuta et al. have shown that CD8+ CTL clones specific for HER2-expressing cancer cell lines can be generated from peripheral blood lymphocytes of volunteers with HLA-A2402 *(130)*. Furthermore, it has also been shown that CTL derived against a Her2/neu HLA-A2 peptide from HLA-A2 patients, with cancer overexpressing HER2/neu, can recognize autologous and allogeneic tumor cells overexpressing HER2/neu in an HLA-A2-restricted fashion. This has been demonstrated from ascitis of patients with pancreatic cancer *(131)* and from tumor-associated lymphocytes in patients with gastric, breast, and ovarian cancers *(122,132–134)*. These results and others demonstrates that HER2/neu is a TAA in cancers that carry the amplified gene.

Clinical trials using Her2/neu antigens as vaccine targets in cancer patients have been initiated. Disis et al. have reported the generation of specific immune responses in patients with advanced ovarian and breast cancers (stage III and IV) after vaccination with Her2/neu peptides. These investigators have found that intradermal injection of multiple 15–18 amino acids HER-2/neu peptides derived from the extracellular domain (ECD) or intracellular domain (ICD) mixed with GM-CSF lead to the generation of specific CD4+ and CD8+ T cell responses *(135,136)*. On the other hand, Zaks et al. *(132)* have found that vaccinating patients with a 9-mer HLA-A2 Her2/neu peptide spanning amino acids 369–377 and administered subcutaneously and with Freund's incomplete adjuvant failed to generate a specific immune response. Therefore, it is very important to be able to determine the proper immunogenic antigen and the route of administration for any of the antigenic oncoproteins tested in clinical trials.

4.7. HPV E6 and E7 Proteins

HPV is a family of double-stranded DNA viruses. HPV is divided into low risk and high risk types. The low risk HPVs lead to the development of benign mainly skin lesions. On the other hand, the high risk types are associated with the development of cancers including, cervical, anogenital, head and neck, and esophageal cancers. Over

95% of cervical cancers contain high risk HPV-DNA, including the most common types, which are HPV-16 and -18. The high risk HPV-DNA integrates into the host genome and overexpresses two of the HPV early genes, E6 and E7. These two genes are critical to the neoplastic transformation process. Whereas E6 binds the tumor suppressor protein p53 and enhances its degradation *(137)*, E7 binds and inactivates the retinoblastoma protein (pRb) *(138)*. Loss of function of these two tumor suppressor genes results in uncontrolled growth and further malignant transformation. Therefore, continued expression of HPV E6 and E7 proteins are necessary for maintenance of the malignant phenotype *(139)*. In turn, this makes the HPV E6 and E7 proteins ideal targets for vaccine development, since they are foreign antigens, unique to cancer cells, and the tumor cells cannot down-regulate these genes to develop resistance.

Epidemiologic evidence suggests that HPV-induced tumors are directly affected by the immune system. Immunocompromised patients, such as renal transplant patients and patients infected with human immunodeficiency virus (HIV), have an increased incidence of premalignant and malignant lesions and a poorer prognosis *(140)*. Furthermore, patients with cervical intraepithelial dysplasia (CIN) lesions, who were found to have lymphoproliferative responses to HPV E6 and/or E7 peptides, were more likely to eliminate HPV-DNA and CIN lesions *(141)*. In a cross-sectional study, Tsukui et al. found an increase correlation between stage of disease (HPV-infiltrating only, low-grade squamous intraepithelial lesion [LSIL], high-grade squamous intraepithelial lesion [HSIL], and invasive cancer) and the IL-2 production in response to a set of E6 and E7 peptides, further suggesting that the presence of immune response might be protective *(142)*.

Immunization experiments have demonstrated that E6 and E7 are immunogens in mice and that the immune responses generated are specific and capable of lysing cells endogenously expressing these oncoproteins with tumors harboring HPV-DNA. Furthermore these immune responses are found to infer protection against tumor challenge. Feltkamp et al. have shown that immunizing mice with APCs expressing the full-length HPV-16 E7 protein leads to an effective protection against transplanted tumor cells expressing the HPV E7 gene. The immunologic response believed to confer this protection is found to be mediated by CD8+ cytotoxic lymphocytes *(143)*. It has also been shown by other investigators that vaccinating mice with HPV-16 E7 peptides, which bound with high affinity to the MHC Class I molecule, induced a CTL-mediated response, which rendered the animals insensitive to subsequent challenge with HPV-16-transformed cells *(144)*.

High affinity binding peptides were identified for most common HLA class I molecules *(145,146)*. These peptides were also found to be immunogenic and could cause regression of transplanted human tumor cells in nude mice *(147,148)*. In human in vitro stimulation experiments, CTLs against the HPV-16 E6 and E7 epitope have been generated from the peripheral blood mononuclear cells of cervical cancer patients *(144)*. These specific CTLs were also found to be able to lyse HPV-16-positive cervical cancer cells *(149)*. This result further demonstrates that HPV E7 protein is endogenously processed and presented on the cell surface of human tumor cells. Furthermore, HPV-16 E6 protein has also been found to contain sequences with HLA class I binding motifs. One of these peptides, E6 (18–26), which is found to be highly bound to HLA-A2, has also been shown to be immunogenic and cause specific regression of transplanted human tumors expressing HPV-16 E6 *(148)*.

Phase I and phase II HPV vaccine clinical trials have been conducted to test the feasibility of administering different HPV antigens in patients with tumors containing the HPV genome. At the National Cancer Institute, we have vaccinated patients with either E6 or E7 HLA-A2 binding peptides, by transfusing peptide-pulsed peripheral blood mononuclear cells (PBMC) intravenously to patients with advanced cervical cancer. We have found that both peptides can generate specific and strong immune responses *(150)*. Muderspach et al. have also found that vaccinating women with high grade cervical or vulvar intraepithelial neoplasia with HLA-A2 E7 peptide alone or in combination with a different HLA-A2 E7 peptides, linked to a helper T cell epitope, resulted in immunological response to both of these peptides. Also, 3 of 18 treated patients cleared their dysplasia after the vaccine, and 6 of these patients had partial colposcopically measured regression of their CIN *(151)*. Furthermore, full-length HPV-16 E7 protein has also been utilized in clinical trials. In a phase I clinical trial, vaccinating normal volunteers with a single dose in a dose-escalating manner using the full-length E7 protein fused to a heat-shock protein (HSP)-E7, investigators found that 4 of 8 subjects developed E7-specific proliferative responses *(152)*. In another trial utilizing the HSP-E7 protein, Palefsky et al. have vaccinated HSIL patients with the fusion protein monthly, for a total of 3 vaccines. Some patients were found to demonstrate down-regulation of their lesions at 3 and 6 mo, respectively *(153)*.

This is a highly active area of cancer vaccine development research. Many companies have generated vaccine reagents that target HPV, including different forms of peptides, full HPV E6 and E7 recombinant proteins, DNA, and viral vectors containing partial sequences of the oncogenes. Some of these reagents have already entered clinical trails for testing, and some are expected to be starting soon.

5. CONCLUSION

We believe that the manipulation of the immune system, directed against specific tumor targets, is one of the most promising strategies in cancer therapy. This therapy is expected to be useful in both the prevention and the treatment of the disease. In this chapter, we have reviewed the state of the art of vaccine development targeting oncogene products (antigenic oncoproteins). As outlined above, research in the area have already proven that the product of some oncogenes form TAAs and that it is possible to generate specific immune responses against these antigens, which are able to distinguish between the altered proteins and their normal counterpart. However, to date, not too many clinical responses have been observed as a result of this type of therapy. Therefore, after proving that specific immune response against oncogene products can be generated, the current research in this area is concentrated on how to translate the immune response seen into a clinical response. Currently, this is done through the following venues: *(i)* identifying improved ways for vaccine delivery and antigen presentation; *(ii)* improving antigen immunogenicity by modifying the antigens or utilizing different combinations cytokines; *(iii)* identifying the appropriate patients cohorts, such as earlier disease and prevention of recurrence; *(iv)* enhancing and expanding the resultant specific immune response by in vitro or in vivo expansion of specific T cells; and *(v)* combining vaccines with other standard modalities. Clearly, there is still a way to go in this exciting area of oncogene targeting, however, I believe that great strides have been made, and we will be seeing a lot of development in this area in the near future.

REFERENCES

1. Uenishi T, Hirohashi K, Tanaka H, Ikebe T, Kinoshita H. Spontaneous regression of a large hepato-cellular carcinoma with portal vein tumor thrombi: report of a case. *Surg Today* 2000; 30:82–85.
2. Hachiya T, Koizumi T, Hayasaka M, et al. Spontaneous regression of primary mediastinal germ cell tumor. *Jpn J Clin Oncol* 1998; 28:281–283.
3. Markowska J, Markowska A. Spontaneous tumor regression. *Ginekol Pol* 1998; 69:39–44.
4. Otley CC, Pittelkow MR. Skin cancer in liver transplant recipients. *Liver Transpl* 2000; 6:253–262.
5. Penn I. Overview of the problem of cancer in organ transplant recipients. *Ann Transplant* 1997; 2:5–6.
6. Konety BR, Tewari A, Howard RJ, et al. Prostate cancer in the post-transplant population. Urologic Society for Transplantation and Vascular Surgery. *Urology* 1998; 52:428–432.
7. Flattery MP. Incidence and treatment of cancer in transplant recipients. *J Transpl Coord* 1998; 8:105–110; quiz 111–112.
8. Sheil AG. Cancer in immune-suppressed organ transplant recipients: aetiology and evolution. *Transplant Proc* 1998; 30:2055–2057.
9. Royal RE, Steinberg SM, Krouse RS, et al. Correlates of response to IL-2 therapy in patients treated for metastatic renal cancer and melanoma. *Cancer J Sci Am* 1996; 2:91.
10. Bourantas KL, Hatzimichael EC, Makis AC, et al. Prolonged interferon-alpha-2b treatment of hairy cell leukemia patients. *Eur J Haematol* 2000; 64:350–351.
11. Parkinson DR, Sznol M. High dose interleukin-2 in the therapy of metastatic renal cell carcinoma. *Semin Oncol* 1995; 22:61–66.
12. Stadler WM, Vogelzang NJ. Low dose interleukin-2 in the treatment of metaststic renal call carcinoma. *Semin Oncol* 1995; 22:67–73.
13. Coley W. Treatment of inoperable malignant tumors with toxins of erysipelas and the bacillus prodigious. *Trans Am Surg Assn* 1894; 12:183–212.
14. Nauts H. Beneficial effects of immunotherapy (bacterial toxins) on sarcoma of the soft tissue, other than lymphosarcoma. End results in 186 determinate cases with microscopic confirmation of diagnosis—49 operable, 137 inoperable. Cancer Research Institute, New York 1975.
15. Coley W. Cancer of the testis; containing a report of 64 cases, with special reference to 12 cases of cancer of the undescended testis. *Trans South Surg Gyn Assn* 1914; 63:35–70.
16. Coley W. Primary neoplasms of the lymphatic glands including Hodgkin's disease. *Ann Surg* 1916; 63:35–70.
17. Coley W, Hoguet J. Melanotic cancer; with a report of ninety cases. *Trans Am Surg Assn* 1916; 34:319–383.
18. Coley W. Multiple myeloma. *Ann Surg* 1931; 93:77–89.
19. Coley W. Endothelioma, or Ewing's tumor. *Am J Surg* 1935; 27:7–18.
20. Roitt BJ I, Male D. Immunology. Mosby International, London, 1998.
21. Prehn R and Main JM. Immunity to methycholanthrene-induced sarcomas. *J Natl Cancer Inst* 1957; 18:769–778.
22. Klein G, Sjogren HO, Klein E, Hellström KE. Demonstration of resistance against methycholanthrene-induced sarcomas in the primary autochthonous host. 1960; 20:1561–1572.
23. Wilkinson KD. Ubiquitination and deubiquitination: Targeting of proteins for degradation by the proteasome [in process citation]. *Semin Cell Dev Biol* 2000; 11:141–148.
24. Rock KL, Rothstein L, Benacerraf B. Analysis of the association of peptides of optimal length to class I molecules on the surface of cells. *Proc Natl Acad Sci USA* 1992; 89:8918–8922.
25. Brodsky FM, Lem L, Bresnahan PA. Antigen processing and presentation [see comments]. *Tissue Antigens* 1996; 47:464–471.
26. Lurquin C, Van PA, et al. Structure of the gene of tum- transplantation antigen P91A: the mutated exon encodes a peptide recognized with Ld by cytolytic T cells. *Cell* 1989; 58:293–303.
27. De Plaen E, Lurquin C, Van PA, et al. Immunogenic (tum-) variants of mouse tumor P815: cloning of the gene of tum- antigen P91A and identification of the tum- mutation. *Proc Natl Acad Sci USA* 1988; 85:2274–2278.
28. Davis MM, Chien Y. Topology and affinity of T-cell receptor mediated recognition of peptide-MHC complexes. *Curr Opin Immunol* 1993; 5:45–49.
29. Hanau D, Saudrais C, Haegel-Kronenberger H, Bohbot A, De La Salle H, Salamero J. Fate of MHC class II molecules in human dendritic cells. *Eur J Dermatol* 1999; 9:7–12.
30. Batalia MA, Collins EJ. Peptide binding by class I and class II MHC molecules. *Biopolymers* 1997; 43:281–302.

31. Wubbolts R, Neefjes J. Intracellular transport and peptide loading of MHC class II molecules: regulation by chaperones and motors. *Immunol Rev* 1999; 172:189–208.

32. Pareja E, Tobes R, Martin J, Nieto A. The tetramer model: a new view of class II MHC molecules in antigenic presentation to T cells. *Tissue Antigens* 1997; 50:421–428.

33. Solheim JC. Class I MHC molecules: assembly and antigen presentation. *Immunol Rev* 1999; 172:11–19.

34. Hanahan D, Weinberg RA. The hallmarks of cancer. *Cell* 2000; 100:57–70.

35. Peoples GE, Goedegebuure PS, Smith R, Linehan DC, Yoshino I, Eberlein TJ. Breast and ovarian cancer-specific cytotoxic T lymphocytes recognize the same HER2/neu-derived peptide. *Proc Natl Acad Sci USA* 1995; 92:432–436.

36. Ropke M, Hald J, Guldberg P, et al. Spontaneous human squamous cell carcinomas are killed by a human cytotoxic T lymphocyte clone recognizing a wild-type p53-derived peptide. *Proc Natl Acad Sci USA* 1996; 93:14704–14707.

37. Theobald M, Biggs J, Dittmer D, Levine AJ, Sherman LA. Targeting p53 as a general tumor antigen. *Proc Natl Acad Sci USA* 1995; 92:11993–11997.

38. Theobald M, Biggs J, Hernandez J, Lustgarten J, Labadie C, Sherman LA. Tolerance to p53 by A2.1-restricted cytotoxic T lymphocytes. *J Exp Med* 1997; 185:833–841.

39. Peace DJ, Chen W, Nelson H, Cheever MA. T cell recognition of transforming proteins encoded by mutated ras proto-oncogenes. *J Immunol* 1991; 146:2059–2065.

40. Yanuck M, Carbone DP, Pendleton DC, et al. A mutant p53 or ras tumor suppressor protein is a target for peptide-induced CD8+ cytotoxic T cells. *Cancer Res* 1993; 53:3257–3261.

41. Khleif SN, Abrams SI, Hamilton JM, et al. A phase I vaccine trial with peptides reflecting ras oncogene mutations of solid tumors. *J Immunother* 1999; 22:155–165.

42. Wolfel T, Hauer M, Schneider J, et al. A p16INK4a-insensitive CDK4 mutant targeted by cytolytic T lymphocytes in a human melanoma. *Science* 1995; 269:1281–1284.

43. Castelli C, Rivoltini L, Andreola G, Carrabba M, Renkvist N, Parmiani G. T-cell recognition of melanoma-associated antigens. *J Cell Physiol* 2000; 182:323–331.

44. Kawakami Y, Robbins PF, Rosenberg SA. Human melanoma antigens recognized by T lymphocytes. *Keio J Med* 1996; 45:100–108.

45. Worley BS, van den Broeke LT, Goletz TJ, et al. Antigenicity of fusion proteins from sarcoma-associated chromosomal translocations. *Cancer Res* 2001; 61:6868–6875.

46. Nevins JR. Cell cycle targets of the DNA tumor viruses. *Curr Opin Genet Dev* 1994; 4:130–134.

47. Levine AJ. The origins of the small DNA tumor viruses. *Adv Cancer Res* 1994; 65:141–168.

48. Arvin AM, Mallory S, Moffat JF. Development of recombinant varicella-zoster virus vaccines. *Contrib Microbiol* 1999; 3:193–200.

49. Liljeqvist S, Stahl S. Production of recombinant subunit vaccines: protein immunogens, live delivery systems and nucleic acid vaccines. *J Biotechnol* 1999; 73:1–33.

50. Restifo NP, Rosenberg SA. Developing recombinant and synthetic vaccines for the treatment of melanoma. *Curr Opin Oncol* 1999; 11:50–57.

51. Rolph MS, Ramshaw IA. Recombinatn viruses as vaccines and immunological tools [see comments]. *Curr Opin Immunol* 1997; 9:517–524.

52. Ciernik IF, Berzofsky JA, Carbone DP. Induction of cytotoxic Tlymphocytes and antitumor immunity with DNA vaccines expressing single T cell epitopes. *J Immunol* 1996; 156:2369–2375.

53. Romani N, Gruner S, Brand D, et al. Proliferating dendritic cell progenitors in human blood. *J Exp Med* 1994; 180:83–93.

54. Steinman RM. The dendritic cell system and its role in immunogenicity. *Annu Rev Immunol* 1991; 9:271–296.

55. Takahashi H, Nakagawa Y, Yokomuro K, et al. Induction of CD8+ CTL by immunization with syngeneic irradiated HIV-1 envelope derived peptide-pulsed dendritic cells. *Int Immunol* 1993; 5:849–857.

56. Celluzzi CM, Mayordomo JI, Storkus WJ, Lotze MT, Falo LD Jr. Peptide-pulsed dendritic cells induce antigen-specific CTL-mediated protective tumor immunity [see comments]. *J Exp Med* 1996; 183:283–287.

57. Mayordomo JI, Loftus DJ, Sakamoto H, et al. Therapy of murine tumors with p53 wild-type and mutant sequence peptide-based vaccines. *J Exp Med* 1996; 183:1357–1365.

58. Hsu FJ, Benike C, Fagnoni F, et al. Vaccination of patients with B-cell lymphoma using autologous antigen-pulsed dendritic cells. *Nat Med* 1996; 2:52–58.

59. Mitsudomi T, Steinberg SM, Nau MM, et al. P53 or Ras gene mutations in non-small lung cancer cell line and their correlation with the presence of ras mutations and clinical features. *Oncogene* 1992; 7:171–180.

60. Mitsudomi T, Steinberg SM, Oie HK, et al. Ras gene mutation in non small cell lung cancer are associated with shortened survival irrespective of treatment intent. *Cancer Res* 1991; 51:4999–5002.

61. Peace DJ, Smith JW, Chen W, et al. Lysis of ras oncogene-transformed cells by specific cytotoxic T lymphocytes elicited by primary in vitro immunization with mutated ras peptide. *J Exp Med* 1994; 179:473–479.

62. Peace DJ, Smith JW, Disis ML, Chen W, Cheever MA. Induction of T cells specific for the mutated segment of oncogenic P21ras protein by immunization in vivo with the oncogenic protein. *J Immunother* 1993; 14:110–114.

63. Abrams SI, Stanziale SF, Lunin SD, Zaremba S, Schlom J. Identification of overlapping epitopes in mutatnt ras oncogene peptides that activate CD4+ an CD8+ T cell responses. *Eur J Immunol* 1996; 26:435–443.

64. Abrams SI, Dobrazanski MJ, Kantor JA, et al. Induction of murine T lymphocyte responses to epitopes of point mutated ras P21. American Association Of Cancer Research, Annual Meeting, Orlando, Florida, 1993.

65. Abrams SI, Dobrazanski MJ, Kantor JA, et al. Activation of murine CD+ T lumphocyte responses to epitopes of point mutated ras p21. *Eur J Immunol* 1995; 25:2588–2597.

66. Fenton RG, Taub DD, Kwak LW, Smith MR, Longo DL. Cytotoxic T-cell response and in vivo protection against tumor cells harboring activated ras proto-oncogenes. *J Natl Cancer Inst* 1993; 85:1294–1302.

67. Skipper J, Stauss HJ. Identification of two cytotoxic T lymphocyte-recognized epotopes in the ras protein. *J Exp Med* 1993; 177:1493–1498.

68. Fossum B, Olsen AC, Thorsby E, Gaudernack G. CD8+ T cells from a patient with colon carcinoma, specific for a mutant p21 ras derived peptide (13Gly—Asp), are cytotoxic towards a carcinoma cell linerbouring the same mutation. *Cancer Immunol Immunother* 1995; 40:165–172.

69. Fossum B, Breivik J, Meling GI, et al. A K-ras 13 Gly→Asp mutation is recognized by HLA-DQ7 restricted T cell in a patient with colorectal cancer: Modifying effect of DQ7 restricted T cell in a patient with colorectal cancer: Modifying effect of DQ7 on established cancer harboring this mutation. *Int J Cancer* 1994; 58:506–511.

70. Fossum B, Gedde-Dahl T III, Breivik J, Eriksen JA, Spurkland A, Thorsby E, et al. p-21 ras-peptide-specific T-cell responses in a patient with colorectal cancer: CD4+ and CD8+ T cells recognize a peptide corresponding to a common mutation. *Int J Cancer* 1994; 56:40–45.

71. Gedde-Dahl TI, Spurkland A, Eriksen JA, Thorsby E, Gaudernack G. Memory T cells of a patient with follicular thyroid carcinoma recognize pepides derived from mutated p21 ras. *Int Immunol* 1992; 4:1331–1337.

72. Gedde-Dahl TI, Fossum B, Eriksen JA, Thorsby E, Guadernack G. T cell clones specific for p-21 ras-derived peptides: characterization of their fine specificity and HLA restriction. *Eur J Immunol* 1993; 23:754–760.

73. Gedde-Dahl T III, Spurkland A, Fossum B, Wittinghofer A, Thorsby E, Gaudernack G. T cell epitopes encompassing the mutational hot spot position 61 of p21 ras. Promiscuity in ras peptide binding to HLA. *Eur J Immunol* 1994; 24:410–414.

74. Smith MC, Pendleton CD, Maher VE, Kelley MJ, Carbone DP, Berzofsky JA. Oncogenic mutations in ras create HLA-A2.1 binding peptides but affect their extracellular antigen processing. *Int Immunol* 1997; 9:1085–1093.

75. Van Elsas A, Nijman HW, Van der Minne CE, et al. Induction and characterization of cytotoxic T-lymphocytes recognizing a mutated p21 Ras peptide presented by HLA-A-201. *Int J Cancer* 1995; 61:389–396.

76. Abrams SI, Khleif SN, Bergmann-Leitner ES, Kantor JA, Chung Y, Hamilton JM, et al. Generation of Stable CD4+ and CD8+ T cell lines from patints immunized with mutated Ras oncogene-derived peptides reflecting codon 12 mutations. *Cell Immunol* 1997; 182:137–151.

77. Wojtowicz M, Hamilton M, Benrnstein S, et al. Clinical Trial of Mutant Ras Peptide Vaccination Along with IL-2 or GM-CSF. *Proc Am Soc Clin Oncol* 2000:1818.

78. Gjertsen MK, Bjorheim J, Saeterdal I, Myklebust J, Gaudernack G. Cytotoxic CD4+ and CD8+ T lymphocytes, generated by mutant p21-ras (12Val) peptide vaccination of a patient, recognize 12Val-dependent nested epitopes present within the vaccine peptide and kill autologous tumour cells carrying this mutation. *Int J Cancer* 1997; 72:784–790.

79. Tsang KY, Nieroda CA, DeFilippi R, et al. Induction of human cytotoxic T cell lines directed against point-mutated p21 ras-derived synthetic peptides. *Vaccine Res* 1994; 3:183–193.

80. Gjertsen MK, Buanes T, Rosseland AR, et al. Intradermal ras peptide vaccination with granulocyte-macrophage colony- stimulating factor as adjuvant: clinical and immunological responses in patients with pancreatic adenocarcinoma. *Int J Cancer* 2001; 92:441–450.

81. Simon RM, Steinberg SM, Hamilton M, et al. Clinical trial designs for the early clinical development of therapeutic cancer vaccines. *J Clin Oncol* 2001; 19:1848–1854.

82. Levine AJ, Momand J, Finlay CA. The p53 tumour suppressor gene. *Nature* 1991; 351:453–456.

83. El-Deiry WS, Tokino T, Velculescu VE, et al. WAF1, a potential mediator of p53 tumor suppression. *Cell* 1993; 75:817–825.

84. Macleod KF, Sherry N, Hannon G, et al. p53-dependent and independent expression of p21 during cell growth, differentiation, and DNA damage. *Genes Dev* 1995; 9:935–944.

85. Michieli P, Chedid M, Lin D, Pierce JH, Mercer WE, Givol D. Induction of WAF1/CIP1 by a p53-independent pathway. *Cancer Res* 1994; 54:3391–3395.

86. Harris CC, Hollstein M. Clinical implications of the p53 tumor-suppressor gene. *N Engl J Med* 1993; 329:1318–1327.

87. Nigro JM, Baker SJ, Preisinger AC, et al. Mutations in the p53 gene occur in diverse human tumour types. *Nature* 1989; 342:705–708.

88. Fearon ER, Vogelstein B. A Genetic model for colorectal tumorigenesis. *Cell* 1990; 61:759–767.

89. Chiba I, Takahashi T, Nau MM, et al. Mutation in the p53 gene are frequent in primary resected non small lung cancer. *Oncogene* 1990:1603–1610.

90. Teneriello MG, Ebina M, Linnoila RI, et al. p53 and Ki-ras gene mutations in epithelial ovarian neoplasms. *Cancer Res* 1993; 53:3103–3108.

91. Greenblatt MS, Grollman AP, Harris CC. Deletions and insertions in the p53 tumor supressor gene in human cancers: Confirmation of the DNA polymerase slippage/misalignment model. *Cancer Res* 1996; 56:2130–2136.

92. Greenblatt MS, Bennett WP, Hollstein M, Harris CC. Mutations in the p53 tumor suppressor gene: clues to cancer etiology and molecular pathogenesis. *Cancer Res* 1994; 54:4855–4878.

93. Oren M, Maltzman W, Levine AJ. Post-translational regulation of the 54K cellular tumor antigen in normal and transformed cells. *Mol Cell Biol* 1981; 1:101–110.

94. Noguchi Y, Chen YT, Old LJ. A mouse mutant p53 product recognized by CD4+ and CD8+ T cells. *Proc Natl Acad Sci USA* 1994; 91:3171–3175.

95. Ciernik IF, Berzofsky J, Carbone DP. Mutant oncopeptide immunization induces CTL specifically lysing tumor cells endogenously expressing the corresponding intact mutant p53. *Hybridoma* 1995; 14:139–142.

96. Noguchi Y, Richards EC, Chen YT, Old LJ. Influence of interleukin 12 on p53 peptide vaccination against established Meth A sarcoma. *Proc Natl Acad Sci USA* 1995; 92:2219–2223.

97. Gabrilovich DI, Cunningham HT, Carbone DP. IL-12 and mutant P53 peptide-pulsed dendritic cells for the specific immunotherapy of cancer. *J Immunother Emphasis Tumor Immunol* 1996; 19:414–418.

98. Lacabanne V, Viguier M, Guillet JG, Choppin J. A wild-type p53 cytotoxic T cell epitope is presented by mouse hepatocarcinoma cells. *Eur J Immunol* 1996; 26:2635–2639.

99. Roth J, Dittmer D, Rea D, Tartaglia J, Paoletti E, Levine AJ. p53 as a target for cancer vaccines: recombinant canarypox virus vectors expressing p53 protect mice against lethal tumor cell challenge. *Proc Natl Acad Sci USA* 1996; 93:4781–4786.

100. Zeh H Jr, Leder GH, Lotze MT, et al. Flow-cytometric determination of peptide-class I complex formation. Identification of p53 peptides that bind to HLA-A2. *Hum Immunol* 1994; 39:79–86.

101. Stuber G, Leder GH, Storkus WT, et al. Identification of wild-type and mutant p53 peptides binding to HLA-A2 assessed by a peptide loading-deficient cell line assay and a novel major histocompatibility complex class I peptide binding assay. *Eur J Immunol* 1994; 24:765–768.

102. Houbiers JG, Nijman HW, van der Burg SH, et al. In vitro induction of human cytotoxic T lymphocyte responses against peptides of mutant and wild-type p53. *Eur J Immunol* 1993; 23:2072–2077.

103. Nijman HW, Houbiers JG, van der Burg SH, et al. Characterization of cytotoxic T lymphocyte epitopes of a self-protein, p53, and a non-self-protein, influenza matrix: relationship between major histocompatibility complex peptide binding affinity and immune responsiveness to peptides. *J Immunother* 1993; 14:121–126.

104. Gnjatic S, Bressac-de Paillerets B, Guillet JG, Choppin J. Mapping and ranking of potential cytotoxic T epitopes in the p53 protein: effect of mutations and polymorphism on peptide binding to purified and refolded HLA molecules. *Eur J Immunol* 1995; 25:1638–1642.

105. Gnjatic S, Cai Z, Viguier M, Chouaib S, Guillet JG, Choppin J. Accumulation of the p53 protein allows recognition by human CTL of a wild-type p53 epitope presented by breast carcinomas and melanomas. *J Immunol* 1998; 160:328–333.

106. McCarty TM, Liu X, Sun JY, Peralta EA, Diamond DJ, Ellenhorn JD. Targeting p53 for adoptive T-cell immunotherapy. *Cancer Res* 1998; 58:2601–2605.

107. Daley GQ, Van Etten RA, Baltimore D. Induction of chronic myelogenous leukemia in mice by the P210bcr/abl gene of the Philadelphia chromosome. *Science* 1990; 247:824–830.

108. Kloetzer W, Kurzrock R, Smith L, et al. The human cellular abl gene product in the chronic myelogenous leukemia cell line K562 has an associated tyrosine protein kinase activity. *Virology* 1985; 140:230–238.

109. Kurzrock R, Gutterman JU, Talpaz M. The molecular genetics of Philadelphia chromosome-positive leukemias. *N Engl J Med* 1988; 319:990–998.

110. Chen W, Peace DJ, Rovira DK, You SG, Cheever MA. T-cell immunity to the joining region of p210BCR-ABL protein. *Proc Natl Acad Sci USA* 1992; 89:1468–1472.

111. Chen W, Qin H, Reese VA, Cheever MA. CTLs specific for bcr-abl joining region segment peptides fail to lyse leukemia cells expressing p210 bcr-abl protein. *J Immunother* 1998; 21:257–268.

112. Bosch GJ, Joosten AM, Kessler JH, Melief CJ, Leeksma OC. Recognition of BCR-ABL positive leukemic blasts by human CD4+ T cells elicited by primary in vitro immunization with a BCR-ABL breakpoint peptide. *Blood* 1996; 88:3522–3527.

113. ten Bosch GJ, Kessler JH, Joosten AM, et al. A BCR-ABL oncoprotein p210b2a2 fusion region sequence is recognized by HLA-DR2a restricted cytotoxic T lymphocytes and presented by HLA-DR matched cells transfected with an Ii(b2a2) construct. *Blood* 1999; 94:1038–1045.

114. Greco G, Fruci D, Accapezzato D, et al. Two brc-abl junction peptides bind HLA-A3 molecules and allow specific induction of human cytotoxic T lymphocytes. *Leukemia* 1996; 10:693–699.

115. Bocchia M, Wentworth PA, Southwood S, et al. Specific binding of leukemia oncogene fusion protein peptides to HLA class I molecules. *Blood* 1995; 85:2680–2684.

116. Bocchia M, Korontsvit T, Xu Q, et al. Specific human cellular immunity to bcr-abl oncogene-derived peptides. *Blood* 1996; 87:3587–3592.

117. Pinilla-Ibarz J, Cathcart K, Korontsvit T, et al. Vaccination of patients with chronic myelogenous leukemia with bcr-abl oncogene breakpoint fusion peptides generates specific immune responses. *Blood* 2000; 95:1781–1787.

118. Goletz TJ, Zhan S, Pendleton CD, Helman LJ, Berzofsky J. Cytotoxic T Cell responses against the EWS/FLI-1 Ewing sarcoma fusion protein and the PAX/FKHR alveolar rhabdomyosarcoma fusion protein. *Proc Am Assoc Cancer Res* 1996:3243.

119. Berchuck A, Kamel A, Whitaker R, et al. Overexpression of HER-2/neu is associated with poor survival in advanced epithelial ovarian cancer. *Cancer Res* 1990; 50:4087–4091.

120. Maguire HC Jr, Greene MI. The neu (c-erbB-2) oncogene. *Semin Oncol* 1989; 16:148–155.

121. Looi LM, Cheah PL. C-erbB-2 oncoprotein amplification in infiltrating ductal carcinoma of breast relates to high histological grade and loss of oestrogen receptor protein. *Malays J Pathol* 1998; 20:19–23.

122. Disis ML, Knutson KL, Schiffman K, Rinn K, McNeel DG. Pre-existent immunity to the HER-2/neu oncogenic protein in patients with HER-2/neu overexpressing breast and ovarian cancer. *Breast Cancer Res Treat* 2000; 62:245–252.

123. Lachman LB, Rao XM, Kremer RH, Ozpolat B, Kiriakova G, Price JE. DNA vaccination against neu reduces breast cancer incidence and metastasis in mice. *Cancer Gene Ther* 2001; 8:259–268.

124. Chen Y, Emtage P, Zhu Q, et al. Induction of ErbB-2/neu-specific protective and therapeutic antitumor immunity using genetically modified dendritic cells: enhanced efficacy by cotransduction of gene encoding IL-12. *Gene Ther* 2001; 8:316–323.

125. Foy TM, Bannink J, Sutherland RA, et al. Vaccination with Her-2/neu DNA or protein subunits protects against growth of a Her-2/neu-expressing murine tumor. *Vaccine* 2001; 19:2598–2606.

126. Wei WZ, Shi WP, Galy A, et al. Protection against mammary tumor growth by vaccination with full-length, modified human ErbB-2 DNA. *Int J Cancer* 1999; 81:748–754.

127. Dakappagari NK, Douglas DB, Triozzi PL, Stevens VC, Kaumaya PT. Prevention of mammary tumors with a chimeric HER-2 B-cell epitope peptide vaccine. *Cancer Res* 2000; 60:3782–3789.

128. Disis ML, Smith JW, Murphy AE, Chen W, Cheever MA. In vitro generation of human cytolytic T-cell specific for peptides derived from the HER-2/neu protooncogene protein. *Cancer Res* 1994; 54:1071–1076.

129. Fisk B, Blevins TL, Wharton JT, et al. Identification of an immunodominent peptide of HER-2 neu protooncogene recognized by ovarian tumor-specific cytotoxic T lymphocytes lines. *J Exp Med* 1995; 181:2109–2117.

130. Ikuta Y, Okugawa T, Furugen R, et al. A HER2/NEU-derived peptide, a K(d)-restricted murine tumor rejection antigen, induces HER2-specific HLA-A2402-restricted CD8(+) cytotoxic T lymphocytes. *Int J Cancer* 2000; 87:553–558.

131. Peiper M, Goedegebuure PS, Izbicki JR, Eberlein TJ. Pancreatic cancer associated ascites-derived CTL recognize a nine-amino- acid peptide GP2 derived from HER2/neu. *Anticancer Res* 1999; 19:2471–2475.

132. Zaks TZ, Rosenberg SA. Immunization with a peptide epitope (p369–377) from HER-2/neu leads to peptide-specific cytotoxic T lymphocytes that fail to recognize HER- 2/neu+ tumors. *Cancer Res* 1998; 58:4902–4908.

133. Tuttle TM, Anderson BW, Thompson WE, et al. Proliferative and cytokine responses to class II HER-2/neu-associated peptides in breast cancer patients. *Clin Cancer Res* 1998; 4:2015–2024.

134. Kono K, Rongcun Y, Charo J, et al. Identification of HER2/neu-derived peptide epitopes recognized by gastric cancer-specific cytotoxic T lymphocytes. *Int J Cancer* 1998; 78:202–208.

135. Disis ML, Grabstein KH, Sleath PR, Cheever MA. Generation of immunity to the HER-2/neu oncogenic protein in patients with breast and ovarian cancer using a peptide-based vaccine. *Clin Cancer Res* 1999; 5:1289–1297.

136. Knutson KL, Schiffman K, Disis ML. Immunization with a HER-2/neu helper peptide vaccine generates HER- 2/neu CD8 T-cell immunity in cancer patients. *J Clin Invest* 2001; 107:477–484.

137. Scheffner M, Werness BA, Huibregtse JM, Levine AJ, Howley PM. The E6 oncoprotein encoded by human papillomavirus types 16 and 18 promotes the degradation of p53. *Cell* 1990; 63:1129–1136.

138. Dyson N, Howley PM, Munger K, Harlow E. The human papilloma virus-16 E7 oncoprotein is able to bind to the retinoblastoma gene product. *Science* 1989; 243:934–937.

139. Nindl I, Rindfleisch K, Lotz B, Schneider A, Durst M. Uniform distribution of HPV 16 E6 and E7 variants in patients with normal histology, cervical intra-epithelial neoplasia and cervical cancer. *Int J Cancer* 1999; 82:203–207.

140. Kadish AS, Ho GY, Burk RD, et al. Lymphoproliferative responses to human papillomavirus (HPV) type 16 proteins E6 and E7: outcome of HPV infection and associated neoplasia. *J Natl Cancer Inst* 1997; 89:1285–1293.

141. Chen L, Thomas EK, Hu SL, et al. Human papillomavirus type 16 nucleoprotein E7 is a tumor rejection antigen. *Proc Natl Acad Sci USA* 1991; 88:110–114.

142. Tsukui T, Hildesheim A, Schiffman MH, et al. Interleukin 2 production in vitro by peripheral lymphocytes in response to human papillomavirus-derived peptides: correlation with cervical pathology. *Cancer Res* 1996; 56:3967–3974.

143. Feltkamp MG, Smits HL, Vierboom MP, et al. Vaccination with cytotoxic T lymphocyte epitope containing peptide protects against a tumor induced by human papillomavirus type 16-transformed cells. *Eur J Immunol* 1993; 23:2242–2249.

144. Evans EM, Man S, Evans AS, Borysiewicz LK. Infiltration of cervical cancer tissue with human papillomavirus-specific cytotoxic T-lymphocytes. *Cancer Res* 1997; 57:2943–2950.

145. Kast WM, Brant RM, Drijfhout JW, et al. Human Leukocyte antigen-A2.1 restricted candidate cytotoxic T lymphocyte epitopes of human papillomaviris the 16 E6 and E7 proteins identified by using the processing-defective human cell line T2. *Immunotherapy* 1993; 14:115–120.

146. Kast WM, Brandt RM, Sidney J, et al. Role of HLA-A motifs in identification of potential CTL epitopes in human papillomavirus type 16 E6 and E7 proteins. *J Immunol* 1994; 152:3904–3912.

147. Ressing ME, Sette A, Brandt RM, et al. Human CTL epitopes encoded by human papillomavirus type 16 E6 and E7 identified through in vivo and in vitro immunogenicity studies of HLA- A*0201-binding peptides. *J Immunol* 1995; 154:5934–5943.

148. Chen L, Mizuno MT, Singhal MC, et al. Induction of cytotoxic T lymphocytes specific for syngeneic tumor expressing the E6 protein of human papillomavirus type 16. *J Immunol* 1992; 148:2617–2621.

149. Alexander M, Salgaller ML, Celis E, et al. Generation of tumor-specific cytolytic T lymphocytes from peripheral blood of cervical cancer patients by in vitro stimulation with a synthetic human papillomavirus type 16 E7 epitope. *Am J Obstet Gynecol* 1996; 175:1586–1593.

150. Wojtowicz M, Hamilton JM, Khong H, et al. Vaccination of cervical cancer patients with papilloma virus type 16 E6 and E7 Peptides. American Society of Clinical Oncology, Atlanta, GA, 1999.

151. Muderspach L, Wilczynski S, Roman L, et al. A phase I trial of a human papillomavirus (HPV) peptide vaccine for women with high-grade cervical and vulvar intraepithelial neoplasia who are HPV 16 positive [in process citation]. *Clin Cancer Res* 2000; 6:3406–3416.

152. Kadish AS, Ho G, Wang Y, et al. Antigen-specific cell mediated immunity in phase I dose-escalation trial of single doses of Hspe7 in healthy volunteers. Thirty-Sixth Annual Meeting of the American Society for Clinical Oncology, New Orleans, LA, 2000. Vol. 19.

153. Palefsky JM, Goldstone LS, Boux LJ, Neefe JR. Pathological response to treatment with HspE7 in anal dysplasia of multiple HPV types. Cancer Vaccine 2000, New York, NY, 2000.

22

Bcl-2 Antisense Oligonucleotides Therapy for Cancer

Targeting the Mitochondria

Finbarr E. Cotter, PhD, FRCP, FRCPATH, and Dean A. Fennell, MD

CONTENTS

1. INTRODUCTION

1.1. Bcl-2 as a Target for Emerging Cancer Therapeutics

Programmed cell death, also termed apoptosis, is the final biochemical pathway underlying the therapeutic efficacy of several cytotoxic therapies for cancer, both in vitro *(1,2)* and in vivo *(3–7)*. Susceptibility to apoptosis is associated with curability *(8,9)*, whereas resistance to apoptotic stimuli significantly reduces efficacy. Neoplastic cells aquire their growth advantage through somatic evolution arising from genome instability *(10)*, a process that results in the expression of anti-death proteins, including those of the Bcl-2 family such as Bcl-2, Bcl-X_1, Mcl-1, Bcl-W, and Survivin *(11–16)*.

The best known death antagonist gene, Bcl-2, was discovered by Yoshidide Tsjuimoto et al. in 1985, following DNA sequence analysis of the chromosomal breakpoint involved in the t(14;18)(q32;21) translocation that occurs in the great majority of follicular non-Hodgkins lymphomas (NHL) *(17)*. Bcl-2 provided researchers with the first example of a human proto-oncogene that contributes to the expansion of neoplastic cells by preventing cell death, rather than accelerating proliferation *(18)*. A diverse

From: *Oncogene-Directed Therapies*
Edited by: J. W. Rak © Humana Press Inc., Totowa, NJ

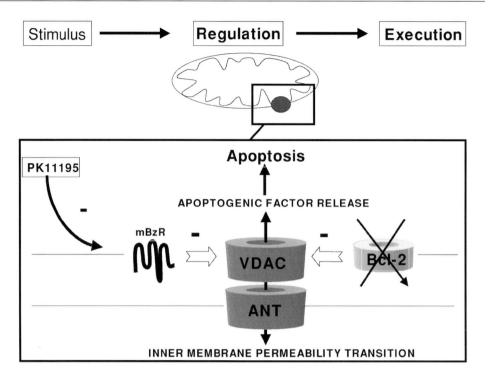

Fig. 1. A schematic representation of the mitochondrial permeability transition pore (MPTP) within the mitochondrial membrane. The VEDAC and ANT portions are within the outer and inner membrane respectively. The Bcl-2 protein and the mitochondrial benzoziazepine receptor (MBZR) keep the MPTP in the closed position. Down regulation of the Bcl-2 protein by antisense oligonucleotides and MBZR ligands such as PK11195 lead to "opening" of the MPTP, release of Cytochrome C into the cytosol and subsequent induction of apoptosis via the Caspase 9 (intrinsic) pathway.

number of malignancies have been shown to exhibit high levels of Bcl-2 expression including melanoma, prostate, and cholangiocarcinoma (Fig. 1), making this protein an attractive candidate for pharmacological inhibition.

1.2. Bcl-2 Blocks Apoptosis by Stabilizing Mitochondrial Membrances

In 1990, Chen-Levy and Cleary, as well as Stanley Korsmeyer's group independently identified Bcl-2 as a 24 to 25-kDa membrane-bound protein localized to mitochondria, implicating an involvement in the regulation of oxidative phosphorylation, electron transport, or metabolite transport. Bcl-2 was the first oncogene discovered to be associated with this organelle *(13,19)*, residing on the cytoplasmic face of the outer mitochondrial membrane and less abundantly at the endoplasmic reticulum and outer nuclear envelope *(11)*.

The first evidence that Bcl-2 function involves modulation of apoptosis, was presented by two groups in 1991 (Korsmeyer and Cory and coworkers) who showed independently that Bcl-2 could protect from multiple forms of apoptotic stimuli in T cells of transgenic mice *(20,21)*. In the thymus, the site of T cell development, Bcl-2 expression is normally localized to the mature thymocytes (which express either the accessory molecule CD8 or CD4) in the medulla. In the transgenic mice, Bcl-2 was redirected to CD4 and CD8 positive cortical immature thymocytes, which are usually susceptible to a high death rate required for self-reactive deletion during immune system ontogeny. Bcl-2 protected the CD4$^+$CD8$^+$ thymocytes from glucocorticoids, radiation, anti-CD3, and γ irradiation-induced apoptosis (20,21). However, Bcl-2 was not able to prevent clonal deletion of T cells recognizing endogenous superantigens.

The ability of Bcl-2 to inhibit γ irradiation-induced apoptosis stimulated investigations by Hockenbery et al. in 1993 based on the then understood mechanism of action of hydroxyl radical production by ionizing radiation (22). It was postulated that because γ irradiation produces reactive oxygen species capable of damaging macromolecules including DNA, proteins, and lipid membranes, and this could be blocked by Bcl-2, that Bcl-2 may in some way be acting as an antioxidant. In their seminal study of Bcl-2 function, Hockenbery et al. demonstrated the ability of Bcl-2 to completely protect against oxidative stress induced by low concentrations (0.25–0.5mM) of hydrogen peroxide. In the same year, Bredesden's group showed that Bcl-2 could block the cytotoxic effects of organic hydroperoxide tert-butylhydroperoxide (23). Importantly, the antioxidant effect of Bcl-2 was shown not to prevent the formation of dangerous production of peroxides during cell treatment with hydrogen peroxide (detected using the oxidation sensitive fluoresence probe 5,6 carboxy-2', 7'-dichlorofluorecein-diacetate), but rather, to block their damaging effects including lipid peroxidation.

Significant advances in the understanding of the mode of biochemical mode of action have been achieved, although the precise mechanism of death suppression remains to be elucidated. Thus, Bcl-2 localizes in the outer mitochondrial membrane to regions of contact between the outer and the inner mitochondrial membrances that are spanned by a multimeric protein complex known as the mitochondiral megachannel, or permeability transition pore complex (PTPC) (Fig. 2). This structure comprises outer membrane porin (voltage dependent anion channel [VDAC]), peripheral benzodiazepine receptor (PBR), while the inner membrane part comprises the adenine nucleotide translocator (ANT), and cyclophilin D. Opening of the PTPC is involved in two critical events associated with apoptosis. Increased outer membrane permeability results in the nonspecific diffusion of intermembrance space pro-apoptotic proteins into the cytoplasm (including cytochrome C and apoptosis-inducing factor), which triggers apoptosis through ATP-dependent activation of death effector serine proteases termed caspases via the formation of a trimeric activation complex with procaspase 9, APAF 1, and cytochrome C. This is often referred to as the mitochondrial caspase 9 pathway.

Increased inner mitochondrial membrane permeability, mediated by opening of the PTPC (high conductance state termed permeability transition), dissipates the proton gradient ($\Delta\Psi_m$) utilized by complex V to generate ATP and serves to uncouple oxidative phosphorylation and increase reactive oxygen species production (24,25). Bcl-2 prevents increases in both outer and inner membrane permeabilization during apoptosis (26,27), a process that is induced by death agonists homologues such as Bax (28–32). Anti-apoptosis activity of Bcl-2 is mediated through direct physical contact with VDAC, via the BH4 domain, and can inhibit cytochrome C release via this conduit (33,34). Bcl-2 is predicted to form a functional cation channel, on the basis of homology with Bcl-X$_L$ structure, determined by X-ray, and also functional single channel conductance studies. Tsujimoto has suggested that Bcl-2 inhibits apoptosis by mediat-

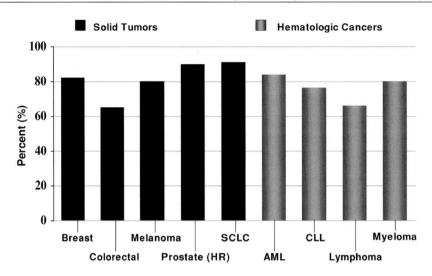

Fig. 2. Percentage of various malignancies presenting with raised Bcl-2 protein levels.

ing proton leak across the outer mitochondrial membrane proton-specific channel that serves to stabilize $\Delta\Psi_m$ *(35)*.

1.3. Bcl-2 Family Tunes Cellular Apoptosis Threshold

The functional antagonism between Bcl-2 and the pro-apoptotic agonists, such as Bax, occurs following their mobilisaton from the cytosol to mitochondrial contact sites during apoptosis *(36,37)*. This has been likened to a cellular rheostat (apopstat); the stoichiometric balance of death agonist to antagonist determining cellular apoptotic threshold *(38)*. Overexpression of either death agonist or antagonist is sufficient to substantially modify cellular apoptosis threshold *(20,21,38–40)*. Conversely, suppression of the expression of an up-regulated death antagonist could potentially impart apoptosis sensitization by altering the cellular apostat.

2. INHIBITION OF POLYPEPTIDE SYNTHESIS AS A STRATEGY FOR MODULATING Bcl-2 ACTIVITY

In 1977, Paterson and colleagues provided the first evidence that formation of an antisense DNA-mRNA heteroduplex could effectively arrest translation in a cell-free system *(41)*. In the following year, Stephenson and Zamecnik reported the first study detailing the inhibition of Rous sarcoma viral replication using a tri-decamer synthetic ASO, d(A-A-T-G-G-T-A-A-A-A-T-G-G), complementary to the reiterated 3′ and 5′ terminal sequences of the virally encoded 35S RNA in infected chick embryo fibroblast cultures *(42,43)*. Evidence for the existence of natural reverse complementary nucleic acids as regulators of prokaryotic gene expression was obtained by Simons and Kleckner in 1983 and by Mizuno et al. in 1984 *(44,45)*. This was later to be reinforced in eukaryotic cells by Izant and Weintraub in 1984 who demonstrated the ability of antisense RNA to regulate gene expression *(46)*. These studies collectively initiated the field of antisense oligonucleotide (ASO) technology, which grew explosively during the last decade.

ASOs exploit Watson-Crick DNA-RNA interactions to selectively bind mRNA, on the basis of sequence. The backbone of these ASOs are usually chemically modified to protect them from nuclease enzyme breakdown. The first generation of modification was to replace the oxygen molecule (phosphodiesters) with a sulfur molecule (phosphorothioates), and it is these that have largely been moved to the clinic. Through selective hybridization and formation of a heteroduplex, gene expression is disrupted at the level of translation. From thermodynamics, Khan and Coulson estimated that at 37°C and physiological ionic strength, a minimum size of 12 bases was required for a phosphodiester oligoucleotide to form a stable heteroduplex with its target. Statistical considerations dictate that a minimum ASO length of between 12 and 15 bases is required to recognize a gene, since there are approximately 3 to 4 billion bp in the human genome with the expectation of any one 17-base sequence occurring only once *(47)*. In a typical interaction between complementary 18-mers, the Gibbs free energy of binding induced by a single mismatch varies from +0.2 to +4.0 kcal/mol/modification at 100 mM NaCl; this implies that a single base mismatch could result in a change in affinity of approximately 500-fold.

2.1. Role of mRNA Structure in ASO Binding

Fresco first showed in 1960 that single-stranded RNA folds back onto itself in structures stabilized by hydrogen bonds between complementary bases *(48)*. The conformational constraints arising from RNA–RNA duplex formation within large RNAs result in the formation of complex 3-dimensional structures. There exist very few well-established tertiary RNA structures. With the development of fast computing technology, it has been possible to design RNA folding algorithms that can predict secondary structures with minimum free energy *(49)*. However, such algorithms are of no use in predicting the conformation adopted by secondary folded RNAs. Tertiary structural prediction has classically relied upon X-ray crystallography. It is the RNA tertiary structure that imposes restrictions on the accessibility of binding sequences for ASOs.

Theoretical binding affinities for single-stranded nucleic acid interactions predicted between DNA and RNA using nearest neighbor rules are very large, yet are measured as several orders of magnitude lower in practice *(50)*. Accessibility of some ASO sequences to their cognate binding sites underlies this discrepancy. Not all sequences bind their RNA due to restrictions of tertiary structure. The design of ASOs, based solely on predicted melting temperature from primary sequence, is essentially an inefficient method with an estimated <25% successes rate *(51)*. Empirical methods have been designed to enable the rapid determination of accessible sites, including degenerate reverse transcription polymerase chain reaction (RT-PCR) with primer extension analysis *(52,53)*, oligonucleotide arrays *(54,55)*, or by using a brute force approach involving synthesis of nonoverlapping ASOs (chromosome walking), and determining mRNA down-regulation in cells *(56)*.

2.2. Degrading the Message: Phosphorothioate ASOs Utilize Nucleases

Several post-hybridization processes are implicated in ASO-mediated translational inhibition and can be classified as either passive (occupancy-mediated disruption of physiological RNA processing) or active (ASO-mediated degradation of target

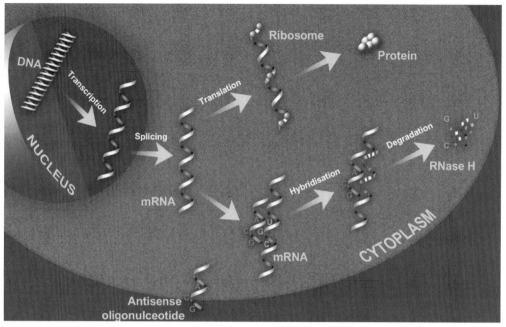

Fig. 3. Schematic representation of the mode of action of antisense oligonucleotides.

mRNA). ASO hybridization with the initiation codon has been an extensively used approach to sterically block the protein and ribosomal interaction necessary for translation. Owing to the conformational heterogeneity in this region between different mRNAs, only a few sequences have been shown to bind to sites to which they were designed. The role of steric translation arrest in ASO action was examined in a cell-free system by Gee et al. *(57)*. A series of high affinity ASOs were designed to target and sterically hinder the ribosomal translation initiation complex associated with translation of the N protein of vesicular stomatitis virus. Only ASOs binding irreversibly to their target (via covalent modification using platinated peptide nucleic acid derivatives) or inducing ribonuclease H (RNaseH)-mediated mRNA degradation were shown to inhibit translation; reversible hydribridization *per se* was not shown to be sufficient in this cell-free system.

RNaseH is a ubiquitous enzyme, which degrades the RNA strand of an RNA–DNA heteroduplex. A considerable amount of evidence supports a role for this protein in mediating the effects of ASOs, including the direct demonstration of RNaseH-mediated target mRNA cleavage by ASOs *(58,59)* (Fig. 3). Several isoenzymes have been identified in eukaryotic cells, and the highest concentrations are localized to the nucleus. Two human RNaseH enzymes have been cloned that exhibit homology to the *Escherichia coli* RNase H1 and H2 proteins *(60,61)*. RNaseH can recognize tetramers *(62)* and a single ribonucleotide in a deoxyribonucleotide sequence hybridizing with its complementary strand *(63)*, but does not recognize oligonucleotides with 2′ sugar modifications (such as 2′-fluoro or 2′-O-methyl) *(64,65)*. Backbone modifications such as phosphorothioates (PS) are good substrates for RNaseH *(66,67)*, whereas methylphosphonates are not *(68)*.

Although phosphorothioate ASO-RNA heteroduplexes are effective RNaseH substrates, the phosphorothioate modification forms relatively less stable duplexes compared with phosphodiester (PO) ASOs. However, 2′ sugar modifications, such as 2′-0-methyl, exhibit a high binding affinity and have been exploited in chimeric molecules possessing a combination of RNaseH activating PS and 2′ sugar modifications to increase binding affinity *(69,70)*.

2.3. ASOs are Large Molecules

PS ASOs retain the negatively charged backbone of unmodified DNA. Cellular uptake precedes initially via an electrostatic interaction with cell surface proteins. This is followed by endocytosis leading to a punctate distribution of ASO in endosomes and lysosomes, where sequestration limits interaction with target mRNA. Direct intracytoplasmic delivery of oligonucleotide by microinjection, results in immediate nuclear trafficking, effectively bypassing the endosomal compartment *(71–73)*. The elimination of the phosphate backbone and associated negative charge in methylphosphonates has been shown to enhance cellular uptake by increasing hydrophobicity *(74)*, but this is associated with a reduction in aqueous solubility and removes RNase H sensitivity. Electrostatic neutralization of the net negative charge associated with PS ASOs can be achieved by complexation with a positively charged hydrophobic lipid such as N-(1-2,3-dioleyoxy)propyl-n,n,n-trimethylammonium (DOTMA), to form a high molecular weight lipoplex. Cationic lipid–ASO preparations were shown by Bennett and coworkers in the early 1990s to be associated with enhanced uptake of ASO, and a consequent enhancement of antisense potency in down-regulating ICAM-1 protein expression *(75)*. Dissociation of the lipoplex occurs prior to entry of the ASO into the nucleus and was first demonstrated by Marcusson et al., who used both fluorescently labeled cationic lipid and ASO to monitor intracellular trafficking *(76)*. These investigators confirmed uptake of lipoplex into endosomal compartment, which counterstained with the endocytic marker TMA-DPH. Fluorescent ASO dissociated from the endosomal lipoplex after 1 h, staining the nucleus and reaching a peak at 4 h (coinciding with maximal protein kinase c-α mRNA reduction). However, fluorescently labeled cationic lipid remained within the endosomal compartment and did not distribute to the nucleus. Bennett and collegues have demonstrated that ASOs undergo nucleocytoplasmic shuttling that is both ATP and temperature sensitive in vivo *(77)*.

Several enhancers of ASO intracellular entry have been developed that enable effective concentrations of oligonucleotide to be in the nanomolar range, and include liposomes *(78)*, streptolysin-O *(79–82)*, dendrimers *(83)*, polycations *(84)*, conjugation with a hydrophobic moiety such as cholesterol *(85)*, peptides *(86)*, aggregation with ligands for cell surface receptors *(87)*, electroporation *(88)*, and cationic porphyrins *(89)*.

2.4. ASO Uptake In Vivo

Few studies have rigorously examined the cellular and subcellular fate of ASOs in vivo, despite numerous reports of in vivo efficacy in the absence of cationic lipid, implying a difference between the trafficking of oligonucleotides in tissue culture vs in vivo. Graham et al. investigated the nuclear, cytosolic, and membrane distribution of a PS ASO in rat liver cells, following administration as an intravenous bolus at a doses of 10 mg/kg and greater *(90)*. Differential uptake of ASO was observed with 80% of total dose to the organ in parenchymal (Kuppfer and endothelial) cells, compared with only 20% in hepatocytes. Although the nonparenchymal cells exhibited nuclear, cytosolic, and membrane levels of ASO, this was not observed in hepatocytes below 25 mg/kg. Following doses higher than 25 mg/kg, nonparenchymal cells exhibited saturation of uptake, while the hepatocytes continued to accumulate ASO at significant levels in the nucleus and other compartments (90). The saturability of binding of ASO in endothelial cells was shown to be associated with polyinosinic acid inhibitable and polyadenylic resistant binding to plasma membrane scavenger receptors SR-AI/II (91). However, in scavenger receptor knock-out mice, ASO was still shown to be taken up by tissues, implicating non-SRAI/II mechanisms (92).

3. ASOs CAN SUPPRESS Bcl-2 EXPRESSION IN VITRO AND IN VIVO

In 1990, Reed and coworkers demonstrated that ASOs, designed to target the mRNA of Bcl-2, could specifically suppress the proliferation of lymphoma and leukemia cells in culture compared with scrambled control oligonucleotides (93). PO and PS and ASOs designed to hybridize with the initiation site of Bcl-2 transcripts (5'-CAG CGT GCT GCG CCA TCC TCC CC-3') were tested with 697 leukemic cell cultures in serum free medium, which was used in the experiments to minimize nuclease activity. Concentration-dependent inhibition of proliferation was shown for the ASO by 24–48 h, which was not seen with either scrambled (containing the same base composition) or the sense controls. PS ASOs exhibited 5- to 10-fold potency compared with PO ASOs. No effects were observed within the first 24–48 h, and the concentration required to achieve marked suppression of cell growth with PS ASOs was approximately 25 μM. These effects were associated with a concentration-dependent reduction in Bcl-2 protein (measured by quantitative immunofluorescence assay) without alteration in human lymphocyte antigen diabetic retinopathy (HLA-DR) control levels, suggesting a specific ASO targeting of Bcl-2; 70% reduction in Bcl-2 was observed by 4 d of culture with a 25 μM concentration of PS ASO.

Kitada et al. demonstrated that enhanced chemosensitivity was associated with antisense down-regulation of Bcl-2 (94). PS and PO Bcl-2 ASOs were delivered to SUDHL4 lymphoma cells expressing Bcl-2 at a high level due to t(14;18)(q21;q32), complexed with cationic lipid (lipofectin) a 1:1 mixture of DOTMA, and dieleoylphosphatidylethanolamine (DOPE). A single treatment of cells with 75–300 nM ASO produced a sequence-specific reduction in the expression of bcl-2 within 24 h, as measured using a semiquantitative RT-PCR assay. Reduction in Bcl-2 expression varied from 66% to as little as 10%, compared to cells treated with control oligonucleotides, and required 72 h as a consequence of the long protein half-life (10–12 h). Although the ASO exhibited negligible cytotoxicity by itself, it enhanced ara-c-, methotrexate-, and dexamethasone-induced cytotoxicity after administration after 2 d of treatment with Bcl-2 ASO.

Further evidence for a sequence-specific effect of Bcl-2 ASO was elegantly demonstrated by Kitada et al., who stably transfected the interleukin 3-dependent cell line 32D.C13 with either Bcl-2 or the viral Bcl-2 homologue BHRF-1, which possesses only 22% homology, but can support survival of the 32D.C13 cell line in the absence of interleukin 3. Bcl-2 ASO, in combination with cytotoxic therapy, produced no significant difference in the 32D-BHRF-1 cells, but significantly enhanced sensitivity in the 32D-Bcl-2 cells. Similar results were obtained by using an antisense Bcl-2 plasmid construct in the t(14;18)(q21;32) lymphoma cell line RS11846, which was chemosensitized in the presence of ara-c following induction of Bcl-2 antisense via the metallothionein promoter. Corroborating evidence for the chemosensitizing potency of ASO-mediated Bcl-2 down-regulation was provided by Campos et al., in CD34 positive acute myeloid leukemia *(95)*. Several in vitro studies have since demonstrated chemosensitizing efficacy associated with Bcl-2 down-regulation in a variety of cell types.

3.1. Experimental Bcl-2 Suppression In Vivo

The ability of Bcl-2 down-regulation to prevent the in vivo formation of t(14;18) human lymphoma xenografts in severe combined immunodeficient (SCID) mice was first reported in 1994 *(96)*. DOHH2 lymphoma cells containing the t(14;18) translocation were treated ex vivo with a 10 μM concentration twice at 48-h intervals, resulting in a reduced Bcl-2 expression as detected qualitatively by immunohistochemistry and quantitatively by flow cytometry. Associated loss of viability (cytotoxicity) post-treatment was observed in DOHH2 cells, but not in NFB1 normal fibroblast cells lacking Bcl-2 expression. The effect of Bcl-2 down-regulation on tumorigenicity was evaluated in SCID mice by generation of xenografts using DOHH2 cells that had been treated in vitro with ASO to prevent engraftment as detected by peripheral blood PCR to t(14;18) (across the IgH promoter/Bcl-2 junction). In contrast, control oligonucleotide pretreated DOHH2 cells went on to produce tumors by 28 d.

The first direct evidence for in vivo chemosensitizing efficacy of Bcl-2 ASO was reported by Jansen et al. *(97)*, who showed that a combination of the ASO G3139 (5′-TCT CCC AGC GTG CGC AT -3′) infused at 5 mg/kg for 14 d in the absence of cationic lipid and dacarbazine (5 d at 80 mg/kg/d injected intraperitoneally) resulted in the eradication of 518A2 melanoma xenografts in SCID mice. Several similar studies have reported similar findings in different model systems *(98–100)*. ASO G3139 has been shown to bind to an accessible region in the Bcl-2 mRNA transcript in its native conformation using an oligonucleotide array (unpublished observation).

4. CLINICAL Bcl-2 ANTISENSE THERAPY

The first reported clinical study of ASO therapy targeted Bcl-2 in patients with NHL *(101)*. Nine patients diagnosed with relapsed NHL of any histological grade, and evidence of high Bcl-2 expression on lymph node biopsy samples, were treated with a continuous subcutaneous infusion of G3139 (Genasense™; Genta Inc, USA), increasing from 4.6 mg/m² to 73.6 mg/m². Two patients showed reduced tumor size visualized by computerized tomography (one complete response and one minor response), and in two of five patients studied, reduction in the expression of Bcl-2 was observed. The study was extended to 21 patients *(102)* and showed Bcl-2 reduction in the blood, bone marrow, or lymph nodes in 7 of the 16 patients assessed, supporting antisense activity of G3139 in the clinical setting. G3139 (Genasense) has subsequently been entered into ongoing randomized phase 3 clinical trials globally for advanced malignant melanoma, myeloma, and chronic lymphatic leukemia (CLL), combining the Bcl-2 antisense with chemotherapy. The antisense is currently administered by continuous intravenous infusions over 5–7 d (doses range from 3–7 mg/kg/d depending on the tumor type) with the aim of reducing Bcl-2 protein levels in the tumor cells before administering the chemotherapy. The CLL studies suggest increased sensitivity to Genasense (O'Brien, American Society of Hematology presentation Dec., 2001) suggesting a dose above 4 mg/kg/d will cause toxicities. Phase 2 trials were for prostate, breast, colon, and acute leukemia. In general, Genasense is a well-tolerated compound with minimal toxicites within the dose range required to produce the required reduction of Bcl-2 protein, making this a promising therapy for the oncology clinic to overcome chemotherapy resistance. The use of chemotherapy after Bcl-2 down-regulation does not appear to produce prolonged marrow suppression, but does give more selective antitumor efficacy.

5. Bcl-2 ANTISENSE OR OLIGONUCLEOTIDE TOXICITY? WHY SEMANTICS MATTERS, AND WHY IT DOES NOT

The polyanionic property of PS ASO, has been shown to be associated with binding to several different types of cell surface protein, including CD11b/CD18/Mac1 *(103)*, basic fibroblast growth factor (bFGF), platelet derived growth factor (PDGF) *(104,105)*. Binding to PDGF and bFGF can block their interaction with their receptors at pharmacologically relevant 50% inhibitory concentrations (IC$_{50}$) of 5 mM and 200 nM, respectively *(106)*. Polyanionic binding to bFGF was exploited by Jansen and coworkers, who showed that melanoma growth in a SCID-hu mouse model could be reduced by a nonantisense mechanism that could be inhibited in vitro by the addition of bFGF at 1 ng/mL *(107)*.

Numerous sequence-dependent nonspecific effects have been reported for PS ASOs. The G-quartet, defined as a series of contiguous guanosine residues, has been shown to be antiproliferative in a sequence-independent manner *(108)*. This implies that for antisense experiments, in which the ASO but not the control oligonucleotide possesses a G-quartet, antisense efficacy could be erroneously interpreted *(106)*. Evidence suggests that sequence-specific antiproliferative effects can be demonstrated in vivo despite the existence of a G-quartet in the ASO, as evidenced by the lack of potency of a Q-quintet containing control oligonucleotide *(109)*. A large body of evidence supports an immune stimulatory role for CpG motifs, in which the 5′ end is flanked by two purines and the 3′ side is flanked by two pyrimidines *(110)*. Oligo CpG regions can potently stimulate NK cell lytic activity and have been shown to be abundant motifs in bacterial DNA *(110,111)*.

ASOs are metabolized by enzymic hydrolysis intracellularly, leading to stepwise release of 5′ monophosphate deoxyriboucleotides (dNMPs). Vaerman et al. have shown that the 3′ sequence of the ASO determines a nonantisense effect associated with antiproliferative activity, with the exception of a terminal cytosine at either the last or penultimate base position *(112)*. The cytotoxicity of released dNMPs varies, such that dCMP is not toxic, whereas dGMP, dTMP, and damp are toxic at 5–10 μM concentration. Furthermore, dCMP can inhibit the toxicity of dGMP, dTMP, and dAMP *(112)*. Thus, despite a substantial body of evidence supporting sequence-specific effects of PS ASOs, with regard to antitumor activity, several factors may interact to mediate antiproliferative effects, thus complicating the interpretation of true antisense activity as the only relevant underlying mechanism. This is clearly important if an agent's dominant mode of action is to be classified as antisense and may impact on efforts to rationally develop more potent anti-Bcl-2 ASOs for therapy. Ethical constraints prevent the clinical evaluation of sequence-specific efficacy, which must be assumed from successful preclinical experiments. This limitation can be partly overcome in some diseases by the quantitative demonstration of protein down-regulation, which is measured in biopsied tissues and is consistent with antisense efficacy *(101,102)*. Conversely, nonantisense oligonucleotide activities that exhibit significant antineoplastic efficacy may be relevant therapeutically and so, exploited; an empiracle perspective in which pharmacodynamics is less important.

Genasense has, to date, been shown to bind specifically to the Bcl-2 mRNA and to selectivly down-regulate bcl-2 protein production in a dose-dependent manner and induce apoptosis on its own and with synergy when chombined with chemotherapy. These effects have been consistent from in vitro to in vivo to the clinic. These findings suggest that in this case, the effects are largely due to a true ASO effect.

6. SUMMARY

Bcl-2, the first mitochondrial oncoprotein, remains a valid target for pharmacological inhibition. ASOs have provided target validation for this molecule in experimental models of cancer, and the protein down-regulating efficacy of clinically administered P ASO has been demonstrated. Several clinical trials are currently in progress to determine the therapeutic effiacacy of the Bcl-2-specific ASO, G3139 (Genasense). Suppression of Bcl-2 gene expression (or its anti-death homologues) may only be the first of several new approaches for inhibiting this protein, which may be anticipated with increased understanding of its biochemical function.

REFERENCES

1. Kaufmann SH. Induction of endonucleolytic DNA cleavage in human acute myelogenous leukemia cells by etoposide, camptothecin, and other cytotoxic anticancer drugs: a cautionary note. *Cancer Res* 1989; 49:5870–5878.
2. Eastman A. Activation of programmed cell death by anticancer agents: cisplatin as a model system. *Cancer Cells* 1990; 2:275–280.
3. Su IJ, Cheng AL, Tsai TF, Lay JD. Retinoic acid-induced apoptosis and regression of a refractory Epstein-Barr virus-containing T cell lymphoma expressing multidrug-resistance phenotypes. *Br J Haematol* 1993; 85:826–828.
4. Midgley CA, Owens B, Briscoe CV, Thomas DB, Lane DP, Hall PA. Coupling between gamma irradiation, p53 induction and the apoptotic response depends upon cell type in vivo. *J Cell Sci* 1995; 108:1843–1848.
5. Potten CS. The significance of spontaneous and induced apoptosis in the gastrointestinal tract of mice. *Cancer Metastasis Rev* 1992; 11:179–195.
6. Meyn RE, Stephens LC, Hunter NR, Milas L. Apoptosis in murine tumors treated with chemotherapy agents. *Anticancer Drugs* 1995; 6:443–450.
7. Gorczyca W, Bigman K, Mittelman A, Ahmed T, Gong J, Melamed MR, et al. Induction of DNA strand breaks associated with apoptosis during treatment of leukemias. *Leukemia* 1993; 7:659–670.
8. Langley RE, Palayoor ST, Coleman CN, Bump EA. Radiation-induced apoptosis in F9 teratocarcinoma cells. *Int J Radiat Biol* 1994; 65:605–610.
9. Lutzker SG, Barnard NJ. Testicular germ cell tumors: molecular understanding and clinical implications. *Mol Med Today* 1998; 4:404–411.
10. Cahill DP, Kinzler KW, Vogelstein B, Lengauer C. Genetic instability and darwinian selection in tumours. *Trends Cell Biol* 1999; 9:M57–M60.
11. Krajewski S, Tanaka S, Takayama S, Schibler MJ, Fenton W, Reed JC. Investigation of the subcellular distribution of the bcl-2 oncoprotein: residence in the nuclear envelope, endoplasmic reticulum, and outer mitochondrial membranes. *Cancer Res* 1993; 53:4701–4714.
12. Chen-Levy Z, Nourse J, Cleary ML. The bcl-2 candidate proto-oncogene product is a 24-kilodalton integral-membrane protein highly expressed in lymphoid cell lines and lymphomas carrying the t(14:18) translocation. *Mol Cell Biol* 1989; 9:701–710.

13. Hockenbery D, Nunez G, Milliman C, Schreiber RD, Korsmeyer SJ. Bcl-2 is an inner mitochondrial membrane protein that blocks programmed cell death. *Nature* 1990; 348:334–336.

14. Boise LH, Gonzalez-Garcia M, Postema CE, Ding L, Lindsten T, Turka LA, et al. Bcl-X, a Bcl-2 related gene that functions as a dominant regulator of apoptotic cell death. *Cell* 1993; 74:597–608.

15. Reynolds JE, Li J, Craig RW, Eastman A. BCL-2 and MCL-1 expression in Chinese hamster ovary cells inhibits intracellular acidification and apoptosis induced by staurosporine. *Exp Cell Res* 1996; 225:430–436.

16. Gibson L, Holmgreen SP, Huang DC, Bernard O, Copeland NG, Jenkins NA, et al. bcl-w, a novel member of the bcl-2 family, promotes cell survival. *Oncogene* 1996; 13:665–675.

17. Tsujimoto Y, Cossman J, Jaffe E, Croce CM. Involvement of the bcl-2 gene in human follicular lymphoma. *Science* 1985; 228:1440–1443.

18. Vaux DL, Cory S, Adams JM. Bcl-2 gene promotes haemopoietic cell survival and cooperates with c-myc to immortalize pre-B cells. *Nature* 1988; 335:440–442.

19. Chen-Levy Z, Cleary ML. Membrane topology of the Bcl-2 proto-oncogenic protein demonstrated in vitro. *J Biol Chem* 1990; 265:4929–4933.

20. Sentman CL, Shutter JR, Hockenbery D, Kanagawa O, Korsmeyer SJ. bcl-2 Inhibits multiple forms of apoptosis but not negative selection in thymocytes. *Cell* 1991; 67:879–888.

21. Strasser A, Harris AW, Cory S. bcl-2 transgene inhibits T cell death and perturbs thymic self-censorship. *Cell* 1991; 67:889–899.

22. Hockenbery DM, Oltvai ZN, Yin XM, Milliman CL, Korsmeyer SJ. Bcl-2 functions in an antioxidant pathway to prevent apoptosis. *Cell* 1993; 75:241–251.

23. Zhong LT, Sarafian T, Kane DJ, Charles AC, Mah SP, Edwards RH, et al. bcl-2 inhibits death of central neural cells induced by multiple agents. *Proc Natl Acad Sci USA* 1993; 90:4533–4537.

24. Zamzami N, Marchetti P, Castedo M, Decaudin D, Macho A, Hirsch T, et al. Sequential reduction of mitochondrial transmembrane potential and generation of reactive oxygen species in early programmed cell death. *J Exp Med* 1995; 182:367–377.

25. Lemasters JJ, Nieminen AL, Qian T, Trost LC, Elmore SP, Nishimura Y, et al. The mitochondrial permeability transition in cell death: A common mechanism in necrosis, apoptosis and autophagy. *Biochim Biophys Acta Bioenerg* 1998; 2:177–196.

26. Decaudin D, Geley S, Hirsch T, Castedo M, Marchetti P, Macho A, et al. Bcl-2 and Bcl-XL antagonize the mitochondrial dysfunction preceding nuclear apoptosis induced by chemotherapeutic agents. *Cancer Res* 1997; 57:62–67.

27. Susin SA, Zamzami N, Castedo M, Hirsch T, Marchetti P, Macho A, et al. Bcl-2 inhibits the mitochondrial release of an apoptogenic protease. *J Exp Med* 1996; 184:1331–1341.

28. Marzo I, Brenner C, Zamzami N, Jurgensmeier JM, Susin SA, Vieira HLA, et al. Bax and adenine nucleotide translocator cooperate in the mitochondrial control of apoptosis. *Science* 1998; 281:2027–2031.

29. Doran E, Halestrap AP. Cytochrome c release from isolated rat liver mitochondria can occur independently of outer-membrane rupture: possible role of contract sites [in process citation]. *Biochem J* 2000; 348:343–350.

30. Halestrap AP, Doran E, Gillespie JP, O'Toole A. Mitochondria and cell death [in process citation]. *FEBS Lett* 2000; 473:285–291.

31. Pastorino JG, Tafani M, Rothman RJ, Marcineviciute A, Hoek JB, Farber JL. Functional consequences of the sustained or transient activation by bax of the mitochondrial permeability transition pore [in process citation]. *J Biol Chem* 1999; 274:31734–31739.

32. Pastorino JG, Chen ST, Tafani M, Snyder JW, Farber JL. The overexpression of Bax produces cell death upon induction of the mitochondrial permeability transition. *J Biol Chem* 1998; 273:7770–7775.

33. Shimizu S, Konishi A, Kodama T, Tsujimoto Y. BH4 domain of antiapoptotic bcl-2 family members closes voltage-dependent anion channel and inhibits apoptotic mitochondrial changes and cell death [in process citation]. *Proc Natl Acad Sci USA* 2000; 97:3100–3105.

34. Shimizu S, Narita M, Tsujimoto Y. Bcl-2 family proteins regulate the release of apoptogenic cytochrome c by the mitochondrial channel VDAC [see comments]. *Nature* 1999; 399:483–487.

35. Shimizu S, Eguchi Y, Kamiike W, Funahashi Y, Mignon A, Lacronique V, et al. Bcl-2 prevents apoptotic mitochondrial dysfunction by regulating proton flux. *Proc Natl Acad Sci USA* 1998; 95:1455–1459.

36. Hsu YT, Wolter KG, Youle RJ. Cytosol-to-membrane redistribution of Bax and Bcl-X(L) during apoptosis. *Proc Natl Acad Sci USA* 1997; 94:3668–3672.

37. Wolter KG, Hsu YT, Smith CL, Nechushtan A, Xi XG, Youle RJ. Movement of Bax from the cytosol to mitochondria during apoptosis. *J Cell Biol* 1997; 139:1281–1292.
38. Korsmeyer SJ, Shutter JR, Veis DJ, Merry DE, Oltvai ZN. Bcl-2/Bax: a rheostat that regulates an anti-oxidant pathway and cell death. *Semin Cancer Biol* 1993; 4:327–332.
39. Sakakura C, Sweeney EA, Shirahama T, Igarashi Y, Hakomori S, Tsujimoto H, et al. Overexpression of bax sensitizes breast cancer MCF-7 cells to cisplatin and etoposide. *Surg Today* 1997; 27:676–679.
40. Kobayashi T, Ruan S, Clodi K, Kliche KO, Shiku H, Andreeff M, et al. Overexpression of Bax gene sensitizes K562 erythroleukemia cells to apoptosis induced by selective chemotherapeutic agents. *Oncogene* 1998; 16:1587–1591.
41. Paterson BM, Roberts BE, Kuff EL. Structural gene identification and mapping by DNA-mRNA hybrid-arrested cell-free translation. *Proc Natl Acad Sci USA* 1977; 74:4370–4374.
42. Stephenson ML, Zamecnik PC. Inhibition of Rous sarcoma viral RNA translation by a specific oligodeoxyribonucleotide. *Proc Natl Acad Sci USA* 1978; 75:285–288.
43. Zamecnik PC, Stephenson ML. Inhibition of Rous sarcoma virus replication and cell transformation by a specific oligodeoxynucleotide. *Proc Natl Acad Sci USA* 1978; 75:280–284.
44. Simons RW, Kleckner N. Translational control of IS10 transposition. *Cell* 1983; 34:683–691.
45. Mizuno T, Chou MY, Inouye M. A unique mechanism regulating gene expression: translational inhibition by a complementary RNA transcript (micRNA). *Proc Natl Acad Sci* USA 1984; 81:1966–1970.
46. Izant JG, Weintraub H. Inhibition of thymidine kinase gene expression by anti-sense RNA: a molecular approach to genetic analysis. *Cell* 1984; 36:1007–1015.
47. Khan IM, Coulson JM. A novel method to stabilise antisense oligonucleotides against exonuclease degradation [published erratum appears in Nucleic Acids Res 1993 Sep 11;21(18):4433]. *Nucleic Acids Res* 1993; 21:2957–2958.
48. Fresco JR. ABM. *Nature* 1960; 188:98.
49. Zuker M. On finding all suboptimal foldings of an RNA molecule. *Science* 1989; 244:48–52.
50. Stull RA, Zon G, Szoka FC Jr. An in vitro messenger RNA binding assay as a tool for identifying hybridization-competent antisense oligonucleotides. *Antisense Nucleic Acid Drug Dev* 1996; 6:221–228.
51. Gewirtz AM, Sokol DL, Ratajczak MZ. Nucleic acid therapeutics: state of the art and future prospects. *Blood* 1998; 92:712–736.
52. Ho SP, Bao Y, Lesher T, Malhotra R, Ma LY, Fluharty SJ, et al. Mapping of RNA accessible sites for antisense experiments with oligonucleotide libraries [see comments]. *Nat Biotechnol* 1998; 16:59–63.
53. Ho SP, Britton DH, Stone BA, Behrens DL, Leffet LM, Hobbs FW, et al. Potent antisense oligonucleotides to the human multidrug resistance-1 mRNA are rationally selected by mapping RNA-accessible sites with oligonucleotide libraries. *Nucleic Acids Res* 1996; 24:1901–1907.
54. Milner N, Mir KU, Southern EM. Selecting effective antisense reagents on combinatorial oligonucleotide arrays. *Nat Biotechnol* 1997; 15:537–541.
55. Southern EM, Milner N, Mir KU. Discovering antisense reagents by hybridization of RNA to oligonucleotide arrays. *Ciba Found Symp* 1997; 209:38–44; discussion 44–46.
56. Monia BP, Johnston JF, Geiger T, Muller M, Fabbro D. Antitumor activity of a phosphorothioate antisense oligodeoxynucleotide targeted against C-raf kinase. *Nat Med* 1996; 2:668–675.
57. Gee JE, Robbins I, van der Laan AC, van Boom JH, Colombier C, Leng M, et al. Assessment of high-affinity hybridization, RNase H cleavage, and covalent linkage in translation arrest by antisense oligonucleotides. *Cell* 1997; 90:405–413.
58. Tidd DM. Ribonuclease H-mediated antisense effects in intact human leukaemia cells. *Biochem Soc Trans* 1996; 24:619–623.
59. Giles RV, Spiller DG, Tidd DM. Detection of ribonuclease. H-generated mRNA fragments in human leukemia cells following reversible membrane permeabilization in the presence of antisense oligodeoxynucleotides. *Antisense Res Dev* 1995; 5:23–31.
60. Wu H, Lima WF, Crooke ST. Molecular cloning and expression of cDNA for human RNase H. *Antisense Nucleic Acid Drug Dev* 1998; 8:53–61.
61. Crooke ST. Molecular mechanisms of action of antisense drugs. *Biochim Biophys Acta* 1999; 1489:31–44.
62. Donis-Keller H. Site specific enzymatic cleavage of RNA. *Nucleic Acids Res* 1979; 7:1233–1246.
63. Eder PS, Walder JA. Ribonuclease H from K562 human erythroleukemia cells. Purification, characterization, and substrate specificity. *J Biol Chem* 1991; 266:23204–23214.

64. Kawasaki AM, Casper MD, Freier SM, Lesnik EA, Zounes MC, Cummins LL, et al. Uniformly modified 2'-deoxy-2'-fluoro phosphorothioate oligonucleotides as nuclease-resistant antisense compounds with high affinity and specificity for RNA targets. *Diabetologia* 1993; 36:696–706.

65. Sproat BS, Lamond AI, Beijer B, Neuner P, Ryder U. Highly efficient chemical synthesis of 2'-O-methyloligoribonucleotides and tetrabiotinylated derivatives; novel probes that are resistant to degradation by RNA or DNA specific nucleases. *Nucleic Acids Res* 1989; 17:8967–8978.

66. Mirabelli CK, Bennett CF, Anderson K, Crooke ST. In vitro and in vivo pharmacologic activities of antisense oligonucleotides. *Nucleic Acids Res* 1989; 17:2517–2527.

67. Cazenave C, Stein CA, Loreau N, Thuong NT, Neckers LM, Subasinghe C, et al. Comparative inhibition of rabbit globin mRNA translation by modified antisense oligodeoxynucleotides. *Nucleic Acids Res* 1989; 17:8207–8219.

68. Maher LJd, Wold B, Dervan PB. Inhibition of DNA binding proteins by oligonucleotide-directed triple helix formation. *Nucleic Acids Res* 1989; 17:4255–4273.

69. Monia BP, Lesnik EA, Gonzalez C, Lima WF, McGee D, Guinosso CJ, et al. Evaluation of 2'-modified oligonucleotides containing 2'-deoxy gaps as antisense inhibitors of gene expression. *J Biol Chem* 1993; 268:14514–14522.

70. Giles RV, Tidd DM. Increased specificity for antisense oligodeoxynucleotide targeting of RNA cleavage by RNase H using chimeric methylphosphonodiester/phosphodiester structures. *J Am Coll Cardiol* 1992; 20:3–16.

71. Chin DJ, Green GA, Zon G, Szoka FC Jr, Straubinger RM. Rapid nuclear accumulation of injected oligodeoxyribonucleotides. *New Biol* 1990; 2:1091–1100.

72. Zabner J, Fasbender AJ, Moninger T, Poellinger KA, Welsh MJ. Cellular and molecular barriers to gene transfer by a cationic lipid. *J Biol Chem* 1995; 270:18997–19007.

73. Shoeman RL, Hartig R, Huang Y, Grub S, Traub P. Fluorescence microscopic comparison of the binding of phosphodiester and phosphorothioate (antisense) oligodeoxyribonucleotides to subcellular structures, including intermediate filaments, the endoplasmic reticulum, and the nuclear interior. *Antisense Nucleic Acid Drug Dev* 1997; 7:291–308.

74. Stein CA, Cohen JS. Oligodeoxynucleotides as inhibitors of gene expression: a review. *Cancer Res* 1988; 48:2659–2668.

75. Bennett CF, Chiang MY, Chan H, Shoemaker JEE, Mirabelli CK. Cationic lipids enhance cellular uptake and activity of phosphorothioate antisense oligonucleotides. *Mol Pharmacol* 1992; 41:1023–1033.

76. Marcusson EG, Bhat B, Manoharan M, Bennett CF, Dean NM. Phosphorothioate oligodeoxyribonucleotides dissociate from cationic lipids before entering the nucleus. *Nucleic Acids Res* 1998; 26:2016–2023.

77. Lorenz P, Misteli T, Baker BF, Bennett CF, Spector DL. Nucleocytoplasmic shuttling: a novel in vivo property of antisense phosphorothioate oligodeoxynucleotides. *Nucleic Acids Res* 2000; 28:582–592.

78. Legendre JY, Szoka FC Jr. Delivery of plasmid DNA into mammalian cell lines using pH-sensitive liposomes: comparison with cationic liposomes. *Pharm Res* 1992; 9:1235–1242.

79. Giles RV, Grzybowski J, Spiller DG, Tidd DM. Enhanced antisense effects resulting from an improved streptolysin-O protocol for oligodeoxynucleotide delivery into human leukaemia cells. *Nucleosides Nucleotides* 1997; 16:7–9.

80. Giles RV, Spiller DG, Grzybowski J, Clark RE, Nicklin P, Tidd DM. Selecting optimal oligonucleotide composition for maximal antisense effect following streptolysin O-mediated delivery into human leukaemia cells. *Nucleic Acids Res* 1998; 26:1567–1575.

81. Spiller DG, Tidd DM. Nuclear delivery of antisense oligodeoxynucleotides through reversible permeabilization of human leukemia cells with streptolysin O. *Antisense Res Dev* 1995; 5:13–21.

82. Broughton CM, Spiller DG, Pender N, Komorovskaya M, Grzybowski J, Giles RV, et al. Preclinical studies of streptolysin-O in enhancing antisense oligonucleotide uptake in harvests from chronic myeloid leukaemia patients. *Leukemia* 1997; 11:1435–1441.

83. Bielinska A, Kukowska-Latallo JF, Johnson J, Tomalia DA, Baker JR Jr. Regulation of in vitro gene expression using antisense oligonucleotides or antisense expression plasmids transfected using starburst PAMAM dendrimers. *Nucleic Acids Res* 1996; 24:2176–2182.

84. Leonetti JP, Degols G, Lebleu B. Biological activity of oligonucleotide-poly(L-lysine) conjugates: mechanism of cell uptake. *Bioconjug Chem* 1990; 1:149–153.

85. Krieg AM, Tonkinson J, Matson S, Zhao Q, Saxon M, Zhang LM, et al. Modification of antisense phosphodiester oligodeoxynucleotides by a 5' cholesteryl moiety increases cellular association and improves efficacy. *Proc Natl Acad Sci USA* 1993; 90:1048–1052.

86. Bongartz JP, Aubertin AM, Milhaud PG, Lebleu B. Improved biological activity of antisense oligonucleotides conjugated to a fusogenic peptide. *Nucleic Acids Res* 1994; 22:4681–4688.

87. Wu GY, Wu CH. Specific inhibition of hepatitis B viral gene expression in vitro by targeted antisense oligonucleotides. *J Biol Chem* 1992; 267:12436–12439.

88. Watson PH, Pon RT, Shiu RP. Inhibition of cell adhension to plastic substratum by phosphorothioate oligonucleotide *Exp cell Res* 1992; 202:391–397.

89. Benimetskaya L, Takle GB, Vilenchik M, Lebedeva I, Miller P, Stein CA. Cationic porphyrins: novel delivery vehicles for antisense oligodeoxynucleotides. *Nucleic Acids Res* 1998; 26:5310–5317.

90. Graham MJ, Crooke ST, Monteith DK, Cooper SR, Lemonidis KM, Stecker KK, et al. In vivo distribution and metabolism of a phosphorothioate oligonucleotide within rat liver after intravenous administration. *J Pharmacol Exp Ther* 1998; 286:447–458.

91. Bijsterbosch MK, Manoharan M, Rump ET, De Vrueh RL, van Veghel R, Tivel KL, et al. In vivo fate of phosphorothioate antisense oligodeoxynucleotides: predominant uptake by scavenger receptors on endothelial liver cells. *Nucleic Acids Res* 1997; 25:3290–3296.

92. Butler M, Crooke RM, Graham MJ, Lemonidis KM, Lougheed M, Murray SF, et al. Phosphorothioate oligodeoxynucleotides distribute similarly in class A scavenger receptor knockout and wild-type mice. *J Pharmacol Exp Ther* 2000; 292:489–496.

93. Reed JC, Stein C, Subasinghe C, Haldar S, Croce CM, Yum S, et al. Antisense-mediated inhibition of BCL2 protooncogene expression and leukemic cell growth and survival: comparisons of phosphodiester and phosphorothioate oligodeoxynucleotides. *Cancer Res* 1990; 50:6944–6948.

94. Kitada S, Takayama S, De Riel K, Tanaka S, Reed JC. Reversal of chemoresistance of lymphoma cells by antisense-mediated reduction of bcl-2 gene expression. *Antisense Res Dev* 1994; 4:71–79.

95. Campos L, Sabido O, Rouault JP, Guyotat D. Effects of BCL-2 antisense oligodeoxynucleotides on in vitro proliferation and survival of normal marrow progenitors and leukemic cells. *Blood* 1994; 84:595–600.

96. Cotter FE, Johnson P, Hall P, Pocock C, al Mahdi N, Cowell JK, et al. Antisense oligonucleotides suppress B-cell lymphoma growth in a SCID-hu mouse model. *Oncogene* 1994; 9:3049–3055.

97. Jansen B, Schlagbauer-Wadl H, Brown BD, Bryan RN, van Elsas A, Muller M, et al. bcl-2 antisense therapy chemosensitizes human melanoma in SCID mice. *Nat Med* 1998; 4:232–234.

98. Klasa RJ, Bally MB, Ng R, Goldie JH, Gascoyne RD, Wong FM. Eradication of human non-Hodgkin's lymphoma in SCID mice by BCL-2 antisense oligonucleotides combined with low-dose cyclophosphamide [in process citation]. *Clin Cancer Res* 2000; 6:2492–2500.

99. Schlagbauer-Wadl H, Klosner G, Heere-Ress E, Waltering S, Moll I, Wolff K, et al. Bcl-2 antisense oligonucleotides (G3139) inhibit Merkel cell carcinoma growth in SCID mice. *J Invest Dermatol* 2000; 114:725–730.

100. Miyake H, Monia BP, Gleave ME. Inhibition of progression to androgen-independence by combined adjuvant treatment with antisense BCL-XL and antisense Bcl-2 oligonucleotides plus taxol after castration in the Shionogi tumor model. *Int J Cancer* 2000; 86:855–862.

101. Webb A, Cunningham D, Cotter F, Clarke PA, di Stefano F, Ross P, et al. BCL-2 antisense therapy in patients with non-Hodgkin lymphoma. *Lancet* 1997; 349:1137–1141.

102. Waters JS, Webb A, Cunningham, D, Clarke PA, Raynaud F, di Stefano F, et al. Phase I clinical and pharmacokinetic study of bcl-2 antisense oligonucleotide therapy in patients with non-Hodgkin's lymphoma [see comments]. *J Clin Oncol* 2000; 18:1812–1823.

103. Benimetskaya L, Loike JD, Khaled Z, Loike G, Silverstein SC, Cao L, et al. Mac-1 (CD11b/CD18) is an oligodeoxynucleotide-binding protein [see comments]. *Nat Med* 1997; 3:414–420.

104. Wellstein A, Zugmaier G, Califano JAd, Kern F, Paik S, Lippman ME. Tumor growth dependent on Kaposi's sarcoma-derived fibroblast growth factor inhibited by pentosan polysulfate. *J Natl Cancer Inst* 1991; 83:716–720.

105. Zugmaier G, Lippman ME, Wellstein A. Inhibition by pentosan polysulfate (PPS) of heparin-binding growth factors released from tumor cells and blockage by PPS of tumor growth in animals. *J Natl Cancer Inst* 1992; 84:1716–1724.

106. Stein CA, Krieg AM. Problems in interpretation of data derived from in vitro and in vivo use of antisense oligodeoxynucleotides [editorial]. *Antisense Res Dev* 1994; 4:67–69.

107. Jansen B, Wadl H, Inoue SA, Trulzsch B, Selzer E, Duchene M, et al. Phosphorothioate oligonucleotides reduce melanoma growth in a SCID-hu mouse model by a nonantisense mechanism. *Antisense Res Dev* 1995; 5:271–277.

108. Yaswen P, Stampfer MR, Ghosh K, Cohen JS. Effects of sequence of thioated oligonucleotides on cultured human mammary epithelial cells. *Antisense Res Dev* 1993; 3:67–77.

109. Higgins KA, Perez JR, Coleman TA, Dorshkind K, McComas WA, Sarmiento UM, et al. Antisense inhibition of the p65 subunit of NF-kappa B blocks tumorigenicity and causes tumor regression. *Proc Natl Acad Sci USA* 1993; 90:9901–9905.

110. Ballas ZK, Rasmussen WL, Krieg AM. Induction of NK activity in murine and human cells by CpG motifs in oligodeoxynucleotides and bacterial DNA. *Blood* 1996; 88:1788–1795.

111. Krieg AM, Yi AK, Matson S, Waldschmidt TJ, Bishop GA, Teasdale R, et al. CpG motifs in bacterial DNA trigger direct B-cell activation. *J Clin Immunol* 1995; 15:284–292.

112. Vaerman JL, Moreau P, Deldime F, Lewalle P, Lammineur C, Morschhauser F, et al. Antisense oligodeoxyribonucleotides suppress hematologic cell growth through stepwise release of deoxyribonucleotides. *Arthritis Rheum* 1985; 28:341–344.

Index